D1146341

Health Authority

Y.H Library

3 8028 99043308 9

OXFORD MEDICAL PUBLICATIONS

COLORECTAL DISEASES
FOR PHYSICIANS AND SURGEONS

Dose schedules are being continually revised and new side effects recognized. Oxford University Press makes no representation, express or implied, that the drug dosages in this book are correct. For these reasons the reader is strongly urged to consult the pharmaceutical company's printed instructions before administering any of the drugs recommended in this book.

COLORECTAL DISEASES
FOR
PHYSICIANS AND SURGEONS

G.T. DEANS MD FRCS
Consultant Surgeon, and Lead Clinician on Cancer Services, Stepping Hill Hospital, Stockport

R.A.J. SPENCE MA MD FRCS
Consultant Surgeon, Belfast City Hospital, and Honorary Lecturer in Surgery,
The Queen's University of Belfast, Belfast

A.H.G. LOVE CBE BSc MD FRCP FRCPI
Professor of Medicine and Head of Clinical Science,
The Queen's University of Belfast, Belfast

Oxford   New York   Tokyo
OXFORD UNIVERSITY PRESS
1998

Oxford University Press, Great Clarendon Street, Oxford OX2 6DP

Oxford   New York
Athens   Auckland   Bangkok   Bogota   Bombay
Calcutta   Cape Town   Dar es Salaam   Delhi
Florence   Hong Kong   Istanbul   Karachi
Kuala Lumpur   Madras   Madrid   Melbourne
Mexico City   Nairobi   Paris   Singapore
Taipei   Tokyo   Toronto   Warsaw
and associated companies in
Berlin   Ibadan

Oxford is a trade mark of Oxford University Press

Published in the United States
by Oxford University Press Inc., New York

© G.T. Deans, R.A.J. Spence & A.H.G. Love, 1998

All rights reserved. No part of this publication may be
reproduced, stored in a retrieval system, or transmitted, in any
form or by any means, without the prior permission in writing of Oxford
University Press. Within the UK, exceptions are allowed in respect of any
fair dealing for the purpose of research or private study, or criticism or
review, as permitted under the Copyright, Designs and Patents Act, 1988, or
in the case of reprographic reproduction in accordance with the terms of
licences issued by the Copyright Licensing Agency. Enquiries concerning
reproduction outside those terms and in other countries should be sent to
the Rights Department, Oxford University Press, at the address above.

This book is sold subject to the condition that it shall not,
by way of trade or otherwise, by lent, re-sold, hired out, or otherwise
circulated without the publisher's prior consent in any form of binding
or cover other than that in which it is published and without a similar
condition including this condition being imposed
on the subsequent purchaser.

A catalogue record for this book is available from the British Library

Library of Congress Cataloging in Publication Data
(Data available)

ISBN 0 19 262704 X

Typeset by EXPO Holdings, Malaysia

Printed in Great Britain by
Butler & Tanner Ltd Frome and London

Acknowledgements

Preparation of a book such as this cannot be undertaken in isolation. It is therefore with the deepest gratitude that we would like to thank all of our colleagues for their advice, support, and patience with us during the writing of this book. We are especially grateful to the following for supplying the figures and sharing their wealth of knowledge on colorectal diseases:

Dr **C. Keeling-Roberts**, Consultant Radiologist, Stepping Hill Hospital, Stockport: Figures 1.11, 1.13, 1.17, 5.7, 5.9, 5.11, 5.13, 6.10, 6.12, 6.14, 6.24, 6.25, 6.29, 6.31, 7.5, 7.7, 7.8, 7.9, 7.11, 7.16, 8.12, 8.14a, 8.14b, 8.15, 10.1, 10.3, 11.10, 11.16, 11.17, 11.20, 11.22, 11.23, 11.26, 12.1, 12.3, 12.11, 12.19, 14.6, 14.7, 14.8, 14.11, 15.7, 16.4, 17.9, 17.11, 17.12, 17.18, 17.19

Dr **R. Hale**, Consultant Pathologist, Stepping Hill Hospital, Stockport: Figures 5.2, 6.6, 6.16, 6.21, 6.22, 7.1, 8.2, 8.10, 8.11, 10.2, 10.5, 11.3, 11.7, 11.8, 11.10, 11.11, 11.12, 11.18, 12.18, 14.1, 14.3a & b, 14.4, 14.5, 14.14, 14.15, 14.16, 15.10, 16.1, 16.5, 17.13, 17.14, 19.5, 19.6, 19.7, 19.9, 19.10, 19.11, 19.13, 19.14

Mrs **M. Harrison**, Medical Artist, Stockport, Cheshire: Figures: 1.1, 1.2, 1.3, 1.4, 1.5, 1.6, 1.7, 1.8, 18.1, 18.2, 18.5, 18.7

Dr **S. Mehta**, Consultant Radiologist, Stepping Hill Hospital, Stockport: Figures 1.18, 12.20, 12.21, 12.22, 18.8a & b.

Professor **T.G. Parks** and Dr **B. Johnston**, Belfast City Hospital and Lagan Valley Hospital, Lisburn, Northern Ireland: All figures for Chapters 3 and 13. Also Figures 18.6, 18.9, 18.10, 18.11, 18.12, 18.16, 19.1, 19.4, 19.10

Dr **T. McIlrath**, Consultant Radiologist, Royal Victoria Hospital, Belfast: Figures 7.10, 7.13, 8.21, 11.24, 11.25, 12.12, 12.13, 12.15, 12.16, 14.9, 14.12, 14.13, 15.8, 17.6

Dr **J. Lawson**, Consultant Radiologist, Belfast City Hospital: Figures 1.12, 1.14, 1.15, 5.10, 6.9, 6.11, 7.6, 8.13, 8.16, 11.26, 12.6, 12.7, 12.17, 15.9, 16.3

Dr **L. Johnston**, Consultant Radiologist, Belfast City Hospital: Figures 5.8, 5.12, 6.13, 6.23, 6.30, 7.15, 8.24, 9.5, 11.21

Dr **J. Laird**, Consultant Radiologist, Royal Victoria Hospital, Belfast: Figures 5.14, 5.27, 6.15, 15.11

Drs **P. Thomas** and **L. Sweeney**, Consultant Radiologists, Royal Belfast Hospital for Sick Children: Figures 2.4 to 2.15 inclusive

Dr **J. Sloan**, Consultant Pathologist Royal Victoria Hospital, Belfast: Figures 5.1, 5.3–5.6, 7.2, 7.3, 8.1, 8.4, 8.5, 8.6, 8.7, 8.8, 8.9, 8.18, 10.7, 10.9, 11.2, 11.9, 15.2, 16.2, 17.8, 17.10, 19.12

Dr **D. Allen**, Consultant Pathologist, Belfast City Hospital: Figures 16.6, 16.7

Mr **S.T. Irwin**, Consultant Surgeon, Belfast City Hospital: Figures 5.17, 5.20, 5.21, 5.23, 5.24, 5.25, 5.26, 12.4, 12.10

Mr **J. Campbell**, Surgical Senior Registrar: Figures 9.7, 9.8, 9.9

Mr **E. Mackle**, Consultant Surgeon, Craigavon Area Hospital, Northern Ireland: Figures 8.22, 9.6

Mr **H. Logan**, Consultant Surgeon, Ulster Hospital: Figure 8.23

Dr **R. Maw**, Consultant Venerologist, Royal Victoria Hospital, Belfast for all the figures in Chapter 4.

Dr. **K. McHugh**, John Radcliffe Hospital, Oxford: Figure 2.5

Dr **H. Appleton**, Public Health Laboratory Service, London: Figure 3.2, 3.3

In addition, we are deeply indebted to Mrs Andrea Pollock for her assistance in typing the manuscript and in checking the references. Finally we would like to thank Oxford University Press for their support and technical expertise in the preparation of this book.

Contents

Dedications

To – Rosalind, Chérie, Adèla, and Robert

G.T.D.

To – Di, Robert, Andrew, and Katherine

R.A.J.S.

Preface

Colorectal diseases remain among the commonest abdominal conditions within the remit of the surgeon, physician, gastroenterologist, radiologist, and pathologist. However, gaps still remain in our knowledge of the pathogenesis, diagnosis, and most appropriate form of treatment, whether medical or surgical, of several colorectal conditions. Diseases of the colon, rectum, and anus can be unforgiving and the penalty for errors in management may be high in terms of patient mortality and morbidity. Thus, the clinician treating patients with colorectal disease needs to have current knowledge of the aetiology, pathology, diagnosis, and treatment, both medical and surgical, to recommend correct and safe management.

Our approach to colorectal diseases is constantly evolving so that the traditional separation of specialties has given way to a unified approach with close liaison between physicians and surgeons often to the point of joint clinics for specific conditions. This blurring of former boundaries has led to a need for those trained in medicine or surgery to be familiar with the therapeutic potential, and limits, of each others specialties. Despite this overlap between disciplines, the current authoritative texts tend to be written for one specialty or the other. Consequently, it is difficult for those in one discipline to keep abreast of developments in other fields that may improve the management of their patients.

This book is aimed at providing physicians and surgeons with a succinct, up-to-date text which contains the essential information of the reference texts of both specialties in a single volume. It is not intended to be all-inclusive by covering every aspect of every colorectal condition; nor is it intended to compete with established texts by including extensive technical or operative details. Such an approach would be out of place in a text aimed at both physicians and surgeons; those requiring such details are referred to the numerous surgical books that address operative technique. Similarly long discussions on the aetiology, pathogenesis, or medical management of colorectal conditions have been avoided. Rather a concise, in-depth discussion is presented of each topic, similar to that obtained from literature review articles.

Each chapter has been written with both physicians and surgeons in mind, in an attempt to make it informative to both parties and aid joint decision-making to the benefit of patients. Each chapter therefore contains a comprehensive illustrated overview of the salient medical and surgical features of the topic discussed. This includes relevant information about the incidence, aetiology, and pathophysiology of each condition. Histopathological appearances are treated in some detail, reflecting their importance in the diagnosis, evaluation, and prognosis of alimentary disease. In the sections on clinical presentation and diagnosis we have attempted to place the rapid technological advances in imaging techniques into perspective. It is hoped that the review of current medical and surgical management will prove particularly beneficial to readers. The principal references for each chapter are highlighted in **bold** text, to allow rapid identification for the reader.

This book therefore aims to present an up-to-date account of the practice of colorectal disease within the limits of our present knowledge, based on scientific evidence rather than on clinical impression and personal bias. The approach of the book is essentially clinical and practical. We hope that it will prove valuable to the practising surgeon and physician. It should also be of value to those who are under the unenviable stresses of study for postgraduate surgical, medical, gastroenterological, radiological, or pathological diplomas and degrees. Above all, we trust that a joint approach of surgeons and physicians will further our understanding of colorectal diseases and benefit the management of our patients.

Stockport G.T.D.
Belfast R.A.J.S.
Belfast A.H.G.L.
1997

1 Colorectal anatomy, physiology, and investigation

Anatomy

The colon is 2 m long. The appendix opens on the posteromedial wall of the caecum, 2–4 cm below the ileocaecal valve and varies widely in length from 2 to 20 cm. The three taeniae coli of the colon converge at the base of the appendix, merging into its longitudinal muscle layer (Figure 1.1). The ascending colon is normally fixed to the posterior and lateral abdominal wall by a peritoneal attachment, although in one-quarter of individuals the peritoneum

forms a mesentery, which may rotate to form a caecal volvulus. The hepatic flexure is supported by the nephrocolic ligament and also, in about one-third of cases, by a cysticoduodenocolic ligament (Figure 1.1). The phrenicocolic ligament ensures that the splenic flexure is the most fixed part of the colon. The line of attachment of the sigmoid mesocolon represents an inverted V. The wide variation in the length, location, and mobility of the sigmoid loop predisposes some individuals to sigmoid volvulus. The rectosigmoid junction is characterized by disappearance of the peritoneal investment, mesentery and appendices epiploicae, a narrowing of the bowel lumen and spreading out of the three longitudinal taenia to form a continuous longitudinal muscle coat for the rectum.

The anatomical anal canal, extending from the dentate line to the anal verge, corresponds to the upper and lower borders of the internal sphincter. However, for surgical purposes, the anal canal can be assumed to extend from the anorectal ring to the anal verge (Figure 1.2). The lower-most edge of the anal canal is marked by the anocutaneous line (of Hilton). The coccyx lies posteriorly and the ischiorectal fossa containing the neurovascular supply to the anus is lateral. The anterior relations in the male are the centre of the perineum, the urethral bulb, and the posterior border of the urogenital diaphragm (the triangular ligament) containing the membranous urethra. In the female the perineal body and lower posterior vagina lie in front of the anus.

The mucosa immediately above the anal valves is usually lined by several layers of columnar cells, becoming a single layer after 1 cm. This zone is termed the 'transitional', 'junctional', or 'cloacogenic zone' as it represents the embryological junction of the endoderm and the ectoderm. The limit of the transitional zone varies from 0.6 cm below to 2 cm above the dentate line. Depending on the patient's age and underlying pathology, this zone may be lined by rectal mucosa, stratified columnar epithelium, transitional epithelium as seen in the urinary tract, squamous epithelium, endocrine cells, or melanin-containing cells. Below the dentate line the anal canal is lined with modified skin devoid of hair and sebaceous or sweat glands (the pectin), while the histological features of normal skin begin just outside the anal orifice.

Up to eight anal glands, lined by stratified columnar epithelium, open into the anal crypts. Up to half of these glands completely cross the internal sphincter to reach the intersphincteric longitudinal muscle. This is of clinical importance in the spread of infection to the submucous and intersphincteric spaces (see Chapter 18).

The internal anal sphincter is continuous superiorly with the circular muscle coat of the rectum while the external anal sphincter is composed of three integrated parts: subcutaneous, superficial, and deep. The overall effect of the external sphincter is a three-loop system which is claimed to maintain anal continence. The top loop is attached to the puborectalis, the middle loop to the coccyx, and the lower loop to the perianal skin (Figure 1.3). In the subcutaneous

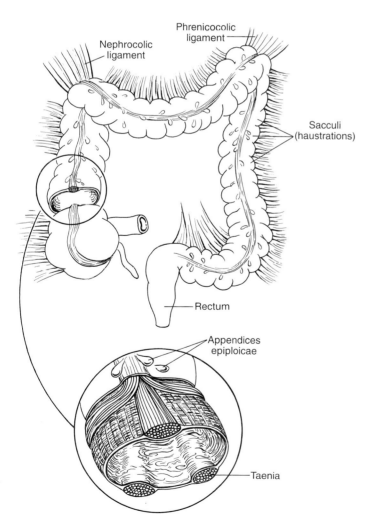

Figure 1.1 Diagram of the principal peritoneal attachments of the colon.

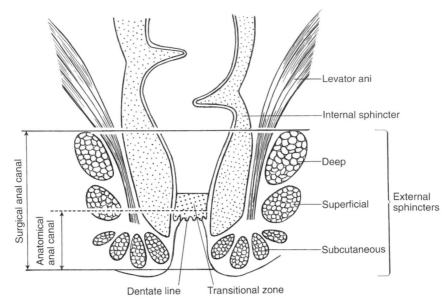

Figure 1.2 The anatomy of the anus and rectum.

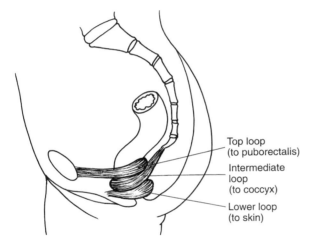

Figure 1.3 The 'three loop' system that maintains anal continence.

portion, the external sphincter is divided into eight to 12 muscle bundles by a fan-shaped expansion of the longitudinal muscle. The longitudinal muscle therefore acts as a skeleton binding the internal and external sphincters, supporting the haemorrhoidal cushions and aiding defecation by everting the anus.

The levator ani muscle forms the majority of the floor of the pelvic cavity. It is composed of three parts. The ileococcygeus runs backwards from the ischial spine and the posterior portion of the fascia covering obturator internus to the coccyx and the anococcygeal raphe. The pubococcygeus arises from the pubis and anterior part of the obturator fascia to the first portion of the coccyx. The puborectalis forms a strong U-shaped loop connecting the rectum to the back of the symphysis pubis and the urogenital diaphragm. The anorectal ring is composed of the upper portion of the internal and external sphincters and the puborectalis sling. It is extremely important to rectal continence. If it is preserved, despite the loss of the rest of the sphincter mechanism, continence will be essentially maintained while its complete division inevitably results in rectal incontinence.

Spaces in relation to the anal canal

Traditionally, there are four spaces around the anal canal: submucous, perianal, ischiorectal, and supralevator. To these have been added the central and intersphincteric space (see Chapter 18). The submucous space lies between the internal sphincter and the mucocutaneous lining of the upper two-thirds of the anal canal. The internal sphincteric space lies between the internal and external sphincters. The perianal space is continuous medially with the lower part of the anal canal and laterally with the subcutaneous fat of the buttocks. The ischiorectal space comprises the upper two-thirds of the ischiorectal fossa. It contains lobulated fat and the inferior haemorrhoidal vessels and nerves. Pus on one side may connect posteromedially with the opposite side via a rectosphincteric space (of Courtney) or extend anteriorly over the urogenital diaphragm. Two potential spaces exist, the supralevator space between the peritoneal floor and the levator ani and a central space lying between the lower end of the longitudinal intersphincteric muscle and the subcutaneous external sphincter. The latter space communicates with all other perianal spaces. The intersphincteric space lies along the longitudinal anal muscle and constitutes the main track for extension of pus along the anal canal.

The blood supply of the colon

The ileocolic artery ends in two caecal branches in 85% of cases, with the superior and inferior colic, appendiceal, ileal, and accessory ileal branches arising separately as collaterals from the main ileocolic stem (Figure 1.4). The blood supply of the appendix is variable, six different patterns of arterial supply having been identified (Kornblith *et al.* 1992). In 80% of individuals several arteries supply the appendix. The principal blood supply is a branch of the lower division of the ileocolic artery, which runs behind the terminal ileum to enter the mesoappendix a short distance from the base of the appendix. It is double in 5% of cases. If it becomes thrombosed as a result of inflammation, gangrene of the distal portion of the appendix ensues. In 40% of cases a recurrent branch arises at the base of the appendix to form a significant anastomosis with a branch of the posterior caecal artery near the base.

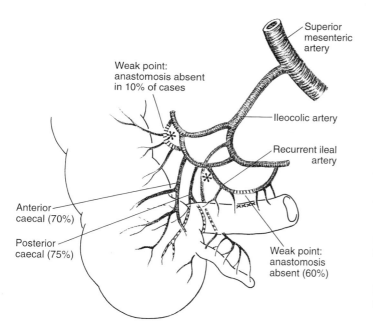

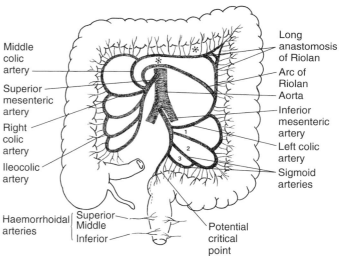

Figure 1.4 The blood supply to the appendix and caecum, showing potential weak points in the arterial anastomoses.

Figure 1.5 The blood supply to the colon showing potential weak points in the arterial system (*).

The right colic artery arises as a branch of a middle colic (52%), directly from the superior mesenteric (38%) or from the ileocolic artery (8%) (Kornblith *et al.* 1992). The middle colic artery arises from the superior mesenteric (44%) or the common right colic middle colic trunk (53%) just below the uncinate process of the pancreas and enters the transverse mesocolon (Figure 1.5). The inferior mesenteric artery gives collaterals only from its left side and ends by dividing into two superior rectal arteries. The first collateral

is the left colic artery. The left colic artery normally bifurcates at the splenic flexure, its right branch joining the middle colic artery and its left branch the marginal artery. In 40% of cases the left colic artery bifurcates 5 cm from the bowel wall so that its left and right branches are not anastomosed but function anatomically as the marginal artery. The marginal artery of Dwight and Drummond is the artery closest to and parallel with the wall of the intestine, which supplies vasa recti to it. It provides a continuous channel of potential collateral blood supply to the gut. Weak points in the colonic marginal arteries are an absent caecocolonic anastomosis (10%) and an absent (7%) or tenuous (33%) anastomosis at the splenic flexure (Kornblith *et al.* 1992) (Figures 1.4 and 1.5). At the

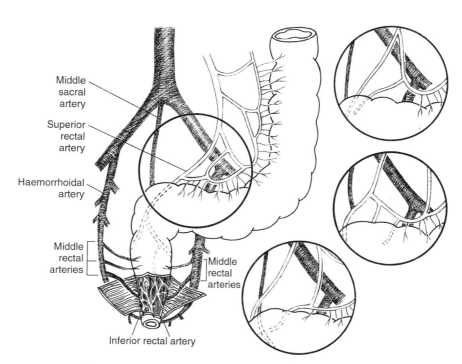

Figure 1.6 Variations in the blood supply of the sigmoid colon and rectum

splenic flexure, there may be no primary or secondary anastomotic arcade linking the left branch of the middle colic artery with the ascending branch of the left colic artery within 5 cm of the colonic wall. To ensure a viable blood supply the left colic artery should always be ligated proximal to its bifurcation.

There are three connections between the superior and inferior mesenteric arteries which may contribute to the collateral circulation when either major vessel is occluded. One is the marginal artery of Drummond. A larger calibre, more centrally placed artery usually represents a direct anastomosis of the middle and left colic arteries. The third connection runs in the base of the mesentery and joins the middle colic artery to the junction of the middle and left colic vessels (the artery of Riolan) (Kornblith *et al.* 1992). Marked dilatation of the latter is apparent angiographically in occlusion of the superior or inferior mesenteric arteries ('the meandering artery of Moskowitz') (Figure 1.5). In major vessel occlusion, collaterals open up with the coeliac axis via aberrantly derived middle colic arteries, the internal and external iliac vessels through rectal, vesical and gluteal branches and with the aorta via the middle sacral and retroperitoneal branches.

Sigmoid arteries arise from all three branches of the left colic, the number of arteries depending on the width and length of the sigmoid mesocolon (Figure 1.6). In 85% of cases two or three arteries are responsible. The descending branch of the inferior mesenteric artery becomes the superior rectal artery which provides the main blood supply to the rectum. After bifurcating its branches enter the rectal wall directly rather than forming arcades. It forms an anastomosis with the middle and inferior rectal arteries, which are derived from the internal iliac artery and supplies blood to the anal margin in up to 90% of individuals. Rectal stumps are therefore normally viable.

The blood supply of the anus is by the inferior haemorrhoidal artery which originates from the internal pudendal branch of the internal iliac artery in Alcock's canal. As it runs medially from the outer walls of the ischiorectal fossa, its branches transverse the sphincters to reach the submucosa and subcutaneous tissues of the anal canal where it communicates with branches from the opposite side. An additional blood supply may come from the middle sacral artery. The levator ani and external sphincter muscles are supplied by branches of the pudendal artery. The insertion of the levator ani is a dividing line for the blood supply to the rectum and anus. Cranially, the superior haemorrhoidal and, distally, the inferior haemorrhoidal artery, respectively, are the principal vessels. The generous blood supply of the inferior haemorrhoidal artery to the anus explains the generally good healing of coloanal anastomoses.

Venous blood from the right half of the colon drains into the superior mesenteric vein which empties directly into the portal vein. Blood from the left colon also goes to the portal vein via the inferior mesenteric, splenic, or superior mesenteric veins. The venous drainage of the anal canal is via the internal submucous haemorrhoidal plexus which drains into the superior rectal vein and from there into the portal system. The external or subcutaneous haemorrhoidal vein drains into the systemic venous circulation by the inferior rectal vein. In normal circumstances there is little communication between these two venous plexuses. However, the absence of valves in the portal system allows the transmission of increased pressure from portal hypertension to the systemic circulation via the connection between these two plexuses.

The arrangement of the lymphatics is uniform throughout the colon. Submucous and subserous lymphatics drain into the epicolic nodes which lie below the serosa and in the appendices epiploicae.

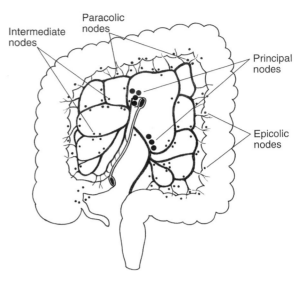

Figure 1.7 The lymphatic drainage of the colon.

These nodes are particularly common in the sigmoid colon. The epicolic nodes drain into the paracolic group along the marginal artery, then into the intermediate nodes along the ileocolic, right, left, and sigmoid colic arteries. From the intermediate nodes, the lymph drains to the principal nodes along the superior and inferior mesenteric arteries and then into the ileolumbar chain and the thoracic duct (Figure 1.7). Lesions arising above the anal verge drain via the mesorectum, superior haemorrhoidal and inferior mesenteric vessels to reach the pre-aortic nodes. Some of the lymph drains laterally from this region via the middle haemorrhoidal vessels and ischiorectal fossa to reach the hypogastric nodes. In contrast, lesions occurring below the anal verge drain principally downward along with lymphatic plexuses in the anal and perianal skin, the anal sphincters, and the ischiorectal fat, eventually to reach the inguinal glands.

Nerve supply

The parasympathetics are thought to accelerate motor and secretory activity of the colon, stimulating peristalsis and opening the rectal sphincter. The parasympathetic innervation of the right colon up to the proximal third of the transverse colon is probably derived from the vagus nerve, that of the left colon from second to fourth sacral nerves. The sympathetic innervation of the colon comes from T_{11}, T_{12}, L_1 and L_2 through the sympathetic chain. The internal anal sphincter is innervated by sympathetic and parasympathetic fibres. The sympathetic fibres arise from the aortic plexus and lumbar splanchnics and run across the common iliac artery as the hypogastric nerves before forming plexuses on either side of the pelvis. These plexuses also receive parasympathetic fibres from the nervi erigentes (S_{2-4}). The voluntary contracting external sphincter is supplied in its anterior two-thirds by the anterior ramus of the external perineal nerve, the inferior haemorrhoidal branch of the internal pudendal and in one-third of cases by a posterior branch arising from the perineal branch of the fourth sacral nerve.

The levator ani is supplied on its pelvic aspect by the fourth sacral nerve and on its perineal aspect by the inferior haemorrhoidal or perineal branches of the pudendal nerves. In two-thirds of cases, two separate nerves arise from the sacral plexus, while in the remaining one-third, a single nerve divides into two branches close to the muscle. Studies on patients with 'chordomas' reveal that it is sufficient to retain only one S_2 nerve root for continence, including the ability to distinguish solid from flatus. Sensory innervation above the dentate line is mediated by the parasympathetic nerves which travel via the inferior haemorrhoidal branches of the pudendal nerve to the sacral roots of S_{234}. However, many encapsulated nerve endings extend into the transitional zone for 0.5–1 cm above the dentate line. This explains why injection or banding of haemorrhoids can be uncomfortable. Below the anal valves, sensation is felt via the inferior haemorrhoidal nerve. However, anal canal discrimination is only preserved if at least both S_2 roots and one S_3 root is intact.

Embryological anomalies

At the sixth gestational week the caecal diverticulum first appears. After the fifth month the distal part of this diverticulum remains rudimentary and forms the vermiform appendix, while the proximal part expands to form the caecum, ascending and transverse colon. The distal portion of the transverse colon to the rectum is derived from the hindgut.

Initially, the gut is a straight tube suspended in a sagittal plane on a common dorsal mesentery. Between the fifth and eighth week the primitive gut elongates on its mesentery about the superior mesenteric artery and then moves 90° counter-clockwise from the sagittal to the horizontal plane (Figure 1.8). At the tenth week the mid-gut loop returns to the peritoneal cavity and rotates 180°

counter-clockwise about the mesenteric root. The final stage of gut rotation consists of the descent of the caecum and fusion of the mesentery. Anomalies may occur at each stage (Table 1.1).

Other embryologically derived abnormalities include colonic atresia. This accounts for only 5% of all gastrointestinal atresias and is probably caused by occlusion of the blood supply to the affected segment during intrauterine development. Congenital diverticula represent minor duplications and often share a common wall with the normal bowel. The lumen of the diverticulum is lined with intestinal (colonic, gastric, or pancreatic) epithelium. In duplication of the entire colon and rectum the two parts lie parallel, sharing a common wall throughout most of their length except in the pelvis. There may be two separate openings but more commonly the accessory lumen, usually the inner loop, ends blindly or drains incompletely through an ectopic opening into the perineum, vagina, or posterior urethra. Abnormalities of the genito-urinary organs occur in half those with colonic duplication. The caecum is almost entirely invested in peritoneum and can be very mobile, causing volvulus.

The rectum and anal canal develop in association with the urogenital system, so that abnormalities in each of these systems often occur together. The urogenital septum separates the cloaca from the segment forming the urinary bladder and urogenital sinus. Abnormal development of the urogenital septum results in the imperforate anus anomalies while persistence of a duct connecting the cloaca to the urogenital septum creates a fistula between the rectum and bladder or urethra (see Chapter 2).

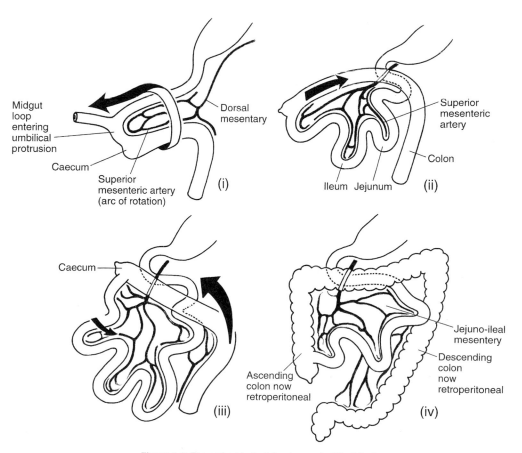

Figure 1.8 The embryological development of the intestine.

Table 1.1 Abnormalities associated with embryological rotation of the gut

Embryological process	Abnormality
Gut undergoes umbilical herniation and first counter-clockwise rotation 5–8 weeks	Situs inversus
	Extroversion of the cloaca
	Duodenal abnormalities
Gut returns to peritoneal cavity and second counter-clockwise rotation 10th week	Non-rotation (caecum in left lower quadrant ± mid-gut volvulus)
	Malrotation (caecum fixed in right upper quadrant ± duodenal constriction)
	Reversed rotation (transverse colon lies behind duodenum and small bowel)
	Internal hernia (small bowel trapped under right colon mesentery)
	Omphalocoele (gut fails to return to peritoneal cavity)
Descent of caecum	Subhepatic caecum
	Mobile caecum
	Overdescent of caecum
	Persistent colonic mesentery
	Common ileocaecal mesentery

Physiology

The principal function of the colon is to absorb water and electrolytes, resulting in a more solid stool. The human colon receives 200–500 ml of fluid per day from the terminal ileum. Depending on consistency, stool contains 60–95% water, the remainder consisting of bacteria, cellular debris, and non-digestible food products. Water reabsorption averages 350 ml/day and is dependent on epithelial electrolyte transport. Almost all of the sodium presented to the colon is actively reabsorbed in the right colon, so that this is also the site of maximum colonic fluid reabsorption. Potassium enters the colon lumen at a rate dependent on sodium absorption. This is mediated by a H^+–K^+-ATPase on the apical membrane which is aldosterone dependent (Watanabe *et al.* 1990). Hypokalaemia may therefore result from repeated tap water enemas while hyperchloraemic acidosis can complicate ureterosigmoid anastomoses. In villous adenomas, colonic fluid loss can be 1–3 litres containing 120–160 mmol of sodium and potassium per day.

Chloride ions are conserved by a process associated with opposite bicarbonate movement. About half of the daily chloride secretion comes from prostaglandins and eicosanoids that originate in the lamina propria. Immune cell products such as immunoglobulin (Ig) E and platelet-activating factor stimulate eicosanoid release and the resulting prostaglandins directly stimulate epithelial cells to secrete chloride (Bern *et al.* 1989). The remainder of the chloride secretion results from activation of the enteric nervous system. Short chain fatty acids, produced by bacterial metabolism of undigested carbohydrate, are the major anions in the colon and therefore also have an important effect on colonic fluid transport. In addition, epithelial fluid and electrolyte transport is under hormonal control, principally from glucocorticoids and mineralocorticoids.

Anal continence

Many factors contribute to the maintenance of anorectal continence. The most important is probably the anorectal angle of 60–105° created between the lower rectum and upper anal canal by the puborectalis sling. Normally, this angle is maintained except on maximal flexion of the hips or during defecation. The anal sphincters aid continence by creating a higher pressure in the anal canal than in the rectum. These pressures are reversed on straining, or performing a Valsalva manoeuvre. The external sphincter induces continence by preventing internal sphincter relaxation and by mechanical compression of the anal canal.

Continence may still be maintained if the striated muscles (puborectalis and the external sphincter) are paralysed so that other factors are important. The internal sphincter contributes 50–60% of the anal pressure at rest. However, the internal sphincter alone cannot completely close the anal canal, an intrasphincteric gap of 7–8 mm remaining. This gap appears to be closed by a combination of the anal cushions, a one-way 'flutter valve' created by the transmission of the intra-abdominal pressure to the side of the anal canal in the region of the anorectal junction and the surface tension of the moist surfaces of the anal canal.

Investigations

Colonoscopy

Colonoscopy is often considered the investigation of choice for assessing the colon, being potentially both diagnostic and therapeutic. It is generally more accurate than barium enema, while also being reproducible, interobserver agreement being almost 100% for lesions over 1 cm and 85% for lesions smaller than this (Hixson

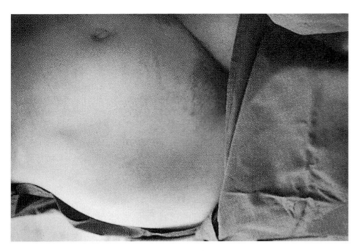

Figure 1.9 Transillumination in the right iliac fossa during colonoscopy signifying the caecum has been reached (see colour plates).

et al. 1991; Norfleet *et al.* 1991). Endoscopic location of polyps or tumours is 85% accurate compared with surgery, with one third of all endoscopic errors occurring in the caecum (Vignati *et al.* 1994; Rex 1995). Colonoscopy is less sensitive than double contrast barium enema at detecting diverticular disease and is claimed to be slower, three times more expensive, and 10 times more dangerous (Dodd 1991). The ability to intubate the caecum is not related to diverticular disease, but is significantly less in women with a history of abdominal hysterectomy (Cirocco and Rusin 1995) (Figure 1.9). Assessment of a previous barium enema is a useful guide to probable technical difficulty of colonoscopy (Saunders *et al.* 1995). In a

recent study 75% of the costs of total colonoscopy would be avoided if only patients presenting with bleeding and inflammatory bowel disease were offered total colonoscopy and patients with radiological abnormalities were treated according to the abnormality (Isbister 1995).

Although colonoscopy is generally safe in both adults and children, the risk of perforation (about 0.3%) is greater than with barium enema (0.04%) (Carpio *et al.* 1989) (Figure 1.10). Colonoscopy should therefore not be performed in those with marked abdominal tenderness or peritonism, but it is safe after recent colonic surgery (Cappell *et al.* 1995). If perforation does occur, patients who are stable and do not have peritonitis or distal obstruction may often be safely treated conservatively with antibiotics (Kavin *et al.* 1992; Weber *et al.* 1993). Serosal burns may occur following 0.5% of polypectomies, being more likely to occur with sessile or thick-stalked polyps (Christie and Marrazzo 1991). Other complications of colonoscopy include delayed massive haemorrhage after the use of hot biopsy forceps in polyps over 5 mm and splenic haematomas (Gores and Simso 1989; Williams 1991). Colonoscopy should be avoided for 3 weeks after myocardial infarction due to the risk of arrhythmias. Patients with valvular heart disease, ascites, immunosuppression, or on peritoneal dialysis require prophylactic antibiotics because of the risk of transient bacteraemia.

The accuracy of colonoscopy can be further increased by 'salvage' (suction-trap aspiration) cytology (Graham *et al.* 1989). For submucosal lesions, sclerotherapy needle aspiration is claimed to be 93% accurate, although deep guillotine biopsy may be even better (Zargat *et al.* 1991). A 'turn and suck' method, in which, with suction applied, the forceps are closed blindly on the mucosa, is claimed to take 50% larger biopsies (Levine and Reid 1991). Dye-laser light transmitted down the endoscope is claimed to discriminate between adenomatous and hyperplastic tissue with a 94% predictive value (von Reuben *et al.* 1993). If patients are going on to surgery, an endoscopically localized lesion may be marked by methylene blue, although this may disappear within 24 h. Indocyanine green may be preferable, lasting up to 7 days (Hammond *et al.* 1989).

The adequate disinfection of colonoscopes is important. Glutaraldehyde (2% alkaline solution) is the only satisfactory disinfectant that destroys all viruses and bacteria. A 4-min soak/channel perfusion is therefore sufficient to eradicate all normal organisms and viruses. In patients sensitized to glutaraldehyde, a bactericidal detergent for 2 min followed by a 70% ethyl alcohol soak for 4 min is an effective alternative. Those at risk of mycobacterial spores, including immunosuppressed patients, require a 60-min soak in glutaraldehyde. The hand controls should also be disinfected by glutaraldehyde or alcohol between cases as contamination of the endoscopist's gloves is common so that the instrument control head is contaminated in one-quarter of cases (Sobala *et al.* 1989).

There is still no ideal bowel preparation (Golub *et al.* 1995). For flexible sigmoidoscopy or limited colonoscopy, two phosphate enemas will frequently clear the bowel up to the hepatic flexure. If full bowel preparation is required iron should be stopped 3–4 days and constipating agents 1–2 days before the examination. A low roughage diet or preferably clear fluids should be commenced 24 h before colonoscopy. Oral lavage regimens are often preferred to purge plus enema as they are quicker, more effective and cause less pain (Berry and DiPalma *et al.* 1994). Sufficient laxative should be given to produce a fluid diarrhoea which shows that colonic residue has been cleared and small bowel contents are present. Mannitol is

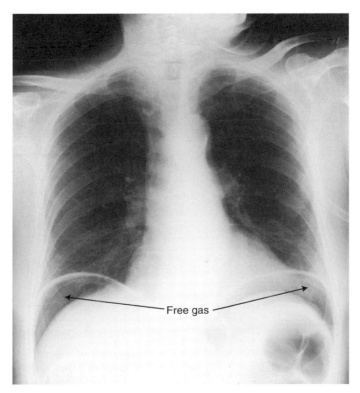

Free gas

Figure 1.10 Erect chest X-ray showing free peritoneal gas from colonic perforation sustained during colonoscopy.

rarely used as the effect of colonic bacteria produces large quantities of hydrogen which makes diathermy or laser unsafe unless carbon dioxide is used. Three to four litres of isotonic saline is effective, but tastes salty. Picolax, which produces both magnesium citrate and bisacodyl by bacterial action, provides 80–90% mucosal visualization provided enough fluid is ingested (Hickson *et al.* 1990). Polyethylene glycol (PEG) is also effective, less than 10% of procedures being abandoned due to inadequate preparation (Rodney *et al.* 1993). However, it is relatively unpalatable, 85% of patients finding it hard to tolerate, with one-quarter vomiting the solution (Hangartner *et al.* 1989). A low sodium PEG preparation is claimed to be as effective while being more palatable to patients (DiPalma and Marshall 1990). Four litres of PEG fluid are required to give adequate visualization in 95% of patients; volumes less than this are generally unsatisfactory (Afridi *et al.* 1995).

The ideal sedative for colonoscopy should be short lasting (15 min) with strong analgesic action but no respiratory effect. Small doses of midazolam are associated with a greater amnesic effect than diazepam. It is claimed that many patients can undergo total colonoscopy without sedation, discomfort only occurring if the endoscopist allows loops (principally sigmoid) to form. However, 15% of examinations done without sedation are terminated because of pain compared with only 5% in sedated patients (Rodney *et al.* 1993). Consequently, the caecum may be reached in only 30–80% of those without sedation compared with over 90% if sedation is used. Against this, if patients are over-sedated complications can occur from excessive force and over-distension of the colon. Approximately half of patients receiving diazepam 5 mg and pethidine 30 mg will develop a PO_2 of under 90% (McKee *et al.* 1991). Hypoxia and hypotension are unpredictable, usually clinically unrecognizable, and often occur after, as well as during, colonoscopy. All patients should receive pulse-oximeter monitoring and elderly patients at least should have low-flow oxygen.

Carbon dioxide clears 100 times faster than air so it is preferable in patients with strictures or functional disorders who are likely to experience pain on distension. In addition, immediate barium enema is more likely to be successful with carbon dioxide insufflation. Many of the potential loops that can form during colonoscopy can be removed by a torque technique so that most experienced endoscopists reach the caecum in 95% of patients (Waye *et al.* 1991). Fluoroscopy can be helpful in colonoscopies that remain difficult despite all attempts to overcome technical problems (Rogers 1990). In cases of severe diverticular disease changing to a paediatric colonoscope or gastroscope allows the scope to be passed beyond the sigmoid in 75–90% of cases (Bat and Williams 1989).

Radiology

Plain radiographs

In the acute abdomen, plain films are the initial, and frequently only, radiological investigation required. Positive findings may be found in half of the cases, although they are frequently non-specific or misleading. The erect chest film is the single most informative radiograph. Supine films should include the inguinal region and diaphragm. In ill patients, the left decubitus (right side up) will demonstrate a small amount of free gas which collects between the liver and the chest wall (Williams and Everson 1997). Fluid levels in the stomach and duodenum are normal, as are little amounts of small intestinal gas. However, a loop which is completely filled with gas should be considered abnormal. The normal bowel wall is less than 2 mm thick and may be assessed when two adjacent loops of

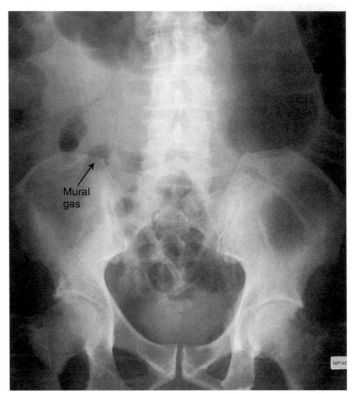

Figure 1.11 Obstructed sigmoid colon tumour causing marked large bowel dilatation. Note gas in the wall of the caecum implying imminent perforation.

bowel are gas-filled. The colon is identified by its peripheral position and the presence of haustra, although these may be absent in the descending and sigmoid colon. Although in elderly patients the colon may reach 15 cm without significant pathology, a diameter of over 5 cm in a patient with colitis signifies toxic megacolon.

In large bowel obstruction, the proximal colon is distended with gas and fluid while the distal bowel is collapsed with no gas in the rectum (Figure 1.11). In chronic obstruction a large amount of faeces builds up in the proximal bowel (Figure 1.12). If the ileocaecal valve is incompetent, the small bowel but not the caecum dilates. The appearances are similar to an ileus, except that there is no gas in the rectum. The risk of perforation is significant if the caecum exceeds 9 cm. Pneumoperitoneum may be suggested by gas in Morrison's pouch, outlining the falciform or umbilical ligaments, in the lesser sac, between loops of bowel, in the subhepatic space, overlying the liver. The properitoneal fat line lies in the flank and outlines the peritoneum. Fat also outlines the liver, spleen kidneys and psoas muscles, so that these structures may be identified in half of plain abdominal radiographs. In patients with suspected inflammatory bowel disease, the insertion of air into the rectum (air enema) can provide valuable information (Lindstrom and Noren 1992). Abnormal features on plain radiographs are listed in Table 1.2.

Barium enema

Bowel preparation for barium enema is often similar to that for colonoscopy, although the time-consuming cleansing enema can be omitted (Hageman and Goei 1993). Single contrast barium enemas consist of a low-density, low-viscosity barium sulphate suspension (Figure 1.13). Double contrast enemas are performed using high-density, high-viscosity barium sulphate suspension with insufflated air (Scullion *et al.* 1995). Double contrast films provide better

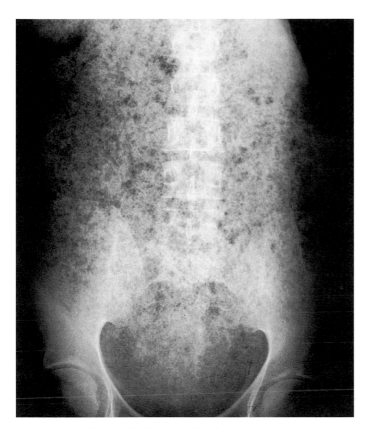

Figure 1.12 Gross faecal loading of the colon.

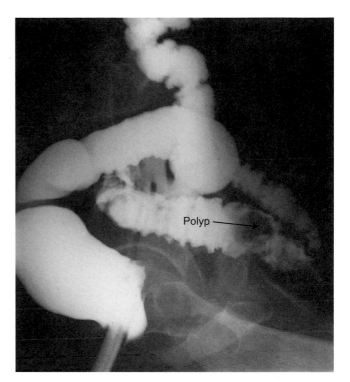

Figure 1.13 Single contrast barium enema showing large polyp in the sigmoid colon.

mucosal detail, especially for polyps less than 1 cm and small ulceration in inflammatory bowel disease (Figures 1.14 and 1.15). However, single contrast enemas are the technique of choice in emergency situations and for debilitated patients who cannot hold the air during the double contrast procedure. If perforation is a possibility a water-soluble enema should be performed. Many patients consider a barium enema significantly less painful than colonoscopy (Steine 1994). A study of tumours identified by colonoscopy but missed on barium enema revealed that all were in the caecum, ascending colon, or sigmoid colon and a review of the

films identified the tumour in three-quarters (Anderson *et al.* 1991). Barium enema is also valuable in investigating the entire colon after flexible sigmoidoscopy and in those in whom total colonoscopy has failed due to diverticular disease (Morosi *et al.* 1991). In patients in

Table 1.2 Abnormal features seen on plain abdominal radiographs

Finding	Abnormality
Fluid levels	*Normal*: stomach, duodenum, 2–3 in small bowel
	Abnormal: More than 3 small bowel fluid levels
	One or more completely gas- or fluid-filled small bowel loops
Gas shadows	Free gas
	Retroperitoneal gas
	Gas in biliary tree, portal vein, bowel wall, abscess, or hernia
Fat lines	Displacement, blurring, effacement
Chest	Elevated diaphragm
Bones	Metastases
	Congenital abnormalities

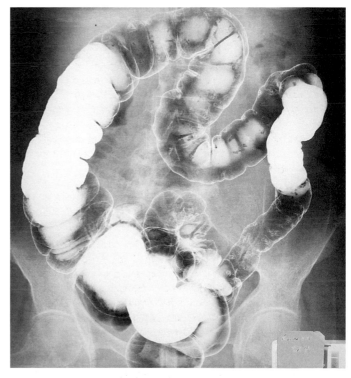

Figure 1.14 The fine mucosal detail obtained by double contrast barium enema in a case of filiform polyposis

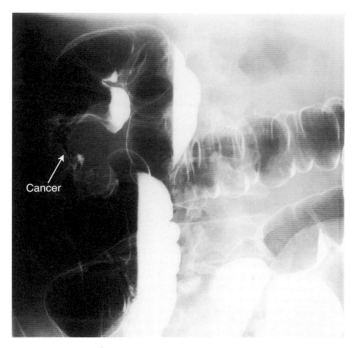

Figure 1.15 Double contrast barium enema showing typical 'apple core' appearances of a colonic carcinoma.

whom standard retrograde studies are unsuccessful, as in severe colonic stenosis, oral barium studies followed through to the colon can provide valuable information (Gotta *et al.* 1990) (Figure 1.16).

Barium enema is a safe and accurate diagnostic study of the colon but, in rare cases, complications may result. Perforation of the bowel is the most frequent serious complication, occurring in 0.02–0.04% of patients (Williams and Harned 1991). Predisposing factors for perforation include reduced tensile strength of the bowel in elderly patients or those receiving long-term steroid therapy, and in disease states such as neoplasm, diverticulitis, inflammatory bowel disease, and ischaemia. Other predisposing factors are recent deep biopsy and polypectomy with electrocautery. Injury to the rectal mucosa or anal canal due to the enema tip or retention balloon is probably the most common traumatic cause of barium enema perforation. Inflation of a retention balloon within a stricture, neoplasm, inflamed rectum, or colostomy stoma is particularly hazardous. Intraperitoneal perforation leads to a severe, acute peritonitis, the ensuing shock of which may be rapidly fatal. If the patient survives, later complications caused by dense intraperitoneal adhesions may develop. Extraperitoneal perforation is usually less catastrophic but may result in pain, sepsis, cellulitis, abscess, rectal stricture, or fistula. Intramural extravasation often forms a persistent submucosal barium granuloma which may ulcerate or be mistaken for a neoplasm. Bacteraemia has been found in up to one-quarter of patients following barium enema and, in rare cases, may cause symptomatic septicaemia (Williams and Harned 1991). Other complications include barium impaction, water intoxication, allergic reactions, and cardiac arrhythmias.

Ultrasound and computerized tomography scanning

Ultrasound is particularly useful in identifying free intraperitoneal fluid, or abdominal abscesses. It is also helpful in equivocal cases of appendicitis, inflammatory bowel disease and pseudomembranous colitis. It may identify colonic conditions, such as carcinoma or diverticulitis, although intraluminal air often prevents adequate pictures. (Figure 1.17). Endorectal ultrasound is useful in staging rectal cancer, while colonoscopic ultrasound (endosonography) is helpful in assessing colon carcinoma or submucosal lipomas (de Lange 1994). Endoanal or endovaginal ultrasound can also assess the anatomy, thickness, function, and abnormalities of the anal sphincters (Sultan

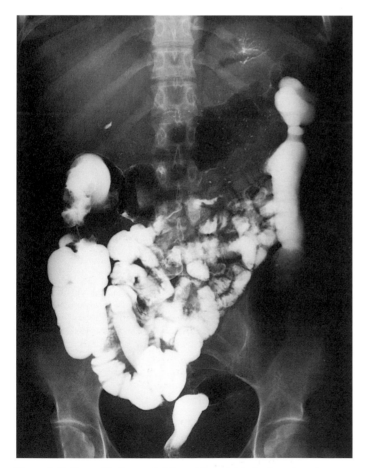

Figure 1.16 Per-oral barium study followed through into the large bowel showing the typical 'hose-pipe' colon of chronic ulcerative colitis.

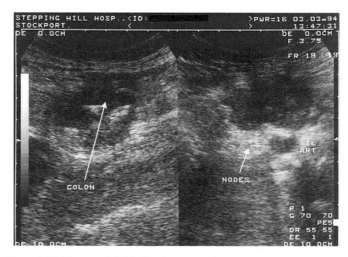

Figure 1.17 Ultrasound of right iliac fossa mass showing the irregular bowel wall of a caecal carcinoma.

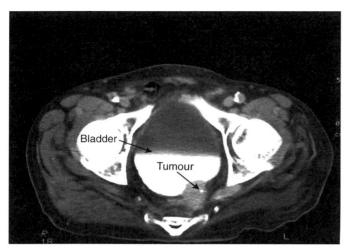

Figure 1.18 Magnetic resonance scan showing recurrent tumour indenting the bladder.

et al. 1994; Van Outryve *et al.* 1994). It is better at evaluating anal anatomy and morphology in defecation disorders than magnetic resonance imaging (Schafer *et al.* 1994).

Ultrasound-guided biopsy and the therapeutic drainage of abscesses are also advantages of the technique. Computerized tomography scanning is beneficial in assessing colonic wall invasion in colorectal cancer and in diagnosing appendicitis. At present the applications of magnetic resonance scanning are limited to the evaluation of colorectal tumours, their recurrence or metastases and to improve the visualization of perianal fistulas (Kraus *et al.* 1994; Myhur *et al.* 1994). (Figure 1.18) The value of techniques such as positron emission tomography remains to be evaluated (Young 1994).

References

Afridi SA, Barthel JS, King PD, Pineda JJ, Marshall JB. Prospective, randomized trial comparing a new sodium phosphate bisacodyl regimen with conventional PEG ES lavage for outpatient colonoscopy preparation. *Gastrointest. Endosc.* 1995; 41: 485–9.

Anderson N, Cook BH, Coates R. Colonoscopically detected colorectal cancer missed on barium enema. *Gastrointest. Endosc.* 1991; 126: 123–7.

Bat L, Williams CB. Usefulness of pediatric colonoscopes in adult colonoscopy. *Gastrointest. Endosc.* 1989; 35: 329–32.

Bern MJ, Sturbaum CW, Karalacin SS, Berschneider HM, Wachsman JT, Powell DW. Immune system control of rat and rabbit colonic electrolyte transport. *J. Clin. Invest.* 1989; 83: 1810–20.

Berry MA, DiPalma JA. Review article: orthograde gut lavage for colonoscopy. *Aliment. Pharmacol. Ther.* 1994; 8: 391–5.

Cappell MS, Ghandi D, Huh C. A study of the safety and clinical efficacy of flexible sigmoidoscopy and colonoscopy after recent colonic surgery in 52 patients. *Am. J. Gastroenterol.* 1995; 90: 1130–4.

Carpio G, Albu E, Gumbs MA, Gerst PH. Management of colonic perforation after colonoscopy: report of three cases. *Dis. Colon Rectum* 1989; 32: 624–6.

Christie JP, Marrazzo J. 'Mini perforations' of the colon, not all postpolypectomy perforations require laparotomy. *Dis. Colon Rectum* 1991; 34: 132–5.

Cirocco WC, Rusin LC. Factors that predict incomplete colonoscopy. *Dis. Colon Rectum* 1995; 38: 964–8.

de Lange EE. Staging rectal carcinoma with endorectal imaging. How much detail do we really need? *Radiology* 1994; 190: 633–5.

DiPalma JA, Marshall JB. Comparison of a new sulfate, free polyethylene glycol electrolyte lavage solution versus a standard solution for colonoscopy cleansing. *Gastrointest. Endosc.* 1990; 36: 285–9.

Dodd GD. Imaging techniques in the diagnsosis of carcinoma of the colon. *Cancer* 1991; 67: 1150–4.

Golub RW, Kerner BA, Wise WE Jr, Meesig DM, Hartmann RF, Khanduja KS, Aguilar PS. Colonoscopic bowel preparations which one? A blinded, prospective, randomized trial. *Dis. Colon Rectum* 1995; 38: 594–9.

Gores PF, Simso LA. Splenic injury during colonoscopy. *Arch. Surg.* 1989; 124: 1342.

Gotta C, Palau GA, Demos TC, Villaveiran RG. Colonic stenosis: use of oral barium when retrograde flow is completely obstructed in barium enema studies. *Radiology* 1990; 177: 703–8.

Graham DY, Tabibian N, Michaletz PA, Kinner BM, Schwartz JT, Heiser MC, *et al.* Endoscopic needle biopsy: a comparative study of forceps biopsy, two different types of needles and salvage cytology in gastrointestinal cancer. *Gastrointest. Endosc.* 1989; 35: 207–9.

Hageman M, Goei R. Cleansing enema prior to double contrast barium enema examination: is it necessary? *Radiology* 1993; 187: 109–12.

Hammond DC, Lane FR, Welk RA, Madura MJ, Borreson DK, Passinault WJ. Endoscopic tattooing of the colon: an experimental study. *Am. Surg.* 1989; 55: 457–61.

Hangartner PJ, Munch R, Meier J, Ammann R, Buhler H. Comparison of three colon cleansing methods: evaluation of a randomised clinical trial with 300 ambulatory patients. *Endoscopy* 1989; 21: 272–5.

Hickson DEG, Cox JGC, Taylor RG, Bennett JR. Enema or Picolax as preparation for flexible sigmoidoscopy? *Postgrad. Med. J.* 1990; 66: 210–11.

Hixson LJ, Fennerty MB, Sampliner RE, Garewal HS. Prospective blinded trial of colonoscopic miss rate of large colorectal polyps. *Gastrointest. Endosc.* 1991; 37: 125–7.

Isbister WH. Colonoscopy: how far is enough? *Aust. N.Z. J. Surg.* 1995; 65: 44–7.

Kavin H, Sinicrope F, Esker AH. Management of perforation of the colon at colonoscopy. *Am. J. Gastroenterol.* 1992; 87: 161–7.

Kornblith PL, Boley SJ, Whitehouse BS. Anatomy of the splanchnic circulation. *Surg. Clin. North Am.* 1992; 72: 1–30.

Kraus BB, Rappaport DC, Ros PR, Torres GM. Evaluation of oral contrast agents for abdominal magnetic resonance imaging. *Magn. Reson. Imaging* 1994; 12: 847–58.

Levine DS, Reid BJ. Endoscopic biopsy technique for acquiring larger mucosal samples. *Gastrointest. Endosc.* 1991; 37: 332–7.

Lindstrom E, Noren B. Air enema revisited in assessment of colitis. *Acta Radiol.* 1992; 33: 360–1.

McKee CC, Ragland JJ, Myers JO. An evaluation of multiple clinical variables for hypoxia during colonoscopy. *Surg. Gynecol. Obstet.* 1991; 173: 37–40.

Morosi C, Ballardini G, Pisani P, *et al.* Diagnostic accuracy of the double contrast enema for colonic polyps in patients with or without diverticular disease. *Gastrointest. Radiol.* 1991; 16: 345–9.

Myhur GE, Myrvold HE, Nilsen G, Thoresen JE, Rinck PA. Perianal fistulas: use of MR imaging for diagnosis. *Radiology* 1994: 191: 545–9.

Norfleet RG, Ryan ME, Wyman JB, Rhodes RA, Nunez JF, Kirchner JP, Parent K. Barium enema versus colonoscopy for patients with polyps found during flexible sigmoidoscopy. *Gastrointest. Endosc.* 1991; 37: 531–4.

Rex DK. Colonoscopy: a review of its yield for cancers and adenomas by indication. *Am. J. Gastroenterol.* 1995; 90: 353–65.

Rodney WM, Dabov G, Orientale E, Reeves WP. Sedation associated with a more complete colonoscopy. *J. Fam. Pract.* 1993; 36: 394–400.

Rogers BHG. Colonoscopy with fluoroscopy. *Gastrointest. Endosc.* 1990; 36: 71–2.

Saunders BP, Halligan S, Jobling C, Fukumoto M, Moussa ME, Williams CB, Bartram CI. Can barium enema indicate when colonoscopy will be difficult? *Clin. Radiol.* 1995; 50: 318–21.

Schafer A, Enck P, Furst G, Kahn T, Frieling T, Lubke HJ. Anatomy of the anal sphincters. Comparison of anal endosonography to magnetic resonance imaging. *Dis. Colon Rectum* 1994; 37: 777–81.

Scullion DA, Wetton CW, Davies C, Whitaker L, Shorvon PJ. The use of air or CO_2 as insufflation agents for double contrast barium enema (DCBE): is there a qualitative difference? *Clin. Radiol.* 1995; 50: 558–61.

Sobala GM, Lincoln C, Axon ATR. Does the endoscope control head need to be cleaned between examinations? *Endoscopy* 1989; 21: 19–21.

Steine S. Which hurts the most? A comparison of pain rating during double contrast barium enema examination and colonoscopy. *Radiology* 1994; 191: 99–101.

Sultan AH, Loder PB, Bartram CI, Kamm MA, Hudson CN. Vaginal endosonography. New approach to image the undisturbed anal sphincter. *Dis. Colon Rectum* 1994; 37: 1296–9.

Van Outryve M, Pelckmans P, Fierens H, Van Maercke Y. Transrectal ultrasonographic examination of the anal sphincter. *Acta Gastroenterol.* 1994; 57: 26–7.

Vignati P, Welch JP, Cohen JL. Endoscopic localization of colon cancers. *Surg. Endosc.* 1994; 8: 1085–7.

von Rueden DG, McBrearty FX, Clements BM, Woratyla S. Photo detection of carcinoma of the colon in a rat model: a pilot study. *J. Surg. Oncol.* 1993; 53: 43–6.

Watanabe T, Suzuki T, Suzuki Y. Ouabain sensitive K-ATPase in epithelial cells from guinea pig distal colon. *Am. J. Physiol.* 1990; 258: G506–11.

Waye JD, Yessaman SA, Lewis BS, Fabry TL. The technique of abdominal pressure in total colonoscopy. *Gastrointest. Endosc.* 1991; 37: 147–51.

Weber DJ, Rodney WM, Warren J. Management of suspected perforation following colonoscopy: a case report. *J. Fam. Pract.* 1993; 36: 567–70.

Williams CB. Small polyps, the virtues and dangers of hot biopsy. *Gastrointest. Endosc.* 1991; 37: 394–5.

Williams SM, Harned RK. Recognition and control of barium enema complications. *Curr. Probl. Diagn. Radiol.* 1991; 20: 123–51.

Williams N, Everson NW. Radiological confirmation of intraperitoneal free gas. *Ann. Roy. Coll. Surg. Engl.* 1997; 79: 8–12.

Young IR. Review of modalities with a potential future in radiology. *Radiology* 1994; 192: 307–18.

Zargat SA, Khuroo MS, Mahajan R, Jan GM, Dewani K, Koul V. Endoscopic fine needle aspiration cytology in the diagnosis of gastro-oesophageal and colorectal malignancies. *Gut* 1991; 32: 745–8.

2 Paediatric conditions

Anorectal malformations

Classification

An international classification of anorectal malformations was devised in 1970 and subsequently revised in 1984 (Santulli 1970; Stephens and Smith 1986). Anomalies are classified as high, intermediate or low depending on the relationship of the bowel to the levator ani (Pena 1995).

High anomalies (normal bowel ends above the levator ani) (Figure 2.1)

1. Anorectal agenesis which includes an absent anal canal with or without a fistula from the distal extremity of the rectum. In the female this fistula is to the vaginal vault (rectovaginal) and in the male either to the prostatic urethra (rectoprostatic–urethral) or the bladder (rectovesical).
2. Rectal atresia. The anal orifice and distal anal canal is present but the proximal canal (embryologically representing the distal extremity of the developing alimentary tract) is absent.

Intermediate anomalies (normal bowel ends at the level of the levator ani) (Figure 2.2)

1. Anal agenesis. The distal two-thirds of the anal canal are absent and the gut ends blindly at the embryological limit of the intestinal endoderm.
2. Anal agenesis (as above) but with a rectobulbar–urethral fistula in the male and a rectovaginal fistula to the lower third of the vagina in the female.

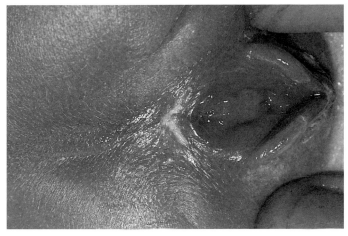

Figure 2.2 Intermediate lesion with rectovestibular fistula. This abnormality should be treated in the same fashion as a high lesion. It is important not to confuse it with an anterior ectopic anus which is a low lesion.

Low anomalies (bowel has a normal relationship to the levator ani) (Figure 2.3)

1. Anal stenosis.
2. Covered anus incomplete with anterior anocutaneous fistula.
3. Anterior ectopic anus.

Pena (1995) has developed an alternative classification orientated towards treatment and prognosis. However, from the practical standpoint of the choice of initial treatment, many surgeons find

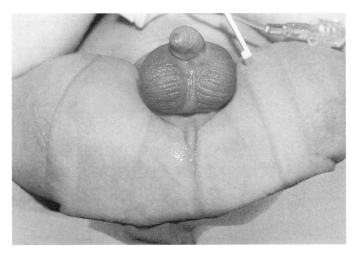

Figure 2.1 High lesion in a boy. Note the absence of an anus and the 'flat perineum' indicating a poor pelvic floor and perianal sphincter complex.

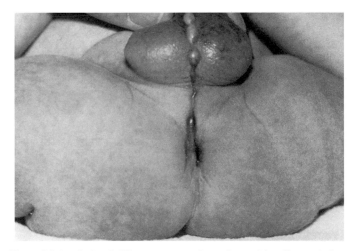

Figure 2.3 Low lesion. In this case a covered anus incomplete with an anterior anocutaneous fistula is clearly seen extending into the scrotum. The anus in this child is normally situated and is surrounded by normal smooth and striated muscle sphincter complexes. Treatment is directed at the anus which is uncovered and if necessary increased in size by performing an anoplasty.

even this classification unnecessarily complex; the distinction between low and high lesions being determined by whether or not meconium can be seen issuing from an orifice in the perineum.

High lesions comprise up to 45% of all anorectal anomalies (Stephens and Smith 1986).

Incidence

The true incidence for anorectal anomalies is difficult to ascertain. Most series report an incidence of about 1 in 4000 live births, with a slight geographical and racial variation. However, if anal stenosis is included, anorectal malformations occur in about 3% of new-borns (Santulli et al. 1970). Males are affected slightly more frequently than females and tend to have supralevator lesions (Stephens and Smith 1971). In contrast, 70–80% of low lesions occur in females.

Family history

A family history is uncommon (Boocock and Donnai 1987). When present this is most often associated with low lesions and may also be associated with chromosome anomalies. A rare autosomal recessive condition, where hereditary multiple atresias involving the gastrointestinal tract from pylorus to rectum which may be associated with immunodeficiency syndrome, has been reported (Moreno et al. 1990).

Associated conditions

Multiple abnormalities in association with anorectal malformation occur in up to 70% of cases (Stephens and Smith 1986). These include the VACTERL (*V*ertebral, *A*norectal, *C*ardiac, *T*racheo-o*E*sophageal fistula, *R*enal and radial *L*imb dysplasia) syndrome, hind-gut duplication cysts, sacrococcygeal teratoma, omphalocoele spinal and cloacal abnormalities (Khoury et al. 1983; Heij et al. 1990; Smith et al. 1992). Some of these are known to be genetically transmitted. Urological anomalies occur in up to 50% of cases, vertebral in up to 30%, and gastrointestinal in 10% (Parrott 1977). Cardiovascular malformations are noted in 10–20% of those with anorectal abnormalities, although in those with synchronous urogenital problems, they are noted in one-third (Teixeira 1983).

Urogenital anomalies are seen in 90% of high anorectal malformations, compared with only 10% of low lesions (Brock and Rich 1987). In females a varying degree of septation or atresia of the vagina is common (30% of cases), uterine abnormalities occur but are less frequent (Hall et al. 1985). Vesico-ureteric reflux is the commonest urological problem and occurs in 40% of the patients, two-thirds of whom will have a neuropathic bladder (Quan and Smith 1973; Ralph et al. 1992). Vertebral anomalies amounting to agenesis may be associated with loss of spinal cord segments, anterior meningocele, enteric duplication cysts and anal or anorectal stenosis. The level of the vertebral aplasia correlates with the motor but not with the sensory level (Carson et al. 1984). Myelography reveals many of these patients have a tethered spinal cord, narrowing of the bony spinal canal, dural sac stenosis or meningocele (Quan and Smith 1973).

Assessment of anorectal anomalies

Clinical

Careful clinical examination will usually indicate whether the defect is a high or low anorectal malformation. A nasogastric tube should be passed to exclude an associated oesophageal atresia. Inspection should be made for meconium discharge from an orifice on the perineum or genitalia or the presence of air or meconium in the urine. A high lesion is indicated by a poorly developed natal cleft (flat bottom) and absence of a skin dimple at the expected site of the anus. This is usually associated with poor muscular contraction in response to perineal cutaneous stimulation. Fistulas should be probed if possible to determine their direction and extent. High lesions run at right angles to the perineal skin whereas low lesions tend to run parallel with it.

Imaging

Echocardiography will usually detect significant associated cardiac abnormalities while abdominal ultrasonography will identify hydronephrosis or hydroureter. These should be routinely performed as a prelude to any operative intervention. Plain abdominal films in the supine, erect, and lateral decubitus positions should be taken and will exclude associated intestinal atresias. Wagensteen–Rice lateral inversion films may assist in determining the level of the malformation in relation to the pelvic floor. Alternatively, prone lateral views with the child's buttocks elevated may be equally effective, without the need to hold the baby upside down for 3 min (Narashimha et al. 1984). Whatever the choice of technique, it is important that these X-rays are taken when the baby is at least 24 h old otherwise gas will not have reached the distal rectum and accurate assessment of the level of the malformation will be impossible. The air bubble is best related to a line drawn on the lateral film from the upper border of the pubis to the last ossified spinal segment (Stephen's line) or to the distance the gas extends below or above the ossified ilium (Santulli's criterion) (de Vries and Cox 1985) (Figure 2.4).

Alternatively, ultrasound assessment of the distance from the perineum to the rectal pouch is simple and non-invasive and is not dependent for accuracy on the age of the child (Donaldson et al.

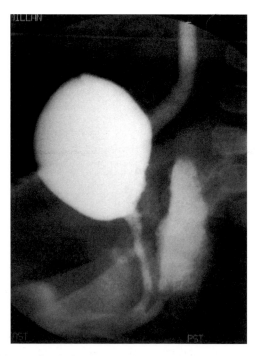

Figure 2.4 Intermediate lesion demonstrating a rectobulbar urethral fistula at micturating cystourethrography. Normally, high and intermediate lesions cannot be demonstrated in boys using this technique and are better shown using a contrast enema or MRI scan.

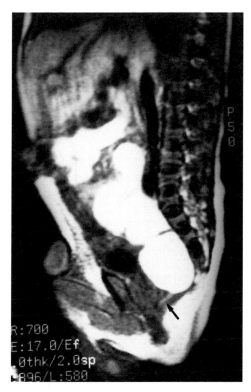

Figure 2.5 High lesion on MRI scan demonstrating a rectovaginal fistula (arrowed). Sacral hypoplasia is shown which may be associated with neuropathic involvement of the bladder and rectum.

1989; Pena 1992; Emblem *et al.* 1994). Computerized tomography (CT) or magnetic resonance (MR) scanning have additional advantages in defining the pelvic musculature and the spinal canal, which are both of importance when considering the long-term prognosis (Leniushkin *et al.* 1992; Doolin *et al.* 1993) (Figure 2.5)

Treatment

Low anomalies

In the covered anus, a membrane of skin obstructs the anus which usually lies in a normal position. This causes progressive abdominal distension with bulging of the membrane of skin. The membrane may be incomplete, creating a small fistula through which a small amount of bowel content is passed. A covered anus is treated by incising the membrane and regularly dilating the lower anal canal. An anoplasty using a Y–V plasty may be necessary if there is a significant persistent anal stenosis. Clinically, this will be apparent if there is difficulty in passing a stool which is often described by parents as narrow or 'toothpaste'-like. Enterocolitis, occasionally fatal, may complicate the condition.

The normal position of the anus can be defined (Upadhyaya 1984). In anterior ectopic anus this is displaced anteriorly but is often surrounded by a normal external anal sphincter complex. This usually requires no surgical treatment providing the anus is not stenosed. However, the anal canal may pass in front of the external anal sphincter which is located in the position of the normally placed anus (Reisner *et al.* 1984). This may contribute to the constipation from which these patients often suffer. Relocation of the anus to a position within the external sphincter complex is a logical form of treatment in these circumstances (Tuggle *et al.* 1990).

While the majority will have a good long-term prognosis, children who have been born with low anorectal malformations will often suffer disabling constipation and/or incontinence even in the absence of anal stenosis (Pena 1992). In these circumstances other strategies such as treatment with aperients or high colonic enemas may be the only alternative to a permanent colostomy.

Intermediate anomalies

From the standpoint of initial management, the distinction between high and intermediate lesions is probably not necessary. Intestinal obstruction is a feature of both requiring a defunctioning colostomy in the first instance followed by definitive surgical correction of the anatomical defect at a later stage. Some rectovestibular intermediate lesions can be confused clinically with an anterior ectopic anus or covered anus. It is most important to make this distinction because these will not be improved by local surgery such as anal dilatation, Y–V plasty, etc. Careful clinical examination will usually make the correct diagnosis but if in doubt, radiological assessment of any opening on the perineum will be of assistance.

When performing a colostomy it is important to prevent overspill from the proximal to the distal limb (Pena 1992). To avoid this a low sigmoid colostomy with the two limbs brought through separate incisions is preferable. This facilitates wash-outs of the distal limb and allows fistulous communications with the genitourinary system to be defined using instillation of contrast (Pena 1992).

Early definitive correction in the neonatal period is tempting because of the relatively limited surgery which is involved and the potential functional advantage for the child (Nixon 1983; Rintala and Lindahl 1995). This should be balanced against the greater difficulty of performing such operations in small babies. The prognosis is similar to that for high lesions (see below).

High anomalies

All high lesions present with early-onset intestinal obstruction, marked abdominal distension and failure to pass meconium. An anus will not be seen on the perineum, although meconium and gas may be expelled from the urethra or vagina indicating a fistulous communication with the rectal stump. Pre-operative assessment for other anomalies such as cardiac defects may cause delay in surgical decompression of the intestine. This is, however, essential for the safety of the child. Generally, the baby will not be compromised if a colostomy is performed within 1 or 2 days of birth.

A sigmoid colostomy is the method of choice in most cases (Pena 1992). In high lesions with a rectovesical fistula, it is usually not possible to achieve sufficient length of intestine to reach the neo-anus without sacrificing the colon and rectum distal to the colostomy site. Therefore, in this situation, a transverse defunctioning loop colostomy is probably the preferred option. Unfortunately, ultrasound scans, straight X-ray of the pelvis, and micturating cysto-urethrography, while useful if a fistula is demonstrated, will often not be helpful. CT and MRI scans of the pelvis (Leniushkin *et al.* 1992) can be of assistance in defining the anatomy. For many children a defunctioning transverse colostomy will be a safer option if there is any doubt concerning the location of the distal fistula. In patients with cloacal abnormalities, the urinary tract is often obstructed. This will require drainage, sometimes by the creation of a temporary vesicostomy.

There is an increasing trend towards definitive surgery perhaps as early as the neonatal period (Nixon 1983). Most believe the definitive operation to correct the high anomaly should be delayed until the child is at least 6 months old (Pena 1992). This allows sufficient time to perform an accurate assessment of the anomaly and simplifies the operation as the structures are larger and more easily identified than in the neonate. Several operative techniques are available (Stephens 1953; Kieswetter 1967; Mollard *et al.* 1978; Pena 1992).

The outcome is critically dependent upon the correct location of the neo-anus in the puborectalis sling. While good results were obtained from these early techniques most now agree that a posterior sagittal approach through the perineum is the safest and most satisfactory (Pena 1992; Rintala and Lindahl 1995). This is based on the principle that the autonomic nerve supply to the pelvis does not cross the mid-line. Better surgical exposure of the fistula is achieved which when divided can be more easily mobilized and brought to the perineum where accurate reconstruction of the sphincters is facilitated. This technique has probably also reduced the risk of damage to the urinary tract and provides better fixation of the rectum reducing the risk of prolapse.

Complications relating to surgery are therefore rare, but faecal incontinence when critically assessed may persist in the majority (Brain and Kiely 1989). These apparently poor functional results may, in some, be related to inadequate anatomical reconstruction of the sphincters, or a primary deficiency of the pelvic floor musculature. Primary correction using a tube created from the perineal skin is claimed to improve continence for solid and liquid faeces and reduce the risk of prolapse (Aluwihare 1989; Yazbeck *et al.* 1992). This provides an innervated skin for the neo-anus whose proximal extremity lies at the level of the levator. Imminent leakage of faecal material from the rectum may therefore be detected and prevented by contraction of the levator. Technically, this procedure is more demanding than the standard posterior sagittal anorectoplasty. A good cosmetic appearance is obtained, but the apparently improved functional results remain unproven. Whichever operation is performed, regular postoperative dilatation of the anus is frequently required for iatrogenic anal stenosis.

Postoperative functional disorders

Those with low anomalies have a surprisingly poor functional outcome with only 60% achieving socially acceptable continence; the majority being afflicted by severe constipation requiring medical treatment on a regular basis (Rintala *et al.* 1992). Almost 40% have additional social and sexual problems.

Fewer than half of those with intermediate or high lesions will have spontaneous bowel movements. This constipation, which is often intractable and unrelated to anal stenosis, is possibly caused by hypomotility induced by chronic bowel dilatation and problems with the external anal sphincter but may also be related to an associated pelvic neuropathy. Evacuation can be stimulated once or twice a day often with the help of irrigation enemas or drugs. Faecal incontinence will affect almost all children and this may complicate an underlying problem of constipation or its treatment. In refractory cases hospitalization will be required for intensive medical treatment or disimpaction.

In resistant cases, further surgery may be necessary. Reoperation may improve the function of some by relocating the neo-anus within the levator sling (Brain and Kiely 1989), while in others resection of the dilated rectum or sigmoid colon with anastomosis of the non-dilated descending colon to the rectal ampulla may be effective

(Cheu and Grosfield 1992; Pena *et al.* 1993). A recent alternative to performing a permanent colostomy is the use of an appendicostomy to deliver proximal colonic enemas (Malone *et al.* 1990). This has the combined effect of treating the underlying constipation while at the same time significantly reducing faecal incontinence. Recent experience of this technique suggests that over 70% will achieve satisfactory control of both of these problems and avoid the necessity for a permanent colostomy.

Many of these children will in addition have urinary incontinence due to an associated neuropathic bladder. This can often be treated using clean intermittent self-catheterization of the bladder. However, some will require surgical intervention in the form of insertion of an artificial urinary sphincter, bladder augmentation, or urinary diversion.

The severe psychosocial implications of the disease mean that most children in the long term are significantly handicapped by the condition.

Hirschsprung's disease

Historical

Hirschsprung first described a syndrome which we now recognize as being caused by aganglionosis in 1887 (Hirschprung 1887). Swenson and Bill were the first to report a surgical cure for Hirschsprung's disease, which they recognized as being caused by aganglionosis (Swenson and Bill 1948) (Figure 2.6).

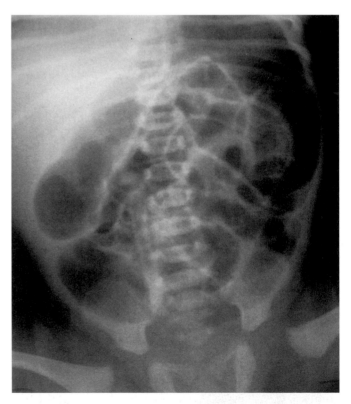

Figure 2.6 Straight abdominal X-ray in Hirschsprung's disease demonstrating absence of gas in the rectum and distended loops of small intestine. This appearance at 24–48 h of life is suggestive, but not diagnostic, of Hirschsprung's disease.

Pathology and pathophysiology

The ganglion cells of the intrinsic enteric nervous system are absent in the affected contracted distal zone, while the nerve plexii, whose cell bodies lie outside the intestine, are hypertrophied and contain increased concentrations of neurotransmitter substances and their degradation enzymes. Particularly, acetylcholinesterase (ACHE) is greatly increased in all plexii of the affected gut. This has been used as a diagnostic tool for assessing mucosal biopsies (Schofield *et al.* 1990). These intrinsic cell bodies are essential to the normal propagation and control of intestinal peristalsis. Inhibitory reflexes which are normally mediated through the adrenergic and cell bodies of the intrinsic enteric nervous system are absent in aganglionosis. Nitric oxide may play a part (Tomita *et al.* 1995). Thus in Hirschsprung's disease there is a failure of propagation of peristalsis and relative spasm of the affected gut. Intestinal obstruction proximal to the abnormal aganglionic zone causes dilatation and hypertrophy of the muscle fibres of the otherwise normal gut. The zone between the collapsed aganglionic and the dilated normally innervated intestine shows a change in calibre which has been referred to as the transitional zone. This too may also be abnormally innervated (Figure 2.7).

The internal anal sphincter, which represents the distal limit of the smooth muscle of the intestinal tract, is always affected. Aganglionosis can affect a variable distance from the anus. Hirschsprung's disease may be classified depending on the position of the transitional zone as ultra-short, short, or long disease.

Incidence

The incidence of Hirschsprung's disease is 1 in 5000 births. Male to female ratio is 4:1. As the affected segment becomes longer, the male predominance is less marked, being 12:1 for rectal disease, 3:1 when the sigmoid colon is affected and 2:1 for total colonic involvement.

Ultra-short segment disease is said to exist only affecting the internal anal sphincter. It is claimed to account for 10% of children with constipation (Figure 2.8).

In 45% of cases, the transitional zone is situated in the rectum, in the sigmoid colon in 30%, the descending colon in 20%, and the transverse or ascending colon in 5%.

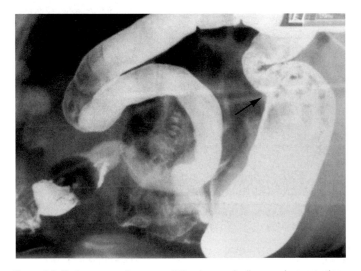

Figure 2.7 Barium enema in a case of Hirschsprung's disease, demonstrating the transitional zone in the descending colon (arrowed).

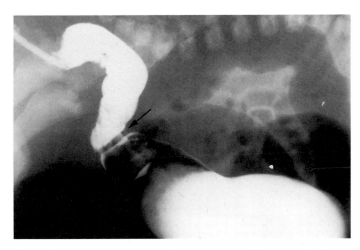

Figure 2.8 Barium enema demonstrating short segment Hirschsprung's disease with the transitional zone in the lower rectum indicated by the arrow.

Rarely, the whole intestine in involved and this is usually incompatible with survival. This relative distribution of the transitional zone has remained unchanged over the last 25 years (Harrison *et al.* 1986).

Aetiology

It is thought that aganglionosis is caused by a failure of the normal distal migration of enteric neuroblasts derived from the cephalad neural crest, along the developing intestinal tract. This conveniently explains why skip lesions probably do not occur. The migration hypothesis is supported by the association of Hirschsprung's disease with abnormalities derived from the neural crest such as autonomic or cardiac anomalies (Waardenburg's syndrome). The factors which affect this migration are unclear but are probably related to substrate failure necessary for the well-being of these migrating ganglion cell precursors rather than direct inhibition of the neuroblasts themselves. While most cases do not have affected family members, about 30% of those suffering from long segment disease, have relatives with aganglionosis. A genetic component is supported by the association with Down's syndrome in 10% of cases. The risk to siblings is 1 in 20 for brothers, 1 in 100 for sisters, and 1 in 10 for long segment disease, irrespective of sex. It is suggested that a recessive gene with variable penetrance may be responsible.

Clinical presentation

Intestinal obstruction

The majority of patients will present in the neonatal period with a history of failure to pass meconium during the first 48 h of life and signs of low intestinal obstruction (Teitelbaum 1995). The anus appears to be small and may be mistaken for anal stenosis. The baby is usually otherwise well (Figure 2.9).

A minority will present at a later date with a history of chronic constipation, abdominal distension, and failure to thrive. This often becomes apparent at the time of weaning. Rectal examination may reveal a dilated rectum and this will often produce explosive passage of stool (Luukkonen *et al.* 1990). These patients will often give a history of episodes of gross abdominal distension, general malaise, and explosive foul smelling diarrhoea indicating recurrent enterocolitis.

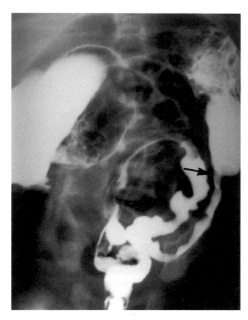

Figure 2.9 Barium enema in a case of Hirschsprung's disease, demonstrating the transitional zone in the rectosigmoid region. Note the contracted distal aganglionic segment (arrowed).

Enterocolitis

The aetiology of this potentially lethal complication is uncertain. Distal intestinal obstruction appears to be a major aetiological factor (Figure 2.10). Ischaemic, bacterial and recently, viral causes, have been implicated (Imamura *et al.* 1992). It is characterized by marked abdominal distension, vomiting, profuse watery diarrhoea, and signs of septicaemia, which is often rapidly fatal. Pathologically, there is widespread superficial mucosal loss with little inflammatory

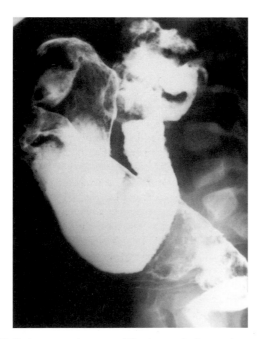

Figure 2.10 Barium enema in a case of Hirschsprung's disease demonstrating a transitional zone in the rectum. Note the distended rectosigmoid and the irregular mucosal pattern indicating ulceration and oedema associated with enterocolitis.

infiltrate. *Clostridium difficile* toxins are elevated, while in those who have undergone surgery a form of diversion colitis may occur causing repeated bacteraemia, abdominal pain, and bleeding (Drut and Drut 1992; Ordein *et al.* 1992).

Volvulus

Occasionally, colonic volvulus may occur, particularly if the diagnosis of Hirschsprung's disease is delayed late into childhood (Neilson and Youssef 1990).

Diagnosis

Rectal biopsy provides definitive diagnostic evidence of Hirschsprung's disease. These were traditionally assessed by haematoxylin and eosin (H&E) staining on full-thickness biopsies. However, it is now recognized that elevation of the mucosal ACHE activity is characteristic of Hirschsprung's disease and reliable results can be obtained from rectal suction biopsies performed without anaesthetic (Nixon 1985; Kurer *et al.* 1986). Two mucosal biopsies should be taken from the posterior wall of the rectum below the peritoneal reflection at sites 5–10 mm and 30–50 mm proximal to the dentate line. Diagnostic accuracy is 97% with ACHE histochemistry compared with 75% with H&E staining (Athow *et al.* 1990). ACHE stains are generally reliable, although misleading results are obtained in 10% of cases (Athow *et al.* 1990). When available immunocytochemistry staining for neuron-specific enolase may provide important additional information. This will demonstrate the ganglion cells in the normal proximal segment and abnormal nerve trunks in the aganglionic segment. Specific monoclonal antibodies such as D7, 3G6, 2F11 and protein gene product 9.5 are alternatives.

It should be remembered that there is a normal hypoganglionic zone at the distal extremity of the intestine which has to be distinguished from aganglionosis. In doubtful cases, full thickness biopsies still have a place. Some patients who have ultra-short segment disease may be treated by rectal myectomy/biopsy without colostomy (Ohi *et al.* 1990). In addition this type of biopsy material which contains both mucosa and muscle, provides additional information which may be of importance in distinguishing aganglionosis from NID (a related affection of the enteric nervous system).

If a laparotomy is required then biopsies should be taken distal to the macroscopic transitional zone to confirm the diagnosis, and at several points proximally which should be marked with unabsorbable suture material for future reference. If frozen section facilities exist then this can confirm the appropriate site for the enterostomy in normally innervated gut.

Plain radiographs will demonstrate signs of intestinal obstruction with a gasless rectum. If anal manipulation has occurred these X-rays become unreliable. Barium enema studies are helpful, although specificity is only about 75%. These are best performed without preparation. Typical barium enema appearances on unprepared bowel are of a normal-sized rectum with dilated proximal bowel. When present, a rectosigmoid transition zone or cone, is the single most reliable radiographic sign of Hirschsprung's disease. However, its absence does not exclude the condition (Rosenfield *et al.* 1984). The appearances of a cone can be misleading in long segment or in ultra-short segment disease (Nagasaki *et al.* 1984). Retention of barium seen on radiographs obtained 24 h after a barium enema is highly significant but is not as specific as a transitional zone when this is identified.

Reflex inhibition of the internal anal sphincter occurs following stimulation of the rectum is mediated by the ganglion cells of the intrinsic enteric nervous system and is absent in aganglionosis. Anorectal manometry measures this reflex by using a system of balloons placed in the anal canal and rectum. It has an overall accuracy for diagnosing Hirschsprung's disease of 90%, a sensitivity of 80%, a specificity of 97%, a positive predictive value of 94%, and negative predictive value of 88% (Low *et al.* 1989). Resting pressures lie within the upper range of normal, with enhanced waves in the internal sphincter. In most cases of short segment disease and one-fifth of long segment cases there is a baseline rise with increase in amplitude of superimposed rhythmical waves with rectal distension. The recto-anal inhibitory response is absent in 96% of those with Hirschsprung's disease, compared with less than 10% of normal children (Nagasaki *et al.* 1989).

Differential diagnosis

In the new-born period, aganglionosis has to be distinguished from intestinal atresia, meconium ileus and the intestinal dysfunction associated with prematurity. Clinically, these children present in a very similar fashion with low intestinal obstruction and failure to pass meconium. Biopsy remains the definitive diagnostic tool but age-related change in the morphology is sometimes difficult to interpret (Low *et al.* 1989). If there is any doubt these should be repeated some months later when the micro-anatomy has matured and is easier to define.

In older children the clinical history is usually typical of aganglionosis but may be confused with idiopathic constipation. In the latter, the child will have thrived and the stool is usually hard, bulky, and often associated with soiling of the perianal region. This is related to reflex anal dilatation in response to chronic rectal over-filling. In aganglionosis of the usual distribution, the rectum will be empty but rectal loading does not exclude ultra-short segment disease. The transitional zone is usually easily demonstrated in rectosigmoid disease but ultra-short segment aganglionosis will be indistinguishable from idiopathic constipation.

Intestinal neuronal dysplasia (NID)

There has been considerable debate as to whether this condition is the cause of a functional disorder similar to Hirschsprung's disease (Koletzko *et al.* 1993; Milla and Smith 1993). Some believe that this problem can result in a functional disorder similar to that of aganglionosis. Others argue that there is no clear correlation between the anatomical abnormality of neuronal dysplasia and the functional disorder of the intestine. It is possible that at least in some, NID can be secondary to other local problems such as chronic sepsis.

In this condition there are abnormal ganglion cells in the submucous and myenteric plexuses (Smith 1993). These ganglia may be abnormally distributed within the muscle layers rather than between them. The similarity of intestinal symptoms in MEN II B and NID paediatric patients suggests that the two disorders could be the result of mutations affecting the same domain of the RET proto-oncogene (Martucciello *et al.* 1994). Increase in ACHE staining in the lamina propria is usually not as marked as in Hirschprung's disease. Two types of NID are thought to exist: type A related to intestinal spasticity and type B to adynamic bowel. Type A accounts for 15% of cases, type B for 70%, the remaining 15% representing a combination of the two types. In older children NID is sometimes associated with gross megarectum with or without megacolon or unexplained colonic obstruction.

NID can be associated with Hirschsprung's disease and clinical, radiological, and histological distinction between the two diseases if one exists can be difficult. As in Hirschsprung's disease, the recto-anal inhibitory reflex is often absent. The consensus is that when NID is identified in association with a functional disorder, the histologically abnormal segment should be excised in a similar fashion to aganglionosis. If, however, the condition occurs in association with Hirschsprung's disease, good results have been obtained by only resecting the aganglionic segment provided the bowel affected by neuronal dysplasia has shown to be functionally satisfactory. If children do not show an improvement of colon dysmotility, extended resection is recommended.

Treatment

The 5% of patients with very mild disease may be successfully managed conservatively using regular enemas. Short or ultra-short segment disease may also respond to conservative treatment or a sphincterotomy combined with biopsy myectomy.

Most cases will present with intestinal obstruction and require urgent decompression in order to avoid the potentially life-threatening complication of enterocolitis. A suction rectal biopsy and other investigations will have confirmed the presence of aganglionosis. However, the extent of the disease will need to be confirmed at laparotomy when further full thickness biopsies can be taken from above, at and below any apparent transitional zone. These biopsy sites are closed with non-absorbable suture material so that the site can be identified at a later stage when definitive surgical correction is undertaken. If possible the specimens should be processed using frozen section after appropriate ACHE staining. A temporary stoma (usually a defunctioning transverse colostomy) can then be planned with confidence at the correct level based upon the histology. This relieves acute obstruction and allows time to confirm the diagnosis so that definitive surgery can be deferred if necessary until about 1 year.

The definitive procedure performed should be chosen to address the individual requirements of that patient, dependence on a single operation for all patients being inappropriate (Harrison *et al.* 1986).

Swenson's operation (Swenson and Bill 1948)

The rectum is mobilized as far as the pelvic floor from above. It is important to keep the dissection as close to the gut as possible in order to reduce as far as possible the risk of damage to the pelvic nerves. The distal extremity of the normally innervated intestine is then prolapsed through the anus with the rectum, which is inverted. The rectum is excised obliquely at the dentate line. This ensures that the upper third of the internal sphincter has been excised. The normal intestine is anastomosed to the anal skin and the suture line is pulled back into the pelvis. Complications include anastomotic breakdown with infection and fistula and stricture formation. The risk of these may be reduced by a proximal stoma (Nixon 1985). Neuropathic bladder has been reported in some children post-operatively presumably caused by damage to pelvic nerves during the mobilization of the rectum.

There are potential advantages for the child in performing the definitive corrective surgery in the new-born period after the diagnosis has been made and without a covering colostomy. Swenson's operation is ideal for this purpose providing there is confidence that the diagnosis is correct. However, for many units, there is sufficient doubt that this single stage correction is safe and the child is best treated initially using a colostomy. Laparoscopic Swenson's operation has been proposed which may reduce unnecessary morbidity (Curran and Raffensberger 1994). Although poor control may occur during childhood, long-term functional results are generally good and social continence in adulthood is possible in the majority (Nixon 1985).

Duhamel's operation (Duhamel 1983)

The potential advantage of this operation is that deep dissection in the pelvis is restricted to the mid-line posteriorly. Thus the risk of damage to pelvic nerves is reduced and long-term functional results are good (Heij *et al.* 1995). The operation leaves the aganglionic rectum (which has usually been resected just above the peritoneal reflection) in place (Jung 1995). A space is developed in the mid-line posteriorly as far as the anal canal. A vertical incision is then made in the mid-line posteriorly at the dentate line extending for approximately 3 cm. The upper one-third of the internal sphincter is divided with the smooth muscle of the rectum. Care is taken to avoid damaging the striated anal sphincter complex. The normally innervated intestine can then be pulled through the space behind the rectum and out of the anal canal through the incision in the rectal wall posteriorly. The anastomosis of the ganglion-containing gut to the aganglionic rectum is usually performed front to back using a stapling device which at the same time divides the septum between the rectum in front and the normal intestine behind. The undivided fibres of the internal sphincter can cause persistent obstructive symptoms and at least two-thirds of the smooth muscle sphincter should be divided. Anastomotic leakage is uncommon but dilatation of the pouch may be sufficient to require resection. The operation may be performed laparoscopically (Smith *et al.* 1994).

Long segment disease can also be treated using a modification of this technique. An increased length of the distal aganglionic segment is retained to utilize its fluid absorption capacity, which is normal. The resection point is best placed in or around the mid-descending colon. An extended side to side anastomosis is then performed to complete the operation in the usual fashion.

For short segment disease, there are excellent functional results with almost complete continence and a low morbidity and mortality (Coran 1990).

Soave's operation

This operation was devised in an attempt to avoid damage to the pelvic nerves. The rectal mucosa is removed as far as the dentate line of the anal canal, leaving the aganglionic muscle cuff *in situ*. Ganglion-containing intestine is pulled through this muscle cuff to the anal canal where a cutaneous full thickness anastomosis is performed. There is a significant risk of infection between the cuff and the pulled-through colon, but this can be reduced by using a defunctioning colostomy. These patients will often develop strictures and will tend to have poor continence relating to immobility of the levator and sphincter muscles because of secondary fibrosis (Morikawa *et al.* 1989). However, long-term results and continence are good, improving with time so that by 10 years after operation, 90% of patients will have satisfactory social continence.

Total colonic aganglionosis

This condition presents special problems. Many patients have delayed diagnosis and pull-through procedures often result in loose diarrhoea and incontinence (Levy and Reynolds 1992). Various pull-through techniques are described all of which utilize aganglionic intestine as a means of absorbing fluid from the stool. These are usually staged procedures covered by an enterostomy. A minority will achieve a stool frequency and consistency in the long term, on an unrestricted diet, which is socially acceptable. Growth and development are usually normal providing the aganglionic zone does not extend high in the small intestine. Pouch procedures are not appropriate in this circumstance because of the abnormal function of the internal sphincter.

If incontinence is socially crippling then most will opt for a permanent enterostomy.

Long-term prognosis

Large series have shown that in the long term there is little to choose between the various operative techniques employed for definitive correction. Growth and development is almost invariably normal. Excellent functional results with approximately 90% continence can eventually be expected in short segment disease (Morikawa *et al.* 1989). Constipation and incontinence is one problem for a few but these symptoms can usually be controlled with appropriate use of aperients and or enemas. The recent innovation of the ACE procedure (antegrade continence enema) (Malone *et al.* 1990) which uses an appendicostomy as a means of delivering enema fluid to the proximal colon has avoided a permanent colostomy in 70% of cases where this would otherwise have been necessary (Dick *et al.* 1996).

Constipation

Failure to pass a regular stool becomes pathological when it is persistent and unrelieved by dietary or simple laxative manipulation. Constipation and soiling occurs in 2% of children over the age of 4 years. Approximately 10% of paediatric surgical admissions for acute abdominal pain and 5% of out-patient attendances have this problem (McClung *et al.* 1993). Males are more commonly affected than females by a ratio of 3:1.

The identifiable causes of constipation include: incorrect diet, inappropriate toilet training, endocrine conditions (hypothyroidism, hyperparathyroidism), cystic fibrosis, lead poisoning, and drug ingestion (Murray *et al.* 1992). Anal causes include anal stenosis, anteriorly ectopic anus, and anal fissure. Hirschsprung's disease, neuronal dysplasia, or Chagas' disease are causes affecting the myenteric plexus (Krishnamurthy *et al.* 1993), while muscular atrophy in the rectum has also been incriminated (Kubota *et al.* 1992). For greater than 90% of cases there is no identifiable cause. While most of this group will be easily controlled by appropriate medical management many have a functional disorder which is similar to aganglionosis.

Clinical presentation

Most children have been well until potty training at about 2 years of age. Typically, the child has then started to pass large, firm, painful stools with decreasing frequency. Dyschizia and the passage of blood with defecation usually indicates the presence of a fissure *in ano*, which may perpetuate the problem by reinforcing the desire to voluntarily inhibit the call to defecation. This leads to desiccation and bulking of the stool which when eventually passed will cause more pain and fissuring. The parents of these children will often give a typical history of the child running away to hide, holding their bottom, and becoming agitated as if in discomfort. In these circumstances, if a stool has not been passed for several days the parents will usually give a history of perianal soiling and staining of the child's pants. This is thought to be caused by reflex inhibition of the internal sphincter whose primary role is to prevent leakage of flatus and liquid or semi-liquid stool. When the rectum becomes chronically filled with a faecal bolus the internal sphincter becomes permanently inhibited. Compared with the normal situation the rectum is only filled just prior to defecation and the sphincter is in a state of tonic contraction. Reflex inhibition of the internal sphincter is mediated through the intrinsic ganglion cell bodies of the enteric nervous system, as a consequence, a history of soiling usually excludes conditions affecting the myenteric plexus such as aganglionosis. In younger children, the problem will usually settle with appropriate treatment. However, a small number will have persistent problems which will often deteriorate. These are often pre-adolescent or adolescent girls and some will go on to develop major incapacitating symptoms as adults.

Investigations

In obese or fractious children where abdominal examination is difficult, assessment of the degree of faecal loading may only be possible using a straight X-ray of the abdomen. Barium enema examination is generally of little value. However, in those with an atypical presentation, it may be worth undertaking this investigation as part of the protocol to exclude aganglionosis or similar conditions affecting the enteric nerve plexii. Manometry may be used to differentiate children with functional faecal retention from those with neuropathy or myopathy of the colon (Di Lorenzo et al. 1993). Some parameters of anorectal motility (threshold volume, amplitude of threshold inhibitory anal reflex) differ markedly from controls (Cucchiara et al. 1984). Rectal compliance is significantly higher in children with faecal soiling than in those with constipation without soiling or healthy controls. This may facilitate a greater stimulation of the rectal stretch receptors which probably lie in the muscularis mucosae and initiate the recto-anal reflex. The threshold of the inhibitory reflex and of the recto-anal reflex are not helpful in defining chronic constipation. Difficulties with standardizing the stimulus using a system of rectal balloons has meant that the results of manometry in constipated children have been unreliable. The technique of electromanometry of the anorectum overcomes some of these problems by using an electrical stimulus and appears to be useful in excluding aganglionosis (Cucchiara et al. 1984). Total gastrointestinal transit time is significantly longer in constipated children compared with those with normal bowel habit.

Treatment

If there is an underlying cause then this should be treated. Otherwise, the majority will usually respond to conservative management with aperients, high-fibre diet, and bowel training techniques, provided the child complies (McClung et al. 1993). Some children will require suppositories or enemas, although rectal medication should be avoided if possible, particularly in those with a history of fissure. In these circumstances, an anal stretch can be performed under a general anaesthetic and if necessary this can be combined with a rectal biopsy. At 1 year, half will have normal bowel function, recovery rates being similar for boys and girls (Loening-Baucke 1989). Two-thirds of children with soiling can also be successfully managed by medical treatment and toilet training. In successfully treated children, soiling disappears, gastrointestinal transit times return to normal and anorectal variables change significantly (Cucchiara et al. 1984). Treatment failure is sig-

nificantly related to severe constipation, abnormal contraction of the external sphincter and pelvic floor during attempted defecation, and an inability to defecate the 100 ml balloon in less than 1 min (Loening-Baucke 1989). Intractable cases may respond to prokinetic drugs such as cisapride, controlling encopresis and allowing reduction of other medication (Murray et al. 1990; Longo and Vernava 1993). Biofeedback may be a useful adjuvant to conventional medical management, yielding a short-term cure rate of 70% and a long-term cure rate at 12 months of 90% (Benninga et al. 1993). A small number will be resistant to all medical treatment and may require surgical intervention. Rectal myotomy will provide biopsy material to exclude aganglionosis or NID. It will also usually improve symptoms at least in the short term. In refractory cases the ACE procedure (Malone et al. 1990) may be necessary in order to avoid more radical solutions (such as partial colectomy) to an otherwise intractable problem.

Rectal prolapse

Rectal prolapse in children most frequently presents before the age of 2 years. This occurs most often during or immediately after defecation and is usually an isolated episode. Usually, this is associated with only mild discomfort but its appearance is alarming for parents who frequently do not understand what has occurred. Infrequently the problem recurs on a regular basis.

Most cases of rectal prolapse are partial thickness and are between 1 and 3 cm in length, with mucosal folds radiating from the anal orifice and no groove between the prolapse and the anal skin. Less commonly, full thickness rectal intussusception occurs. This needs to be distinguished from the more common ileocolic intussusception. The latter will usually be associated with signs of intestinal obstruction whereas rectal prolapse will not. It can be demonstrated that as the anal canal relaxes prior to defecation the rectum (either partial or full thickness) prolapses through the anus (Suzuki et al. 1989). The degree to which this occurs will depend upon the mobility of the rectal wall and the underlying cause. Once prolapse has occurred several times the peri-rectal tissues become mobile thus permitting further episodes to occur with greater ease.

Chronic relaxation of the internal anal sphincter and raised intra-abdominal pressure are the most important predisposing factors. In 30% of children with prolapse there will be a history of straining at stool due to constipation. Chronic cough will elevate intra-abdominal pressure and prolapse is often seen in whooping cough and children with cystic fibrosis. This latter condition accounts for up to 10% of cases of rectal prolapse, while prolapse occurs in 10–20% of those with cystic fibrosis. Less frequently, relaxation of the internal sphincter, related to diarrhoeal states, can be a cause, particularly if this is chronic and associated with weight loss for example in gluten enteropathy. Rarely, prolapse occurs when the pelvic floor is deficient, for example in patients suffering from myelomeningocele or ectopia vesicae or following pull-through for anorectal malformations.

Most children who have had one or two episodes of prolapse can be cured by treating constipation if this is the underlying cause. Otherwise, or if this is recurrent, up to 90% of cases can be successfully treated by injection sclerotherapy or a perianal Thiersch stitch (Groff and Nagaraj 1990). Rarely, more aggressive surgical procedures are required which either fix the rectum in the pelvis or excise the redundant rectum.

Necrotizing enterocolitis (NEC)

NEC is the commonest acquired gastrointestinal emergency which occurs in neonatal intensive care units (Jirka 1993) (Figure 2.11). Eighty per cent of all affected children will be less than 34 weeks gestation and weigh less than 2000 g at birth (MacKendrick and Caplan 1993). However, up to 20% of affected babies will be full-term infants. It occurs in 5–10% of all very low birth weight infants (less than 1000 g) (Lui *et al.* 1992). The mean gestational age of those developing NEC is about 30 weeks and the mean birth weight about 1000 g. There is a 2:1 male to female ratio and 95% will have been fed orally before presentation (Covert *et al.* 1989). Most commonly the signs of NEC develop on the third day of life, but approximately 15% of cases will occur on the day of birth (Thilo *et al.* 1984). The disease has been recognized up to 3 months of age or older (Moss and Adler 1982). It occurs almost exclusively in neonatal intensive care units (NICU) where its frequency is approximately 12% (Holman *et al.* 1989). While NEC is uncommon, it is an important cause of morbidity and mortality. Approximately 6% of all neonatal deaths and 15% of those dying after the first week of life are caused by it (Brans *et al.* 1982). In all affected children, mortality is reported to be between 10 and 40%, increasing to more than 50% in high-risk babies (Cikrit *et al.* 1984). In the United States, NEC accounts for 3000–4000 deaths each year (McKeown *et al.* 1992).

Pathology

Macroscopic appearance

The most frequently affected parts are the terminal ileum and ascending and transverse colon. The descending colon and rarely, the greater part of the small intestine and stomach are also affected. NEC is primarily a mucosal disease which extends well beyond the margins of apparently normal intestine on the serosal surface (Richter *et al.* 1993). In the majority of cases, blebs of gas (pneumatosis intestinalis) are visible under the visceral peritoneum and these often extend into the mesentery.

Microscopic appearance

The capillary bed of the submucosal vascular plexus demonstrates plugging with platelet aggregates, which is associated with engorgement of more proximal vessels and distal venous thrombosis (Kosloske and Musemeche 1989). This process is primarily a microvascular as opposed to a macrovascular disease and the main mesenteric vessels are usually patent. The affected intestinal mucosa is oedematous and haemorrhagic with ulceration in more severe cases.

Bacteria can usually be identified early in the disease in the mucosa and deeper layers. However, at this stage, there is a notable absence of infiltration of the bowel wall with inflammatory cells. The serosa will usually be oedematous but may be haemorrhagic or show signs of transmural infarction in severe cases (Richter *et al.* 1993). Gas is often visible in the interstitial tissue and possibly also in the lymphatics of the bowel wall (Kosloske and Musemeche 1989) (Figure 2.12).

In most cases the inflammatory response will resolve without trace but where there has been significant tissue loss caused by necrosis, repair often results in fibrosis which may cause stenosis of the lumen. This process may take at least 3–4 months to become established and has implications for the long-term management of these cases.

Risk factors

There are many pre- and postnatal risk factors associated with NEC. These include: prematurity, low birth weight, previous oral feeding, low Apgar score at birth, hypoglycaemia, polycythaemia, respiratory support, congenital heart disease, umbilical vessel catheterization, and sepsis among others (Anderson and Kliegman 1991; Shanbhogue *et al.* 1991). However, using methods of multivariance analysis the only significant independent risk indicators appear to be low birth weight, prematurity, and oral feeding prior to the onset of disease (Walther *et al.* 1989).

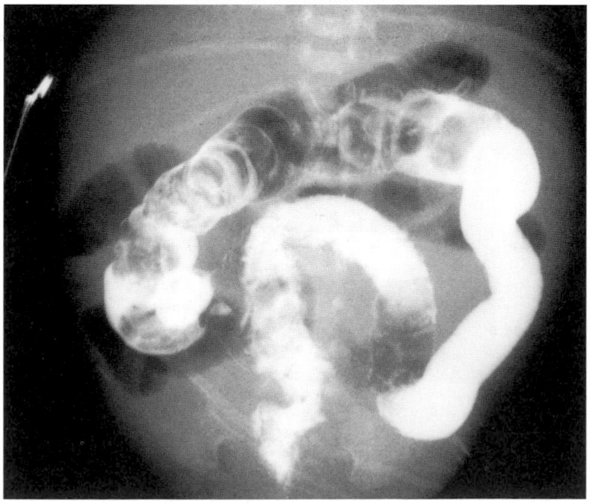

Figure 2.11 Barium enema in a child with early necrotizing enterocolitis. Note the mucosal irregularity in the rectum and sigmoid indicating ulceration.

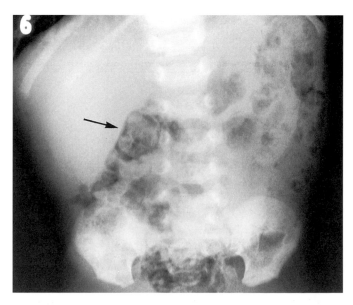

Figure 2.12 Necrotizing enterocolitis demonstrating typical pneumatosis coli. Note the intramural gas in cross-section indicated by the arrow.

Aetiology

No single mechanism accounts for the pathogenesis of NEC. The common feature is a process initiated by mucosal injury, which progresses to either mild or fulminant NEC depending on local circumstances.

Free radicals

In animal models, toxic free radicals of oxygen are released in the intestine in response to reduced intraluminal pH, hypoxia, hypovolaemia, occlusion/reperfusion injury, and cold stress (Caplan and Hseuh 1990). These are known to cause lipid peroxidation and thus damage cell membranes and increase vascular permeability. In NEC, there is good clinical and laboratory evidence that local production of free radicals then causes the release of the cytokines and vasoactive factors (Caplan and MacKendrick 1993). Complex feedback mechanisms between these factors cause a cascade of events which eventually results in bacterial translocation from the lumen, thrombosis of intramural vessels, and transmural infarction typical of NEC.

Infective agents and toxins

At birth, the neonatal intestine is sterile and becomes colonized with increasing age in response to several factors (Stevenson 1989). Full-term and premature infants colonize differently, due to differences in immunological status and feeding practices.

Epidemiologically, two different types of NEC are recognized. Eighty per cent are of the sporadic type, as compared with the rarer epidemic form, which clusters both in time and space (Zabielski et al. 1989). The epidemic form appears to occur by nosocomial spread from child to child within the unit (Rotbart et al. 1988) and the incidence can be reduced by strict infection control measures. While occasional outbreaks of NEC occur, the vast majority are sporadic cases where no specific pathogen has been identified (Mollitt et al. 1991). At least in some, these bacteria, by releasing toxins, may have initiated the disease, while in others, the organisms have translocated into the bowel wall following some other cause of mucosal injury.

Ninety per cent of affected children will have pneumatosis intestinalis (Kliegman and Fanaroff 1982). This gas has been shown to contain hydrogen, and biologically this can only have been derived from the fermentation of carbohydrate by bacteria which have translocated from the lumen into the bowel wall (Bousseboua et al. 1989).

Short chain fatty acids (SCFAs)

It is known that normal colonic commensals can ferment malabsorbed carbohydrate with the production of gas and the SCFAs, acetic, lactic, butyric, and proprionic acids (Jenkins 1989). Only two-thirds of the carbohydrate load ingested by a normal neonate is absorbed by the small intestine. This percentage is less in premature infants where there is a tendency towards disaccharidase deficiency. In babies who have developed NEC the stool will usually contain fatty acids and have a pH <5. Experimental evidence suggests that an intraluminal pH <5 is associated with mucosal damage and may further inhibit SCFA absorption (Garstin et al. 1987).

Enteral feeds

Fresh breast milk is thought to confer protection to the breast-fed infant (Review article, Nutr. Rev. 1989). This probably has two components. First, breast milk induces colonization of the neonatal intestine with bifidobacter, which reduces the risk of subsequent colonization by pathogens. Secondly, inappropriate colonization with these pathogens is inhibited by the immune globulin and white cell content of fresh breast milk (Caplan and MacKendrick 1993). There is also evidence which suggests that immune complexes to cow's milk casein can be formed in premature infants who are fed formula feeds (Clark et al. 1988). Prenatal treatment of the fetus using steroids feeds given to the mother may reduce absorption of these complexes and decrease the incidence of the disease (Caplan and MacKendrick 1993).

Overfeeding and use of hyperosmolar feeds may overwhelm the absorptive capacity of the intestine. Both are known to increase the risk of NEC in susceptible infants.

Mucosal blood flow

Feeding has been shown to increase both the oxygen consumption of the intestine and its blood flow. In premature infants reflex vasodilatation of mucosal blood vessels which accompanies feeding does not occur as readily as mature babies, increasing the risk of mucosal ischaemia (Crissinger and Burney 1992).

Circulatory redistribution of volume can also lead to relative ischaemia of the intestinal mucosa. This can occur with congenital heart disease, exchange transfusion, hyperviscosity, umbilical catheterization, respiratory distress, and a low Apgar score at birth (Hebra et al. 1993).

Raised intraluminal pressure

Mucosal ischaemia is known to occur with raised intraluminal pressure. This may be caused by either intestinal obstruction or increased gas production. Premature infants often demonstrate delay in gastrointestinal transit which may be related to immaturity of intramural nerve plexus function (Garstin and Boston 1987). Increased hydrogen production in the intestine has been shown to occur just prior to the onset of NEC. If this is sufficiently rapid, the evolved gas cannot be cleared and the intraluminal pressure must therefore increase.

Diagnosis

Clinical features

Clinically, NEC is associated with lethargy, feeding intolerance, ileus, gastric and abdominal distension, bilious vomiting, and bloody stools. The most frequent signs are abdominal distension (80%), diffuse tenderness (45%), bloody stools (40%), and absent peristalsis (40%) (Kurscheid and Holschneider 1993). Typically, this occurs in a premature baby who has already been established on formula feeds and who has been making good progress.

There may be a wide range of clinical manifestations, from a mild disturbance of intestinal function to a rapidly fulminant course characterized by signs of peritonitis, septicaemia and shock (Figure 2.13).

Bell suggested a classification of NEC, which has proven valuable not only in terms of diagnosis but also of treatment (Bell et al. 1978).

Stage I

These infants, will develop a mild systemic illness, associated with temperature instability, apnoea, bradycardia, and general lethargy. There may be a minor degree of abdominal distension associated with vomiting and/or increased prefeed gastric residues. Stage I, has been called 'suspected NEC' and many children who demon-

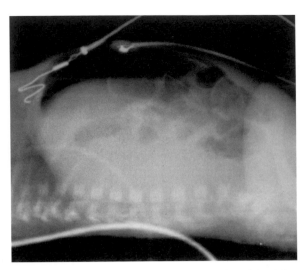

Figure 2.13 Necrotizing enterocolitis. Lateral decubitus view of the abdomen demonstrating free perforation with gas visible anteriorly.

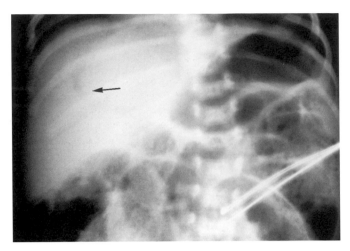

Figure 2.14 Necrotizing enterocolitis demonstrating gas in the portal vein indicated by the arrow.

strate these clinical signs will be suffering from the much more common feeding intolerance associated with prematurity or low birth weight. However, those who demonstrate these clinical characteristics, should be regarded as at risk of developing more fulminant disease and treated accordingly.

Stage II

These babies have profound systemic illness, with mild metabolic acidosis and thrombocytopenia. Abdominal distension is apparent and bowel sounds are absent. Many will demonstrate abdominal tenderness and some will have oedema and cellulitis of the abdominal wall particularly around the umbilicus. There will be definite X-ray findings of NEC with pneumatosis intestinalis with or without free gas in the peritoneal cavity or gas in the portal vein.

Stage III

This is associated with severe life-threatening generalized sepsis. In addition, to the features of stage II disease, the baby will demonstrate hypotension, metabolic acidosis, hyponatraemia, jaundice, and intravascular coagulation. There will be signs of generalized peritonitis, with marked abdominal tenderness and distension and these will usually be associated with radiological signs of perforation and ascites. Neonates with stage III disease have a mortality of over 80%.

X-ray findings

Specific X-ray findings are best demonstrated by sequential examination of at-risk children.

In stage I disease plain radiographs usually reveal abnormal gas shadows in the bowel wall with dilated loops of bowel separated by oedema occurring in up to half of cases (Kurscheid and Holschneider 1993). However, in equivocal cases, the sensitivity and specificity of plain radiographs are both only about 50% (Kao *et al.* 1992). A double contrast enema may be of help in identifying those with early disease who will demonstrate mucosal oedema and perhaps ulceration (Kao *et al.* 1992).

Pneumatosis intestinalis is generally regarded as pathognomonic of NEC. It is usually seen in the more severe stages II and III of the condition but can sometimes be present in stage I disease. In less than 10% of confirmed cases this sign will not be present (Kliegman and Fanaroff 1982). It appears as crescents or haloes around the gas

shadow of the lumen (when viewed in cross-section at right angles to the luminal axis of the intestine) or a more diffuse 'ground glass' appearance.

The interface between loops of bowel is increased in peritonitis and intestinal oedema (Kurscheid and Holschneider 1993). Fixed distension of loops usually indicates necrosis and free gas, perforation (Buchheit and Stewart 1994). Gas can be seen in the portal vein in 10% of cases (Kurscheid and Holschneider 1993) (Figure 2.14). Both ascites and portal vein gas are usually associated with stage III disease and are generally regarded as indications for surgical intervention (Black *et al.* 1989).

Abdominal ultrasound scan

Accurate localization of oedema of affected intestine, fluid in the abdominal cavity and Morrison's pouch, and gas in the liver, is possible using this technique (Avni *et al.* 1991). Sonographic evidence of portal venous gas occurs in 20–50% of cases although its absence does not exclude NEC (King and Shuckett 1992). In addition, real-time Doppler flow techniques may demonstrate altered haemodynamics of septicaemic shock with opening of the ductus arteriosus and loss of end-diastolic or reversal of flow in the superior mesenteric artery (Kempley and Gamsu 1992).

Stool reducing substances

Malabsorption of carbohydrate has been shown significantly to increase prior to the onset of NEC. Sequential testing of the stool using 'Clinitest' tablets seems to have a reported positive predictive value for NEC of approximately 70% (Book *et al.* 1976).

Breath hydrogen

Hydrogen, a product of bacterial fermentation of malabsorbed carbohydrate is absorbed and can be measured in the expired gas. This can be measured using a simple non-invasive test by sampling air from the oropharynx during the expiratory phase of respiration (Cheu *et al.* 1989). High excretion occurs up to 28 h before the earliest clinical signs of NEC.

Markers of mucosal damage

Intestinal fatty acid binding protein (I-FABP) is a sensitive biochemical marker for early intestinal mucosal injury due to mesenteric ischaemia and may prove a valuable test, along with T-cryptantigen determination (Gollin and Marks 1993).

Markers of cytokine activation

Thromboxane A_2 is a major metabolite of arachidonic acid. It has a short half-life and its more stable metabolite thromboxane B_2 is excreted and can be measured in the urine. Elevated levels of urinary thromboxane have been documented to occur in NEC (Hyman et al. 1987).

Plasma interleukin-6 and tumour necrosis factor are non-specific and will be elevated in the presence of sepsis from other causes. The former has been shown to be of greater value in predicting NEC affected babies than the latter.

Treatment

Prophylaxis

Avoidance of situations which are known to predispose to NEC will reduce the risk of development of the condition. Prenatal use of steroids given to the mother has been shown reduce the incidence of NEC (Halac et al. 1990). Postnatal steroids do not decrease the incidence but improve the outcome of NEC. Postnatally, 'stress' situations should be avoided which would otherwise predispose to shunting of blood away from the new-born intestine. These include hypothermia, hypoxaemic or hypercarbia, metabolic acidosis, hypovolaemia, and pain. Drugs such as methylxanthines or prostaglandin antagonists, are known to have an adverse effect upon intestinal blood flow and should be administered with caution (Canarelli et al. 1993). Strict infection control measures within the NICU, will reduce the risk of nosocomial colonization with pathogens.

Mothers should be encouraged to provide fresh breast milk. This contains protective white cells and immunoglobulin (Ig) A and promotes more appropriate gut colonization. Enteral feeding should be introduced cautiously in at-risk babies. These should be fed breast milk by preference, formula feeds being withheld, or introduced very gradually (Pohlandt 1990). Early introduction of high volume feeds, particularly with hyperosmolar solutions should be avoided. Storage of human milk for too long or exposing formula feeds to light during tube feeding potentiates lipid peroxidation and may increase the risk of developing NEC (van Zoeren Grobben et al. 1993). If necessary, total or supplemental parenteral nutrition should be employed to maintain adequate calorie intake.

Oral IgA appears to reduce the risk of developing NEC while the administration of an iron chelating agent has been shown to have a beneficial effect on both survival and histology (Lelli et al. 1993).

After the onset of NEC

Stage I disease

Continuance of oral feeding is likely to cause progression of the disease in children who have NEC. On the other hand, there are many babies who have clinical features of stage I NEC who are better treated by continuing with oral feeds.

When a firm diagnosis of NEC is established oral feeds should be discontinued and nasogastric decompression of the stomach and parenteral antibiotics against both aerobic and anaerobic organisms commenced. Total parenteral nutrition will be necessary to maintain the acute metabolic demands of the individual (Wesley 1992).

Stage II disease

The systemic affects of sepsis such as endotoxic shock and disseminated intravascular coagulation need to be corrected aggres-

sively, if necessary delaying surgical intervention even if this is indicated.

A falling platelet count, rising or falling white blood cell count, left shift in the myeloid series, persistently or progressively low pH, increasing frequency of apnoea or bradycardia, abdominal mass or abdominal skin erythema indicate clinical deterioration and impending gangrene (Buchheit and Stewart 1994). Perforation or gas visualized in the portal vein, are both indications for operation, providing the child is stable and has responded to resuscitation measures. In the absence of signs of perforation or gas in the portal vein affected children can be treated conservatively as in stage I.

Stage III disease

These children who are profoundly unwell, usually have extensive transmural infarction and perforation and will suffer a high mortality. The same general principles apply as with stage II disease. Intensive cardiopulmonary resuscitation will be required before operative intervention is considered. The child may be too unwell to tolerate open laparotomy initially and simple decompression of the abdomen by using a drain inserted under local anaesthesia is the best treatment in the short term (Takamatsu et al. 1992).

Operation

Approximately half of the recognized cases of NEC will come to surgery (Jackman et al 1990). However, there has been much debate as to the appropriate surgical approach in these circumstances (Buchheit and Stewart 1994).

Peritoneal drainage

Open laparotomy may carry a greater risk than simple drainage of the abdominal cavity for many small premature infants (Takamatsu et al. 1992). This is effective in stabilizing 80% of small and/or very ill babies with a NEC perforation, the overall survival rate being over 50%. One-third of such cases are successfully treated by drainage alone. The objective is to reduce peritoneal soiling and decompress the abdomen. This reduces the source of continuing sepsis, reduces diaphragmatic splinting and improves ventilation.

Simple drainage should not be regarded as an alternative to open surgery which will be required in most cases after the child's general condition improves. It has been suggested that simple peritoneal drainage is appropriate for children with congenital cyanotic heart disease or where the birth weight is less than 1000–1500 g (Takamatsu et al. 1992).

Laparotomy

Expediency in the interests of safety for the child will usually mean some form of limited primary operation with reconstruction at a later stage (Illing et al. 1991).

Primary resection and direct end-to-end anastomosis of healthy bowel is possible. However, in order to obtain a safe primary anastomosis, extensive resection of potentially viable gut will be necessary. As a rule, resection and primary end-to-end anastomosis should only be performed if this can be done safely and without risking intestinal failure due to short gut.

In most circumstances, the duration of surgery should not be prolonged and if resection is required, the proximal and distal limbs should be exteriorized at the limits of viability (as judged on the serosal surface), rather than performing an anastomosis (Cikrit et al. 1984). It is an advantage when subsequently closing this enterostomy, if the two stomata are placed together, thus avoiding two separate abdominal incisions (Illing et al. 1991).

If extensive necrosis is not apparent, a proximally based defunctioning enterostomy (usually in the terminal ileum), can be performed without resection even in the presence of perforation. This avoids extensive mobilization and reduces the necessity for excision of potentially viable intestine.

Reintroduction of feed

If refeeding is started prematurely there is a 5% risk of recurrence of NEC and should therefore be delayed for at least one week. A formula containing short chain carbohydrate, peptones, or amino acids and medium chain triglycerides may be more readily absorbed in those with malabsorption.

Closure of the enterostomy

Reconstruction should only be undertaken after patency of the distal intestine has been determined by a contrast enema (Radhakrishnan et al. 1991). This should be delayed for at least 3–4 months, during which time most secondary strictures (which occur in up to 30% of cases), will have developed (Walsh et al. 1988). However, if fluid losses are high, restoration of intestinal continuity should be considered sooner. Delayed stricturing is uncommon. Occasionally, persistent strictures require resection, stricturoplasty, or proximal diversion (Radhakrishnan et al. 1991). Alternatively, they may be treated by balloon dilatation (Peer et al. 1993) (Figure 2.15).

Prognosis

NEC is still a serious condition associated with an overall mortality rate of 20–40% (Kurscheid and Holschneider 1993). Death is related to the severity of the disease, perforation, low Apgar scores within the first minute, and very low weight rather than surgery itself (St Vil et al. 1992). For infants weighing less than 1000 g the risk of death is 50%, being 25% for those weighing 1000–1500 g, and 20% for infants over 1500 g. (Ricketts and Jerles 1990). Infants with diffuse disease or perforation who do not undergo surgery have a particularly poor prognosis. Only about half of the survivors enjoy good health (Jackman et al. 1990).

Mental and motor development is abnormal in 33–50% of patients, with severe developmental delay occurring in about 20% (Walsh et al. 1989). These are related to the severity of the disease.

Significant long-term complications include failure-to-thrive in about 20% which is directly related to the length of ileal resection. Normal gastrointestinal status returns in 75% of cases while 10% will have persistent significant dysfunction requiring treatment (Kurscheid and Holschneider 1993).

NEC is the commonest cause of short bowel syndrome in children, accounting for half of all cases. This complication will develop in about 10% of those undergoing surgery for NEC and may require long-term, often home-based, parenteral nutrition (Jackman et al. 1990). About three-quarters of these patients can eventually be weaned from the parenteral nutrition as the remaining small intestine adapts with time. Despite significant morbidity, the overall survival of those with dysfunction is over 90% (Warner and Ziegler 1993).

Recurrent episodes of NEC may occur, most often a month after the initial episode (Stringer et al. 1993). There is no consistent association between recurrent NEC and the type or timing of enteral feeds, the anatomical site, or treatment of the original attack. The mortality of recurrent NEC is similar to that for the primary disease (Stringer et al. 1993).

References

Aluwihare A. Imperforate anus in male children: a new operation of primary perineal rectourethroanoplasty. *Ann. R. Coll. Surg. Engl.* 1989; 71: 14–9.

Anderson DM, Kliegman RM. The relationship of neonatal alimentation practices to the occurrence of endemic necrotizing enterocolitis. *Am. J. Perinatol.* 1991; 8: 62–7.

Athow AC, Filipe MI, Drake DP. Problems and advantages of acetylcholinesterase histochemistry of rectal suction biopsies in the diagnosis of Hirschsprung's disease. *J. Pediatr. Surg.* 1990; 25: 520–6.

Avni EF, Rypens F, Cohen E, Pardou A. Peri-cholecystic hyper-echogenicities in necrotizing enterocolitis: a specific sonographic sign? *Pediatr. Radiol.* 1991; 21: 179–81.

Bell MJ, Ternberg JL, Feigin RD, et al. Neonatal necrotizing enterocolitis: therapeutic decisions based upon clinical staging. *Ann. Surg.* 1978; 187: 1–6.

Benninga MA, Buller HA, Taminiau JA. Biofeedback training in chronic constipation. *Arch. Dis. Child.* 1993; 68: 126–9.

Black TL, Carr MG, Korones SB. Necrotizing enterocolitis: improving survival within a single facility. *South Med. J.* 1989; 82: 1103–7.

Boocock GR, Donnai D. Anorectal malformations: familial aspects and associated anomalies. *Arch. Dis. Child.* 1987; 62: 576–9.

Book LS, Herbst JJ, Jung AL. Carbohydrate malabsorption in necrotizing enterocolitis. *Pediatrics* 1976; 57: 201–4.

Bousseboua H, Coz YL, Dabard J, et al. Experimental cecitis in gnotobiotic quails monoassociated with *Clostridium butyricum* strains isolated from patients with neonatal necrotizing enterocolitis and from healthy newborns. *Infect. Immun.* 1989; 57: 932–6.

Brain AJ, Kiely EM. Posterior sagittal anorectoplasty for reoperation in children with anorectal malformations. *Br. J. Surg.* 1989; 76: 57–9.

Brans YW, Escobedo MB, Hayashi RH, Huff RW, Kagan Hallet KS, Ramamurthy RS. Perinatal mortality in a large perinatal center: five year review of 31 000 births. *Am. J. Obstet. Gynecol.* 1982; 148: 284–9.

Brock WA, Rich M. Anorectal malformations: urological implications. Associated genito urinary malformations. *Dialog. Paediatr. Urol.* 1987; 10: 5–7.

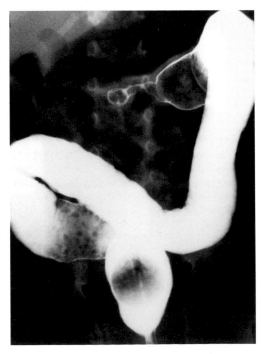

Figure 2.15 Barium enema of a child 3 months post-necrotizing enterocolitis. Note the stricture in the transverse colon

Buchheit JQ, Stewart DL. Clinical comparison of localized intestinal perforation and necrotizing enterocolitis in neonates. *Pediatrics* 1994; 93: 32–6.

Canarelli JP, Poulain H, Clamadieu C, Ricard J, Maingourd Y, Quintard JM. Ligation of the patent ductus arteriosus in premature infants—indications and procedures. *Eur. J. Pediatr. Surg.* 1993; 3: 3–5.

Caplan MS, Hsueh W. Necrotizing enterocolitis: role of platelet activating factor, endotoxin, and tumor necrosis factor. *J. Pediatr.* 1990; 117: S47–51.

Caplan MS, MacKendrick W. Necrotizing enterocolitis: a review of pathogenetic mechanisms and implications for prevention. *Pediatr. Pathol.* 1993; 13: 357–69.

Carson JA, Barnes PD, Tunell WP, et al. Imperforate anus: the neurologic implication of sacral abnormalities. *J. Pediatr. Surg.* 1984; 19: 838–42.

Cheu HW, Brown DR, Rowe MI. Breath hydrogen excretion as a screening test for the early diagnosis of necrotizing enterocolitis. *Am. J. Dis. Child.* 1989; 143: 156–9.

Cheu HW, Grosfeld JL. The atonic baggy rectum: a cause of intractable obstipation after imperforate anus repair. *J. Pediatr. Surg.* 1992; 27: 1071–3.

Cikrit D, Castandrea J, West KW, Schreiner RL, Grosfeld JL. Necrotizing enterocolitis: factors affecting mortality in 101 surgical cases. *Surgery* 1984; 96: 648–55.

Clark DA, Fornabaio DM, McNeill H, Mullane KM, Caravella SJ, Miller MJS. Contribution of oxygen derived free radicals to experimental necrotizing enterocolitis. *Am. J. Pathol.* 1988; 130: 537–42.

Coran AG. A personal experience with 100 consecutive total colectomies and straight ileoanal endorectal pull throughs for benign disease of the colon and rectum in children and adults. *Ann. Surg.* 1990; 212: 242–7.

Covert RF, Neu J, Elliott MJ, Rea JL, Gimotty PA. Factors associated with age of onset of necrotizing enterocolitis. *Am. J. Perinatol.* 1989; 6: 455–60.

Crissinger KD, Burney DL. Influence of luminal nutrient composition on hemodynamics and oxygenation in developing intestine. *Am. J. Physiol.* 1992; 263: G254–60.

Cucchiara S, Coremans G, Staiano A, et al. Gastrointestinal transit time and anorectal manometry in children with fecal soiling. *J. Pediatr. Gastroenterol. Nutr.* 1984; 3: 545–50.

Curran TJ, Raffensberger JG. The feasibility of laparoscopic Swenson pull through. *J. Pediatr. Surg.* 1994; 29: 1273–5.

de Vries PA, Cox KL. Surgery of anorectal anomalies. Surg. Clin. North Am. 1985; 65: 1139–67.

Di Lorenzo C, Flores AF, Reddy SN, Snape WJ Jr, Bazzocchi G, Hyman PE. Colonic manometry in children with chronic intestinal pseudo obstruction. *Gut* 1993; 34: 803–7.

Dick AC, McCallion WA, Brown S, Boston VE. Antegrade colonic enemas. *Br. J. Surg.* 1996; 83: 642–3.

Donaldson JS, Black CT, Reynolds M, Sherman JO, Shkolnik A. Ultrasound of the distal pouch in infants with imperforate anus. *J. Pediatr. Surg.* 1989; 24: 465–8.

Doolin EJ, Black CT, Donaldson JS, Schwartz D, Raffensperger JG. Rectal manometry, computed tomography, and functional results of anal atresia surgery. *J. Pediatr. Surg.* 1993; 28: 195–8.

Drut R, Drut RM. Hyperplasia of lymphoglandular complexes in colon segments in Hirschsprung's disease: a form of diversion colitis. *Pediatr. Pathol.* 1992; 12: 575–81.

Duhamel B. Surgical treatment of anal incontinence in children. *Ann. Gastroenterol. Hepatol.* 1983; 19: 147–150.

Emblem R, Diseth T, Morkrid L, Stien R, Bjordal R. Anal endosonography and physiology in adolescents with corrected low anorectal anomalies. *J. Pediatr. Surg.* 1994; 29: 447–51.

Garstin WHI, Boston VE. Assessment of hindgut function in premature infants. *J. Pediatr. Surg.* 1987; 22: 353–5.

Garstin WHI, Kenny BD, McAneaney D, Boston VE. The role of intraluminal tension and pH in the development of necrotising enterocolitis: an animal model. *J. Pediatr. Surg.* 1987; 22: 205–7.

Gollin G, Marks WH. Elevation of circulating intestinal fatty acid binding protein in a luminal contents initiated model of NEC. *J. Pediatr. Surg.* 1993; 28: 367–70.

Groff DB, Nagaraj HS. Rectal prolapse in infants and children. *Am. J. Surg.* 1990; 160: 531–2.

Halac E, Halac J, Begue EF, et al. Prenatal and postnatal corticosteroid therapy to prevent neonatal necrotizing enterocolitis: a controlled trial. *J. Pediatr.* 1990; 117: 132–8.

Hall JW et al. The genital tract in female children with imperforate anus. *Am. J. Obstet. Gynecol.* 1985; 151: 169–71.

Harrison MW, Deitz DM, Campbell JR, Campbell TJ. Diagnosis and management of Hirschsprung's disease. A 25 year perspective. *Am. J. Surg.* 1986; 152: 49–56.

Hebra A, Brown MF, Hirschl RB, et al. Mesenteric ischemia in hypoplastic left heart syndrome. *J. Pediatr. Surg.* 1993; 28: 606–11.

Heij HA, Moorman Voestermans CG, Vos A, Kneepkens CM. Triad of anorectal stenosis, sacral anomaly and presacral mass: a remediable cause of severe constipation. *Br. J. Surg.* 1990; 77: 102–4.

Heij HA, de Vries X, Bremer I, Ekkelkamp S, Vos A. Long term anorectal function after Duhamel operation for Hirschsprung's disease. *J. Pediatr. Surg.* 1995; 30: 430–2.

Hirschsprung H. Stuhltrageit Neugeborener in Folge von Dilatation und Hypertrophie des Colons. *Jahrb. Kinderheilkd.* 1887; 27: 1–7.

Holman RC, Stehr Green K, Zelasky MT. Necrotizing enterocolitis mortality in the United States 1979–85. *Am. J. Public Health* 1989; 79: 987–9.

Hyman PE, Abrams CE, Zipser RD. Enhanced urinary immunoreactive thromboxane in neonatal necrotizing enterocolitis: a diagnostic indicator of thrombotic activity. *Am. J. Dis. Child.* 1987; 141: 686–9.

Illing P, Hecker WC, Holzer KH, von Kooten HJ. Surgical therapy of neonatal necrotizing enterocolitis. *Chirurg* 1991; 62: 42–6.

Imamura A, Puri P, O'Brian DS, Reen DJ. Mucosal immune defence mechanisms in enterocolitis complicating Hirschsprung's disease. *Gut* 1992; 33: 801–6.

Jackman S, Brereton RJ, Wright VM. Results of surgical treatment of neonatal necrotizing enterocolitis. *Br. J. Surg.* 1990; 77: 146–8.

Jenkins DJA. The link between colon fermentation and systemic disease. *Am. J. Gastroenterol.* 1989; 84: 1362–4.

Jirka JH. Necrotizing enterocolitis. *Nebr. Med. J.* 1993; 78: 95–7.

Jung PM. Hirschsprung's disease: one surgeon's experience in one institution. *J. Pediatr. Surg.* 1995; 30: 646–51.

Kao SC, Smith WL, Franken EA Jr, Sato Y, Sullivan JH, McGee JA. Contrast enema diagnosis of necrotizing enterocolitis. *Pediatr. Radiol.* 1992; 22: 115–7.

Kempley ST, Gamsu HR. Superior mesenteric artery blood flow velocity in necrotising enterocolitis. *Arch. Dis. Child.* 1992; 67: 793–6.

Khoury MJ, Cordoro JF, Greenberg F, James LM, Erickson JD. A population study of the VACTERL Association: evidence for it's etiologic heterogeneity. *Pediatrics* 1983; 71: 815–20.

Kieswetter WB. Imperforate anus II. The rationale and technique of the sacro-perineal operation. *J. Pediatr. Surg.* 1967; 2: 106–10.

King S, Shuckett B. Sonographic diagnosis of portal venous gas in two pediatric liver transplant patients with benign pneumatosis intestinalis. Case reports and literature review. *Pediatr. Radiol.* 1992; 22: 577–8.

Kliegman RM, Fanaroff AA. Neonatal necrotizing enterocolitis in the absence of pneumatosis intestinalis. *Am. J. Dis. Child.* 1982; 136: 618–20.

Koletzko S, Ballauff A, Hadziselimovic F, Enck P. Is histological diagnosis of neuronal intestinal dysplasia related to clinical and manometric findings in constipated children? Results of a pilot study. *J. Pediatr. Gastroenterol. Nutr.* 1993; 17: 59–65.

Kosloske AM, Musemeche A. Necrotizing enterocoitis of the neonate. Clin. Perinatol. 1989; 16: 97–111.

Krishnamurthy S, Heng Y, Schuffler MD. Chronic intestinal pseudo-obstruction in infants and children caused by diverse abnormalities of the myenteric plexus. *Gastroenterology* 1993; 104: 1398–408.

Kubota M, Nagasaki A, Sumitomo K. Manometric evaluation of children with chronic constipation using a suction stimulating electrode. *Eur. J. Pediatr. Surg.* 1992; 2: 287–90.

Kurer MHJ, Lawson JON, Pambakian H. Suction biopsy in Hirschsprung's disease. *Arch. Dis. Child.* 1986; 61: 83–4.

Kurscheid T, Holschneider AM. Necrotizing enterocolitis (NEC)—mortality and long term results. *Eur. J. Pediatr. Surg.* 1993; 3: 139–43.

Lelli JL Jr, Pradhan S, Cobb LM. Prevention of postischemic injury in immature intestine by deferoxamine. *J. Surg. Res.* 1993; 54: 34–8.

Leniushkin AI, Pankevich TL, Lukin VV. Computed tomography of the pelvis in pediatric proctology. *Khirurgiia Mosk.* 1992; 11–12: 45–9.

Levy M, Reynolds M. Morbidity associated with total colon Hirschsprung's disease. *J. Pediatr. Surg.* 1992; 27: 364–6.

Loening Baucke V. Factors determining outcome in children with chronic constipation and faecal soiling. *Gut* 1989; 30: 999–1006.

Longo WE, Vernava AM, 3d. Prokinetic agents for lower gastrointestinal motility disorders. *Dis. Colon. Rectum* 1993; 36: 696–708.

Low PS, Quak SH, Prabhakaran K, Joseph VT, Chiang GS, Aiyathurai EJ. Accuracy of anorectal manometry in the diagnosis of Hirschsprung's disease. *J. Pediatr. Gastroenterol. Nutr.* 1989; 9: 342–6.

Lui K, Nair A, Giles W, Morris J, John E. Necrotizing enterocolitis in a perinatal centre. *J. Paediatr. Child Health* 1992; 28: 47–9.

Luukkonen P, Heikkinen M, Huikuri K, Jarvinen H. Adult Hirschsprung's disease. Clinical features and functional outcome after surgery. *Dis. Colon Rectum* 1990; 33: 65–9.

MacKendrick W, Caplan M. Necrotizing enterocolitis. New thoughts about pathogenesis and potential treatments. *Pediatr. Clin. North Am.* 1993; 40: 1047–59.

Malone PS, Ransley PG, Kiely EM. Preliminary report: the antegrade continence enema. *Lancet* 1990; 336: 1217–18.

Martucciello G, Caffarena PE, Lerone M, Mattioli G, Barabino A, Bisio G, Jasonni V. Neuronal intestinal dysplasia: clinical experience in Italian patients. *Eur. J. Pediatr. Surg.* 1994; 4: 287–92.

McClung HJ, Boyne LJ, Linsheid T, Heitlinger LA, Murray RD, Fyda J, Li BU. Is combination therapy for encopresis nutritionally safe? *Pediatrics* 1993; 91: 591–4.

McKeown RE, Marsh TD, Amarnath U, Garrison CZ, Addy CL, Thompson SJ, Austin JL. Role of delayed feeding and of feeding increments in necrotizing enterocolitis. *J. Pediatr.* 1992; 121: 764–70.

Milla PJ, Smith VV. Intestinal neuronal dysplasia. *J. Pediatr. Gastroenterol. Nutr.* 1993; 17: 356–7.

Mollard P, Marechal JM, Jaubert de Beaujeu M. Surgical treatment of high imperforate anus with definition of the puborectalis sling by the perineal approach. *J. Pediatr. Surg.* 1978; 13: 499–504.

Mollitt DL, String DL, Tepas JJ 3d, Talbert JL. Does patient age or intestinal pathology influence the bacteria found in cases of necrotizing enterocolitis? *South Med. J.* 1991; 84: 879–82.

Moreno LA, Gottrand F, Turck D, Manouvrier Hanu S, Mazingue F, Morisot C, *et al.* Severe combined immunodeficiency syndrome associated with autosomal recessive familial multiple gastrointestinal atresias: study of a family. *Am. J. Med. Genet.* 1990; 37: 143–6.

Morikawa Y, Matsufugi H, Hirobe S, Yokoyama J, Katsumata K. Motility of the anorectum after the Soave Denda operation. *Prog. Pediatr. Surg.* 1989; 24: 67–76.

Moss TJ, Adler R. Necrotizing enterocolitis in older infants. Children, and adolescents. *J. Pediatr.* 1982; 100: 764–6.

Murray RD, Li BU, McClung HJ, Heitlinger L, Rehm D. Cisapride for intractable constipation in children: observations from an open trial. *J. Pediatr. Gastroenterol. Nutr.* 1990; 11: 503–8.

Murray RD, Qualman SJ, Powers P, Caniano DA, McClung HJ, Ulysses B, *et al.* Rectal myopathy in chronically constipated children. *Pediatr. Pathol.* 1992; 12: 787–98.

Nagasaki A, Ikeda K, Hayashida Y. Radiologic diagnosis of Hirschsprung's disease utilizing rectosphincteric reflex. *Pediatr. Radiol.* 1984; 14, 384–387.

Nagasaki A, Sumitomo K, Shono T, Ikeda K. Anorectal manometry after Ikeda's Z shaped anastomosis in Hirschsprung's disease. *Prog. Pediatr. Surg.* 1989; 24: 59–66.

Narashimha RLL, Prasad GR, Kotariya S, Mitra S, Pathak IC. Prone cross table lateral view: an alternative to the invertogram in imperforate anus. *Am. J. Roentgenol.* 1984; 140: 227–9.

Neilson IR, Youssef S. Delayed presentation of Hirschsprung's disease: acute obstruction secondary to megacolon with transverse colonic volvulus. *J. Pediatr. Surg.* 1990; 25: 1177–9.

Nixon HH. A different approach to the treatment of anorectal agenesis. *Rev. Pediatr.* 1983; 19: 455–8.

Nixon HH. Hirschsprung's disease: progress in management and diagnostics. *World J. Surg.* 1985; 9: 189–202.

Ohi RJ, Tseng SW, Kamiyama T, Chiba T. Two point rectal mucosal biopsy for selection of surgical treatment of Hirschsprung's disease. *J. Pediatr. Surg.* 1990; 25: 527–30.

Ordein JJ, Di Lorenzo C, Flores A, Hyman PE. Diversion colitis in children with severe gastrointestinal motility disorders. *Am. J. Gastroenterol.* 1992; 87: 88–90.

Parrott TS. Urological implications of imperforate anus. *Urology* 1977; 10: 407–13.

Peer A, Klin B, Vinograd I. Balloon catheter dilatation of focal colonic strictures following necrotizing enterocolitis. *Cardiovasc. Intervent. Radiol.* 1993; 16: 248–50.

Pena A. Current management of anorectal anomalies. *Surg. Clin. North Am.* 1992; 72: 1393–416.

Pena A. Anorectal malformations. *Semin. Pediatr. Surg.* 1995; 4: 35–47.

Pena A, Amroch D, Baeza C, Csury L, Rodriguez G. The effects of the posterior sagittal approach on rectal function (experimental study). *J. Pediatr. Surg.* 1993; 28: 773–8.

Pohlandt F. Prevention and treatment of necrotizing enterocolitis in the newborn infant from the pediatric point of view. *Z. Kinderchir.* 1990; 45: 267–72.

Quan L, Smith DW. The VATER Association. *J. Pediatr. Surg.* 1973; 82: 104–7.

Radhakrishnan J, Blechman G, Shrader C, Patel MK, Mangurten HH, McFadden JC. Colonic strictures following successful medical management of necrotizing enterocolitis: a prospective study evaluating early gastrointestinal contrast studies. *J. Pediatr. Surg.* 1991; 26: 1043–6.

Ralph DJ, Woodhouse CR, Ransley PG. The management of the neuropathic bladder in adolescents with imperforate anus. *J. Urol.* 1992; 148: 366–8.

Reisner SH, Sivan Y, Nitzan M, Merlob P. Determination of anterior displacement of the anus in newborn infants and children. *Pediatrics* 1984; 73; 216–17.

Review article. Immunoglobulin feeding prevents necrotizing enterocolitis in formula fed very low birthweight infants. *Nutr. Rev.* 1989; 47: 186–8.

Richter A, Gortner L, Moller JC, Tegtmeyer FK. Pathogenetic concepts of neonatal necrotizing enterocolitis. *Klin. Pediatr.* 1993; 205: 317–24.

Ricketts RR, Jerles ML. Neonatal necrotizing enterocolitis: experience with 100 consecutive surgical patients. *World J. Surg.* 1990; 14: 600–5.

Rintala RJ, Lindahl H. Is normal bowel function possible after repair of intermediate and high anorectal malformations? *J. Pediatr. Surg.* 1995; 30: 491–4.

Rintala RJ, Mildh L, Lindahl H. Fecal continence and quality of life in adult patients with an operated low anorectal malformation. *J. Pediatr. Surg.* 1992; 27: 902–5.

Rosenfield NS, Ablow RC, Markowitz RI, *et al.* Hirschsprung disease: accuracy of the barium enema examination. *Radiology* 1984; 150: 393–400.

Rotbart HA, Nelson WL, Glade MP, *et al.* Neonatal rotavirus associated necrotizing enterocolitis: case control study and prospective surveillance during and outbreak. *J. Pediatr.* 1988; 112: 87–93.

Santulli, AJ. Anorectal anomalies: a suggested international classification. *J. Paediatr. Surg.* 1970; 5, 281–7.

Schofield DE, Devine W, Yunis EJ. Acetylcholinesterase stained suction rectal biopsies in the diagnosis of Hirschsprung's disease. *J. Pediatr. Gastroenterol. Nutr.* 1990; 11: 221–8.

Shanbhogue LK, Tam K, Lloyd DA. Necrotizing enterocolitis following operation in the neonatal period. *Br. J. Surg.* 1991; 78: 1045–7.

Smith BM, Steiner RB, Lobe TE. Laparoscopic Duhamel pull-through procedure for Hirschsprung's disease in childhood. *J. Laparoendosc. Surg.* 1994; 4: 273–6.

Smith NM, Chambers HM, Furness ME, Haan EA. The OEIS complex (omphalocele exstrophy imperforate anus spinal defects): recurrence in sibs. *J. Med. Genet.* 1992; 29: 730–2.

Smith VV. Intestinal neuronal density in childhood: a baseline for the objective assessment of hypo and hyperganglionosis. *Pediatr. Pathol.* 1993; 13: 225–37.

St Vil D, LeBouthillier G, Luks FI, Bensoussan AL, Blanchard H, Youssef S. Neonatal gastrointestinal perforations. *J. Pediatr. Surg.* 1992; 27: 1340–2.

Stephens FD. Imperforate rectum: a new surgical technique. *Med. J. Aust. N.Z.* 1953; 2: 202–3.

Stephens FD, Smith ED. Classification, identification and assessment of surgical treatment of anorectal anomalies. *Paediatr. Surg. Int.* 1986; 1, 200–16.

Stephens FD, Smith ED. *Anorectal malformations in children.* Chicago: Yearbook Medical, 1971.

Stevenson DK. Breath hydrogen in preterm infants. *Am. J. Dis. Child.* 1989; 143: 1262–3.

Stringer MD, Brereton RJ, Drake DP, Kiely EM, Capps SN, Spitz L. Recurrent necrotizing enterocolitis. *J. Pediatr. Surg.* 1993; 28: 979–81.

Suzuki H, Amano S, Matsumoto K, Tsukamoto Y. Anorectal motility in children with complete rectal prolapse. *Prog. Pediatr. Surg.* 1989; 24: 105–14.

Swenson O, Bill AH. Resection of the rectum and rectosigmoid with preservation of sphincter for benign spastic lesions producing megacolon. *Surgery* 1948; 24: 212–20.

Takamatsu H, Akiyama H, Ibara S, Seki S, Kuraya K, Ikenoue T. Treatment for necrotizing enterocolitis perforation in the extremely premature infant (weighing less than 1000 g). *J. Pediatr. Surg.* 1992; 27: 741–3.

Teitelbaum DH. Hirschsprung's disease in children. *Curr. Opin. Pediatr.* 1995; 7: 316–22.

Teixeira OHP. Cardiovascular anomalies with imperforate anus. *Arch. Dis. Child.* 1983; 58: 747–9.

Thilo EH, Lazarte RA, Hernandez JA. Necrotizing enterocolitis in the first 24 hours of life. *Pediatrics* 1984; 73. 476–80.

Tomita R, Munakata K, Kurosu Y, Tanjoh K. A role of nitric oxide in Hirschsprung's disease. *J. Pediatr. Surg.* 1995; 30: 437–40.

Tuggle DW, Perkins TA, Tunell WP, Smith EI. Operative treatment of anterior ectopic anus: the efficacy and influence of age on results. *J. Pediatr. Surg.* 1990; 25: 996–7.

Upadhyaya P. Mid-anal sphincteric malformation, cause of constipation in anterior perineal anus. *J. Pediatr. Surg.* 1984; 19: 183–6.

van Zoeren Grobben D, Moison RM, Ester WM, Berger HM. Lipid peroxidation in human milk and infant formula: effect of storage, tube feeding and exposure to phototherapy. *Acta. Paediatr.* 1993; 82: 645–9.

Walsh MC, Kliegman RM, Fanaroff AA. Necrotizing enterocolitis: a practitioner's perspective. *Pediatr. Rev.* 1988; 9: 219–26.

Walsh MC, Kliegman RM, Hack M. Severity of necrotizing enterocolitis: influence on outcome at 2 years of age. *Pediatrics* 1989; 84: 808–14.

Walther FJ, Verloove Vanhorick SP, Brand R, Ruys JH. A prospective survey of necrotising enterocolitis in very low birthweight infants. *Paediatr. Perinat. Epidemiol.* 1989; 3: 53–61.

Warner BW, Ziegler MM. Management of the short bowel syndrome in the pediatric population. *Pediatr. Clin. North Am.* 1993; 40: 1335–50.

Wesley JR. Efficacy and safety of total parenteral nutrition in pediatric patients. *Mayo Clin. Proc.* 1992; 67: 671–5.

Yazbeck S, Luks FI, St Vil D. Anterior perineal approach and three flap anoplasty for imperforate anus: optimal reconstruction with minimal destruction. *J. Pediatr. Surg.* 1992; 27: 190 4.

Zabielski PB, Groh Wargo SL, Moore JJ. Necrotizing enterocolitis: feeding in endemic and epidemic periods. *J. Parenter. Enteral. Nutr.* 1989; 13: 520–4.

3 Infections and the colon

Infectious diarrhoea

Incidence and transmission

World-wide, infections of the intestine are the commonest conditions affecting the gastrointestinal tract (Farthing *et al.* 1993). Even in Western countries, most patients with diarrhoea seeking medical advice will prove to have an infective cause (Fry 1990). However, the condition is much more frequently seen in developing countries. Whereas European children experience one episode of infective diarrhoea per year, the average in Africa is nine attacks per year (World Health Organization 1990; Guandalini 1989).

Transmission of diarrhoeal agents is by the faeco-oral route and may be either direct or indirect (Table 3.1). Direct contact includes the fingers, lips, or via fomites, such as feeding utensils and clothing. Anal and oral transmission is important among homosexual men (Gracey 1993). Indirect transmission is via contaminated food and water, insect vectors, infected animals or airborne droplets. Institutionalization and areas of overcrowding, poor hygiene, and inadequate sanitation predispose to infection as does the use of contaminated water or inappropriately treated food substances. One specific example is the association between the mass production of poultry and eggs and the increasing incidence of both *Salmonella* species and *Campylobacter jejuni* infections (Baird-Parker 1990; Skirrow 1991). Children have a high incidence of diarrhoea particularly when attending day-care or pre-school centres (Goodman *et al.* 1984). Foreign travel to underdeveloped countries is associated with a 30% risk of infective diarrhoea (Farthing *et al.* 1992).

Table 3.1 Methods of transmission for agents causing diarrhoea

Direct transmission	Indirect transmission
Fingers	Contaminated food and water
Feeding utensils	Insect vectors
Clothing	Infected animals
Sexual transmission	Airborne droplets

Another major risk factor is impaired immunological function. Childhood malnutrition is the commonest cause of this world-wide. In Western countries, the immunocompromise is most commonly seen in the elderly, those on steroids, and more recently, patients with AIDS. Those with AIDS are at increased risk of both faeco-oral contamination during sexual activity and direct transmission during anal intercourse of agents causing proctitis and an associated diarrhoea.

Aetiology

Bacterial agents account for approximately one-third of cases of diarrhoea in the industrialized world and more than one-half in tropical regions where enterotoxigenic *Escherichia coli* (ETEC) is prevalent (DuPont 1994). In Western countries *Shigella, Salmonella, Campylobacter, Yersinia enterocolitica,* and *Clostridium* species are most frequently implicated. Other, rarer, bacterial diarrhoeal agents include *Aeromonas, Pleisciomonas,* and *Vibrio* species. The relative frequency of the different isolates reported to the Communicable Disease Surveillance Centre for England and Wales in 1991 is shown in Table 3.2 (Farthing *et al.* 1993). Rotavirus is the commonest viral pathogen in infective diarrhoea and is especially prevalent in cases involving infants under the age of 1 year. Other viral agents include Norwalk and Norwalk-like viruses, caliciviruses and astroviruses.

Table 3.2 The relative frequency of the different isolates reported to the Communicable Disease Surveillance Centre for England and Wales in 1991

Infectious agent	Frequency of occurrence
Campylobacter spp.	> 30 000
Salmonella spp. (excludes typhi, paratyphi, and arizonae)	> 20 000
Shigella spp.	> 10 000
All others	< 5000

Patients returning from abroad have a different spectrum of pathogens. They should be investigated for ETEC, which accounts for 40% of cases, and *V. cholera*, while 5% will have a protozoal pathogen such as *Entamoeba histolytica* or *Giardia lamblia*. Patients with impaired immunity may develop *Mycobacterium avium intracellulare*, cytomegalovirus, herpes simplex, *Cryptosporidium* species and other parasites.

Pathophysiology and pathology

Organisms may cause diarrhoea by release of enterotoxin or by damage to the gut wall from direct invasion or mechanical disruption of the mucosa (Table 3.3). These categories are not mutually exclusive, some organisms being both invasive and secretors of an enterotoxin (Fry 1990). The most comprehensively studied enterotoxin releasing organism is *V. cholera*. By a series of enzyme activation and receptor binding, a high intracellular concentration of cyclic adenosine monophosphate is produced and chloride ions secreted. These ions are followed by sodium ions and water, resulting in large volumes of isotonic solution flowing into the gut lumen (Booth and McNeish 1993). Another mechanism of toxigenic diarrhoea is via the ingestion of preformed toxins, as is seen in

Table 3.3 Pathogenesis of diarrhoea for different organisms

Non-invasive organisms	Invasive organisms
Escherichia coli (enterotoxic)	*E. coli* (enteroinvasive)
Vibrio cholera	*Campylobacter*
Rotavirus	*Salmonella* spp.
Norwalk virus	*Shigella* spp.
Adenovirus	
Yersinia enterocolitica	
Pseudomembranous colitis	

Staphylococcus aureus and *Bacillus cereus* food poisoning. Vomiting is then a major symptom in addition to the diarrhoea.

Organisms that damage the gut wall as part of the diarrhoeal illness do so by adhering to the epithelium, invading the cells and translocating from the epithelial cells (Farthing *et al.* 1993). Enteropathic *E. coli* (EPEC) attach themselves to the mucous membrane, disrupting the brush border and reducing the absorptive surface (Knutton *et al.* 1987). Typically invasive organisms are *Salmonella*, *Shigella*, and *Campylobacter* species, *E.histolytica*, and enteroinvasive *E. coli* (EIEC). Such organisms invade the epithelial cells and multiply within them, releasing cytotoxins which lead to cell death. This destruction causes inflammation and ulceration of the epithelium. Generally, there is complete resolution of the histological changes within a few weeks of the elimination of the infection translocation through the lamina propria and into the lymphatic system occurs with *Salmonella* species, *Y. enterocolitica*, and *Campylobacter* species This may cause both local inflammation of the lamina propria and generalized bacteraemia.

The mechanism by which viruses cause diarrhoea is less well understood. From work done on the rotavirus in pigs, it appears that they disrupt the normal process of enterocyte renewal, resulting in an increased number of undifferentiated secretory cells and fewer differentiated adsorptive cells.

Clinical presentation

Depending upon the predominant underlying pathophysiology, two typical patterns present: watery diarrhoea or dysentery. Watery diarrhoea is seen with those organisms which secrete enterotoxins and do not damage the epithelial cells. The volume of diarrhoea may vary from a few loose stools to greater than 20 expulsions of watery faeces in a 24-h period. The illness is usually self-limiting and in the majority causes no significant dehydration. Occasionally, severe dehydration is seen, for example, with *V. cholera*. The commonest causes are ETEC, viral pathogens, and *V. cholera*.

Dysentery is the presence of blood and mucus in the diarrhoea and is associated with invasive organisms. It may present as the second part of a bi-phasic illness, with watery diarrhoea being the initial presentation. Stools may be of small volume and associated with tenesmus and faecal urgency. In severe cases, the disease may become fulminant with development of toxic megacolon. The commonest causes in Europe and North America are *C. jejuni* and *Salmonella* and *Shigella* species. Additional systemic features such as arthralgia, rashes, haemolytic–uraemic syndrome, and organomegaly may be present. The most important assessment in the management of such patients is the degree of dehydration which indicates the volumes and route of rehydration required.

In addition to a description of the diarrhoea, other important factors can be gleaned from the history. Such factors include a dietary history, evidence of foreign travel or recent antibiotic therapy, other associated cases, and homosexual activity. Other specific clinical features may point towards a particular diagnosis, for example haemolytic uraemic syndrome with enterohaemorrhagic *E. coli* (EHEC).

Diagnosis

The vast majority of infective diarrhoeal illnesses are benign and self-limiting. A specific diagnosis is therefore not required in every case. This is particularly relevant considering the cost of stool culturing per positive result has been estimated at £600–£750 (Guerrant *et al.* 1985). Laboratory investigation is therefore only appropriate for those with significant disease. This includes patients with dysentery, those with a severe initial presentation of watery diarrhoea, and individuals in whom the symptoms have persisted longer than 5–7 days. A stool examination for leucocytes will indicate an invasive-type organism causing the diarrhoea if polymorphonuclear leucocytes are present. Stool culture is only positive in 15% of cases (DuPont 1994). To optimize results, at least three specimens should be obtained and all sent immediately to the laboratory at room temperature. Special culture techniques will be required if a fungal or viral aetiology is suspected. Examination for parasites is only recommended when: (i) the diarrhoea has persisted for more than 14 days; (ii) the patient is a homosexual male; (iii) there has been travel to relevant countries, such as those where it is not recommended to drink untreated water; or (iv) the patient is in regular contact with a child day-care centre. Three samples of stools should be examined for cysts, larvae, ova, and trophozoites.

Proctosigmoidoscopy may be helpful as a normal mucosa in the presence of watery diarrhoea points towards a toxigenic organism. Mucosal inflammation indicates an invasive pathogen while the finding of yellow/white plaques (pseudo-membranes) gives a rapid diagnosis of infection with *Clostridium difficile* (Counihan and Roberts 1993). Rectal biopsy rarely identifies a specific pathogen. However, it may be of benefit in discriminating between acute ulcerative colitis and an infective colitis (Figure 3.1a,b). In the acute stage, ulcerative colitis patients may have extension of the plasmacytosis into the mucosal base with distortion of crypt architecture (Nostrant *et al.* 1987). If there is any doubt, a repeat biopsy 6–10 weeks later is indicated, as an infective cause will have by then resolved in contrast to the persistent symptoms of untreated ulcerative colitis (Mandal and Schofield 1992). Sigmoidoscopy/colonoscopy and biopsy are of particular importance in the homosexual patient when additional specific pathogens should be sought.

Serology is generally unhelpful; however, there are individual exceptions such as the antibody titres to *E.histolytica* and *Y. enterocolitica* and the immunoglobulin (Ig) M antibody to *G. lamblia* (Arvind *et al.* 1988; Farthing 1990). *Clostridium difficile* is usually diagnosed by identifying the toxin from stool samples. The best technique is by using tissue culture methods and neutralization of the toxin if present. Where this is not available, alternative techniques include counter-immunoelectrophoresis (CIE), enzyme-linked immunosorbent assay (ELISA), and latex particle agglutination. Although all are less sensitive methods, the ELISA technique appears the best of the three. Diagnostic modalities for the future include the development of DNA probes which in addition to

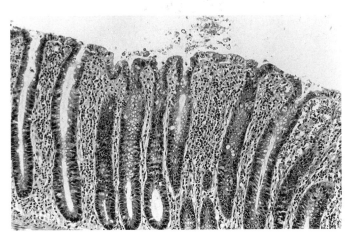

(a)

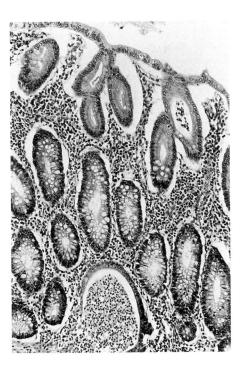

(b)

Figure 3.1 (a) Infective colitis. There is some surface debris with a mixed acute and chronic inflammatory reaction including some emigrating polymorphs in the lamina propria (×73). (b) Ulcerative colitis. In comparison with (a) there is distortion and branching of glands, mucin depletion a large crypt with a dilated gland (×73).

identifying the organism have the capacity to predict its virulence (Char and Farthing 1991).

Treatment

Oral rehydration therapy

The most important aspect of therapy is the maintenance of an adequate fluid and electrolyte balance. In most cases this is achieved by encouraging the patient to drink more, for example, fruit juices and soups. Others will require formal oral rehydration therapy (ORT) and a minority, intravenous fluid replacement.

In developing countries where malnutrition is common and *V. cholera* a likely pathogen, the optimal electrolyte concentration is about 90 mmol Na$^+$/l (Anonymous 1992). However, in Europe and North America, solutions containing sodium concentrations of 40–60 mmol/l are generally used (Elliott *et al.* 1989; DuPont 1994) to avoid hypernatraemia. In addition to glucose-based ORT, cereal-based ORT has been developed with the aim of providing sufficient calories for the malnourished. It has the further benefit, unlike the glucose-based solution, of reducing the volume of faecal losses (Molla *et al.* 1989). Breast feeding of infants with diarrhoea should be continued throughout the illness. Despite the availability and benefit of ORT solutions, they are poorly utilized and the majority of diarrhoeal episodes inappropriately treated even within Europe (Guandalini 1989).

Non-specific therapy

Bismuth subsalicylate acts as an antisecretory agent and reduces the number of stools and the duration of the illness by 50% (DuPont *et al.* 1977). The antimotility agent loperamide, which also has antisecretory properties, is significantly more effective than bismuth, reducing the diarrhoea by 80% (Johnson *et al.* 1986; DuPont *et al.* 1990). However, antidiarrhoeal agents should not be used in patients with dysentery or with a fever because of the danger that they may increase the risk of toxic megacolon in patients with invasive pathogens (DuPont and Hornick 1973). The appropriate role for these drugs is in treating mild diarrhoeas which originate in developed nations. Other than this they should be used with caution.

Antibiotic therapy

Not all patients require antibiotic therapy. When it is given, it may be on an emperical basis or related to specific, identified pathogens. There are three possible situations in which emperical therapy may be started without a definite diagnosis. First, it is appropriate for a febrile dysenteric illness, the appropriate treatment being ciprofloxacin 250 mg twice daily for 3 days. Secondly, trials of antibiotics in travellers' diarrhoea have demonstrated that they reduce the severity and duration of the illness (Farthing *et al.* 1993). Again ciprofloxacin 250 mg, b.d. for 3 days is appropriate medication. The third scenario for emperical treatment is that of diarrhoea persisting for longer than 14 days and the suspicion of a parasitic pathogen. The appropriate therapy is metronidazole 250 mg, q.i.d. for 7–10 days. While metronidazole can be used in children, ciprofloxacin cannot and for children with travellers' diarrhoea or dysentery, trimethoprim plus erythromycin is the appropriate treatment. Antimicrobial therapy for identified infective agents is discussed in the sections on the individual pathogens.

Prevention

Careful attention to personal hygiene and choice of food consumed is the mainstay of diarrhoeal prevention. There is also a case for antibiotic prophylaxis in certain instances. It has been suggested that when travel to a high-risk area for less than 3 weeks is being undertaken, prophylaxis is appropriate for those who already have impaired health and for those in whom an episode of diarrhoea would significantly affect the purpose of the travel (Farthing 1994). In particular, individuals with achlorhydria, whether due to pernicious anaemia or pharmacologically induced, should be considered for prophylaxis as should those with inflammatory bowel disease. In such cases a 4-fluoroquinolone such as ciprofloxacin, appears to be the most effective, reducing episodes of travellers' diarrhoea by more than 85% (Farthing 1994). Before prescribing prophylaxis for the traveller, he/she must be fully informed of the small but definite risk of adverse effects from the antibiotic. This also applies to travellers planning to self-administer antibiotics if they get an episode of diarrhoea. The role for vaccination is considered in the specific sections relating to the individual pathogens.

Specific causes of diarrhoea

Bacteria

Campylobacter jejuni

This is a Gram-negative curved bacilli. Of the subspecies *jejuni*, *fetus*, and *intestinalis*, *C. jejuni* are the most frequent cause of human disease. Animals and improperly cooked food, especially chicken are the primary sources of infection. Infections are commonest during the summer months. The incubation period is 2–5 days.

Campylobacter is the commonest bacterial cause of diarrhoea in the developed world (greater than 15%). Fever and diarrhoea occur in 90%, abdominal pain in 70% and blood in the stool in 50% (Puylaert *et al.* 1997). Influenza-like symptoms are common and may precede the diarrhoea. Reiter's syndrome is a recognized association (Saari and Kauranen 1980). Diagnosis is by culture on selective media. Dark field microscopy of fresh stool for curved, motile rods is specific but has a low sensitivity. Treatment consists of ciprofloxacin for adults, erythromycin for children (Pichler *et al.* 1987).

Salmonella species (non-typhoid strains)

This is a Gram-negative bacilli. Of the 2000 serotypes, 40 account for 90% of human disease and are aggregated into groups A–E. Different strains have different degrees of virulence. *Salmonella* species are found in eggs, chicken, other animals, and water. The incubation period is 12–48 h.

Fifty per cent of patients will have the classical bloody diarrhoea. However, the diarrhoea may initially not be blood-stained. Abdominal pain is a predominant feature. Differentiation from ulcerative colitis is vital as administration of steroids may cause silent perforation and septicaemia in salmonella-infected patients (Dronfield *et al.* 1974). The diarrhoeal/dysenteric illness may progress to bacteraemia and Gram-negative sepsis resulting in localized infection of any organ of the body (Goldberg and Rubin 1988). A sterile reactive arthritis may follow 1–2 weeks after the infection. In approximately 0.5% of infected individuals an asymptomatic carrier state results. This is regardless of whether the infection was symptomatic or asymptomatic (Musher and Rubenstein 1973). Chronic carrier status is more likely in patients with gallstones. Diagnosis is by stool culture, blood cultures being positive during bacteraemia.

Antibiotics are not generally indicated in the treatment of salmonella infection as they increase the incidence and duration of the carrier state (Aserkoff and Bennett 1969). Indications for treatment are septicaemia, the extremes of age, immunocompromised patients and those with prostheses, risk of endocarditis, or haemolytic anaemia (Griffiths and Gorbach 1993). Where possible, antibiotic sensitivity should be obtained because of increasing resistance to many antibiotics (DuPont and Hornick 1973). Before sensitivities are available, ciprofloxacin is a reasonable choice with a third generation cephalosporin such as cefotaxamine being used in children (Farthing *et al.* 1993). Typhoid fever, caused by *Salmonella typhi* is largely an ileal disease, not affecting the colon. It is not further discussed.

Shigella species

This is caused by Gram-negative bacilli of the species *S. dysenteriae*, *S. flexneri*, *S. boydii*, or *S. sonnei*. *Shigella sonnei* is the commonest cause of diarrhoea in the developed world and *S. flexneri* the commonest in the developing world. Infection with *S. dysenteriae* causes the severest diarrhoea of the *Shigella* infections . Humans and some other primates are the only natural host, person to person contact being the commonest form of transmission. An oral innoculum of as few as 10 bacteria is capable of producing infection, as *Shigella* in the lag growth phase are resistant to the acidic environment of the stomach (Gordon and Small 1993). Because of the high numbers of bacteria shed by the patient and the low numbers required for infection, secondary cases are very common. The incubation period is 1–5 days.

Watery diarrhoea and abdominal pain often precede the dysentery. Fever and grossly bloody stools are slightly more common in *Shigella* dysentery than in other types of dysentery. Complications include toxic megacolon, haemolytic–uraemic syndrome, hypoglycaemia with seizures, leukaemoid reaction with white cell counts of over $50\,000/\mu$l and a post-infectious arthritis. Diagnosis is by stool culture on selective media.

Antibiotics are not usually required. Because of increasing resistance to ampicillin and trimethoprim–sulphamethoxazole, ciprofloxacin is the appropriate antibiotic for adults when indicated, with a single dose sufficing (Williams and Richards 1990). In children, ampicillin or the trimethoprim–sulphamethoxazole combination can be given.

Yersinia enterocolitica

These are Gram-negative coccobacilli which are derived from contaminated water, milk, and animals, either pets or as sources of food. The incubation period is 4–10 days.

Fever, abdominal cramps, and diarrhoea persist for an average of 2 weeks, longer than most other infective diarrhoeas (Puylaert *et al.* 1997). Bowel necrosis and metastatic infection are uncommon sequelae. A polyarticular, sterile arthritis associated with erythema nodosum or erythema multiforme can occur. Reactive arthritis in 2% and classical Reiter's syndrome have also been reported. *Yersinia* infection may also be associated with chronic abdominal symptoms (Saebo and Lassen 1992). Abdominal ultrasound scan may help discriminate *Yersinia* infection from acute appendicitis which it may mimic (Puylaert *et al.* 1989). Stool culture on selective media or cultures from blood, peritoneal fluid, or mesenteric nodes may be used to make the diagnosis. A fourfold rise in antibody titres taken 10 days apart or a titre of greater than or equal to 1/160, followed by a subsequent fall, indicates invasive disease.

Yersinia enterocolitica expresses a beta-lactamase making it resistant to penicillins and third-generation cephalosporins. Antibiotic therapy is only indicated for severe disease or evidence of extraintestinal infection. When antibiotics are required, chloramphenicol has been of proven benefit and the 4-quinolones are likely to be the drugs of choice in the future (Hoogkamp-Korstanje 1987).

Escherichia coli

Escherichia coli are Gram-negative coccobacilli. They are the commonest type of aerobic gut flora but certain strains are recognized as being pathogenic. These may be divided into ETEC, EIEC, EPEC, EHEC, and enteroadherent (EAEC). Such strains are derived from infected foodstuffs and water with an incubation period of 1–2 days.

ETEC account for 40% of tropical and travellers' diarrhoea (Farthing 1994). They secrete an endotoxin which induces watery diarrhoea. Clinical features are generally mild and self-limiting. EIEC invade colonic epithelial cells in a similar fashion to *Shigella* species to cause dysentery. ETEC adhere to the mucosal surface, efface the microvillae and increase intracellular calcium, producing a diarrhoea with mucus but no blood. It particularly affects infants and those attending day-care facilities. EHEC is now recognized as one of the commonest causes of infective colitis in western Europe and North America, the strain *E. coli* O157: H7 in particular being responsible for outbreaks of haemorrhagic colitis (Acheson and Keusch 1994; Cimolai *et al.* 1997). This is characterized by mucosal ulceration and marked submucosal oedema and haemorrhage causing bowel wall thickening (Ilnyckyj *et al.* 1997). Infection with EHEC is associated with severe abdominal pain but little pyrexia. Haemolytic–uraemic syndrome and thrombotic thrombocytopenic purpura may also occur (Bitzan *et al.* 1993). The source is usually of animal origin, e.g. hamburgers. EAEC may account for up to 30% of travellers' diarrhoea when no other pathogen is isolated (Mathewson *et al.* 1986).

Diagnosis is by stool culture on selective media. Differentiation of some types (e.g. ETEC) from the normal gut *E. coli* is made by the response to specific antitoxins. For other types (e.g. EPEC) a specific pattern of localized adherence can be seen on tissue culture cells (Scaletsky *et al.* 1985). As treatment is not generally indicated, specific diagnostic tests are not essential for the management of the individual patient. However, routine testing for EHEC has been recommended both to alert the physician to the possibility of the haemolytic–uraemic syndrome and to provide epidemiological information (Acheson and Keusch 1994)·

In general, antibiotics are not indicated. In the case of EHEC, antibiotics have been claimed to improve symptoms (Martin *et al.* 1990) but at the expense of possibly precipitating haemolytic–uraemic syndrome (Carter *et al.* 1987). In severe cases which merit antibiotics, ampicillin or ciprofloxacin are the drugs of choice and neomycin for infants with EPEC.

Vibrio cholera

This is a Gram-negative rod which is derived from contaminated water and foodstuffs especially seafood. Humans are the only known host. Person to person spread is rare. The incubation period is 2–3 days.

The majority of *V. cholera* infections are asymptomatic (>80% for the classical biotype and >95% for the El Tor biotype). These asymptomatic cases facilitate the spread of the disease. When the disease is symptomatic, it may be severe enough to cause diarrhoeal loss of 1 litre/h and death within several hours. The term 'rice water' to describe the diarrhoea relates to small flecks of mucus in otherwise clear fluid. Other clinical features relate to the degree of dehydration and loss of circulatory volume. In endemic regions, it is primarily a disease of children, in other areas it affects all ages. Diagnosis is made by dark field stool microscopy which may reveal the highly motile cholera vibrios. Alternatively, stool culture on thiosulphate–citrate–bile salts–sucrose (TCBS) agar can be used. Specific agglutination/haemagglutination patterns may then identify the specific biotype.

Antibiotics are of benefit, but are of secondary importance to fluid replacement. For adults the treatment is tetracycline 250 mg, q.i.d. for 2–5 days. For children and pregnant women furazolide is preferable. Tetracycline given to family members of infected individuals significantly reduces the secondary attack rate. A parenteral cholera vaccine is available which provides modest protection for a few months. Work is currently ongoing into the development of a live oral vaccine (Levine *et al.* 1988).

Aeromonas species

Like the *V. cholera*, these are members of the Vibrionaceae family. They are ubiquitous in water, even surviving in chlorinated water. Relatively recently recognized as a diarrhoeal pathogen, it predominantly affects children under the age of 2 years. It may cause either watery diarrhoea or dysentery. Both are usually mild. Diagnosis is by stool culture on selective media. Antibiotics are indicated for those with dysentery or chronic diarrhoea. Trimethoprim–sulphamethoxazole is the drug of choice or the 4-fluroquinolones for the septicaemic patient.

Plesiomonas shigilloides is also a member of the Vibrionaceae family. It is a rarer isolate than *Aeromonas* and little information is available on it.

Viruses

Rotavirus

Rotavirus is an RNA virus, a member of the Reoviridae family. Of the seven subgroups (A–G), groups A, B, and C have been isolated in humans with group A being by far the commonest by far (Figure 3.2). Infection occurs from contaminated water and person to person contact (42% of one study were hospital acquired) (Noone and Banatvala 1983). In temperate climates, infection normally occurs during the winter months. The incubation period is 1–4 days.

Rotavirus is the commonest cause of diarrhoeal illness in children under the age of 2 years in both developed and developing countries (Cook *et al.* 1990). Adults can also be infected, often in relation to foreign travel. The clinical spectrum varies from no symptoms at all to the occasional case of fatal gastroenteritis. Most cases present

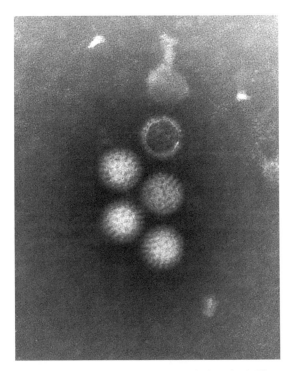

Figure 3.2 Electron micrograph of a rotavirus, negatively stained with phosphoungstic acid (×200 000).

with diarrhoea, usually in association with both pyrexia and vomiting. The respiratory tract can also be involved (Zheng *et al.* 1991). All symptoms normally resolve within 3–4 days. The diagnosis is made from stool samples using commercially available kits based on ELISA or latex agglutination techniques. These have a predictive value of over 90% (Christensen 1989).

Treatment consists of rehydration by oral and, if required, intravenous routes. Temporary disaccharide/monosaccharide intolerance may be helped by altering the carbohydrate content of the diet. The development of a vaccine has been frustrated to date by the ability of the rotaviruses to reassort genes during a mixed infection.

Norwalk virus and other caliciviruses

These are RNA viruses. Norwalk, Norwalk-like, and Caliciviruses are all members of the Caliciviridae family (Figure 3.3) (Greenberg and Matsui 1992). Infection is by direct transmission or ingestion of contaminated water and food. The incubation period is 12–48 h.

Unlike rotavirus, Norwalk, and Norwalk-like viruses predominantly affect older children and adults. However, the other caliciviruses more often affect young children (Schwab and Shaw 1993). Symptoms are generally mild and self-limiting within 2–3 days. In addition to diarrhoea and vomiting, fever, respiratory symptoms, and 'flu-like' symptoms may occur. Electron microscopy of stool samples is the main method of diagnosis. Detection of antigens or antibodies by ELISA, radio-immunoassay, and polymerase chain reaction is possible. None of these techniques are readily available for clinical service. Treatment is the same as for rotavirus.

Enteric adenoviruses

These are DNA viruses, specific serotypes of which cause gastroenteritis. Infection is by direct person to person transmission. The incubation period is 8–10 days.

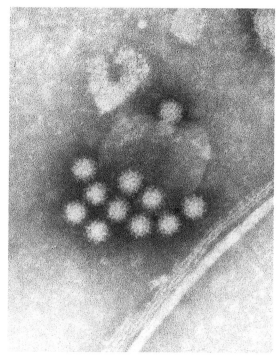

Figure 3.3 Electron micrograph of a Norwalk-like virus, negatively stained with phosphoungstic acid (×200 000).

Enteric adenovirus infection is predominantly a disease of infants and young children, being the second commonest cause of infantile diarrhoea after rotavirus. The disease may be prolonged with diarrhoea lasting up to 12 days (Uhnoo *et al.* 1990). Vomiting and pyrexia may also occur. Diagnosis is only possible in specialized research laboratories. Treatment is the same as for rotavirus.

Other recognized viral causes of diarrhoea include the astrovirus and coronavirus.

Parasitic infections

Entamoeba histolytica

Entamoeba histolytica is a pseudopod-forming protozoan. Infection occurs from ingestion of cysts in contaminated food and water or by direct person to person contact. Sexual transmission among homosexual men is an important source of infection (Phillips *et al.* 1981). The incubation period is long, there being 1–4 months between infection and clinical presentation.

Entamoeba histolytica preferentially affects the caecum and the rectosigmoid area. Initially, there is a mild, non-specific proctitis/colitis, with small groups of neutrophils in the lamina propria and surface epithelium. The organisms are present only on the surface.

Organisms penetrate the lamina propria by separating the intracellular junctions to involve all layers of the intestinal wall, producing an amoebic ulcer; this is surrounded by a dense inflammatory infiltrate and covered with a fibrinoid exudate containing organisms. The colonic ulceration may become chronic and result in stricture formation.

It is estimated that 500 million individuals world-wide are infected with *E. histolytica*, 90% of these being from the developing world (Guerrant 1986). Carriage rates in Europe and North America are nearly 1 in 20, with the immunosuppressed and malnourished being particularly vulnerable (Farthing 1993). Up to 90% of cases are asymptomatic. Symptomatic cases of intestinal disease may present acutely with dysentery progressing to toxic megacolon. Typically, there is no pyrexia. An alternative presentation of intestinal disease is with intermittent episodes of diarrhoea, passage of mucus rectally, mild pyrexia, and symptoms of malaise. Such patients may progress to the formation of both strictures and abdominal masses (amoebomas). Non-colonic presentation may be with a liver abscess which may rupture into the pleural or peritoneal cavities or erode into the hepatic vein (Figure 3.4).

Diagnosis is by stool examination for cysts or trophozoites. At least three fresh samples should be examined microscopically within 1 h using a saline wet mount. Endoscopy in acute amoebic colitis reveals small (1–5 mm) ulcers. There may be adjacent normal mucosa but often the findings are indistinguishable from ulcerative colitis. Scrapings from the edge of an ulcer may be taken and examined in a similar fashion to stool examination. Alternatively, histological staining of the biopsy may show amoeba (Figure 3.5a,b). Tests are available for measuring anti-*E. histolytica* antibodies. However, they are only positive in 70–80% of patients with amoebic colitis and they can remain positive for a long period of time. Their role in the individual patient is mainly when there has been a failure to detect the amoeba by another means (Arvind *et al.* 1988). An ELISA test for faecal antigen is being developed which may also aid diagnosis (Grundy *et al.* 1987).

Treatment consists of metronidazole 400 mg, t.d.s. for 5–10 days. In cases of toxic megacolon and perforation, subtotal colectomy and

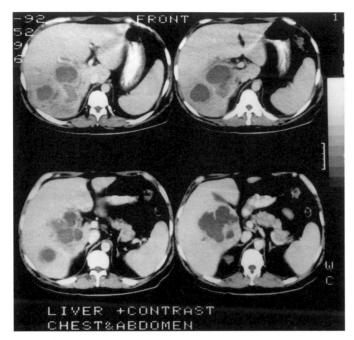

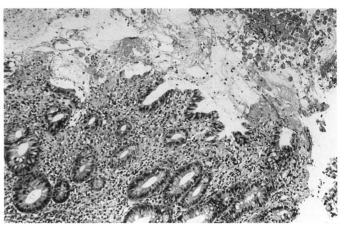

(a)

Figure 3.4 Computerized tomography of an amoebic abscess. There is a well-defined area of low attenuation in the right lobe of liver and a larger one in the caudate lobe which appears septated. These areas have low attenuation values in keeping with a fluid centre and show rim enhancement in keeping with a well formed abscess membrane.

ileostomy is the treatment of choice. Surgery may also be required for stricture formation.

Giardia lamblia

This is a protozoa which is also known as *G. intestinalis*. It is derived from contaminated food or water and by person to person spread including sexual intercourse. The incubation period is 1–3 weeks.

Most infected individuals are asymptomatic. Among symptomatic cases, watery diarrhoea, abdominal distension and weight loss are typical features. In the majority, symptoms resolve within 6 weeks, even without treatment. Some cases present as a chronic diarrhoea state which may be associated with malabsorption. In young children, infection is associated with failure to thrive (Farthing *et al.* 1986). Diagnosis is by faecal microscopy for cysts or trophozoites. Duodenal biopsy or aspirate may also be used (Figure 3.6). Anti-Giardia IgG may persist for years after the initial infection; however, IgM is specific for current infection (Sullivan *et al.* 1991). ELISA tests for faecal antigens are also available (Addiss *et al.* 1991).

Metronidazole is the drug of choice, the adult dose being 2 g as a single dose for 3 days. Drug resistance can be a problem and treatment failure occurs in up to 30% of cases. For treatment failure or proven resistance tinidazole, mepacrine, and furazolidine are alternatives. They may also be used in combination (Crouch *et al.* 1990).

Infectious diarrhoea in the immunocompromised host

The same organisms which cause diarrhoea in the immunocompetent host may also do so in the immunocompromised individual. However, some such as *Salmonella* and *Giardia* are particularly prone to infect the immunosuppressed. Organisms which are not

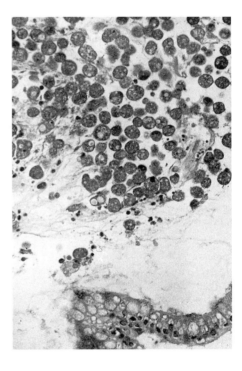

(b)

Figure 3.5 (a) Amoebic dysentery (colon). There is early mucosal erosion and eosinophils are present in the lamina propria. Numerous amoeba are present in the surface debris. (low power ×73). (b) Amoebic dysentery (colon). Amoebae in the surface debris. (high power ×180).

normally pathogens may produce diarrhoea in those with impaired immune function, more than one infective organism being detected in 20% of patients. Sexually acquired proctitis can cause low volume diarrhoea, while the HIV virus itself may be a cause of diarrhoea. In the investigation of such patients examination and culture of three stool samples and histological assessment of a rectal biopsy are the most useful tests (Rene *et al.* 1988; Connolly *et al.* 1990). If these tests are negative, gastroscopy and duodenal biopsy or aspirate should be performed as this is the only means of diagnosing *Microsporidia* species.

Cryptosporidia species account for up to 50% of cases of diarrhoea in patients with AIDS (Connolly *et al.* 1988). Faeco–oral and venereal spread are important means of transmission. However, *Cryptosporidia* may also be transmitted by infected drinking water so

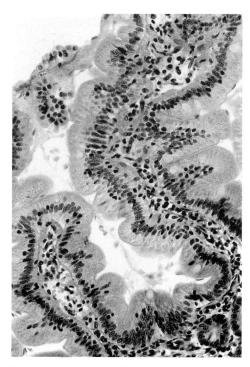

Figure 3.6 Giardiasis (jejunum). The villi appear normal but numerous Giardia can be seen in the intervillous spaces (×190).

that immunocompromised patients should boil water used for drinking (Mayon-White and Frankenberg 1989). Watery diarrhoea, dehydration, and weight loss are predominant features (Connolly *et al.* 1988). Diagnosis is made by stool microscopy after concentration techniques and modified Ziehl–Neelsen staining. The protozoa may be detected histologically in rectal and duodenal biopsies (Figure 3.7).

The inflammation is often mild, limited to a few plasma cells and eosinophils in the lamina propria. However, more severe inflammation can occur with heavier cell infiltrates, cryptitis, and apoptotic bodies. Organisms can be seen in groups on the epithelial surface or within crypts.

There is no effective antiprotozoal agent. Both macrolide antibiotics (Moskovitz *et al.* 1988) and zidovudine (Greenberg *et al.* 1989) may reduce the diarrhoea temporarily but it tends to recur. Antidiarrhoeal agents may give useful symptomatic relief. Other protozoal agents include *Isospora belli*, *Microsporidia* species, and *Blastocystis hominis*. In the treatment of *Microsporidia* species metronidazole or albendazole may be of benefit.

Cytomegalovirus may cause both proctitis and colitis with dysentery (Figure 3.8). It can be associated with significant abdominal pain and may progress to perforation or toxic megacolon (Jacobson *et al.* 1988). The diagnosis is made by histological demonstration of inclusion bodies in the tissue (Figure 3.9). Treatment is with ganciclovir, although relapse is frequent. Herpes simplex virus may cause proctitis with bloody diarrhoea and symptoms of tenesmus and incomplete evacuation (Goodell *et al.* 1983). This responds well to acyclovir. In the immunocompromised host, infections with cytomegalovirus and herpes simplex virus typically cause punched-out ulcers, which vary in size from minute to greater than 5 mm. The surrounding mucosa is oedematous. The characteristic feature of cytomegalovirus colitis is the presence of intranuclear inclusion bodies within macrophages. In herpes simplex virus infection, giant cells are present at the edge of the ulcers. When no other pathogen can be demonstrated, the HIV virus itself may be a pathogen causing an enteropathy (Klein *et al.* 1984).

Salmonella infection is 20 times more common in patients with AIDS and is more severe than in those with normal immune function (Bodey and Fainstein 1986). *Mycobacterium avium-intracellulare* may cause diarrhoea in patients with AIDS. It may be cultured from stool or jejunal biopsy. Histological findings may resemble Whipple's disease with large foamy macrophages present on rectal (and jejunal) biopsy (Roth *et al.* 1985). Ziehl Neelsen staining reveals acid-fast organisms in approximately one-quarter of cases. A

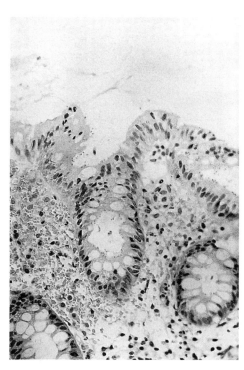

Figure 3.7 Cryptosporidiosis (colon). Numerous round organisms line the luminal borders of the crypts and mucosal surface (×190).

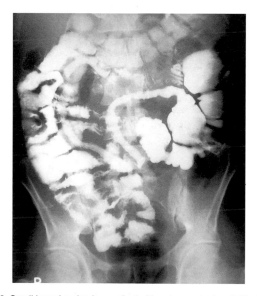

Figure 3.8 Small bowel series in a patient with cytomegalovirus ileitis. There are a number of long strictures in the ileum with separation of the loops caused by their thickened oedematous walls. The terminal ileum displays rose-thorn transmural ulceration and thickening of its folds.

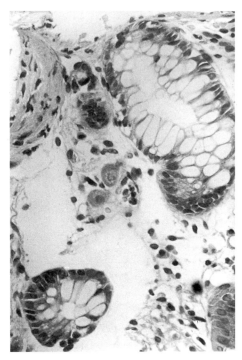

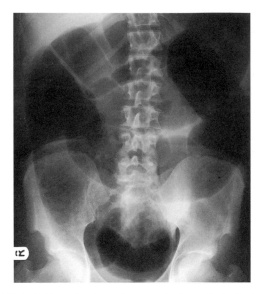

Figure 3.10 Plain X-ray showing toxic megacolon in a patient with clostridium difficile colitis.

Figure 3.9 Cytomegalovirus infection (colon). Cytomegalic inclusions which appear to be mainly within endothelial cells in a rectal biopsy (×300).

combination such as ethambutol, rifabutin, and clofazimine may be effective. Monotherapy is not recommended (Gazzard and Blanshard 1993).

Pseudomembranous colitis and antibiotic-associated colitis

Clostridium difficile is a Gram-positive spore-forming organism. Infection is derived from the environment, domestic animals, and healthy infants. Within health care facilities, hand carriage between patients is an important factor (Johnson *et al.* 1990). The incubation period is variable. In the majority, the onset of diarrhoea is within 5–10 days of commencing antibiotic therapy. However, in a significant minority of cases it does not begin until up to 6 weeks after cessation of antibiotics.

There is a spectrum of disease ranging from pseudomembranous colitis, through antibiotic-associated colitis (with no pseudo-membranes), to antibiotic-associated diarrhoea. Antibiotic-associated diarrhoea is characterized by diarrhoea and crampy abdominal pain occurring within the first week of commencing antibiotic therapy. Colonic biopsy is normal and the symptoms resolve on cessation of the antibiotics. Twenty per cent of these patients will have *C. difficile* cytotoxin in their stools. In addition to the absence of pseudomembranes, antibiotic-associated colitis is also different from pseudomembranous colitis in that the cytotoxin will be present in the faeces of 100% of patients with the latter diagnosis in contrast to 60–75% of those with antibiotic-associated colitis.

Almost all antibiotics have been implicated in the development of pseudomembranous colitis and antibiotic-associated colitis but the commonest culprits are clindamycin, ampicillin, amoxycillin, and cephalosporins (Anonymous 1994). Chemotherapy (Nielsen *et al.* 1992), gastrointestinal motility agents (McFarland *et al.* 1990), and gastrointestinal surgery (Bartlett 1990) have also been implicated as causative factors. Recent evidence suggests that *C. difficile* is also a

diarrhoeal pathogen in the absence of any of these factors (Griffiths and Gorbach 1993). In addition to diarrhoea, which may be watery or dysenteric, abdominal cramps, high pyrexia, and marked leuco-cytosis (greater than $50\,000/\mu\mathrm{l}$) are common. Toxic megacolon and colonic perforation can also occur (Figure 3.10).

Pathology

The histological appearance of colonic biopsies range from normal in patients with antibiotic-associated diarrhoea to complete mucosal ulceration and necrosis in severe pseudomembranous colitis. In early pseudomembranous colitis and antibiotic-associated colitis, 'summit lesions' can be identified histologically (Coyne *et al.* 1997). The terminology arises from the presence of small superficial erosions, with a 'luminal spray' of mucus, polymorphs, and nuclear debris appearing to flow out of the erosion (Figure 3.11).

Classical pseudomembranous colitis is seen histologically at the plaque stage. Because the intervening mucosa can often be normal, the plaques themselves must be biopsied. This reveals focal groups

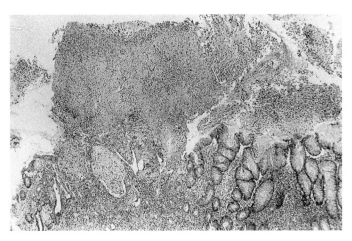

Figure 3.11 Pseudomembranous colitis (colon). Mushroom-like mass of mucin and neutrophils attached to the mucosa, which is only slightly inflamed (×26).

of disrupted crypts with a covering layer of mucin, fibrin, and polymorphs.

Diagnosis

Tissue culture of the stool provides a cytopathic toxin. Diagnosis is made by demonstrating the neutralization of this toxin on exposure to specific clostridia antitoxin. Stool culture on selected media can also be performed. These tests can be falsely negative and require a 1–2 day incubation period. When an immediate diagnosis is desirable, endoscopy should be performed. The finding of yellow-white pseudomembranes is characteristic but not universal and in 30% of cases pseudomembranes are absent in the rectum but present more proximally. They have the appearance of raised plaques which can be as small as 3–4 mm. Intervening mucosa may be hyperaemic and oedematous but can also be normal. Pseudomembranes may coalesce and the involved segment of the colonic mucosa slough.

Treatment

Patients with *C. difficile* in diarrhoeal faeces, especially if incontinent, should be treated with enteric isolation precautions (McFarland *et al.* 1989). They should be nursed and examined using disposable gloves with careful hand washing after patient contact.

Pseudomembranous colitis is treated initially by stopping the offending antibiotic and ensuring adequate fluid replacement. If it is felt necessary to maintain the current antibiotic this can be continued alongside the treatment for pseudomembranous colitis. However, remission of diarrhoea is considerably more rapid if the offending antibiotic can be stopped (Tedesco *et al.* 1974). Vancomycin 125 mg q.i.d. given orally for 10–14 days is currently the drug of choice. However, oral metronidazole is as effective and is considerably cheaper (Bartlett 1990). It can be given in a dosage of 250 mg q.i.d. for 10–14 days. Oral vancomycin is poorly absorbed and its mechanism of action is by achieving high concentrations within the faeces in the colon. Intravenous vancomycin is therefore not useful. By contrast metronidazole is absorbed and reaches the colon via the bloodstream. In patients with toxic megacolon or who are otherwise unable to take oral medication 125 mg metronidazole intravenously every 6 h is the appropriate therapy. Persistence of diarrhoea while on vancomycin or metronidazole suggests that there is an additional cause for the illness other than pseudomembranous colitis.

Relapse occurs in 10–20% of cases and will respond to repeat therapy with the same antibiotic. An additional or alternative therapy for episodes of relapse is the use of cholestyramine to bind the toxin. Four grams t.i.d. is effective in mild colitis. If given along with vancomycin or metronidazole, the antibiotic in addition to the toxin, will be bound to the resin. Administration of the two therapies should be separated by several hours. Despite this pseudomembranous colitis is still associated with a 10–20% mortality, the elderly and debilitated being particularly vulnerable (Anonymous, 1994).

Tuberculosis

Incidence

From the introduction of antituberculous therapy in the early 1950s until the 1980s the annual incidence of tuberculosis declined steadily in the developed world. However, since the 1980s the number of cases has risen steadily due to both an increase in the

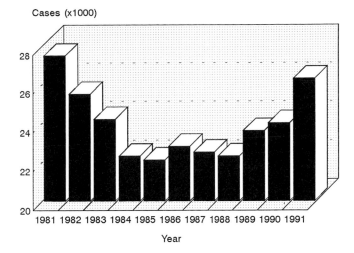

Cases (x1000)

Figure 3.12 Incidence of tuberculosis in the USA, 1981–91 (×1000).

numbers of immigrants and the spread of the AIDS virus (Figure 3.12) (Jereb *et al.* 1991). Globally, half the world's population is infected with *Mycobacterium tuberculosis* (Daniel 1991). Abdominal tuberculosis has become a rare form of tuberculosis since the introduction of pasteurization for milk. Peritoneal and intestinal sites each account for approximately half the cases, the ileocaecal region being the commonest area for intestinal disease (Marshall 1993). When associated with HIV disease, tuberculosis infection is four times more likely to involve extrapulmonary sites and the extent of involvement is more severe (Balthazar *et al.* 1990; Bargallo *et al.* 1992; Marshall 1993). Colonic tuberculosis is equally prevalent in males and females and may affect any age.

Transmission

Colonic tuberculosis may occur: (i) via swallowing infected sputum in patients with active pulmonary disease; (ii) by haematogenous spread from miliary tuberculosis or a silent bacteraemia with acute pulmonary disease; (iii) by direct spread from adjacent organs, e.g. the genitourinary tract; or (iv) by ingestion of contaminated milk.

Pathology

There are classically three types of intestinal lesions: ulcerative, hypertrophic, or a combination of these two. Ulcers are typically small and transverse with raised, sharp edges (Shah *et al.* 1992). They may become circumferential, forming strictures as they heal. Fibroblastic hypertrophy results in thickening of the gut wall and is particularly seen in the ileocaecal region (Balthazar *et al.* 1990).

Clinical features

Symptoms typically will have been present for several months. Abdominal pain occurs in 90% and may be generalized and dull, or cramping in nature. Weight loss occurs in 74% and anorexia in 60%. Physical examination may be entirely normal or an abdominal mass (58%) or ascites (10%) may be present (Shah *et al.* 1992). Complications include obstruction, perforation, and fistula formation (Marshall 1993, Monkemuller and Lewis 1996).

Diagnosis

A Mantoux test is positive in 70–90% of patients. Two situations limit the usefulness of the test. In developing countries the test will be positive in a number of patients who have been exposed to

Table 3.4 Differentiating abdominal tuberculosis from Crohn's disease

	Tuberculosis	Crohn's disease
Sociogeographic	Third World countries	North America/Europe
Associated disease	Alcoholism/AIDS	—
Examination	Chest disease	Perianal disease
Chest X-ray	Abnormal	Normal
Abdominal imaging/gross pathology	Transverse strictures	Longitudinal strictures
Granulomata	Caseating	Non-caseating
Biopsy staining	Acid-fast bacilli	No acid-fast bacilli

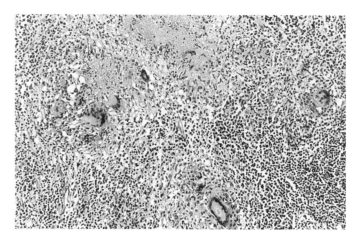

Figure 3.14 Tuberculosis (colon). The mucosa is extensively ulcerated and replaced with inflammatory cells in which granulomata with Langhans-type giant cells and central caseation are seen (×26).

M. tuberculosis in childhood, while in severe disease the test may be negative. Nevertheless, a strongly positive Mantoux test suggests the diagnosis of active tuberculosis (Tandon 1993).

A chest X-ray will reveal active pulmonary tuberculosis in one-fifth of cases. Another 20% may have evidence of old disease (fibrosis or calcification). Barium enema and computerized tomography imaging can be helpful. No feature on barium enema is diagnostic of tuberculosis, the differential diagnosis including Crohn's disease, colonic malignancy, and abdominal lymphoma (Table 3.4). However, in the appropriate clinical context, the demonstration of shallow transverse ulcers, ileocaecal valve deformity, stricturing, and retraction of the bowel all point towards tuberculosis (Figure 3.13) (Radhika *et al.* 1989). Computerized tomography may reveal thickening of the ileocaecal valve and medial wall of the caecum and low-density lesions within areas of lymphadenopathy in keeping with caseous necrosis (Balthazar *et al.* 1990).

Colonoscopy and histology are important diagnostic tools in colonic tuberculosis giving a positive diagnosis in 80% of cases (Shah *et al.* 1992). Nodular mucosa with areas of ulceration is the commonest finding. This may occur segmentally within the colon and not be confined to the ileocaecal region. Biopsy material can be stained to demonstrate acid-fast bacilli as well as looking for the typical histological changes. Areas of biopsy should include the base of the ulcer when searching for granulomas (Figure 3.14) (Shah *et al.* 1992).

Culture of stool and biopsy material can be performed, but rarely is of benefit over colonoscopy and biopsy (Shah *et al.* 1992; Marshall 1993). Ultrasonically guided biopsy of intra-abdominal lymph nodes may help to distinguish tuberculosis from lymphoma (Radhika *et al.* 1989).

Laparotomy has been advocated as a last resort for making the diagnosis in some patients when malignancy cannot be excluded. An alternative approach is the therapeutic trial of antituberculous therapy. If tuberculosis is present, a response will occur within 7–10 days (Shah *et al.* 1992; Tandon 1993).

Treatment

Combination chemotherapy taken regularly with adequate supervision is the key to curing tuberculosis. The recommended therapy is a 9-month course of rifampicin (10–20 mg/kg, up to 600 mg) and isoniazid (5–10 mg/kg, up to 300 mg) with a third drug added for the first 3 months. The third drug may be ethambutol, streptomycin, or pyrazinamide (Snider *et al.* 1985). For abdominal tuberculosis 6 months of therapy may be sufficient (Tandon 1993). Patients should be carefully monitored for side-effects of the medication, of which hepatitis is the most common. A rise in transaminases of less than twofold is often seen and does not require a change of treatment. If the diagnosis of abdominal tuberculosis is correct, a significant response to therapy can be expected within 2 weeks. Fever and abdominal pain may disappear within the first few days of commencing therapy.

Tuberculous strictures and masses causing intestinal obstruction will resolve without surgery (Anand *et al.* 1988). Surgery is indicated for complications such as complete obstruction or perforation. Conservative operations such as stricturoplasty are preferable for small bowel strictures but resection is generally required when the

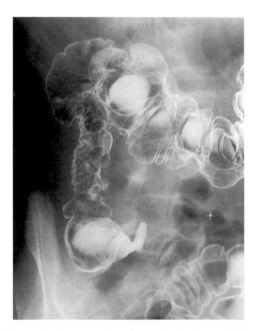

Figure 3.13 Barium enema tuberculosis. The ascending colon is shortened and the caecum elevated. There are numerous transmural ulcers on the lateral side and several pseudosaccules on the medial side. The mucosa assumes a granular appearance with tiny collections of barium lying in the ulcers.

strictures are in the large bowel. Where possible, surgery should be preceded by 6 weeks of antituberculous therapy (Pujari 1979).

Intestinal parasites

Parasitic diseases of the colon can be divided into protozoa and helminths. Protozoal infections include *E. histolytica*, *G. lamblia*, and Cryptosporidiae species and are discussed in the sections on infectious diarrhoea. Helminths may be subdivided into round worms, tape worms, and flukes. The round worms discussed include *Strongyloides stercoralis*, *Trichuris trichiura*, and *Enterobius vermicularis*. Hookworms and *Ascaris lumbricoides* affect predominantly the small bowel and are not discussed further; neither are the tapeworms. The most important fluke to affect the colon is the *Schistosomiasis* group.

Round worms (nematodes)

Strongyloides stercoralis

Although most common in tropical areas, this small nematode occurs world-wide. It may live in the environment, producing rhabditiform (free-living) larvae (Figure 3.15). However, these may become filariform (infective) larvae which invade the skin or mucosal surfaces. These larvae proceed to the lungs where they induce an eosinophilic pneumonitis. They develop into adult worms which penetrate the alveoli/bronchioles to be coughed up and swallowed. In the small intestine the female burrows into the mucosa to lay 30–40 eggs per day. Eggs develop into rhabditiform larvae and both these and adult males (which do not invade the mucosa) are passed in the faeces. Occasionally, the transformation to the filari-

form larvae may occur within the large bowel prior to excretion. These larvae burrow into the colonic mucosa to cause ongoing auto-infection and hyperinfection to non-intestinal sites (Gill and Bell 1979). The immunosuppressed, those with AIDS or a malignancy, and institutionalized patients are at increased risk of hyperinfection (Genta 1989). In addition to invasion through the skin, infection can also occur sexually either during rectal intercourse or oral–anal exposure (Phillips *et al.* 1981).

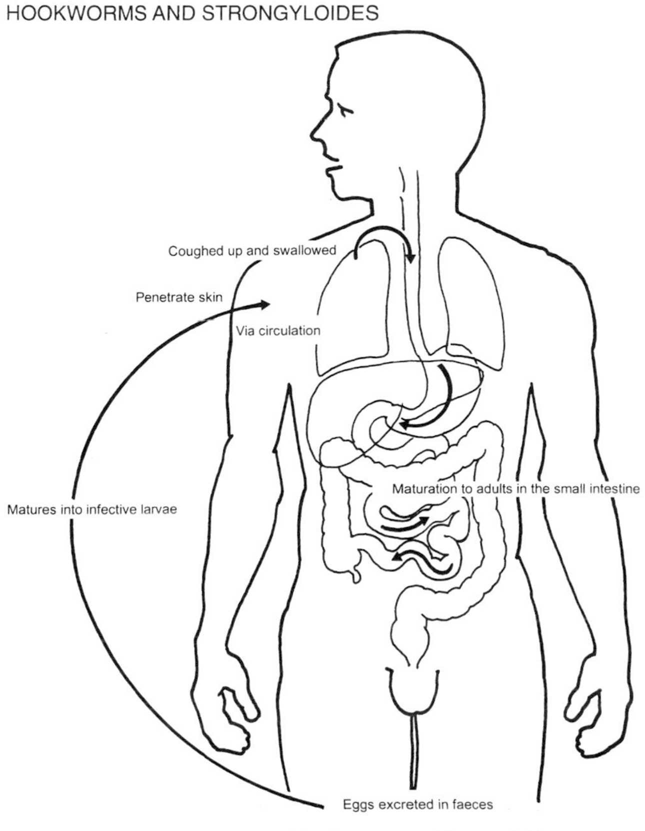

At the time of skin invasion, petechiae, urticaria, and a maculo-papular rash occur. Pulmonary symptoms are present in half of those infected. Intestinal infestation is usually asymptomatic but diarrhoea, non-specific abdominal pain, weight loss, iron deficiency anaemia, and pruritus ani may occur.

Larvae may be seen in the stools in approximately 30% of cases. However, examination of duodenal secretions, either by aspirate or using a weighted string, is significantly more likely to be positive (Owen 1993). A mild (8–10%) eosinophilia is usually present but this may increase to 50% in severe infections. Iron deficiency anaemia may also be present. Barium studies and mucosal biopsies are generally unhelpful.

Strongyloides should always be treated, even if asymptomatic, because of the risk of hyperinfection. Thiabendazole (25 mg/kg daily for 3–8 days) is the treatment of choice, although ivermectin is also effective (Naquira *et al.* 1989).

Whip worm (*Trichuris trichiura*)

Although predominantly a tropical disease, *T. trichiura* is found world-wide, particularly in areas of poor sanitation. It has been estimated to infest more than 2 million people in the USA and world-wide is the third commonest gastrointestinal worm infestation after ascariasis and hookworm (Warren and Mahmoud 1976). The egg requires a 3–5 week period in the environment for the embryo to reach the infective stage. Once ingested on contaminated material, stomach acid dissolves the egg to release the larva into the small bowel. The larva migrates to the caecum and heavy infections may involve the entire colon, each female worm laying 6000 eggs per day.

The thin end of the adult worm is attached to the mucosa, penetrating as deep as the submucosa. Despite this invasion, there is generally little mucosal inflammation. With heavy infections a colitis and proctitis can occur.

The majority of infestations are asymptomatic. Heavier worm burdens may cause colitis, appendicitis or rectal prolapse. Direct faecal examination or use of concentration techniques demonstrate the barrel-shaped eggs. At colonoscopy the worms can be seen attached to the mucosa by their whip-like thin end. Treatment is only required for those with heavy infestations and symptoms. Mebendazole 100 mg, b.d. for 3 days is the treatment of choice.

Pin worm (*Enterobius vermicularis*)

This is the most prevalent nematode in Europe and North America, affecting up to 40 million individuals (Banwell and Variyam 1993). Infestation occurs by the faeco-oral route. The eggs hatch in the small bowel and develop into adult worms in the large bowel. The female worm deposits the eggs in the perianal area, often at night. This causes intense pruritus ani. Transfer of infection to other individuals occurs via poor hygiene and hand contamination, contact with soiled clothing, and oral–anal contamination during sexual activity.

Adult worms attach to the caecal mucosa but can also be found in the lumen of the appendix in resected specimens. The female worm lays her eggs on the perianal skin, the eggs causing an intense pru-

HOOKWORMS AND STRONGYLOIDES

Coughed up and swallowed

Penetrate skin

Via circulation

Matures into infective larvae

Maturation to adults in the small intestine

Eggs excreted in faeces

Figure 3.15 Life cycle of hookworms and *Strongyloides*.

ritus. The worm itself may become embedded in the submucosa causing an inflammatory reaction.

When symptomatic, the commonest feature is pruritus ani, particularly at night. Infestation may also cause appendicitis and peritonitis. Eggs from the unwashed perineal area may be obtained by pressing a cellophane tape against the area. The eggs may then be demonstrated by examining the tape under a microscope. This technique should be repeated several times if negative and if positive; other family members should also be examined (Gill and Bell 1979). The treatment of choice is a single dose of mebendazole (100 mg) or pyrantel pamoate (11 mg/kg, to a maximum of 1 g) with a repeat dosage in 2 weeks. All family members and regular sexual partners should be treated at the same time (Owen 1993).

Trematodes (flukes): schistosomiasis

Schistosomiasis affects 200 million individuals throughout the world (Webbe 1981). It is caused by *Schistosoma mansoni*, *S. japonicum*, and *S. haematobium*. A snail host releases cercariae (infective forms) into water. If contact with human skin is made within 48 h, the cercariae invade the host and eventually reach the portal bed of the liver where they mature into adults (Figure 3.16). They migrate into the mesenteric vasculature predominantly affecting the small intestine (*S. japonicum*), descending colon (*S. mansoni*), and bladder and rectum (*S. haematobium*). Eggs are deposited in the gut wall. Half will erode into the lumen and be excreted. Enzymes released to facilitate this erosion provoke an inflammatory response with ulceration and haemorrhage.

Light microscopy of biopsy material may reveal eggs in the mucosa and submucosa of the rectum (*S. mansoni*) and right colon

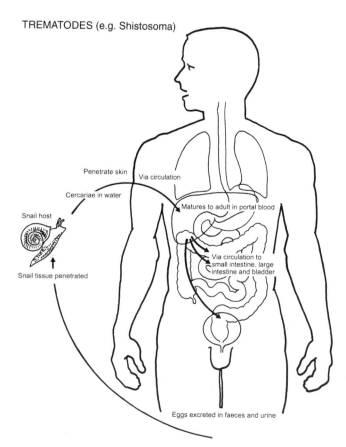

Figure 3.16 Life cycle of trematodes.

(*S. japonicum*). Often they are seen as a calcified shell surrounded by a rim of collagen. At other sites or in other cases, a granulomatous reaction can occur with the egg surrounded by lymphocytes, macrophages, and giant cells.

With skin invasion, and especially on repeated exposures, a hypersensitivity reaction with pruritus and a papular rash occurs. Four to six weeks later the eggs begin to be deposited in the intestinal submucosa and to erode through into the lumen. This causes abdominal cramps and diarrhoea which may be bloody. A serum sickness-type illness occurs with influenza-like symptoms, spiking fever, urticaria, and oedema. Hepatomegaly, lymphadenopathy, and splenomegaly occur. The liver becomes increasingly involved with ova regularly being transported into the portal vein to become entrapped causing progressive fibrosis. With time polypoid lesions develop on the mucosa of the intestine. They may ulcerate and bleed, form a focus for intussusception or cause intestinal obstruction. Bilharziomas may also occur, typically in the serosa. These represent a localized inflammatory reaction to heavy egg deposits.

In the acute stage, ova can be seen in the faeces, especially by using concentration techniques. Examination of a rectal or colonic biopsy under a microscope may also demonstrate the ova. Sigmoidoscopy or colonoscopy in the acute stage demonstrates a small area of ulceration and haemorrhage. There may also be a 'sandpaper' appearance of calcified ova in the submucosa. Eosinophilia (10–75%) is present in peripheral blood. Anti-schistosome antibody is usually elevated (Gazzinelli *et al.* 1985).

Oxamniquine (15 mg/kg for adults) is effective as a single dose against *S. mansoni*. In Africa higher doses are required. Metrifonate (7.5 mg/kg) given every fortnight for three doses is effective only against *S. haematobium*. Praziquantel acts effectively against all *Schistosoma* species, the dose being species dependent (Davis and Wegner 1979).

Chagas' disease

This disease is caused by *Trypanosoma cruzi*. The parasite is injected into humans by a bite from an insect vector. It is a widespread disease of South America affecting seven million people in Brazil alone (Habr-Gama 1993). Its effects on the colon are due to long-standing infection causing progressive damage to the autonomic nervous system. This results in megacolon. The greater cause of morbidity and mortality in this disease is the effect on the heart, and in particular the high incidence of heart block. The diagnosis is made by a complement fixation test. The management is as for other causes of megacolon and volvulus (see Chapter 13).

References

Acheson DWK, Keusch GT. The shigella paradigm and colitis due to enterohaemorrhagic *Escherichia coli*. *Gut* 1994; 35: 872–4.
Addiss DG, Mathews HM, Stewart JM, *et al.* Evaluation of a commercially available enzyme-linked immunosorbent assay for *Giardia lamblia* antigen in stool. *J. Clin. Microbiol.* 1991; 29: 1137–42.
Anand BS, Nanda R, Sachdev GK. Response of tuberculous stricture to antituberculous treatment. *Gut* 1988; 29: 62–9.
Anonymous. The management of acute diarrhea in children: oral rehydration, maintenance, and nutrition therapy. *MMWR* 1992; 41: 1–20.
Anonymous. Antibiotic-associated colitis. *Curr. Prob. Pharmacovigilance* 1994; 20: 7.

Arvind AS, Shetty N, Farthing MJG. Serodiagnosis of amoebiasis. *Serodiag. Immunother.* 1988; 2: 79–84.

Aserkoff B, Bennett JV. Effect of antibiotic therapy in acute salmonellosis on the fecal excretion of salmonellae. *N. Engl. J. Med.* 1969; 281: 636–40.

Baird-Parker AC. Foodborne salmonellosis. *Lancet* 1990; 336: 1231–5.

Balthazar EJ, Gordon R, Hulnick D. Ileocecal tuberculosis: CT and radiologic evaluation. *Am. J. Roentgenol.* 1990; 154: 499–503.

Banwell JG, Variyam EP. Worm infestations. In: Bouchier IAD, Allan RN, Hodgson HJF, Keighley MRB, eds. *Gastroenterology— clinical science and practice*, 2nd edn. London: WB Saunders, 1993: 1401–18.

Bargallo N, Nicolau C, Luburich P, Ayuso C, Cardenal C, Gimeno F. Intestinal tuberculosis in AIDS. *Gastrointest. Radiol.* 1992; 17: 115–8.

Bartlett JG. *Clostridium difficile*: clinical considerations. *Rev. Infect. Dis.* 1990; 12 (Suppl. 2): S243–51.

Bitzan M, Ludwig K, Klemt M, Konig H, Buren J, Muller-Wiefel DE. The role of *Escherichia coli* O 157 infections in the classical (enteropathic) haemolytic uraemic syndrome: results of a Central European, multicentre study. *Epidemiol. Infect.* 1993; 110: 183–96.

Bodey GP, Fainstein V. Infections of the gastrointestinal tract in the immunocompromised patient. *Annu. Rev. Med.* 1986; 37: 271–81.

Booth IW, McNeish AS. Mechanisms of diarrhoea. *Baillières Clin. Gastroenterol.* 1993; 7: 215–42.

Carter AO, Borczyk AA, Carlson JA, *et al.* A severe outbreak of *Escherichia coli* O157: H7-associated hemorrhagic colitis in a nursing home. *N. Engl. J. Med.* 1987; 317: 1496–500.

Char S, Farthing MJ. DNA probes for diagnosis of intestinal infection. *Gut* 1991; 32: 1–3.

Christensen ML. Human viral gastroenteritis. *Clin. Microbiol. Rev.* 1989; 2: 51–89.

Cimolai N, Blair GK, Murphy JJ, Fraser GG. Impact of infection by vero-toxigenic Escherichia coli O157:H7 on the use of surgical services in a children's hospital. *Canadian J. Surg.* 1997; 40: 28–32.

Connolly GM, Dryden MS, Shanson DC, Gazzard BG. Cryptosporidial diarrhoea in AIDS and its treatment. *Gut* 1988; 29: 593–7.

Connolly GM, Youle M, Gazzard BG. Diclazuril in the treatment of severe cryptosporidial diarrhoea in AIDS patients. *AIDS* 1990; 4: 700–1.

Cook SM, Glass RI, LeBaron CW, Ho MS. Global seasonality of rotavirus infections. *Bull. WHO* 1990; 68: 171–7.

Counihan TC, Roberts PL. Pseudomembranous colitis. *Surg. Clin. North Am.* 1993; 73: 1063–74.

Coyne JD, Dervan PA, Haboubi NY. Involvement of the appendix in pseudomembranous colitis. *J. Clin. Path.* 1997; 50: 70–1.

Crouch AA, Seow WK, Whitman LM, Thong YH. Sensitivity *in vitro* of *Giardia intestinalis* to dyadic combinations of azithromycin, doxycycline, mefloquine, tinidazole and furazolidone. *Trans. R. Soc. Trop. Med. Hyg.* 1990; 84: 246–8.

Daniel TM. Tuberculosis. In: Wilson JD, Braunwald E, Isselbacher KJ, *et al.*, eds. *Harrison's principles of internal medicine*, 12th edn. New York: McGraw-Hill, 1991: 637–45.

Davis A, Wegner DH. Multicentre trials of praziquantel in human schistosomiasis: design and techniques. *Bull. WHO* 1979; 57: 767–71.

Dronfield MW, Fletcher J, Langman MJ. Coincident salmonella infections and ulcerative colitis: problems of recognition and management. *Br. Med. J.* 1974; 1: 99–100.

DuPont HL. Review article: infectious diarrhoea. *Aliment. Pharmacol. Ther.* 1994; 8: 3–13.

DuPont HL, Hornick RB. Adverse effect of lomotil therapy in shigellosis. *JAMA* 1973; 226: 1525–8.

DuPont HL, Sullivan P, Pickering LK, Haynes G, Ackerman PB. Symptomatic treatment of diarrhea with bismuth subsalicylate among students attending a Mexican university. *Gastroenterology* 1977; 73: 715–8.

DuPont HL, Flores Sanchez J, Ericsson CD, *et al.* Comparative efficacy of loperamide hydrochloride and bismuth subsalicylate in the management of acute diarrhea. *Am. J. Med.* 1990; 88: 15–9S.

Elliott EJ, Cunha-Ferreira R, Walker-Smith JA, Farthing MJ. Sodium content of oral rehydration solutions: a reappraisal. *Gut* 1989; 30: 1610–21.

Farthing MJ. Immunopathology of giardiasis. *Springer Semin. Immunopathol.* 1990; 12(2–3): 269–82.

Farthing MJ. Intestinal parasites. *Baillières' Clin. Gastroenterol.* 1993; 7: 333–64.

Farthing MJ. Travellers' diarrhoea. *Gut* 1994; 35: 1–4.

Farthing MJ, Mata L, Urrutia JJ, Kronmal RA. Natural history of *Giardia* infection of infants and children in rural Guatemala and its impact on physical growth. *Am. J. Clin. Nutr.* 1986; 43: 395–405.

Farthing MJ, Du Pont HL, Guandalini S, Keusch GT, Steffen R. Treatment and prevention of travellers' diarrhoea. *Gastroenterol. Int.* 1992; 5: 162–75.

Farthing MJ, Katelaris PH, Dias J, Munzer D, Popovic O. Bacterial and parasitic intestinal infections in Europe. *Gastroenterol. Int.* 1993; 6: 149–66.

Fry RD. Infectious enteritis. A collective review. *Dis. Colon Rectum* 1990; 33: 520–7.

Gazzard B, Blanshard C. Diarrhoea in AIDS and other immuno-deficiency states. *Baillières' Clin. Gastroenterol.* 1993; 7: 387–419.

Gazzinelli G, Lambertucci JR, Katz N, Rocha RS, Lima MS, Colley DG. Immune responses during human *Schistosomiasis mansoni*. XI. Immunologic status of patients with acute infections and after treatment. *J. Immunol.* 1985; 135: 2121–7.

Genta RM. Global prevalence of strongyloidiasis: critical review with epidemiologic insights into the prevention of disseminated disease. *Rev. Infect. Dis.* 1989; 11: 755–67.

Gill GV, Bell DR. *Strongyloides stercoralis* infection in former Far East prisoners of war. *Br. Med. J.* 1979; 2: 572–4.

Goldberg MB, Rubin RH. The spectrum of *Salmonella* infection. *Infect. Dis. Clin. North Am.* 1988; 2: 571–98.

Goodell SE, Quinn TC, Mkrtichian E, Schuffler MD, Holmes KK, Corey L. Herpes simplex virus proctitis in homosexual men. Clinical, sigmoidoscopic, and histopathological features. *N. Engl. J. Med.* 1983; 308: 868–71.

Goodman RA, Osterholm MT, Granoff DM, Pickering LK. Infectious diseases and child day care. *Pediatrics* 1984; 74: 134–9.

Gordon J, Small PLC. Acid resistance in enteric bacteria. *Infect. Immun.* 1993; 61: 364–7.

Gracey M. Infectious diarrhoea. Transmission and epidemiology. *Baillières Clin. Gastroenterol.* 1993; 7: 195–214.

Greenberg H, Matsui S. Astroviruses and caliciviruses: emerging enteric pathogens. *Infect. Agents Dis.* 1992; 1: 71–91.

Greenberg RE, Mir R, Bank S, Siegal FP. Resolution of intestinal cryptosporidiosis after treatment of AIDS with AZT. *Gastroenterology* 1989; 97: 1327–30.

Griffiths JK, Gorbach SL. Other bacterial diarrhoeas. *Baillières Clin. Gastroenterol.* 1993; 7: 263–305.

Grundy MS, Voller A, Warhurst D. An enzyme-linked immunosorbent assay for the detection of *Entamoeba histolytica* antigens in faecal material. *Trans. R. Soc. Trop. Med. Hyg.* 1987; 81: 627–32.

Guandalini S. Overview of childhood acute diarrhoea in Europe: implications for oral rehydration therapy. *Acta Paediatr. Scand. Suppl.* 1989; 364: 5–12.

Guerrant RL, Shields DS, Thorson SM, Schorling JB, Groschel DH. Evaluation and diagnosis of acute infectious diarrhea. *Am. J. Med.* 1985; 78: 91–8.

Guerrant RL. Amebiasis: introduction, current status, and research questions. *Rev. Infect. Dis.* 1986; 8: 218–27.

Habr-Gama A. Chagas' disease. In: Bouchier IAD, Allan RN, Hodgson HJF, Keighley MRB, eds. *Gastroenterology—clinical science and practice*, 2nd edn. London: WB Saunders, 1993: 1468–77.

Hoogkamp-Korstanje JA. Antibiotics in *Yersinia enterocolitica* infections. *J. Antimicrob. Chemother.* 1987; 20: 123–31.

Ilnyckyj A, Greenberg H, Bernstein CN. Escherichia coli O157:H7 infection mimicking Crohn's disease. *Gastroenterol.* 1997; 112: 995–9.

Jacobson MA, O'Donnell JJ, Porteous D, Brodie HR, Feigal D, Mills J. Retinal and gastrointestinal disease due to cytomegalovirus in patients with the acquired immune deficiency syndrome: prevalence, natural history, and response to ganciclovir therapy. *Q. J. Med.* 1988; 67: 473–86.

Jereb JA, Kelly GD, Dooley SW Jr, Cauthen GM, Snider DE Jr. Tuberculosis morbidity in the United States: final data, 1990. *MMWR* 1991; 40: 23–7.

Johnson PC, Ericsson CD, DuPont HL, Morgan DR, Bitsura JA, Wood LV. Comparison of loperamide with bismuth subsalicylate for the treatment of acute travelers' diarrhea. *JAMA* 1986; 255: 757–60.

Johnson S, Gerding DN, Olson MM, *et al.* Prospective, controlled study of vinyl glove use to interrupt *Clostridium difficile* nosocomial transmission. *Am. J. Med.* 1990; 88: 137–40.

Klein RS, Harris CA, Small CB, Moll B, Lesser M, Friedland GH. Oral candidiasis in high-risk patients as the initial manifestation of the acquired immunodeficiency syndrome. *N. Engl. J. Med.* 1984; 311: 354–8.

Knutton S, Lloyd DR, McNeish AS. Adhesion of enteropathogenic *Escherichia coli* to human intestinal enterocytes and cultured human intestinal mucosa. *Infect. Immun.* 1987; 55: 69–77.

Levine MM, Kaper JB, Herrington D, *et al.* Safety, immunogenicity, and efficacy of recombinant live oral cholera vaccines, CVD 103 and CVD 103-HgR. *Lancet* 1988; ii: 467–70.

Mandal BK, Schofield PF. ABC of colorectal diseases. Tropical colonic diseases. *Br. Med. J.* 1992; 305: 638–41.

Marshall JB. Tuberculosis of the gastrointestinal tract and peritoneum. *Am. J. Gastroenterol.* 1993; 88: 989–99.

Martin DL, MacDonald KL, White KE, Soler JT, Osterholm MT. The epidemiology and clinical aspects of the hemolytic uremic syndrome in Minnesota. *N. Engl. J. Med.* 1990; 323: 1161–7.

Mathewson JJ, Johnson PC, DuPont HL, Satterwhite TK, Winsor DK. Pathogenicity of enteroadherent *Escherichia coli* in adult volunteers. *J. Infect. Dis.* 1986; 154: 524–7.

Mayon-White RT, Frankenberg RA. 'Boil the water'. *Lancet* 1989; ii: 216.

McFarland LV, Surawicz CM, Stamm WE. Risk factors for *Clostridium difficile* carriage and *C. difficile*-associated diarrhea in a cohort of hospitalized patients. *J. Infect. Dis.* 1990; 162: 678–84.

McFarland MV, Mulligan ME, Kwok RY, *et al.* Nosocomial acquisition of *Clostridium difficile* infection. *N. Engl. J. Med.* 1989; 320: 240.

Molla AM, Molla A, Nath SK, Khatun M. Food-based oral rehydration salt solution for acute childhood diarrhoea. *Lancet* 1989; ii: 429–31.

Monkemuller KE, Lewis JB Jr. Massive rectal bleeding from colonic tuberculosis. *Am. J. Gastroenterol.* 1996; 91: 1439–41.

Moskovitz BL, Stanton TL, Kusmierek JJ. Spiramycin therapy for cryptosporidial diarrhoea in immunocompromised patients. *J. Antimicrob. Chemother.* 1988; 22 (Suppl. B): 189–91.

Musher DM, Rubenstein AD. Permanent carriers of nontyphosa salmonellae. *Arch. Intern. Med.* 1973; 132: 869–72.

Naquira C, Jimenez G, Guerra JG, *et al.* Ivermectin for human strongyloidiasis and other intestinal helminths. *Am. J. Trop. Med. Hyg.* 1989; 40: 304–9.

Nielsen H, Daugaard G, Tvede M, Bruun B. High prevalence of *Clostridium difficile* diarrhoea during intensive chemotherapy for disseminated germ cell cancer. *Br. J. Cancer* 1992; 66: 666–7.

Noone C, Banatvala JE. Hospital acquired rotaviral gastroenteritis in a general paediatric unit. *J. Hosp. Infect.* 1983; 4: 297–9.

Nostrant TT, Kumar NB, Appelman HD. Histopathology differentiates acute self-limited colitis from ulcerative colitis. *Gastroenterology* 1987; 92: 318–28.

Owen RL. Parasitic diseases. In: Sleisenger MH, Fordtran JS, eds. *Gastrointestinal disease. Pathophysiology/diagnosis/management*, 5th edn. Philadelphia: WB Saunders, 1993: 1190–224.

Phillips SC, Mildvan D, William DC, Gelb AM, White MC. Sexual transmission of enteric protozoa and helminths in a venereal-disease-clinic population. *N. Engl. J. Med.* 1981; 305: 603–6.

Pichler HE, Diridl G, Stickler K, Wolf D. Clinical efficacy of ciprofloxacin compared with placebo in bacterial diarrhea. *Am. J. Med.* 1987; 82: 329–32.

Pujari BD. Modified surgical procedures in intestinal tuberculosis. *Br. J. Surg.* 1979; 66: 180–1.

Puylaert JB, Vermeijden RJ, van der Werf SD, Doornbos L, Koumans RK. Incidence and sonographic diagnosis of bacterial ileocaecitis masquerading as appendicitis. *Lancet* 1989; ii: 84–6.

Puylaert JB, Van der Zant FM, Mutsaers JA. Infectious ileocecitis caused by Yersinia, Campylobacter, and Salmonella: clinical, radiological and US findings. *Eur. Radiol.* 1997; 7: 3–9.

Radhika S, Gupta SK, Chakrabarti A, Rajwanshi A, Joshi K. Role of culture for mycobacteria in fine-needle aspiration diagnosis of tuberculous ymphadenitis. *Diagn. Cytopathol.* 1989; 5: 260–2.

Rene E, Marche C, Chevalier T, *et al.* Cytomegalovirus colitis in patients with acquired immunodeficiency syndrome. *Dig. Dis. Sci.* 1988; 33: 741–50.

Roth RI, Owen RL, Keren DF, Volberding PA. Intestinal infection with *Mycobacterium avium* in acquired immune deficiency syndrome (AIDS). Histological and clinical comparison with Whipple's disease. *Dig. Dis. Sci.* 1985; 30: 497–504.

Saari KM, Kauranen O. Ocular inflammation in Reiter's syndrome associated with *Campylobacter jejuni* enteritis. *Am. J. Ophthalmol.* 1980; 90: 572–3.

Saebo A, Lassen J. Acute and chronic gastrointestinal manifestations associated with *Yersinia enterocolitica* infection. A Norwegian 10-year follow-up study on 458 hospitalized patients. *Ann. Surg.* 1992; 215: 250–5.

Scaletsky IC, Silva ML, Toledo MR, Davis BR, Blake PA, Trabulsi LR. Correlation between adherence to HeLa cells and serogroups, serotypes, and bioserotypes of *Escherichia coli*. *Infect. Immun.* 1985; 49: 528–32.

Schwab KS, Shaw RD. Infectious diarrhoea. Viruses. *Baillières' Clin. Gastroenterol.* 1993; 7: 307–31.

Shah S, Thomas V, Mathan M, *et al.* Colonoscopic study of 50 patients with colonic tuberculosis. *Gut* 1992; 33: 347–51.

Singh V, Kumar P, Kamal J. Prakash V, Vaiphei K, Singh K. Clinicocolonoscopic profile of colonic tuberculosis. *Am. J. Gastroenterol.* 1996; 91: 565–8.

Skirrow MB. Epidemiology of *Campylobacter enteritis*. *Int. J. Food Microbiol.* 1991; 12: 9–16.

Snider DE Jr, Cohn DL, Davidson PT, Hershfield ES, Smith MH, Sutton FD Jr. Standard therapy for tuberculosis 1985. *Chest* 1985; 87 (Suppl. 2): 117–24S.

Sullivan PB, Neale G, Cevallos AM, Farthing MJ. Evaluation of specific serum anti-Giardia IgM antibody response in diagnosis of giardiasis in children. *Trans. R. Soc. Trop. Med. Hyg.* 1991; 85: 748–9.

Tandon RK. Abdominal tuberculosis. In: Bouchier IAD, Allan RN, Hodgson HJF, Keighley MRB, eds. *Gastroenterology—clinical science and practice*, 2nd edn. London: WB Saunders, 1993: 1459–68.

Tedesco FJ, Barton RW, Alpers DH. Clindamycin-associated colitis: a prospective study. *Ann. Intern. Med.* 1974; 81: 429.

Uhnoo I, Svensson L, Wadell G. Enteric adenoviruses. *Baillières' Clin. Gastroenterol.* 1990; 4: 627–42.

Warren KS, Mahmoud AA. Algorithms in the diagnosis and management of exotic diseases. IX. Trichuriasis. *J. Infect. Dis.* 1976; 133: 240–3.

Webbe G. The six diseases of WHO. Schistosomiasis: some advances. *Br. Med. J.* 1981; 283: 1104–6.

Williams HM, Richards J. Single-dose ciprofloxacin for shigellosis. *Lancet* 1990; 335: 1343–4.

World Health Organization. *Programme for control of diarrhoeal diseases: interim programme report 1990*. Geneva: World Health Organization, 1990: 34–6.

Zheng BJ, Chang RX, Ma GZ, *et al.* Rotavirus infection of the oropharynx and respiratory tract in young children. *J. Med. Virol.* 1991; 34: 29–37.

4 Sexually transmitted diseases

There are many preconceived ideas which can be detrimental to the diagnosis, management, and prevention of anorectal sexually transmitted diseases (STDs). When confronted with any perianal, anal canal, or rectal disorder, STDs or other possible relationship to sexual practices must be considered. To assess the likelihood of STDs, a sensitively taken history is invaluable, but even in the most careful hands, important aspects of sexual history may be withheld due to fear or embarrassment. The history of sexual practices should include not only that of insertive anal sexual intercourse, but also anogenital contact, oro-anal sex, digital manipulation of the anus by self or partner, and the use and sharing of 'sex toys'. Many homosexual men do not regularly have anal intercourse (Davies *et al.* 1992). In a large national study in Great Britain a history of anoreceptive sexual intercourse was recorded in 13% of women (Wellings *et al.* 1994). Oro-anal sex, while a more common gay male sexual practice, is also a part of some heterosexual males' and females' sexual repertoire. The practice of digital stimulation by self or partner is an historical point often not asked. In two studies using anonymous questionnaires taken from sexually transmitted disease clinic attenders with a history of genital warts, 37% and 21%, respectively, of females and 27% and 37% of males gave a history of receptive anodigital sex by self or partner (Sonnex *et al.* 1991; Armstrong *et al.* 1994).

In addition to these factors, accidental transmission of infection from one anatomical site to another is not uncommon.

This is especially seen in females, in for example, infected discharge spreading across the perineum to infect the anus in gonorrhoea and chlamydia infections.

For examination of the anus and distal rectum good illumination preferably using an illuminated proctoscope is essential. A high index of suspicion needs to be maintained as seemingly innocuous lesions may be due to STDs such as herpes simplex or syphilis. Looking for signs of receptive anal sex such as decreased anal tone, contraction followed by relaxation of the anal sphincter to palpation, and the ability to maintain the anus in a dilated condition (the '0' sign) may be of interest, but should not be relied on to arouse suspicion of STDs in the light of the foregoing. The use of anal manometry may be helpful in the diagnosis of loss of anal tone. In homosexual men who have regular anoreceptive sexual intercourse, maximum anal resting pressure is found to be lowered. Voluntary anal squeeze pressure is normal in continent men, but those who are incontinent have a significantly reduced maximum squeeze pressure (Miles *et al.* 1993). An increased incidence of episodes of faecal incontinence without alteration of bowel habit is noted in homosexual men. In the event that a diagnosis of possible STD is made, the relevant investigations as related subsequently should be performed, but it should always be borne in mind that STDs are often multiply transmitted (Aral *et al.* 1990) and that referral for a full screen to a genitourinary medicine department is advisable. This is especially important in respect of partner notification, counselling, education, and prevention. These aspects are particularly relevant

Table 4.1 Sexually transmissible anorectal and enteric infections

Bacteria
  Treponema pallidum
  Neisseria gonorrhoea
  N. meningitides
  Chlamydia trachomatis D–K
  C. trachomatis L 1–3
  Haemophilus ducreyi
  Calymmatobacterium granulomatis

Virus
  Herpes simplex virus
  Human papilloma virus
  Human immunodeficiency virus

Fungus
  Candida spp.

Protozoa
  Giardia lamblia
  Entamoeba histolytica

Helminths
  Enterobius vermicularis
  Strongyloides stercoralis

Enteric bacterial pathogens
  Shigella spp.
  Salmonella spp.
  Campylobacter spp.

Syphilis

when considering anorectal disease in the era of HIV/AIDS as receptive anal intercourse is known to be the highest risk sexual practice for the acquisition of HIV (Winklestein *et al.* 1987) and the presence of other STDs (Table 4.1) are seen to enhance both transmission and acquisition of HIV (Plummer *et al.* 1991).

Syphilis

Aetiology and diagnosis

The cause of syphilis is the *Treponema pallidum*, a member of the spirochete family. Other treponemes causing non-venereally transmitted disease in humans are *T. pertenue* (Yaws) and *T. carateum* (Pinta). These latter are endemic in Africa, the Middle East, Asia, and South America, and will give positive serological tests for syphilis.

Treponema pallidum cannot be cultured in artificial media or tissue cultures. Lesions of primary and secondary syphilis contain numerous spirochetes, and examination of serous exudate expressed from the base of such lesions will usually reveal the characteristic spirochetes under dark field illumination. Non-treponemal spirochetes may contaminate ulcers of a non-syphilitic nature especially in lesions of the anorectal area and an experienced microscopist is needed to differentiate these. Histologically, the primary chancre shows epidermal hyperplasia with an intense lymphohistiocytic and neutrophil infiltrate in the dermis. Lesions of secondary syphilis show a predominance of plasma cells, lymphocytes, and histiocytes extending deeply into the dermis. *Treponema pallidum* may be seen in tissue sections using silver staining, or immunofluorescent techniques.

The Venereal Disease Research Laboratory (VDRL) and the Rapid Plasma Reagent (RPR) tests use cardiolipin antigen to detect anti-lipid antibodies formed against lipoidal material from damaged cells and lipids from the surface of *T. pallidum*. Biologically false positive reactions are not uncommon for a variety of reasons (Hook and Marra 1992). These tests usually become positive within 1–2 weeks after the appearance of the primary chancre, and will almost always be positive in secondary syphilis. If treated early, they will revert to negative. In the natural course of disease, they will tend to become more weakly reactive and may even be negative in late disease. The finding of a positive non-specific test should always be confirmed using a specific test. The specific tests use extracted *T. pallidum* antigens. The two most commonly used are the *T. Pallidum* haemagglutination test (TPHA) and the fluorescent *Treponemal* antibody absorbed (FTA-abs). These become positive earlier than the non-specific tests and unless treated very early will usually remain reactive throughout the rest of the patient's life. Although less common, biologically false positive reactions can also occur.

Epidemiology

An estimated 15 million cases of syphilis occur each year worldwide. In England the number of cases of infectious syphilis reported each year from STD clinics dropped from 1934 in 1983 to 337 in 1993. The ratio of male to female acquired cases had dropped from 8:1 in 1983 to 2:1 in 1993 (DH Statistics Division 2B 1994) which probably reflects the change in sexual practices in the homosexual community in response to the advent of HIV disease.

In the USA reports of infectious syphilis in homosexual men dropped in the mid-1980s as a result of changes in sexual behaviour (Rolfs *et al.* 1990*a*). In contrast, the incidence rose markedly in heterosexual men and women and this has been linked to concomitant epidemics of illegal drug use, in particular, 'crack' cocaine (Rolfs *et al.* 1990*b*).

At a time when infectious syphilis has become much less common in the developed world surgeons must remain alert to the possibility of syphilis as misdiagnosis can lead to unfortunate consequences not least being subsequent transmission to sexual partners (Maw 1981).

Clinical features

The primary chancre forms at the site of inoculation, and is usually a painless ulcer with a raised, firm edge. The lesion will usually appear between 9 and 90 days after infection depending on inoculum size. The regional lymph nodes are usually enlarged and nontender. Perianal or anal canal lesions may be painful due to superinfection. Other causes of painful lesions may be dual infection with herpes simplex or *Haemophilus ducreyi*. Perianal (Figure 4.1)

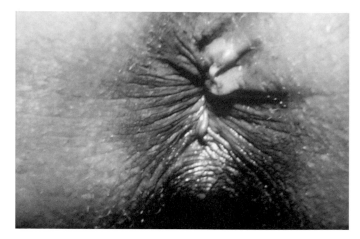

Figure 4.1 Primary chancre at the anal margin.

and anal canal lesions are most common in homosexual men but may also occur in women following anal intercourse. Lesions in the anal canal may have the appearance of anal fissures (Figure 4.2). Uncommonly, lesions may present as a large anal mass, or a rectal ulcer and can be mistaken for carcinomas (Marino 1964; Drusin *et al.* 1977), subsequently undergoing surgical procedures as such (Drusin *et al.* 1976). Lesions of the anus and rectum are often asymptomatic resulting in a delay of diagnosis until the secondary stage or later. Primary lesions may occur outside the anogenital area, especially on the lips and the buccal cavity. Those of the pharynx and tonsils may be painful. Left untreated primary lesions will usually heal without scarring within a few weeks. Manifestations of secondary syphilis occur between 6 weeks and 6 months after the primary lesion has appeared. This systemic illness with multisystem manifestations is frequently manifested by symmetrically distributed maculopapular rashes often affecting the palms of the hands and

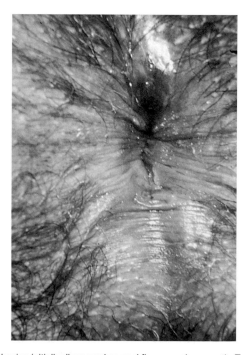

Figure 4.2 Lesion initially diagnosed as anal fissure, subsequently *Treponema pallidum* demonstrated on dark ground microscopy.

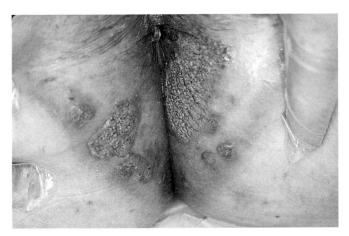

Figure 4.3 Coalescent, wart-like lesions of condylomata lata in secondary syphilis

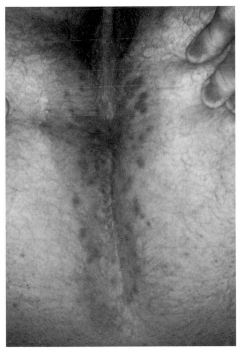

Figure 4.4 Flat, wart-like, perianal condylomata lata of secondary syphilis.

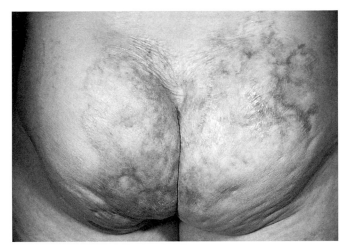

Figure 4.5 Extensive scarring of buttocks as a result of infiltrating syphilitic gummata.

Treatment

The *T. pallidum* organism has not developed resistance to penicillin. Regimens should be chosen in accord with the stage of disease.

Suitable alternative antibiotic regimens are available for those allergic to penicillin. Follow up and contact tracing should be supervised by a specialist in STDs.

Gonorrhoea

Aetiology and diagnosis

Neisseria gonorrhoea (the gonococcus) is the causative organism of gonorrhoea. It is a Gram-negative coccobacillus, kidney-shaped, arranged in pairs, with the long axes parallel and the concave borders apposed to one another. *Neisseria meningitides* accounted for 12% of the *Neisseria* species isolated from the anus in one study making formal identification necessary—not only for correct diagnosis but also to avoid the distress of misdiagnosis which may result in medico-legal action.

Microscope slides for Gram staining should be prepared from affected sites. The characteristic, intracellular Gram-negative diplococci are seen in 95% of males with acute gonococcal urethritis, but this drops to 50–65% of genital tract smears from females (Oates and Csonka 1990). Of smears taken from the anus and rectum in homosexual men the sensitivity was found to be 53% in swabs taken blindly but rose to 79% if using an anoscope to visualize areas of inflammation and purulent discharge (Williams *et al.* 1981). Proctoscopy and culture are therefore essential to ensure the most efficient diagnosis.

Neisseria gonorrhoea is a fastidious organism requiring inoculation onto media containing blood or serum and incubation at a temperature of 36–37°C in a moist carbon dioxide enriched atmosphere for growth. Oxidase positive colonies should be positively identified as *N. gonorrhoea* and antibiotic sensitivity testing performed. There is no reliable serological test for gonorrhoea. Histological changes from the distal rectum are not pathognomonic, showing a picture similar to that of other causes of bacterial proctitis.

soles of the feet. One variety of the rashes of secondary syphilis are the so-called condylomata lata (Figures 4.3 and 4.4) because of the flat warty appearance. These appear in warm, moist areas of the body, especially in the anal and perianal regions. They are broad-based, reddish-brown or grey, granulomatous, superficial coalescent and papular lesions. In appearance, they are smoother and flatter than viral warts, being more suggestive of granulation tissue. Condylomata lata are teeming with *T. pallidum* and are highly infectious. Secondary lesions of the rectal mucosa include lobulated masses, polyps, ulceration, and non-specific erythema.

Late manifestations of syphilis in the form of gummata in the anus are extremely rare but may be mistaken for an anal tumour. Perianal skin may be involved in infiltrating gummatous lesions, resulting in extensive scarring (Figure 4.5).

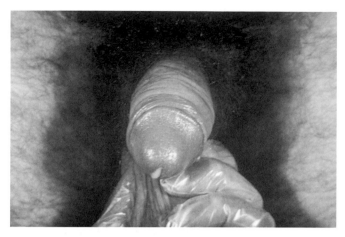

Figure 4.6 Purulent urethral discharge due to gonorrhoea. Patient also has bilateral tinea cruris.

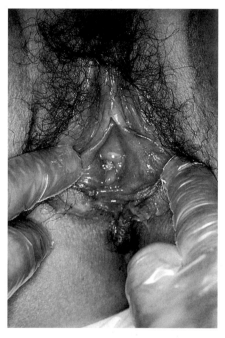

Figure 4.7 Purulent urethral discharge in female with gonorrhoea. Presence of genital warts should also be noted.

Transmission and epidemiology

Neisseria gonorrhoea is a strictly human pathogen. Transmission from an infected male to female has been estimated at between 60 and 90% (Evans 1976; Chippenfield and Catterall 1976; Barbour *et al.* 1976), while that to a male from an infected female is lower at 30–50% (Holmes *et al.* 1970). Rectal infection in males is always the result of anal intercourse but 25–50% of females infected with gonorrhoea will have rectal infection most caused by spread of infected discharge across the perineum probably infecting the rectal mucosa at defecation, although some may be due to rectal intercourse (Battacharya and Jepphcot 1974).

There are an estimated 66 000 000 new cases of gonorrhoea each year world-wide. In recent years there has been a fall in cases of gonorrhoea reported in the Western world. The number of cases diagnosed in genitourinary medicine clinics in England has dropped from 48 393 in 1983 to 11 803 in 1993, the lowest number of cases ever recorded (DH Statistics Division 2B 1994). In the same period reported cases in the USA fell from 900 435 in 1983 to 439 673 in 1993 (Centers for Disease Control and Prevention, December 1994). The fall has been particularly dramatic in homosexual men as a result of safer sexual practices, but fears have been expressed that young homosexual men may not identify themselves as being at risk and may once again be following high-risk sexual practices (Evans *et al.* 1993).

Clinical features

The most common manifestation of gonorrhoea in men is urethritis, which is usually symptomatic, with symptoms of a purulent urethral discharge (Figure 4.6), frequency, and dysuria occurring 3–10 days after infection. In females the endocervical canal and urethra (Figure 4.7) are most commonly infected, but is asymptomatic in approximately 70% of cases. Symptoms may include vaginal discharge, frequency, dysuria, and abdominal pain suggests infection of the upper genital tract. Rectal infection in homosexual men is symptomatic in 18–34% cases, but in only 5% of females (Morse *et al.* 1989). The gonococcus does not infect the anal canal but causes inflammation of the rectal mucosa; it does not spread into the sigmoid colon. If symptoms occur, they may be mucopurulent anal discharge which may be blood-stained, pruritus, anal pain, and tenesmus. On proctoscopy, mucopus may be seen in the anal canal or on the rectal mucosa (Figure 4.8), with an underlying inflammatory response

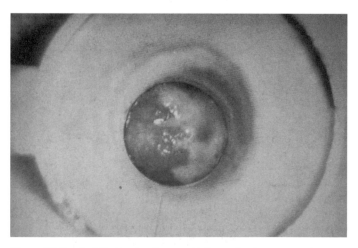

Figure 4.8 Purulent discharge and mucosal inflammation in gonococcal proctitis.

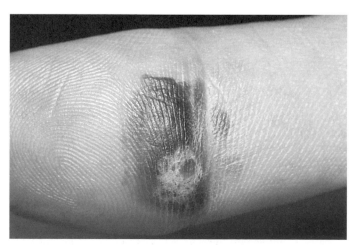

Figure 4.9 Cutaneous lesion of disseminated gonorrhoea.

being apparent. The mucosa may be friable with contact bleeding, and sometimes may have a granular appearance, but the rectal mucosa may appear quite normal. Occasionally, disseminated *N. gonorrhoea* infection may occur characterized by typical skin lesions (Figure 4.9) tenosynovitis, arthritis, and rarely endocarditis or meningitis.

Treatment

Owing to the widespread development of antibiotic resistant strains of *N. gonorrhoea*, it is necessary to be familiar with the local patterns of resistant strains before making treatment decisions. In the UK the vast majority of strains currently isolated are still penicillin sensitive and a single dose of amoxycillin 3 g plus probenecid 1 g will result in cure in the vast majority of cases.

Chlamydia trachomatis infections

Aetiology and diagnosis

Chlamydia trachomatis is an obligate intracellular parasite which has both an extracellular (elementary body) and intracellular (reticulate body) phase in its life cycle, and hence it cannot be grown in artificial media. It can be grown in tissue culture, but many antigen detection methods using enzyme-linked immunosorbent assay (ELISA), monoclonal antibody immunofluorescence, polymerase chain reaction, and ligase chain reaction techniques are now available. Reports of ligase chain reaction testing for diagnosis using urine samples from both men and women are very encouraging (Lee *et al.* 1995). There are three distinct serotype groups of *Chlamydia trachomatis*: types L.1–L.3 being the cause of lymphogranuloma venereum; types A–C, causing blinding trachoma eye disease; and types D–K, the cause of anogenital disease, inclusion conjunctivitis in neonates and adults, and upper respiratory tract infection and pneumonia in infants. Serological tests using micro-immunofluorescence are not regarded as helpful in everyday clinical practice because of problems with sensitivity and genus specificity. The complement fixation test for lymphogranuloma venereum is sensitive, but not specific, although a negative result can help to rule out the diagnosis in early disease but the test may revert to negative in late disease.

Chlamydia trachomatis infection, types D–K

Chlamydia trachomatis infections of the anogenital tract are the most common STD in the Western world.

The infection accounts for 30–50% of non-gonococcal urethritis in men (Csonka 1990). There were 100 820 cases of non-gonococcal urethritis genital tract infections recorded in Genitourinary Medicine Clinics in England in 1993 (DH Statistics Division 2B 1994) and an estimated 3–4 million *C. trachomatis* infections in the USA in 1990 (Zehnilman 1992). It results in significant serious morbidity and *C. trachomatis* is among the most common causes of pelvic inflammatory disease and infertility in the Western world (Cates 1984).

Clinical manifestations

In males, *C. trachomatis* infection will most commonly present with symptoms of urethral discharge (Figure 4.10), dysuria, and fre-

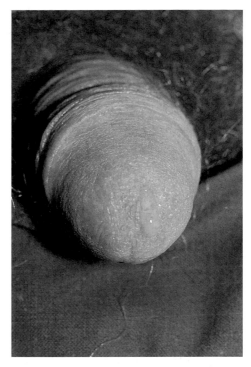

Figure 4.10 Mucopurulent urethral discharge of *C.trachoma* urethritis.

quency. These tend to be less severe than in gonorrhoea, but the two cannot be differentiated clinically and many infected males will be asymptomatic (Bowie 1990). In females the infection is usually of the endocervix giving a mucopurulent discharge in under 40%, and of the urethra giving frequency and dysuria in a minority of those infected, and these are all too easily misinterpreted as other genitourinary problems by both patient and doctor. Pelvic inflammatory disease resulting in infertility, chronic pelvic pain, and menstrual disorders are common, but upper genital tract infection is often silent, making contact tracing and epidemiological treatment cornerstones for the prevention of morbidity (Stamm and Holmes 1990).

As in gonorrhoea, infection of the rectal mucosa is transmitted to this site by anal intercourse in homosexual males and heterosexual females. In females, accidental infection also occurs due to spread of infected discharge from the genitals. The resulting proctitis is often silent but may result in mucopurulent anal discharge, rectal pain,

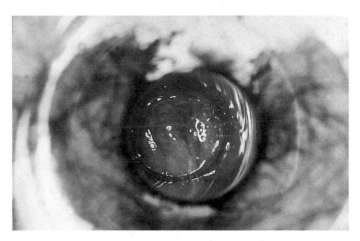

Figure 4.11 Inflamed rectal mucosa due to *C.trachoma* (see colour plates).

tenesmus, constipation, or diarrhoea. Proctoscopic examination may reveal an inflamed mucosa (Figure 4.11) with mucopus and contact bleeding, but in most cases only a mild proctitis is seen (Quinn *et al.* 1981). Diagnosis should be made using either culture or monoclonal antibody immunofluorescent tests. The ELISA test is not suitable for use in diagnosis of *C. trachomatis* from the rectum.

In 1–2% of cases, Reiter's disease may occur with manifestations of circinate balanitis (Figure 4.12), painless oral ulceration (Figure 4.13), keratoderma blenorrhagica (Figure 4.14), conjunctivitis (Figure 4.15), anterior uveitis, arthritis, and rarely cardiac conduction defects and neurological disorders.

Treatment

Chlamydia trachomatis is sensitive to tetracyclines and macrolides such as erythromycin; new generation macrolides such as azithromycin have made 'one shot' treatments for uncomplicated chlamydial infections a realistic possibility (Waugh 1991).

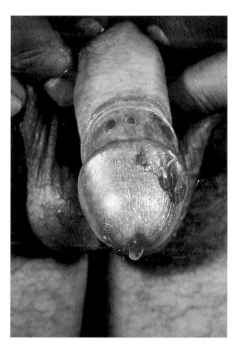

Figure 4.12 Painless, erosive lesions of circinate balanitis.

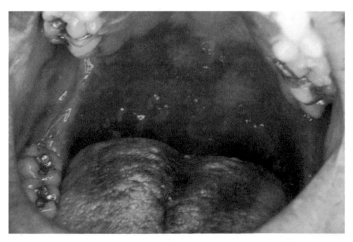

Figure 4.13 Painless, erosive lesions of oral mucosa in Reiter's disease.

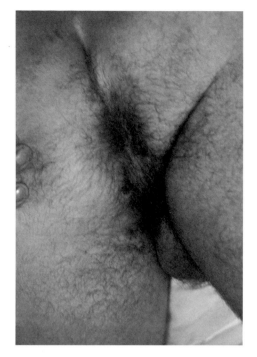

Figure 4.14 Perianal keratoderma blenorrhagica lesions.

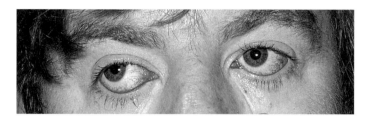

Figure 4.15 Bilateral conjunctivitis in Reiter's disease.

Lymphogranuloma venereum

Epidemiology and diagnosis

Lymphogranuloma venereum (LGV) is transmitted by sexual intercourse. It is principally a disease of central Africa, Asia, and South America, and may be contracted by travellers in these regions. It is rarely seen in the UK, with less than 100 cases per year, since 1983, and in the USA less than 500 cases per year have been reported since 1977 (Centers for Disease Control and Prevention 1994). Diagnosis in the acute stage should be by tissue culture from material taken from genital lesions, swabs from the rectum in the case of proctitis, and aspirated material from lymph nodes. Modern tests such as polymerase chain reaction will improve the diagnosis of this and other anogenital ulcerative diseases (Joseph and Rosen 1994). Serological diagnosis has been discussed in relation to *Chlamydia trachoma* infections.

Pathogenesis

Infection of the anogenital region is followed by systemic spread which localizes in the lymphatics and lymph nodes of the genitalia and rectum. An acute inflammatory response of the lymph nodes

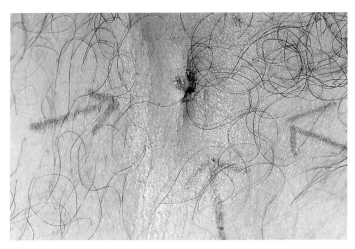

Figure 4.16 Lymphogranuloma venereum lesion of anal margin resembling encrusted herpes simplex lesion.

leads to local invasion which may result in multifocal abscesses, with suppuration and formation of fistulae. A direct infection of the rectal mucosa occurs in homosexual men (Quinn *et al.* 1981) resulting in an acute non-granulomatous inflammation in some cases.

Clinical manifestations

The initial lesion occurs at the site of inoculation after 1–4 weeks. It is usually a painless, papular lesion (Figure 4.16) which ulcerates and heals within 2–5 days. The lesion may be mistaken for herpes simplex and cultures should be taken to try to differentiate the two. An acute proctitis with inflammation and a bloody purulent discharge may be seen as a result of anal intercourse. Proctoscopy may reveal inflammation of the rectal mucosa with punctate haemorrhage

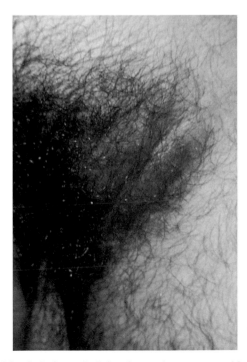

Figure 4.17 Inguinal adenopathy in lymphogranuloma venereum 'sign of the groove'.

and mucopurulent discharge. One to 6 weeks after the primary lesion has healed the regional lymph nodes become enlarged, inflamed, and fluctuant. In approximately 20% of cases, enlargement of both femoral and inguinal nodes occurs, this resulting in the so-called 'sign of the groove' (Figure 4.17)—said to be pathgnomonic of LGV (Schachter 1977). Systemic manifestations may include fever, headache, pneumonitis, hepatitis, meningo-encephalitis, erythema nodosum, and erythema multiforme. Untreated, the early disease will run its course in 6–8 weeks and many cases will resolve completely. Late manifestations which may occur up to 20 years later are due to scarring of the lymphatics and chronic inflammation. These can lead to local lymphoedema, ulceration, and perianal and perineal abscess formation. Chronic inflammation with cicatricial scarring of the rectum and colon can lead to stricture formation, extending from about 2–5 cm from the anal verge (Perine and Osoba 1990). Radiologically, the left colon may give a featureless appearance similar to that of ulcerative colitis or strictures resembling the skip lesions of Crohn's disease. Carcinoma has been reported in the strictures due to LGV in 2–5% of cases (Levin 1964).

Treatment

Treatment is with tetracycline therapy, or if the patient is allergic, macrolides using the erythromycin group. New generation long acting macrolides can be used, although these are expensive for use in developing countries. In late disease, following antibiotic therapy, surgery may involve dilatation of strictures or resection of these accompanied by colostomy.

Chancroid

Aetiology and diagnosis

Chancroid is caused by *H. ducreyi*, which is a Gram-negative bacillus. The organism may be seen on Gram stain smears taken from the undermined edge of ulcers, but this lacks specificity and sensitivity. Infected material from ulcers or aspiration from bubos should be inoculated on to enriched blood and chocolate agar plates. Culture confirmation is obtained in up to 60% of cases (Schmid *et al.* 1989). More recently, diagnosis has been shown to be enhanced using polymerase chain reaction techniques (Johnson *et al.* 1994). Histological sections from ulcers have been described as showing three zones: a superficial one demonstrating necrotic tissue, fibrin, neutrophils, and numerous Gram-negative coccobacilli; a middle zone with oedema and neovasoformation at right angles to the surface of the ulcer; and a deep zone showing a dense, infiltrate of neutrophils, plasma cells, and fibroblastic proliferation (Sheldon and Heyman 1946).

Epidemiology

It is estimated that there are 9 million new cases of chancroid per year world-wide. It is principally seen in developing countries and is associated with poor socio-economic conditions, and with men who use prostitutes (Blackmore 1985). Less than 100 cases per year are reported annually in the UK (DH Statistics Division 2B 1994), but in the USA the incidence rose from under 1000 cases per year in 1980 to over 5000 cases per year in 1987—most cases occurring in

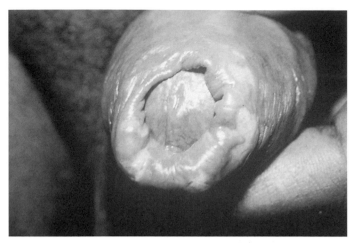

Figure 4.18 'Rosette' of chancroid lesions of the prepuce.

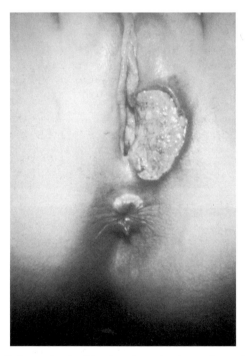

Figure 4.19 Large ulcer involving the vulva and perineum due to chancroid.

the black and Hispanic male population, with a male to female ratio of 4:1, although world-wide the ratio is of the order of 10:1 (Schmid *et al.* 1989). In the last decade an increase has been seen in diagnosis in heterosexual men and women in the USA, which has been attributed to the use of crack cocaine (Martin and Di Carlo 1994). The disease in homosexual men has not been adequately studied.

Clinical manifestations

After inoculation, there is a 4–10-day incubation period. The initial lesion is an erythematous papule, which may go unnoticed, forming at the site of inoculation. This leads to painful ulceration secondary to thrombotic occlusion of underlying dermal vessels. Genital ulcers (Figure 4.18) characteristically have an irregular margin described as 'beefy' and granular, but they are not indurated. Fifty per cent of patients develop unilateral or bilateral inguinal adenopathy. These glands are usually painful, and bubo formation may occur, and subsequently suppurate, resulting in fistulae and sometimes secondary

ulceration. Occasionally, a transient chancre lasting 4–6 days (chancre mou volant) occurs but the patient subsequently develops painful inguinal adenopathy, and this may lead to diagnostic difficulties. Perianal and anal ulceration (Figure 4.19) occurs as a result of anal intercourse in homosexual men, but in females lesions may be the result of auto-inoculation. Hypertrophic lesions in the perianal region (pseudo-granuloma inguinale) may occur (Kraus *et al.* 1982). Tissue destruction is usually minimal but healing may take months to years. There have been reports of rectovaginal fistula formation. Differentiation from syphilis and LGV needs to be made. Mixed infection can occur and initial ulceration due to chancroid may later develop into a typical syphilitic lesion (ulcus mixtum). Lymphadenopathy caused by LGV usually occurs after the healing of the painless anogenital lesion, whereas in chancroid, painful ulceration, inguinal adenopathy, and bubo formation coexist.

Treatment

Resistant strains of *H. ducreyi* to penicillins, sulphonamides, and tetracyclines are increasingly common.

Current treatment regimens consist of using macrolides, cephalosporins and Co-trimoxazole.

Granuloma inguinale (Donovanosis)

Granuloma inguinale is caused by the *Calymmatobacterium granulomatous*. The organism is best demonstrated by staining material from ulcers with Leishmann's, Wright's or Giemsa stain, so-called Donovan bodies being seen in the cytoplasm of mononuclear cells.

Epidemiology

This is a disease of tropical regions, especially the Caribbean, India, New Guinea, and central Australia. Although 90% of lesions occur in the anogenital region and primary perianal regions are most commonly seen in homosexual men (Davis 1970), there is no consensus that the infection is sexually transmitted. There is speculation that the organism may be carried in the gastrointestinal (GI) tract, and that contamination of abraded skin in the perianal and genital regions may occur from the bowel (Robertson *et al.* 1980).

Clinical manifestations

The incubation period is not known as the means of transmission are uncertain. The initial lesion is a papular or nodular lesion which may be intensely pruritic. This is followed by abscess formation, leaving a granulomatous ulcer (Figure 4.20). The regional lymph nodes are not enlarged. Lesions may remain static over years, but there may be extensive tissue destruction (Figures 4.21 and 4.22), with fibrous scarring and lymphoedema. Rarely lesions of the liver, spleen, and bone have been reported. Treatment is with tetracyclines or ampicillin.

Candidiasis

Candidiasis is caused by yeasts of the *Candida* species, most commonly *Candida albicans*, but also *C. tropicalis* and *Torulopsis glabrata*. The yeasts are common commensals in warm, moist areas of the

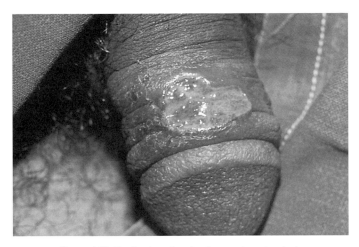

Figure 4.20 Penile ulceration due to granuloma inguinale.

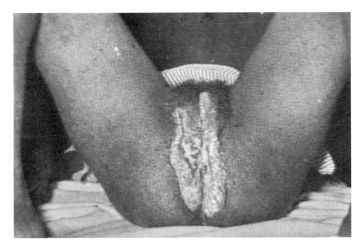

Figure 4.21 Massive destruction of perianal and vulval tissue due to granuloma inguinale.

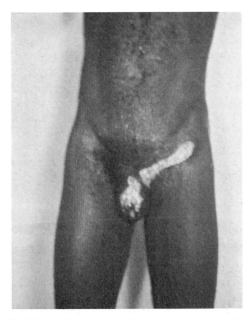

Figure 4.22 Total destruction of penis, with extensive inguinal involvement due to granuloma inguinale.

body, especially around the anogenital region, and carriage in the rectum is common. Predisposing factors to clinical disease are obesity, diabetes mellitus, and immunodeficient states, such as AIDS. It has also been associated with patients on total parenteral nutrition.

Clinical manifestations

Candidiasis commonly affects the genital and perianal skin (Figure 4.23) concurrently in both sexes. Candida lesions present between the buttocks perianally, and in the natal cleft, with pruritic lesions starting as pustules on an erythematous base which coalesce. Typically, satellite lesions are seen away from the main body of the rash. Maceration is commonly seen at the border of an inflamed area with fissuring and epithelial erosions in the perianal region.

Diagnosis

The typical Gram-positive hyphae with budding spores may be seen on Gram staining of swabs taken from the lesions. Culture on Sabourd's medium should be carried out on swabs or scrapings.

Treatment

Treatment consists of general hygiene measures and the use of local application of Imidazole creams or oral Azol therapy such as fluconazole or itraconazole, although resistance to these agents is now emerging in patients with AIDS and oral candidiasis (Sangeorzan *et al.* 1994).

Herpes simplex virus infections

Aetiology and diagnosis

Herpes simplex is a double-stranded DNA virus which can be grown in tissue culture. Two types herpes simplex virus (HSV) 1

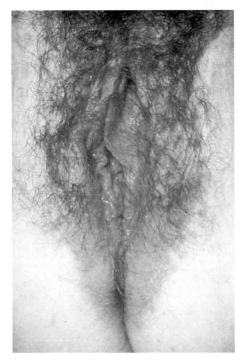

Figure 4.23 Vulval and perianal acute candidiasis. Note the satellite lesions at the margin (see colour plates).

and HSV 2 which are biologically and antigenically distinct can infect the anogenital region.

The gold standard of diagnosis is isolation in tissue culture. Swabs from suspected lesions should be inoculated into a virus transport medium which should be stored at 4°C if there is to be any delay in transportation to the virus laboratory. Alternative methods of diagnosis are antigen detection methods such as direct immunofluorescence test or ELISA technique. Electron microscopy is held to be an insensitive method of detection for genital lesions (Brown *et al.* 1979). Serological testing presents many difficulties and is not generally used for diagnosis of individual cases. Biopsy of rectal lesions may show diffuse ulceration with lymphocytic infiltration. Intranuclear inclusions may be seen in 40% of cases if multiple biopsies are taken (Goodell *et al.* 1983).

Epidemiology

HSV 1 was traditionally described as the cause of oropharyngeal disease and HSV 2 the cause of anogenital disease. Over the last three decades orogenital sex has become a much more common sexual practice and some authors have recently reported up to 70% isolation of HSV 1 from genital lesions (Tayal and Pattman 1994), probably reflecting these changes of sexual practice and a lack of awareness that 'cold sores' on the lips can result in 'herpes' on a partner's genitals.

The number of new infections of genital herpes reported from genitourinary medicine clinics in England and Wales has risen from 16 534 to 25 502 between the years 1983 and 1993 (DH Statistics Division 2B 1994). Serological surveys from several Western countries have shown a seroprevalence of HSV 2 specific antibodies in 7–20% of the adult population. One large study in the USA of 4201 adult participants in the second National Health and Nutrition Examination Survey in the USA found a seroprevalence of 16.4% (Johnston *et al.* 1989). Viral shedding in women without genital symptoms has been detected in 1.6–8.0% of women attending STD clinics (Corey *et al.* 1993). These among other facts underline the proposition that HSV 2 is a much underestimated infection which is most often sexually transmitted from an asymptomatic partner (Mertz *et al.* 1992).

Natural history

Infection of skin and mucosal surfaces occurs through a breach in the epithelium. The virus infects terminal ends of sensory nerves and travels along the nerve sheath to lodge in the dorsal root ganglia of the sacral plexus where latency is established. Reactivation with new lesion formation in those with clinical disease occurs on average of five to six times per year. Recurrences become less frequent over time (Corey *et al.* 1993), and HSV 1 lesions of the genitals relapse much less frequently than those caused by HSV 2 (Lafferty *et al.* 1989).

Clinical manifestations

Primary anogenital herpes—that is in persons never previously infected with either HSV 1 or HSV 2—has an incubation period of 2–12 days. Typically, the lesions manifest as vesicles which break down to form painful ulcers. Lesions may be widespread throughout the anogenital region (Figure 4.24), and untreated will usually heal in 3–4 weeks. Anorectal herpes is often extremely painful with associated tenesmus, haematochezia and anal discharge. Proctoscopy may reveal a diffuse inflammation of the rectal mucosa, usually involving only the first 10 cm of the rectum or sometimes the appearance may be that of discrete ulceration of the mucosa. Sacral radiculopathy secondary to acute herpetic proctitis resulting in urinary retention, constipation, and impotence has been described (Samarasinghe *et al.* 1979).

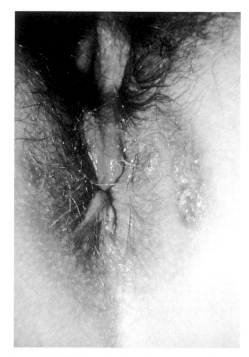

Figure 4.24 Vulval and perianal herpes simplex lesions.

Constitutional symptoms are commonly seen and these include fevers, malaise, and headache (Corey *et al.* 1993). Non-primary episodes of anogenital herpes and recurrences tend to be much less severe and lesions may be discrete (Pannuti *et al.* 1997).

Treatment

Treatment of primary anogenital herpes is with acyclovir, the usual dose being 200 mg orally five times per day for 5 days.

Severe cases with systemic manifestations may need hospitalization, and intravenous therapy. Urinary retention may respond to analgesia and instructing the patient to pass urine in a warm bath, but suprapubic bladder aspiration may be necessary. Urinary retention should not be managed with catheterization of the urethra, as the infection may be spread to the urethral mucosa, with subsequent trauma on removal of the catheter. Recurrent episodes may be able to be managed with symptomatic therapy, but those with frequent recurrences can be placed on suppressive therapy, using starting doses of acyclovir of 400 mg, b.d. or 200 mg, q.i.d., the dose being titrated to give maximum control of breakthrough episodes. Resistant strains to acyclovir are now well recognized (Lehrman *et al.* 1986).

Recently, the acyclovir analogue Famciclovir has been licensed for treatment in the UK and this may allow less frequent dosing for initial and prophylactic treatment. Clinical trials of vaccines are currently under way.

Human papilloma virus lesions (anogenital warts)

Aetiology and diagnosis

Anogenital warts are caused by the human papillomavirus (HPV). This is a double-stranded DNA virus which cannot be grown in cell cultures, but with the use of molecular biology techniques a greater understanding of the epidemiology and spectrum of disease has been obtained. Over 70 types of HPV have now been described. Those causing anogenital lesions are usually found to be types 6 or 11, being detected in up to 90% of lesions. These types are not associated with malignant transformation, but others principally HPV 16 and 18 are highly associated with anogenital tract malignancy, and may be found in 10% of anal warts (Von Krogh *et al.* 1989). HPV infection usually affects squamous epithelial cells, but some types affecting the anogenital region are mucosotrophic and are seen to infect cuboidal cells of the rectum and colon (de Villiers 1989), anal warts are characterized by a marked acanthosis and surface hyperkeratosis with koilocytosis, dilated vessels and some degree of inflammation of basal cells.

Epidemiology

Anogenital warts behave epidemiologically as a STD with two-thirds of sex partners of those with warts developing lesions within 8 months (Oriel 1971). It is now recognized that a wide spectrum of anogenital papillomavirus disease exists ranging through latent, subclinical, and clinical disease, with overt warts being only the tip of the iceberg (Von Krogh 1989). Many partners of those with genital warts are found on investigation to have subclinical disease (Von Krogh 1989). Human papillomavirus infection of the anogenital region has been described as the most common STD in the world, with an estimated lifetime risk of up to 79% acquisition of at least one anogenital HPV type (Syrjanen 1990). The distribution of both clinical and subclinical infection across the anogenital areas is widespread in both heterosexuals and homosexuals. Perianal and anal canal warts are more common in homosexual men (Oriel 1971), but these lesions are frequently seen in heterosexual men and women. One study found the presence of perianal and anal warts in 47% and 31% of heterosexual women and men with genital warts, and an additional 32% and 43%, respectively, had colposcopic appearance of subclinical diseases (Sonnex *et al.* 1991). Studies have shown no statistical difference in the sexual practices of anal intercourse and anodigital insertion into the anal canal in heterosexual men and women with or without anal canal lesions (Sonnex *et al.* 1991; Armstrong *et al.* 1994).

Clinical presentation

Only one-quarter of patients notice a perianal lesion at the time of presentation. Most frequent presenting symptoms were bleeding (85%), pruritus (45%), and anal discomfort (45%). Lesions may be of three morphological types: (i) 'classical' condyloma acuminata, described as soft, fleshy, with a spiky surface—seen most commonly in warm, moist areas such as the sub-preputial sac, the vulva (Figure 4.25), and intertriginous areas; (ii) papular lesions seen on fully keratinized regions of the anogenital area such as the penile shaft or the perianal skin (Figure 4.26); and (iii) Macular lesions which may be seen on naked eye, but frequently are only visible after applying 5% acetic acid and viewing the area with a colposcope. Most exophytic lesions are easily identified on clinical examination as warts but should there be any doubt, condylomata lata lesions of secondary syphilis can be diagnosed by immediate dark field examination and syphilis serology tests will be positive. A biopsy may be needed if the lesions are atypical, and is essential if there is any possibility of malignant transformation. Discharge is not usually associated with anal warts, and may suggest associated proctitis, possibly due to another STD or the presence of an anal fistula.

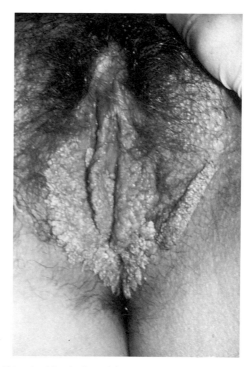

Figure 4.25 Extensive 'classical' condylomata acuminata of vulva and perianal region.

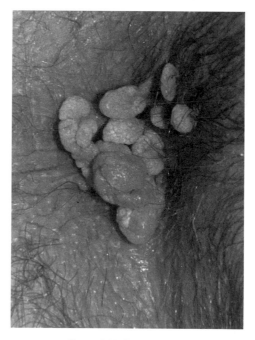

Figure 4.26 Perianal warts.

Treatment

All treatment modalities are associated with a high incidence of relapse and new lesion formation. Commonly used methods of treatment include electrocautery, excision, cryotherapy, laser, chemical application with Podophyllin, purified Podophyllotoxin, and trichloracetic acid (Kraus and Stone 1990)

Anal warts in children

Although anal warts may be the result of vertical transmission at birth, from digital HPV types or other accidental methods of transmission, the finding of anal warts in children should arouse the suspicion of possible sexual abuse. There have been widely different assessments of the incidence of such warts secondary to sexual abuse (Handley *et al.* 1993), but referral to a specialist is recommended for social and clinical investigation (Figures 4.27 and 4.28) (Oriel 1988).

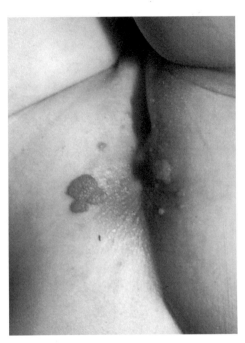

Figure 4.27 Perianal warts in a child.

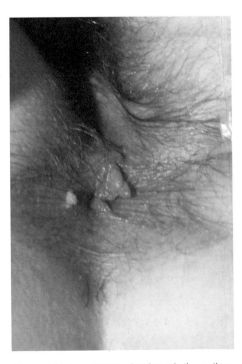

Figure 4.28 Concurrent perianal wart in the mother.

Enteric infections

Oro-anal sex results in the sexual transmission of a number of intestinal infections, and hence are more commonly seen in homosexual men (McLean 1990). An appropriately taken sexual history will enable the examining doctor to give appropriate advice on future avoidance of such infections and request for partners to be investigated.

Protozoans

Giardia lamblia may result in asymptomatic colonization of the bowel but can cause nausea, flatulence, crampy abdominal pain, and diarrhoea. In chronic infection weight loss may occur due to malabsorption in a small number of cases. Diagnosis is made by identifying cysts in specimens of fresh faeces, but may need duodenal aspirate or jejunal biopsy to make a diagnosis. Treatment is with metronidazole, 2 g orally for 3 days, or tinidazole 2 g stat. repeated 1 week later. *Entamoeba histolytica* infects the large intestine and can give mild to severe, sometimes bloody diarrhoea. Proctocolitis can occur, but most organisms excreted by homosexual men are found to be non-pathogenic types, and it has been debated if therapy is necessary in the asymptomatic person. Diagnosis is made by identifying cysts in fresh faeces samples, or from rectal biopsies. In symptomatic individuals, treatment is recommended with metronidazole, 800 mg three times daily for 10 days, or tinidazole 2 g stat. followed by 500 mg three times daily for 1 week (McLean *et al.* 1990).

Helminths

Oro-anal sex can result in the sexual transmission of both *Enterobius vermicularis* (threadworm, pinworm) and possibly *Strongyloides stercoralis*, principally in homosexual men. *Enterobius vermicularis* can be a cause of inflammation of the rectum, perianal excoriation, and pruritus ani. The worms may be seen on proctoscopic examination or on microscopic examination of clear adhesive tape which has been applied to the anal margin overnight. Ulceration of the colon can be caused by *S. stercoralis*. Both of these infestations can be treated with mebendazole.

Bacteria

Enteric bacterial pathogens such as *Shigella* and *Salmonella* species and *Campylobacter jejuni* may be sexually transmitted by oro-anal sex, and can result in enteric infection and proctocolitis. Diagnosis is made by stool culture and treatment is with appropriate antibiotic therapy.

Human immunodeficiency virus disease

Introduction

The first cases of what is now known as the acquired immune deficiency syndrome (AIDS) were described in 1981 (Gottlieb *et al.* 1981; Masur *et al.* 1981), although it is now clear that this disease existed in a sporadic form for some time prior to this (Huminer *et al.* 1987). The aetiological agent first detected in 1984 is now called the human immunodeficiency virus (HIV). The spectrum of disease from initial virus infection to late HIV disease has been classified by the Centers for Disease Control (CDC) Atlanta (MMWR 1986). In the USA this has been superseded by the 1993 revised system of classification (Centers for Disease Control and Prevention 1992). In the UK and Europe, persons infected with HIV are diagnosed as having AIDS if they fulfil the criteria for a diagnosis of an AIDS indicator disease as described in the CDC Surveillance Case Definitions for AIDS 1993 (Centers for Disease Control and Prevention 1992). The additional definition of persons infected with HIV and having a T-helper lymphocyte count of under $200 \times 10^6/\mu$l now used in the USA as defining AIDS has not been adopted as yet in the UK and Europe. AIDS indicator diseases vary in their incidence throughout the world. Among the most commonly seen in the UK are *Pneumocystis carinii* pneumonia (PCP), Kaposi's sarcoma (KS), systemic manifestations of candidiasis, persistent herpes simplex infections, persistent diarrhoea due to cryptosporidiosis, cytomegalovirus (CMV) disease, atypical mycobacterial infections, and cerebral and non-Hodgkin's lymphomas.

Aetiology

AIDS is caused principally by the human immunodeficiency virus type 1 (HIV-1). A small proportion of cases is caused by a related, less virulent virus, HIV-2, first reported from Senegal in 1985 (Barin *et al.* 1985), causing AIDS principally in West Africa. There is approximately 60% homology between the core antigens of HIV-1 and HIV-2 but the envelope antigens are unrelated. HIV-1 is a retrovirus made up of an outer lipid envelope through which the transmembrane glycoprotein (gp) 41 is attached to the external gp 120. HIV attaches on to cells it infects by a short conserved sequence on the gp 120. Internally, there are structural polypeptides principally P17 surrounding the core P24 and two identical linear molecules of RNA (Figure 4.29). The genome contains the three basic genes of retroviruses; GAG encoding for the core nucleocapsid polypeptides, ENV encoding for the surface proteins, and POL which gives rise to the viral reverse transcriptase, protease, integrase, and ribonuclease enzymes. HIV-1 is a member of the Lentivirinae subfamily of retroviruses which have considerably more complex genomes, HIV-1 containing at least seven additional genes to the three essential genes of the retrovirus. These additional genes control factors such as latency, activation, and production of the virus within the host cell.

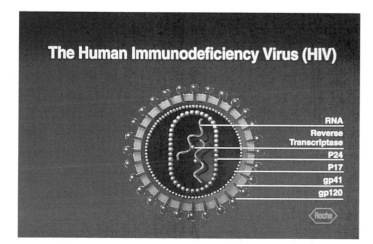

Figure 4.29 Diagrammatic representation of HIV (slide produced by Roche Pharmaceuticals).

Pathogenesis

The major target for HIV infection are cells expressing the CD4 epitope on their surface, this acting as a receptor for the HIV envelope associated external glycoprotein, gp 120. CD4 epitopes are present in particularly high concentrations on T-helper/inducer lymphocytes CD4+ lymphocytes, cells of the macrophage monocyte lineage and Langerhans'/dendritic cells. HIV-1 may also infect cells of the gut epithelium, the bone marrow progenitors, and glial cells in the central nervous system (Castro *et al.* 1988). On entry into the infected cell the viral reverse transcriptase enzyme initiates transcription of a DNA copy of the RNA genome. This proviral DNA becomes integrated into the host cell DNA. Subsequent activation of cellular replication results in reassembly of viral particles with resulting new virions budding through the cell surface. The principal effect of HIV-1 infection on the immune system is the destruction of CD4+ T lymphocytes. These cells have a central role in the immune response interacting with macrophages, other T lymphocytes, B cells, and natural killer cells, either by direct contact or via lymphokines such as interferons and interleukin 2. The end result of the CD4 cell loss and other immune dysfunction which occurs is a state of profound immunosuppression, resulting in manifestations of HIV disease and AIDS.

The precise mechanisms by which HIV-1 causes its pathogenic effects are still matters for intense research and debate. One of the puzzles in the natural history of HIV disease was the seemingly prolonged latent period between infection and late disease during which it had been thought that viral replication was relatively quiescent but recent publications (Wei Xiping *et al.* 1995; Ho *et al.* 1995) have suggested that far from remaining latent there is a continuous dynamic process in which it is calculated that up to 10^8 virus particles are produced per day and that 2×10^7 CD4 cells are destroyed everyday. It is speculated that this continuous battle leads to the eventual exhaustion of the immune system's ability to respond to such an onslaught. If confirmed, these contributions to our understanding of the disease process will be a major step forward.

Epidemiology

The known routes of HIV transmission are by sexual intercourse and receipt of infected blood from sharing needles by injecting drug users, blood transfusion, and previously by infected blood products. The highest risk sexual practice is anoreceptive intercourse (Winklestein *et al.* 1987).

By the end of 1994, sexual intercourse between men had accounted for 60% of the 23 104 of HIV infections reported in the UK (Communicable Disease Report 1995). World-wide, heterosexual intercourse is estimated to account for at least 60% of the world's HIV infection, and in the UK the number of HIV infections acquired by heterosexual intercourse is seen to have risen from 200 in 1988 to over 600 in 1994 (Communicable Disease Report 1995).

The link between HIV transmission and other STDs is now apparent (Plummer *et al.* 1991), with both ulcerative and inflammatory STDs increasing the risk of acquiring HIV infection. Ulcerative disease provides a portal of entry for HIV, and inflammatory disease by recruiting activated T lymphocytes to the urogenital tract resulting in transport of HIV to the region, or an increased likelihood of acquiring HIV from infected material introduced into the genitals at sexual intercourse.

Besides blood and genital secretions, HIV has been isolated in low titres from other body fluids such as saliva, tears, urine, amniotic fluid, and cerebrospinal fluid, but it is generally believed that the amount of virus present in these fluids constitutes an extremely low risk of infection as a result of exposure to these.

In the health care setting, the principal cause for concern is exposure to potentially infected blood. Although there have been a few cases of infection as a result of contamination of open wounds by infected blood, the principal mode of transmission among health care workers has been transcutaneous injuries with hollow bore needles (Heptonstall *et al.* 1993). It has been estimated that the risk of infection after such an injury is 0.4%. In comparison, seroconversion occurs in about 25% of those exposed to needlestick injuries from patients positive for the e antigen of hepatitis B. The risk to surgeons can be directly equated to the prevalence of HIV in the patient population. In areas of high seroprevalence such as California, the risk of seroconversion of a surgeon has been estimated as one infection every 8 years (Gerberding *et al.* 1990). In a low seroprevalence area based on a surgeon performing 500 operations per year, an estimated risk of seroconversion of one in 800 over a career life span of 30 years has been calculated (Leentvaar-Kuijpers *et al.* 1988).

Studies examining the risks of needlestick injuries during operative procedures have shown that nurses and medical students are at greatest risk, followed by house staff and phlebotomists. The frequency of needlestick injuries exposing surgeons to risk of blood-borne infection has been estimated to occur in between 2% and 15% of operative procedures. The median rate of needlestick injuries to surgeons during operation has been calculated to be eight per 1000 operating hours. The risk to surgeons can be reduced by the use of disposable gowns and instruments, double gloving, wearing visors, and possibly by laparoscopic techniques. With the use of double gloves, a puncture rate of 11% of the outer and 2% of the inner glove was reported. It has been stated that approximately 40% of needlestick injuries could be prevented if existing hospital control procedures were followed. The most common occasions in which needlestick injuries were seen to occur were in resheathing needles and incorrect disposal of needles.

The risk of transmission of HIV from an infected health care worker to a patient during surgical procedures is unknown. There has been one well publicized case of a Florida dentist who, on the basis of evidence from phylogenetic analysis of HIV sequences, appears to have infected five of his patients (Ou *et al.* 1992). There is no other published case of transmission from a health care worker to a patient. In an analysis of 19 000 patients exposed to potential risk from infected health care workers none was identified as having been infected (Robert *et al.* 1993).

In the event of exposure to possible infected material by a health care worker or patient, the advice should be the same. San Francisco General Hospital (SFGH) have developed a useful model of management based on the perceived risk to the injured party on a basis of whether the injury was a definite exposure to HIV infected material, the type of injury and the volume of material involved (Gerberding 1995). Any wounds should be immediately cleaned, disinfected, and encouraged to bleed. The injured party should be counselled as to the likely risk of the exposure, and a discussion as to whether to immediately commence prophylaxis with zidovudine should be held. Because of the difficulties in carrying out a controlled study for those exposed to HIV, it has not been possible to evaluate the efficacy of such prophylaxis. Theoretically, the use of zidovudine, if initiated within 24 h of exposure, could prevent establishment of infection. In saying that, there have been a number of incidents recorded when such prophylaxis has failed (Tokars *et al.* 1993).

The decision as to whether to take zidovudine prophylaxis should be taken by the injured party, but useful guidelines as to recommendations are those of the SFGH (Gerberding 1995) which can be summarized as: (i) massive exposure warrants strong encouragement; (ii) iv definite parenteral exposure use is endorsed; (iii) possible parenteral exposure use is not routinely recommended but available on request; and (iv) doubtful or non-parenteral exposure use is discouraged.

If zidovudine prophylaxis is instituted, it should be at standard dosages, e.g. 200 mg t.i.d. for 2–6 weeks. Careful haematological monitoring should be undertaken. Prophylaxis is not routinely recommended for pregnant women. It is advisable that a baseline blood test for HIV is taken, as in the event of seroconversion it is necessary from a compensation point of view to be able to show the person was HIV negative at the time of injury. For all of these events, adequate expert counselling is necessary, and a discussion as to the possible need for safer sex practices during follow-up is required. The following of guidelines for the reduction of risk to health care workers (Centers for Disease Control and Prevention 1989), and the adequate sterilization of instrumentation, are essential, and all health care workers should be instructed in these. The principle on which these are founded are that blood and all bodily fluids are potentially infective material. Therefore, contact with blood, stools, or other materials with skin and mucous membrane is to be avoided. This will mean that those involved in invasive procedures should wear a protective smock, protective eyewear, and two pairs of latex gloves. Smoke from electrocautery, despite the fact that there is no evidence for transmission of HIV by inhalation, should be evacuated using high-powered suction devices, and the operators should wear masks capable of filtering out particles as small as 0.3 μm. Non-disposable metal instruments should be cleaned immediately with detergent, and then subjected to gas sterilization. Endoscopes should be rinsed and cleaned with detergent followed by immersion in 2% gluteraldehyde for 20 min before the next examination. Despite the fact that HIV is inactivated within minutes other pathogens such as mycobacteria may contaminate instruments.

Diagnosis and testing

Following HIV infection the first event to occur is that of viraemia but routine tests for HIV virus isolation or sensitive antigen detection methods are not available at this point in time. Routine testing for HIV infection relies on the detection of antibodies to the virus. Seroconversion usually occurs between 4 and 8 weeks following infection, although delayed seroconversion of 2 years or more has been recorded. Antibodies against the external gp 120 and the transmembrane gp 41 are initially detected and these are followed by

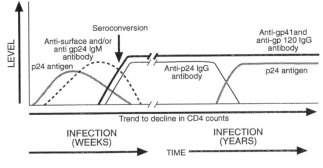

Figure 4.30 Serological markers of HIV infection

antibodies against the core protein P24. Later immunoglobulin (Ig) G and IgM antibodies against all the components of the virus can be detected (Figure 4.30). Poor prognosis has been associated with a poor antibody response to the P24 protein in the early phase of infection or persistence of P24 antigen. Falling levels of antibody to P24 have been associated with advancing immunodeficiency. Tests employed to detect HIV antibodies include ELISA, Western blotting, and gel agglutination. In the UK, if a screening ELISA test is positive the serum is tested by two alternative ELISA methods and a repeat sample is taken for confirmation assays.

The testing of patients for HIV has aroused considerable controversy especially the ethical issue of requiring informed consent for such testing. In practice this presents little problem if the patient is provided with adequate information and, where appropriate, pre-test counselling. In the event of a patient whose history or clinical condition suggests the need for HIV testing and the patient refuses, he/she should be informed that any procedures would be performed as if a test had proved positive.

Laboratory markers of disease progression commonly employed are the counting of CD4 helper/inducer lymphocytes and CD8 cytotoxic/suppressor lymphocytes. Shortly after infection with HIV, a marked fall of CD4 cells may be seen which usually recovers within a matter of weeks. A rise in CD8 cells may be seen at this stage. Long-term follow-up monitoring of lymphocyte cell counts shows a gradual decline in CD4 cell numbers and in those with counts of under 200/mm an AIDS-defining disease can be expected within 3 years. In late-stage disease, CD8 cells are seen to fall also. Another surrogate marker of disease progression used is measurement of beta-2 microglobulin concentrations, this is seen to rise in situations of high cell turnover and death. Levels of over 5.0 mg/ml are associated with a poor prognosis with progression to an AIDS-defining disease being seen within 3–5 years (Banatvala 1992). Increased levels of serum neopterin associated with cellular activation has also been correlated with advancing clinical HIV disease (Fahey et al. 1990).

HIV disease

The stages of HIV disease are divided into four categories by the Communicable Disease Centers of Atlanta, USA (Table 4.2). The seroconversion illness first recognized in 1985 has been reported to occur with variable numbers of patients. The onset is usually within 2–4 weeks of acquiring the virus. The illness is characterized by the development of a flu-like illness with features resembling glandular fever. Symptoms include fever, sore throat, oral ulceration, macular rash mostly on the torso, arthralgia, myalgia, nausea, vomiting, diarrhoea, and neurological symptoms. There have been reports of both oral and oesophageal candidiasis (Pedersen et al. 1987) and pneumocystis carinii pneumonia (PCP) (Vento et al. 1993) at this stage, secondary to a profound depletion of circulating CD4 cells which can occur in this illness. The length and severity of the seroconversion illness has been shown to have prognostic significance, in that, statistically there is a more rapid progression to late-stage disease in those with a more severe and lengthy illness (Pedersen et al. 1989). This has been attributed to the possible acquisition of a more virulent virus and possible different individual responses to infection. It should be noted that the HIV antibody test may not become reactive until some weeks after the onset of the seroconversion illness and therefore, adequate serological follow-up of persons suspected of having this manifestation is essential. This illness may last up to several weeks, after which the person becomes asymptomatic in common with the majority of persons who initially contract HIV. Many persons who are otherwise asymptomatic will be found to have generalized lymphadenopathy. Lymph nodes are characteristically rubbery in consistency, painless and symmetrically distributed, usually involving axillary, cervical, and submandibular nodes. The person is said to have persistent generalized lymphadenopathy (PGL) (Centers for Disease Control and Prevention 1986) if lymph nodes for which no other cause is found are present at two or more sites outside the inguinal area are over 1 cm in diameter and persist for longer than 3 months. The finding of PGL does not infer any prognostic significance in these cases but interestingly the disappearance of lymph nodes is a poor prognostic sign as this has been shown to be coincidental with the breakdown of lymph node architecture seen in advanced disease (Chadburn et al. 1989). It is not necessary to routinely biopsy glands in PGL but should they be asymmetrical, become rapidly enlarging or painful, these may be indications for biopsy. Progression to late manifestations of HIV disease stage IV is very variable in individual cases. It has been estimated that 50% of persons infected with HIV will have developed an AIDS diagnosis within 11 years of infection. The clinical onset of late-stage disease can usually be correlated with a progressive decline in CD4 helper cell numbers detected in the laboratory. Skin and oral manifestations may be the first to become apparent and are useful indicators for diagnosis of HIV infection. Characteristic skin signs include Kaposi's sarcoma (KS) (Figure 4.31), generalized ichthyosis, seborrhoeic dermatitis (Figure 4.32), persistent and severe herpes simplex infection (Figure 4.33), herpes zoster

---

Table 4.2 Centers for Disease Control and Prevention Classification for HIV infections

Group I   Acute infection
Group II   Asymptomatic infection
Group III   Persistent generalized lymphadenopathy
Group IV   Other disease:
  Subgroup A Constitutional disease
  Subgroup B Neurological disease
  Subgroup C Secondary infectious diseases
    Category C-1 Specified secondary infectious diseases listed in the CDC surveillance definition for AIDS
    Category C-2 Other specified secondary infectious diseases
  Subgroup D Secondary cancers
  Subgroup E Other conditions

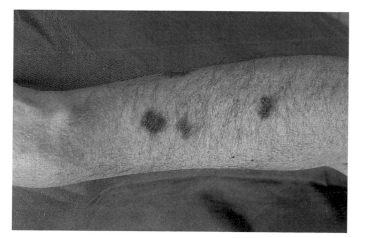

Figure 4.31 Kaposi's sarcoma lesions of arm.

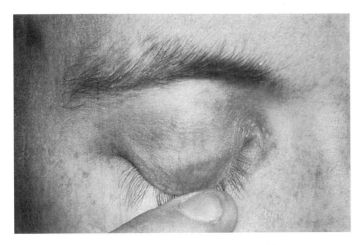

Figure 4.32 Seborrhoeic dermatitis of eyelid.

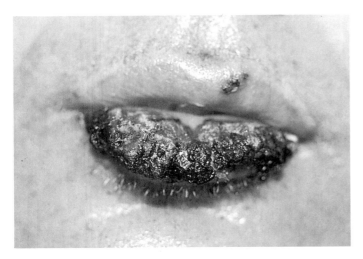

Figure 4.33 Herpes simplex virus infection of lip in HIV positive man.

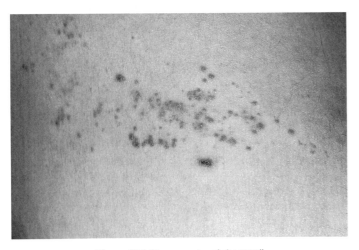

Figure 4.34 Herpes zoster of chest wall

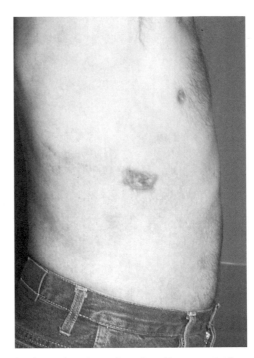

Figure 4.35 Persistent ulceration and scarring of herpes zoster 8 months after initial lesions.

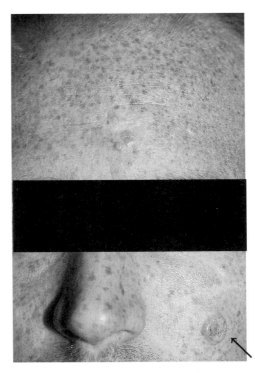

Figure 4.36 Molluscum contagiosum of face (arrowed).

infection (Figures 4.34 and 4.35), and fungal infections including those of nail beds. Facial molluscum contagiosa (Figure 4.36) and warts are seen frequently.

Oral candidiasis (Figure 4.37) is particularly characteristic and HIV should be strongly suspected in those with no other pre-disposing cause for this. Hairy leucoplakia (Figure 4.38), a corrugated white lesion, usually seen on the lateral border of the tongue but also seen at other sites in the oral cavity, is caused by Epstein–Barr virus and is characteristic of HIV disease (Hollander *et al.* 1986). Other oral lesions include KS (Figure 4.39), ulceration due to herpes simplex, CMV, and non-specific aphthous ulcers. Gingivitis and dental abscesses are common.

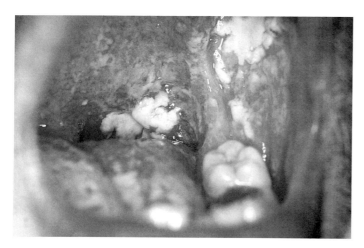

Figure 4.37 Oral candidiasis.

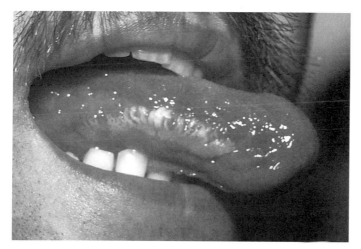

Figure 4.38 Hairy leucoplakia of lateral border of tongue.

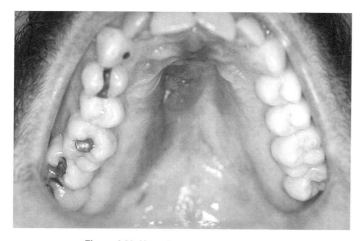

Figure 4.39 Kaposi's sarcoma of hard palate.

festations as described. The clinical diagnosis of AIDS is made with the onset of one of a multiplicity of infective or malignant AIDS defining diseases (Centers for Disease Control and Prevention 1987). The incidence of AIDS-defining disease varies throughout the world because of differences in endemic infections. In the Western world the commonest diagnosis has been that of PCP, but this condition is becoming less common with the use of effective prophylaxis in individuals known to be infected with HIV. Prophylaxis against PCP should be recommended if the patient's T4 helper cell count falls below $200 \times 10^6/l$. Two commonly employed regimens are 960 mg co-trimoxazole, once daily, or inhaled Pentamidine 300 mg, monthly. Other common opportunistic infections are CMV disease, principally retinitis and colitis, atypical mycobacterial infections and *M. tuberculosis* is seen to be rising in African communities as a result of the HIV epidemic. Neurological diseases both secondary to HIV infection and other causes are very common in late disease. They include dementia, meningoencephalitis, encephalopathy, peripheral neuropathy, and myositis. Studies have revealed almost 90% of patients having neurological disease on post-mortem studies (Lantos *et al.* 1989). There is a marked increase of malignancies in AIDS, characteristically KS, which usually has its onset in the skin, but widespread systemic disease occurs. In addition, non-Hodgkin's lymphomas and primary cerebral lymphomas occur, and these are seen to be increasing in patients whose survival is being prolonged by antiviral and prophylactic therapy.

The gastrointestinal tract in HIV disease

The clinical stage of HIV infection at which intestinal mucosal immunity fails is by definition when opportunistic infection occurs. The pathophysiology of intestinal disease is not yet fully understood but two main mechanisms have been postulated. The first is reduced intestinal immunity resulting in chronic opportunistic infections which themselves cause altered intestinal function. The second is that HIV *per se* affects the intestinal mucosa causing malfunction. The mechanisms by which this occurs may be the result of either direct infection of mucosal epithelial cells or macrophages within the mucosa by HIV. Reports have documented the presence of the HIV genome in both epithelial argentochromaffic cells and macrophages (Griffin 1990). In addition profound degeneration of intrinsic jejunal autonomic neurones has been demonstrated but the functional significance of this denervation is as yet unknown.

Anal and rectal disease in HIV

Examination should be carried out with good illumination and the use of an illuminated anoscope. Sigmoidoscopy may also be necessary. An adequate level of anaesthesia should be provided for the procedures involved and appropriate protection provided for all operative staff. The position, size, and depth of all ulceration should be noted. Investigations on samples taken from ulcers should include dark ground microscopy, virus cultures for herpes simplex virus, and CMV, India ink staining for *Cryptococcus neoformans*, staining and culture for mycobacteria. Biopsies should be taken of ulcers for histology. Pre-operative assessment as to the clinical stage of disease should include full blood picture, serum albumin, serum protein, T4 lymphocyte count, T4/T8 ratio, coagulation studies, and chest X-ray. Procedures on extensively ulcerated, infected, and abscess lesions should be covered with antibiotic therapy. Anal manometry can be used to assess suitability if lateral sphincterotomy is contemplated.

The onset of constitutional symptoms (CDC IVA) previously referred to as the AIDS-related complex (ARC) often precedes an imminent AIDS-defining condition. Features include fever, night sweats, diarrhoea for which no infective cause is found, weight loss, lymphadenopathy, hepatosplenomegaly, oral candida, and oral hairy leucoplakia. These patients will often have skin and oral mani-

Anorectal surgery in HIV disease

The results of early surgical series gave depressing results. Of 51 patients undergoing 73 procedures including biopsy, incision and drainage of abscesses, sphincterotomy, fistulotomy, and haemorrhoidectomy, wound healing took place in only 12% under 1 month, a further 12% at 1–6 months and over 6 months 13%. Forty-three per cent of patients had died within 6 months, mostly with unhealed wounds (Wexner *et al.* 1986). Similar early poor results were reported by other authors (Moening *et al.* 1990; Wolokomir *et al.* 1990). With improved antiviral therapy and more accurate staging, diagnosis and treatment, Schmitt and Wexner have subsequently reported a much improved healing rate following anorectal procedures (Schmitt *et al.* 1993). This improved outcome has been confirmed in other studies (Carr *et al.* 1989; Safavi *et al.* 1991).

Anal fissure

The commonest cause of anal ulceration in HIV disease is a typical benign fissure (Figure 4.40) as described for non-HIV infected persons (Gottesman 1995). The fissures are usually located in the anteroposterior ventral axis of the anus. Fissures, like lesions at other sites, should be carefully assessed for other aetiologies. Benign fissures have been attributed to hypertonicity of the internal anal sphincter and often associated with the passage of hard stools (Northmann and Schuster 1974) but in HIV positive persons they are commonly seen in patients with chronic diarrhoea. Fissures located posteriorly may be the result of anoreceptive intercourse or chronic diarrhoea. The association with diarrhoea may affect the decision to carry out internal spincterotomy as it may result in incontinence in those with chronic diarrhoea. In an early series of patients operated on for anorectal disease, eight patients had a sphincterotomy, all of whom had some degree of incontinence postoperatively (Wexner *et al.* 1986). Treatment should be with bulking agents and topical anaesthetics. Open lateral internal sphincterotomy is recommended in the event that these measures fail.

Fistulo in ano and abscesses

Fistulo-in-ano and ischiorectal abscesses are commonly seen in HIV positive patients. Fistulo-in-ano have been classified into four types based on their complexity (Parks *et al.* 1976). In his review of the subject in HIV positive patients, Gingold (1991) has found that complex fistula and more extensive abscess formation are more common in HIV disease. He describes the HIV positive patient with an ischiorectal abscess as a true surgical emergency because of the risks of septicaemia, Fournier's gangrene, and other septic complications, making immediate drainage essential. He recommends a simple catheter drainage using a 10 Fr mushroom catheter for uncomplicated abscesses but for more complicated ones, multiple looped Penrose drains are recommended. For supralevator abscesses, a 12 Fr Pezzer catheter inserted through the levator ani musculae and brought out through the perianal skin is recommended. Extra sphincteric tracts can be drained by heavy silk setons tied loosely. If the internal opening of the process can be identified, he recommends that the proximal 1 cm of the tract is unroofed and this can avoid the need for a separate fistulotomy at a later date. The procedures should be covered with broad-spectrum antibiotics and culture of the pus taken at operation sent for identification of organisms and sensitivities. Antibiotics should be continued until induration resolves which should hopefully be within 2–3 weeks.

Herpes virus infections

Evidence of HSV infection has been found in up to 95% of homosexual men with AIDS (Nerurkar *et al.* 1983; Rogers *et al.* 1983); hence ulceration due to HSV has been observed commonly in persons with HIV disease. Perianal ulceration may show typical discrete ulcers but often lesions are coalescent and persistent (Siegal *et al.* 1981) (Figure 4.41), but extensive ulceration of the anal canal does not seem to occur (Gottesman 1995). Proctitis and ulceration may occur with involvement of the rectum and distal colon being seen. These may be accompanied by anorectal pain, tenesmus, constipation, inguinal adenopathy, urinary retention, and sacral paraesthesia. Diagnosis should be by biopsy and viral culture.

CMV has been described as causing perianal ulcers (Horn and Hood 1990).

Non-specific ulceration and AIDS

AIDS specific ulcers are described as occurring more in the proximal anal canal and are longer and wider than benign fissures. These

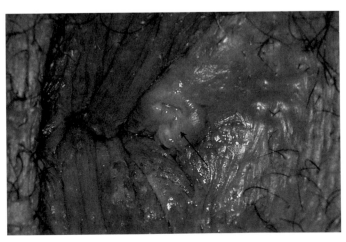

Figure 4.40 Benign anal fissure in HIV disease (arrowed).

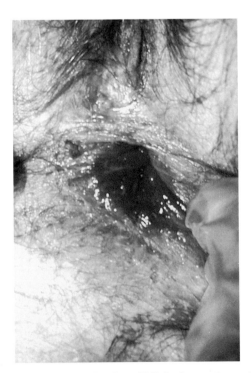

Figure 4.41 HSV ulceration of anal canal initially diagnosed as anal fissure.

lesions may erode across all mucosal and sphincteric planes into the superficial and deep post-anal spaces. Pain occurs secondary to the fissure formation and the pressure of the collection of pus and stool in the cavities produced, which are usually single and in the posterior quadrant of the anus. The aetiology of these lesions is as yet unknown, although HIV has been implicated (Gottesman 1995). Gottesman has recommended operative debridement of the ulcer with marsupialization and intralesional injection of a depo-steroid preparation (80 mg/ml). This procedure gave significant pain relief in 95% of 30 patients treated thus. If there is severe erosive ulceration associated with faecal incontinence, consideration should be given to performing a diverting colostomy to provide relief and aid healing.

Other causes of ulceration

Other causes of anorectal ulceration described include *M. tuberculosis*, that can be the cause of superficial ulceration which is described as circumferential with the long axis perpendicular to the lumen. Only 10–40% of these patients will have a positive PPD test (Chaisson *et al.* 1987). The diagnosis is best made by culture and biopsy. *Entamoeba histolytica* is an occasional cause of ulceration and a few cases of ulceration due to *C. neoformans* have been described. The possibility of primary syphilitic ulceration should always be borne in mind and specimens should be taken for dark ground microscopy from any suspicious lesions. Serological tests for syphilis may be negative at this stage.

Human papilloma virus (HPV) infection and anal cancer in HIV disease

It has been recognized that homosexual men are more likely to manifest warts perianally than on the penis (Oriel 1971). HPV infection of the anal canal is detected more commonly in HIV-positive homosexual men than in those who are HIV negative (Caussy *et al.* 1990). This may be due to loss of immune control and hence greater replication rather than a higher incidence of infection. Detection of anal HPV is also seen to be increased in HIV-positive women (Williams *et al.* 1994). The presence of anal warts in HIV-positive persons presents a number of problems. Treatment with podophyllin is best avoided in view of concerns that it may promote malignant transformation (Wade and Ackerman 1984). It has been recommended that in CDC stage II disease, debulking using cryotherapy, electrocautery or excision is used and that relapses are controlled with these methods (Scholefield and Northover 1991). Relapse is extremely common and total eradication is unlikely. In CDC stage IV disease, lesions are often widespread and delayed, wound healing has been noted (Croxon *et al.* 1984), although more recently improved results have been achieved with surgery.

As for carcinoma of the cervix, a strong link has been established between the detection of HPV types 16 and 18 and the finding of dysplasia in the anal canal. In those with HIV disease, dysplasia has been found in 29% in the anal canal (Crook *et al.* 1992) and men with CDC stage IV disease have been found to have an exceedingly high prevalence of HPV DNA detected and abnormal anal cytology (Palefsky *et al.* 1990). The natural history of these lesions is not as yet known but an increased incidence of squamous cell carcinoma of the anus in men with AIDS has been confirmed (Melbye *et al.* 1993), being found to be 40 times greater than the general population and this has led to the suggestion that screening of both men and women who are at increased risk of anal intraepithelial neoplasia

should be considered (Palefsky 1994). Further investigation of abnormal cytology can be performed with the application of 5% acetic acid to the anal canal and examining the area with a colposcope. Suspicious lesions should be biopsied. It has been recommended that medium- or high-grade dysplastic lesions or anal intraepithelial neoplasia (AIN) grades II or III are treated with excision biopsy and electrocautery (Palefsky 1994). In the event of malignant transformation radiotherapy is the recommended treatment.

Kaposi's sarcoma (KS)

KS is a tumour probably of vascular endothelial origin commonly seen in patients with AIDS. It is more frequent, not only in HIV-positive homosexual men but also in those who are HIV negative, and this has led to speculation that it may have an infective aetiology, possibly a sexually transmitted virus (Friedman-Kien *et al.* 1990). A newly identified human herpesvirus type 8 has recently been described as having a possible aetiological role in KS. Although more commonly seen in T-helper cell depleted patients KS can occur at any stage of HIV disease.

Flexible sigmoidoscopy of the GI tract of 50 AIDS patients with nodular cutaneous KS lesions revealed KS-like lesions in 40%, although not all were confirmed on biopsy (Saltz *et al.* 1984). This may be because the lesions are submucosal and the biopsies taken were not deep enough to sample the lesion (Friedman *et al.* 1985). KS is commonly found on autopsy in the GI tract in persons dying of AIDS (Friedman *et al.* 1985), although lesions are usually asymptomatic. Digital examination of the anus and rectum may reveal KS lesions but small lesions of the large bowel will not be seen on barium studies, although larger ones may be seen as target lesions with central umbilicated ulceration (Cello 1988). Very occasionally GI haemorrhage, perforation, or obstruction have been reported, necessitating acute surgical intervention. Asymptomatic GI lesions do not need treatment. Large symptomatic lesions of the GI tract have been treated successfully with Nd/YAG laser photocoagulation (Metroka and Vallejo 1991).

Non-Hodgkin's lymphoma

There is an increased incidence of non-Hodgkin's lymphoma (NHL) in patients with AIDS usually when there is severe CD4 helper cell depletion. GI tract NHL may present in a non-specific fashion with unexplained fever, night sweats, and weight loss and should be thought of in the context of HIV disease. More specific symptoms of GI tract bleeding, bowel obstruction, perirectal ulceration, or abscess formation may occur. Organomegaly with or without ascites may be seen (Smith *et al.* 1992). A rise in serum lactic dehydrogenase and uric acid may be clues to the diagnosis. Further investigation using endoscopy with biopsy, CT scan, gallium scan, and biopsy of enlarged nodes are indicated. Aggressive chemotherapy has given poor results to date but subsets may have a better prognosis. Evaluation and management should be by a specialist unit (Mayer and Wanke 1994).

Other tumours

A possible association with AIDS has been noted for adenocarcinoma of the colon and rectum and also Hodgkin's disease.

Large bowel disease

In patients with AIDS in the Western world, 30–50% are reported to have diarrhoeal illnesses. This rises to 90% in developing countries (Smith *et al.* 1992). A careful clinical history of symptoms and signs will be helpful in differentiating small and large bowel disease. Diarrhoea associated with large bowel disease is characteristically small volume, frequent and regular, associated with pain, fever and bloody or mucoid stools and an increase in faecal leucocytes may be seen (Mayer and Wanke 1994). Pathogens associated with large bowel diarrhoea may also cause disease of the small bowel. Bacterial causes include *Salmonella*, *Shigella*, *Campylobacter*, *M. tuberculosis*, and *Mycobacterium avium intracellulare* and these organisms may be associated with a bacteraemia indicating the need for blood cultures on investigations. Protozoans such as *G. lamblia* and *E. histolytica* are not found more commonly in HIV disease in homosexual men. *Cryptosporidia* is usually associated with small bowel disease in severely immunocompromised patients (Nime *et al.* 1976) but has been described as causing colitis (Connolly *et al.* 1988). Other significant protozoans causing diarrhoea in HIV disease are microsporidium, cyclospora, and isospora, which are usually associated with small bowel disease. Endemic mycoses of histoplasmosis and coccidoidomycosis may be causes of diarrhoea in the USA and South America. The most significant virus infection of the large bowel in late HIV disease is CMV. CMV is a cause of colitis with ulceration (Figure 4.42) and inflammation seen on sig-

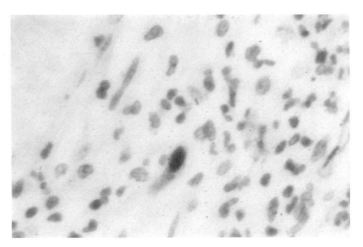

Figure 4.44 Immunohistochemical staining showing characteristic owl's eye inclusion of cytomegalovirus.

moidoscopy or colonoscopy. As the identification of CMV in stools, urine, and blood is common in late HIV disease, the diagnosis needs to be confirmed by histology of biopsy material (Figures 4.43 and 4.44). In a review of 55 HIV-infected patients with diarrhoea on initial colonoscopy, ulcerative or inflammatory lesions were found in nine (16%) of the patients. Colonic cultures for CMV were positive in 15 (27%) but histological confirmation was obtained in only four (7%) of patients. Treatment for CMV has been limited to intravenous therapy with ganciclovir or foscarnet with the need for long-term maintenance in relapsing cases. Recently, an oral preparation of ganciclovir has become available in the UK. Many patients have diarrhoea secondary to their medication and this should be reviewed. Patients on antibiotic therapy may develop diarrhoea due to *C. difficile*.

Investigation of large bowel disease should commence with stool examination for faecal leucocytes, *C. difficile* toxin, bacteriological, and parasitological studies. Up to six stool specimens may need to be sent for investigations. Furthermore, investigation should include rigid sigmoidoscopy with biopsy, colonoscopy with biopsy and double contrast barium enema (DCBE), and blood cultures. A series of 58 CDC stage IV patients with a history of diarrhoea over 1 month who had investigations of stools, sigmoidoscopy, colonoscopy, and DCBE performed, sigmoidoscopy provided a diagnosis in 31 patients. No extra information was provided by DCBE and only one extra diagnosis by colonoscopy (Connolly *et al.* 1990). DCBE was seen to miss four of six patients with KS and seven of 10 patients with CMV. A more aggressive approach to diagnosis has been advocated (Smith *et al.* 1992) but the cost-effectiveness of such an approach has been questioned (Johanson *et al.* 1990). A useful algorithm approach to the diagnosis of diarrhoea has been described (Mayer and Wanke 1994).

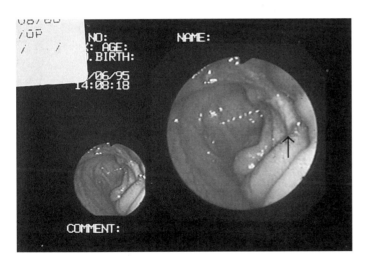

Figure 4.42 Cytomegalovirus ulceration of colon on sigmoidoscopy (arrowed). (See colour plates).

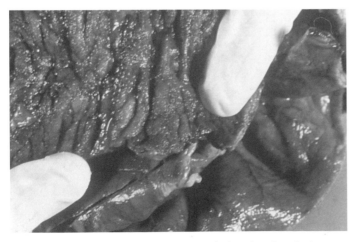

Figure 4.43 Autopsy specimen of cytomegalovirus ulceration of colon.

References

Aral SO, Holmes KK. Epidemiology of sexual behaviour and sexually transmitted diseases. In: Holmes KK, Mardh P-A, Sparling PF, Wiesner PJ, eds. *Sexually transmitted diseases.* New York: McGraw-Hill, 1990: 19–36.

Armstrong D, Crowe G, Dinsmore W, Maw R. Relation of anal warts to anal sexual practices. *Venereology* 1994; 7: 110–12.

Barbour D, Nayyar K, Phillips J, Barron J. Diagnosis of gonorrhoea in women. *Br. J. Vener. Dis.* 1976; 52: 326–8.

Barin F, M'Boup S, Denis F, *et al*. Serological evidence for virus-related to Simian T lymphotrophic retrovirus III in residents of West Africa. *Lancet* 1985; ii: 1387–9.

Battacharya MN, Jepphcot AE. Diagnosis of gonorrhoea in women. Role of rectal sample. *Br. J. Vener. Dis.* 1974; 50: 109–12.

Blackmore CA. An outbreak of chancroid in Orange County, California: descriptive epidemiology and disease control measures. *J. Infect. Dis.* 1985; 151: 840–44.

Bowie WR. Urethritis in males. In: Holmes KK, Mardh P-A, Sparling PF, Wiesner PJ, eds. *Sexually transmitted diseases*. New York: McGraw Hill, 1990: 627–39.

Brown ST, Zaidi A, Filker R. Sensitivity and specificity of diagnostic tests for genital infections with herpes virus hominis. *Sexual Transm. Dis.* 1979; 6: 10–13.

Carr ND, Mercey D, Slack WW. Non-condylomatous perianal disease in homosexual men. *Br. J. Surg.* 1989; 76: 1064–8.

Castro BA, Cheng-Mayer C, Evans LA, *et al*. HIV heterogeneity and viral pathogenesis. *AIDS* 1988; 2: S17–27.

Cates W Jr. Sexually transmitted organisms and infertility: the proof of the pudding. *Sex Transm. Dis.* 1984; 11: 113–6.

Caussy D, Goedert JJ, Palefsky J, *et al*. Interaction of human immunodeficiency and papilloma viruses: association with anal epithelial abnormality in homosexual men. *Int. J. Cancer* 1990; 46: 214–19.

Cello JP. Gastrointestinal tract manifestations of AIDS. Management of HIV infections and their complications. *Infect. Dis. Clin. North Am.* 1988; 2: 387–96.

Centers for Disease Control and Prevention. Classification system for human T-lymphotropic virus type III/lymphadenopathy associated virus infection. *MMWR* 1986; 35: 334–9.

Centers for Disease Control and Prevention. Revision of the CDC surveillance case definition for acquired immunodeficiency syndrome. *MMWR* 1987; 36: 1–15S.

Centers for Disease Control and Prevention: Guidelines for prevention of transmission of human immunodeficiency virus and hepatitis B virus to health care and public safety workers *MMWR* 1989: 38 (No. S6); 3–37.

Centers for Disease Control and Prevention. Revised classification system for HIV infection and expanded surveillance definition for AIDS among adolescents and adults. *MMWR* 1992; 41 (RR-17): 1–19.

Centers for Disease Control and Prevention. *Sexually Transmitted Disease Surveillance 1993 Division of STD/HIV Prevention*. Centers for Disease Control and Prevention, Atlanta, USA, December 1994.

Chadburn A, Metroka C, Mouradian J. Progressive lymph node histology and its prognostic value in patients with acquired immunodeficiency syndrome and AIDS-related complex. *Hum. Pathol.* 1989; 20: 579–87.

Chaisson RE, Schecter GF, Theucr CP, *et al*. Tuberculosis in patients with the acquired immunodeficiency syndrome: clinical features, response to therapy and survival. *Ann. Rev. Respir. Dis.* 1987; 136: 570–4.

Chippenfield EJ, Catterall RD. Reappraisal of gram staining and culture techniques for the diagnosis of gonorrhoea in women. *Br. J. Vener. Dis.* 1976; 52: 36–9.

Classification system for human T-lymphotropic virus type II/lymphadenopathy—associated virus infections. *MMWR* 1986; 35: 34.

Communicable Disease Report HMSO, London 1995; Vol. 5, No. 3: 13–16.

Connolly GM, Dryden MS, Shanson DC, Gazzard BG. Cryptosporidial diarrhoea in AIDS and its treatment. *Gut* 1988; 29: 593–7.

Connolly GM, Forbes A, Gleeson JA, Gazzard BG. The value of barium enema and colonoscopy in patients infected with HIV. *AIDS* 1990; 4: 687–9.

Corey L, Adams HG, Brown ZA, Holmes KK. Genital herpes simplex virus infections: clinical manifestations, course and complications. *Ann. Intern. Med.* 1993; 98: 958–72.

Crook T, Wrede D, Tidy JA, Mason WP, Evans DJ, Vousden KH. Clonal p53 mutation in primary cervical cancer: association with human-papillomavirus-negative tumours. *Lancet* 1992; 339: 1070–3.

Croxon T, Chabon AB, Rorat E, Barash IM. Intraepithelial carcinoma of the anus in homosexual men. *Dis. Colon Rectum* 1984; 27: 325–30.

Csonka GW. Non gonococcal urethritis and post gonoccocal urethritis. In: *Sexually transmitted diseases—a textbook of genitourinary medicine*. Bates JK, Csonka GW (Eds) Baillière Tindall, London 1990: 40–51.

Davies PM, Weatherburn P, Hunt AJ, Hickson FC, McManus TJ, Coxon AP. The sexual behaviour of young gay men in England and Wales. *AIDS Care* 1992; 4: 259–72.

Davis CM. Granuloma inguinale: a clinical, histological and ultrastructural study. *JAMA* 1970; 211: 632–6.

de Villiers EM. Heterogeneity of the human papillomavirus group. *J. Virol.* 1989; 63: 4898–903.

DH Statistics Division 2B 1994. *New cases seen at Genito Urinary Medicine Clinics in England; 1993.* Annual figures: summary of information from Form KC60. HMSO, London.

Drusin LM, Singer C, Valenti AJ, Armstrong D. The role of surgery in primary syphilis of the anus. *Ann. Surg.* 1976; 184: 65–7.

Drusin LM, Singer C, Valenti AJ, Armstrong D. Infectious syphilis mimicking neoplastic disease. *Arch. Intern. Med.* 1977; 137: 156–60.

Evans BA. Detection of gonorrhoea in women. *Br. J. Vener. Dis.* 1976; 52: 40–2.

Evans BG, Catchpole MA, Heptonstall J, *et al*. Sexually transmitted diseases and HIV-1 infection among homosexual men in England and Wales. *Br. Med. J.* 1993; 306: 426–8.

Fahey JL, Taylor JMG, Detels R, *et al*. The prognostic value of cellular and serologic markers in infection with human immunodeficiency virus type 1. *N. Engl. J. Med.* 1990; 322: 166–72.

Friedman SL, Wright TL, Altman DF. Gastrointestinal Kaposi's sarcoma in patients with acquired immunodeficiency syndrome—endoscopic and autopsy findings. *Gastroenterology* 1985; 89: 102.

Friedman-Kien AE, Saltzman BL, Cao Y, Niestor MS, Mirabile M, Li J. Kaposi's sarcoma in HIV-negative homosexual men. *Lancet* 1990; i: 168–9.

Gerberding JL. *Limiting the risks of health care workers. The medical management of AIDS.* WB Saunders, Philadelphia: 1995: 89–99.

Gerberding JL, Littell C, Karkington A, *et al*. Risk of exposure of surgical personnel to patients' blood during surgery at San Francisco General Hospital. *N. Engl. J. Med.* 1990; 322: 1788–93

Gingold BS. Anal and perianal sepsis. In: *Anorectal disease in AIDS*. Edward Arnold, London. 1991: 130–40.

Goodell SE, Quinn TC, Mkrtichian E, *et al*. Herpes simplex virus proctitis in homosexual men. Clinical, sigmoidoscopic and histopathological features. *N. Engl. J. Med.* 1983; 308: 868–71.

Gottesman L. Ulcerative disease of the anorectum in AIDS. *Int. J. STD AIDS* 1995; 6: 4–6.

Gottlieb M, Schroff R, Schanker H, *et al*. *Pneumocystis carinii* pneumonia and mucosal candidiasis in previously healthy homosexual men. *N. Engl. J. Med.* 1981; 305: 1425–31.

Handley J, Dinsmore WW, Maw R, *et al*. Anogenital warts in pre-pubertal children: sexual abuse or not? *Int. J. STD AIDS* 1993; 4: 271–9.

Heptonstall J, Porter K, Gill ON. *Occupational transmission of HIV. Summary of published reports—September 1993*. Internal report of the PHLS, available from PHLS AIDS Centre at CDSC.

Ho David D, Neumann Avidan U, Perelson Alan S, *et al*. Rapid turnover of plasma virions and CD4 lymphocytes in HIV-1 infection. *Nature* 1995; 373: 123–6.

Hollander H, Greenspan D, Stringari S, *et al*. Hairy leukoplakia and the acquired immunodeficiency syndrome. *Ann. Intern. Med.* 1986; 104: 892–7.

Holmes KK, Johnson DW, Trostle HJ. An estimate of men acquiring gonorrhoea by sexual contact with infected females. *Am. J. Epidemiol.* 1970; 91: 170–4.

Hook EW, Marra CM. Acquired syphilis in adults. *N. Engl. J. Med.* 1992; 326: 1060–9.

Horn TD, Hood AF. Cytomegalovirus is predictably present in perineal ulcers from immunosuppressed patient. *Arch. Dermatol.* 1990; 126: 642–4.

Huminer D Rosenfeld JB, Pitlick SD. AIDS in the pre-AIDS era. *Rev. Infect. Dis.* 1987; 9: 1102–8.

Johanson JF, Sonnenberg A. Efficient management of diarrhoea in the acquired immunodeficiency syndrome (AIDS). *Ann. Intern. Med.* 1990; 112: 942–8.

Johnson SR, Martin DH, Cammarata C, Morse SA. Development of a polymerase chain reaction assay for the detection of *Haemophilis ducreyi*. *Sex. Transm. Dis.* 1994; 21: 13–23.

Johnston RE, Nahmias AJ, Magder LS, *et al.* A sero-epidemiological survey of prevalence of herpes simplex virus type 2 infection in the United States. *N. Engl. J. Med.* 1989; 321: 7–12.

Joseph AK, Rosen T. Laboratory techniques used in the diagnosis of chancroid, granuloma inguinale, and lymphogranuloma venereum. *Dermatol. Clin.* 1994; 12: 1–8.

Kraus SJ, Stone KM. Management of genital infection caused by human papilloma virus. *Rev. Infect. Dis.* 1990; 12: 620–32.

Kraus SJ, Weisman BJ, Budde JW, Limpakarnjanarat K, Rigau-Perez J, *et al.* Pseudogranuloma inguinale caused by *Haemophilus ducreyi*. *Arch. Dermatol.* 1982; 118: 494–7.

Lafferty WE, Coombs RJ, Benedetti J, *et al.* Recurrences after oral and genital herpes infections and viral type. *N. Engl. J. Med.* 1989; 3016: 1444–9.

Lantos PL, McLaughlin JE, Scholtz CL, Berry CL, Tighe JR. Neuropathology of the brain in HIV infection. *Lancet* 1989; i: 309–11.

Lee HH, Charnesky MA, Schacter J, *et al.* Diagnosis of *Chlamydia trachomatis* in women by ligase chain reaction assay of urine. *Lancet* 1995; 345: 213–16.

Leentvaar-Kuijpers A, Keemanjn Dekker E, *et al.* HIV: occupational risk of surgical specialists and operation room personnel in the St Lucas Hospital in Amsterdam. *Ned. Tijdschr. Geneeskd.* 1988; 133: 2388–91.

Lehrman N, Douglas JM, Corey L, Barry DW. Recurrent genital herpes and suppressive oral acyclovir therapy: relationship between clinical outcome and invitro drug sensitivity. *Ann. Intern. Med.* 1986; 104: 786–90.

Levin I. Lymphogranuloma venereum, rectal stricture and carcinoma. *Dis. Colon Rectum* 1964; 7: 129.

Marino AWM. Proctologic lesions observed in male homosexuals. *Dis. Colon Rectum* 1964; 7: 121.

Martin DH, Di Carlo RP. Recent changes in the epidemiology of genital ulcer disease in the United States. The crack cocaine connection. *Sex. Transm Dis.* 1994; 21: S76–80.

Masur H, Michelis MA, Greene JB, *et al.* An outreach of community acquired *Pneumocystis carinii* pneumonia: initial manifestation of cellular immune dysfunction. *N. Engl. J. Med.* 1981; 305: 1431–8.

Maw RD. Don't forget syphilis. *Ulster Med. J.* 1981; 50: 132–6.

Mayer HB, Wanke CA. Diagnostic strategies in HIV-infected patients with diarrhoea. *AIDS* 1994; 8: 1639–48.

McLean KA. (ed) Homosexually acquired sexually transmitted diseases. *Sexually transmitted diseases: a textbook of genitourinary medicine.* Baillière Tindall, London 1990: 322–9.

Melbye M, Cote T, Biggar RJ, Rabkin C. High incidence of anal cancer among AIDS patients. *X International Conference on AIDS, Berlin, June 1993* (abstract PO-B14-1636).

Mertz GJ, Benedetti J, Ashley R, *et al.* Risk factors for the sexual transmission of genital herpes. *Ann. Intern. Med.* 1992; 116: 197–202.

Metroka CE, Vallejo A. Anorectal neoplasia. In: ed. *Anorectal disease in AIDS.* Edward Arnold, London 1991: 154–66.

Miles AJF, Allen Mersh TG, Wastell C. Effect of ano-receptive intercourse on anal function. *J. R. Soc. Med.* 1993; 86: 144–7.

Moening S, Simonton C, Huber P, *et al.* Presentation and treatment of anorectal disorders in the HIV+/AIDS patient. Presented at the Annual Meeting of the American Society of Colon and Rectal Surgeons, St Louis, MO: April 29–May 4, 1990.

Morse SA, Moreland AA, Thompson SE. In: *Atlas of sexually transmitted disease.* JB Lippincott, Crown Medical Publishing, London 1989: 5–7.

Nerurkar L, Goedert J, Wallen W, *et al.* Study of antiviral antibodies in sera of homosexual men. *J. Fed. Proc.* 1983; 42: 6109.

Nime FA, Burek JD, Page DL, Holscher MA, Yardley JH. Acute enterocolitis in a human being infected with the protozoan *Cryptosporodium*. *Gastroenterology* 1976; 70: 592–8.

Northmann BJ, Schuster MM. Internal anal sphincter derangement with anal fissures. *Gastroenterology* 1974; 67: 216–20.

Oates JK, Csonka GW. In: *Sexually transmitted diseases: a textbook of genitourinary medicine.* Baillière Tindall, London. 1990: 209–26.

Oriel JD. Anal warts and anal coitus. *Br. J. Vener. Dis.* 1971; 47: 373–6.

Oriel JD. Anogenital papillomavirus infection in children. *Br. Med. J.* 1988; 296: 1484–5.

Ou CY, Ciesielski CA, Myers G, *et al.* Molecular epidemiology of HIV transmission in a dental practice. *Science* 1992; 256: 1165–71.

Palefsky JM. Anal human papillomavirus infection and anal cancer in HIV-positive individuals: an emerging problem. *AIDS* 1994; 8: 283–95.

Palefsky JM, Gonzales J, Greenblatt RM, Ahn DK, Hollander H. Anal intraepithelial neoplasia and anal papillomavirus infection among homosexual males with group IV HIV disease. *JAMA* 1990; 263: 2911–16.

Pannuti CS, Cristina M, Finck DS, Grimbaun RS, Sumita LM, Almeida AL, Rezende NF, Gomes MP, Pinho JR, Kirchhoff LV. Asymptomatic perianal shedding of herpes simplex virus in patients with acquired immunodeficiency syndrome. *Arch. Dermatol.* 1997; 133: 180–3.

Parks AG, Gordon PH, Hardcastle JD. A classification of fistulae-in-ano. *Br. J. Surg.* 1976; 63: 1–12.

Pedersen C, Getstoft J, Lindhardt BO, Sindrup J. Candida esophagitis associated with acute human immunodeficiency virus infection. *J. Infect. Dis.* 1987; 156: 529–30.

Pedersen C, Lindhardt BO, Jensen BL, *et al.* Clinical course of primary HIV infection: Consequences for subsequent course of infection. *Br. Med. J.* 1989; 299: 154–7.

Perine PL, Osoba AO. Lymphogranuloma venereum. In: Holmes KK, Mardh P-A, Sparling PF, Wiesner PJ, eds. *Sexually transmitted diseases.* New York: McGraw-Hill, 1990: 195–204.

Plummer FA, Simonsen JN, Cameron DW, *et al.* Other STDs enhancing transmission of HIV co-factors in the male/female transmission of human immunodeficiency virus 1. *J. Infect. Dis.* 1991; 163: 233–9.

Quinn TC, Goodell SE, Mkrtichian E, Schuffler MD, Wang SP, Stamm WE, Holmes KK. *Chlamydia trachomatis* proctitis *N. Engl. J. Med.* 1981; 305: 195–200.

Robert L, Marcus R, Kuch B, *et al.* Update: evaluating the risk of HIV transmission from health care workers to patients. In: *Programme and Abstracts of the Ninth International Conference on AIDS: June 7–11, 1993.* Berlin, Germany Abstract W S-C12–4.

Robertson DHH, McMillan A, Young H. *Clinical practice in sexually transmissible diseases.* Pitman Medical, London. 1980: 377–83.

Rogers MF, Morens DM, Stewart JA, *et al.* National case control study of Kaposi's sarcoma and *Pneumocystic carinii* pneumonia in homosexual men. 2: Laboratory results. *Ann. Intern. Med.* 1983; 99: 151–8.

Rolfs RT, Allyn K, Nakashima MD. Epidemiology of primary and secondary syphilis in the United States, 1981 through 1989. *JAMA* 1990a; 264: 1432–7.

Rolfs RT, Goldberg M, Sharrar RG. Risk factors for syphilis; cocaine use and prostitution. *Am. J. Public Health* 1990b; 80: 853–7.

Safavi A, Gottesman L, Dailey TH. Anorectal surgery in the HIV+ patient: an update. *Dis. Colon Rectum* 1991; 34: 299–304.

Saltz RK, Kurtz RC, Lightdale CJ, *et al.* Kaposi's sarcoma—gastrointestinal involvement correlation with skin findings and immunologic function. *Dig. Dis. Sci.* 1984; 29: 817.

Samarasinghe PL, Oates JK, MacLennan IP. Herpetic proctitis and sacral radiculomyelopathy—a hazard for homosexual men. *Br. Med. J.* 1979; 2: 365–6.

Sangeorzan JA, Bradley SF, He X, *et al.* Epidemiology of oral candidiasis in HIV-infected patients: colonization, infection, treatment, and emergence of fluconazole resistance. *Am. J. Med.* 1994; 97: 339–46.

Schachter J. Lymphogranuloma venereum and other nonocular *Chlamydia trachomatis* infections, In: Hobson D, Holmes KK, eds. *Nongonococcal urethritis and related infections.* Washington: American Society for Microbiology, 1977: 91–7.

Schmid GP, Scholle WO, De Witt WE. *Atlas of sexually transmitted diseases.* J.B. Lippincott, Philadelphia. 1989: 3.1–3.16.

Schmitt SL, Wexner SD, Nogueras JJ, Jagelman DG. Is aggressive management of perianal ulcers in homosexual HIV-seropositive men justified? *Dis. Colon Rectum* 1993; 36: 240–6.

Scholefield JH, Northover JMA. In: , ed. *Anorectal disease in AIDS.* Edward Arnold, London. 1991: 141–53.

Sheldon WH, Heyman A. Studies on chancroid; 1—Observations on the histology with an evaluation of biopsy as a diagnostic procedure. *Am. J. Pathol.* 1946; 22: 415.

Siegal FP, Lopez C, Hammer GS, Brown AE, Kornfield SJ, Gold J, *et al.* Severe acquired immunodeficiency in male homosexuals manifested by chronic perianal ulcerative herpes simplex lesions. *N. Engl. J. Med.* 1981; 305: 1439–44.

Smith PD, Quinn TC, Strober W, Janoff EN, Masur H. Gastrointestinal infections in AIDS. *Ann. Intern. Med.* 1992; 116: 63–77.

Sonnex C, Scholefield JH, Kocjan G, *et al.* Anal human papillomavirus infection in heterosexuals with genital warts: prevalence and relation with sexual behaviour. *Br. Med. J.* 1991; 303: 1243.

Stamm WE, Holmes KK. *Chlamydia trachomatis* infections of the adult. In: Holmes KK, Mardh P-A, Sparling PF, Wiesner PJ, eds. *Sexually transmitted diseases.* New York: McGraw-Hill, 1990: 181–93.

Syrjanen KJ. Natural history of genital human papilloma virus infection papilloma virus. *Report* 1990; 1: 1–5.

Tayal SC, Pattman RS. High prevalence of herpes simplex virus type 1 in female anogenital herpes simplex in Newcastle on Tyne 1982–92. *Int. J. STD AIDS* 1994; 5: 359–61.

Tokars JI, Marcus R, Culver DH, *et al.* Surveillance of human immunodeficiency virus infection and zidovudine use among health care workers after exposure to HIV infected blood: the CDC Co-operative Needlestick Group. *Ann. Intern. Med.* 1993; 118: 913–19.

Vento S, Di Perri G, Garofano T, *et al. Pneumocystis carinii* pneumonia during primary HIV-1 infection. *Lancet* 1993; 342: 24–5.

Von Krogh G, Rylander E. *Genitoanal papilloma virus infection. A survey for the clinician.* Karlstad, Sweden: Conpharm/Kabi, 1989: 69–123.

Wade TR, Ackerman AB. The effects of resin of podophyllin on condyloma accuminatum. *Am. J. Dermatopathol.* 1984; 6: 109–22.

Waugh MA. Azithromycin in sexually transmitted diseases—an overview. *Int. J. STD AIDS* 1991; 2: 246–7.

Wei Xiping, Ghosh Sajal K, Taylor Maria E, *et al.* Viral dynamics in human immunodeficiency virus type 1 infection. *Nature* 1995; 373: 117–22.

Wellings K, Field J, Johnson AM, Wadsworth J. *Sexual behaviour in Britain: the national survey of sexual attitudes and lifestyles.* Penguin Books, London. 1994: 133–77.

Wexner SD, Smithy WM, Milsom JW, Dailey TH. The surgical management of anorectal disease in AIDS and pre-AIDS patients. *Dis. Colon Rectum* 1986; 29: 719–23.

Williams AB, Darragh TM, Vranizan K, Ochia C, Moss AR, Palefsky JM. Anal and cervical human papillomavirus infection and risk of anal and cervical epithelial abnormalities in HIV infected women. *Am. J. Obstet. Gynecol.* 1994; 83: 205–11.

Williams DC, Felman, YM, Riccardi NB. The utility of anoscopy in the rapid diagnosis of asymptomatic anorectal gonnorrhoea in men. *Sex. Transm. Dis.* 1981; 8: 16–17.

Winklestein W, Lyman DM, Padian N, *et al.* Sexual practices and risk of infection by the human immunodeficiency virus. *JAMA* 1987; 257: 321–5.

Wolokomir AF, Barone JE, Hardy HW III, Cottone FJ. Abdominal and anorectal surgery and the acquired immune deficiency syndrome in heterosexual intravenous drug users. *Dis. Colon Rectum* 1990; 33: 267–70.

Zehnilman JM. Update on bacterial sexually transmitted disease. *Urol. Clin. North Am.* 1992; 19: 25–34.

5 Ulcerative colitis

Incidence

Ulcerative colitis indicates either macroscopic or microscopic inflammation and ulceration of the colon or rectum. The reported incidence is variable, which reflects the problem of correctly classifying inflammatory bowel disease on isolated colorectal biopsies (Hanauer 1996). Ulcerative colitis accounts for about 55% and Crohn's disease 35% of patients with inflammatory bowel disease. In 15% of cases the distinction between the two conditions is impossible with the clinical and pathological information available (Moum *et al*. 1997). Such cases are classified as 'indeterminate colitis'. About 20% of patients with inflammatory bowel disease discharged from hospital are therefore incorrectly coded, due to either incorrect initial clinical diagnosis or errors in entering the information into a database. In addition, epidemiological studies can underestimate the prevalence of inflammatory bowel disease by up to 30% (Mayberry *et al*. 1989).

Age and sex distribution

Ulcerative colitis displays a bimodal age distribution which is more marked in Caucasians than other ethnic groups (Probert *et al*. 1992). The peak incidence, accounting for 50% of first attacks, occurs in the 20 to 30-year-old age group. The incidence in this age group is 25 per 10^5 per year. Mean age at diagnosis is therefore about 30 years (Tysk and Jarnerot 1992), being slightly earlier in countries, such as Israel, with a younger general population. The second peak, representing 30% of initial presentations, occurs in those of over 50 years of age. The incidence in children ranges from 1 to 4 per 10^5 per year (Kirschner 1996). Patients who develop symptoms later in life are significantly more likely to be male, have proctosigmoiditis, liver involvement, a protracted initial course, shorter remission, and require steroids more frequently than those with a younger presentation. Suggestions that the complication and mortality rates are higher in those with late-onset disease have not been substantiated (Persson *et al*. 1996).

Reports from most countries suggest that at all ages females are more likely to be affected than males in a ratio of 3 to 2 (Tysk and Jarnerot 1992). The mean age at diagnosis is similar for males and females (Kvist *et al*. 1989).

Geographical and racial distribution

The occurrence of ulcerative colitis varies between countries and races (Table 5.1). Jews are among those most commonly affected but the incidence varies considerably even within the Jewish popu-

Table 5.1 Geographic variation in the incidence and prevalence of ulcerative colitis

	Incidence per 100 000	Prevalence per 100 000	Authors
Europe	1.5–25 (Average 10.5)	20–40	Langholz *et al*. 1992 Vucelic *et al*. 1991 Sola Lamoglia *et al*. 1992
	Higher in Northern than Southern Europe		Moum *et al*. 1996 Tragnone *et al*. 1996 Shivananda *et al*. 1996
United Kingdom			
Caucasians	6		Probert *et al*. 1992
Sikhs	16		Jayanthi *et al*. 1992
Hindus	11		Srivastava *et al*. 1992
Muslims	6		Primatesta and
Bangladeshis	1.3		Goldacre 1995
United States			
Whites	3		Haitt and Kaufman 1988
Non-whites	1.8		Stowe *et al*. 1990
Indians	2		Probert *et al*. 1990 Rajput *et al*. 1992
Japan	2	8–18	Yoshida and Murata 1990 Morita *et al*. 1995
Jews	6	60–120	
USA/Europe	11	95	Odes *et al*. 1989
Israel/Africa/ Asia	6	31	Niv and Abukasis 1991

lation. Reports from Western countries of a prevalence of 230 per 100 000 population and incidence of 15 per 100 000 per year probably reflect referral patterns to specialist units (Tysk and Jarnerot 1992). The prevalence in most European studies varies from 20 to 40 per 100 000 and incidence 1.5 to 7.5 per 100 000 per year (Table 5.1). Ulcerative colitis is extremely rare in the endogenous inhabitants of sub-Saharan Africa. In these developing countries the condition is more frequent in urbanized and well educated inhabitants, reflecting the situation in formerly developing countries of the 1960s.

Time trends

Most European studies show none, or only a slight, increase in the incidence of ulcerative colitis over the last 30 years (Srivastava *et al*.

1992; Stewenius *et al.* 1995). The slight increase is due to improved reporting or an increase in distal disease as the incidence of extensive and total colitis has remained stable (Tysk and Jarnerot 1992). In developing countries, however, there is a definite increase in incidence, related to Westernization of the population.

There is no apparent seasonal variation in the month of diagnosis of ulcerative colitis. However, 80% of relapses of the disease, significantly greater than expected, occur in the Autumn and Spring, relapses being less likely to occur in the summer months (Tysk and Jarnerot 1993, Moum *et al.* 1996).

Aetiology

Immune factors (Table 5.2)

Ulcerative colitis is associated with an altered immune response: type I (hypersensitivity), II (cytotoxicity), and III (immune complex) reactions being involved (Hanauer 1996). The synthesis of immunoglobulin is therefore increased throughout the colon in ulcerative colitis, the changes being more marked than those seen in Crohn's disease (Grzybowska and Kozlowski 1993). The type I reaction is evidenced by increased levels of immunoglobulin (IgE) associated with an accumulation of mast cells and eosinophils at the visible line of demarcation between normal and abnormal mucosa. Evidence that this represents an allergic response to an intestinal or circulating antigen is lacking; patients with ulcerative colitis have no greater incidence of atopic symptoms or C3 complement levels than controls. The synthesis of IgA from active colonic mucosa is up to twice that of normal individuals and is related to disease activity (Bischoff *et al.* 1997). Local IgG and IgM production are also increased, although the correlation with disease activity is variable. The increased production of IgG1 is derived from serum factors while the elevated mucosal IgG3 and IgG4 responses are thought to be characteristic of early disease.

Table 5.2 Aetiological factors in ulcerative colitis

Genetic	Positive family history in 10–20% of patients 15 times increased risk if first-degree relative with ulcerative colitis
Immune	Increase in IgE, IgG, and IgM Enhanced suppressor T-cell activity Altered eicosanoid (PGE$_2$, PGF$_2$ alpha) levels Reactive oxygen metabolite formation
Smoking	Cessation of smoking Risk of smoker to non-smoker = 0.5 : 1 Risk of stopping smoking to non-smoker = 3 : 1 Passive smoking protective
Bacterial	Pathogenic *Escherichia coli* Rarely *Mycobacterium paratuberculosis*
Diet	?allergy to milk proteins Coeliac disease Regular fast food consumption (4 times/week)
Psychological	Not proven Relapse at times of stress
Medications	Non-steroidal anti-inflammatory drugs

The elevated immunoglobulin levels in ulcerative colitis implies polyclonal T-cell activation. There is an alteration in mucosal T-cell function associated with impaired intrathymic T-cell maturation and enhanced suppressor T-cell activity in the peripheral blood. Interleukins and platelet-activating factor levels contribute to this abnormal T-cell proliferation and are related to disease activity (Izzo *et al.* 1992; Bioque *et al.* 1996; Wardle *et al.* 1996). The net effect is an alteration in the suppressor T lymphocytes (T8+ and T9+) and CD56+ cells affecting lymphokine-activated killer cell activity and immunoglobulin synthesis (Haruta *et al.* 1992, Bioque *et al.* 1996, Wardle *et al.* 1996). The local activation of these cells leads to a loss of the CD antigen expression, CD4 and CD8 occurring in 3% of those with ulcerative colitis, 60% of Crohn's disease and 80% of normal colons, respectively. This alteration in cytotoxic lymphocytes and decrease in CD antigen expression implies a weakness in mucosal defence mechanisms, which is related to disease activity and returns to normal after colectomy.

The trigger mechanism which initiates the immunological response in ulcerative colitis is unknown. Although circulating antigens to mucosa, neutrophils, or dietary factors have been implicated, definitive evidence for specific antigens is lacking (Colombel *et al.* 1992; Hibi *et al.* 1993). Some cases have been associated with rheumatoid arthritis, Hashimoto's thyroiditis, or Coombs' positive blood reactions following blood transfusion (Tartter *et al.* 1986). There is, however, no strong evidence that ulcerative colitis is an autoimmune disease, the normal alpha interferon levels being in marked contrast to those found in systemic autoimmune disorders such as systemic lupus erythematosus (Capobianchi *et al.* 1992).

There has been considerable interest in chemotactic mediators of the immune response in ulcerative colitis. The principal inflammatory mediators involved in ulcerative colitis are the eicosanoids, particularly prostaglandins E$_2$ and F$_2$ alpha, 15 hydroxy-eicosatetraenoic acid (HETE) and leukotriene B$_4$. 5-aminosalicylic acid (5-ASA) and dietary manipulation with fish oil alter eicosanoid production, resulting in clinical and histological improvement (Aslan and Triadafilopoulos *et al.* 1992; Stenson *et al.* 1992). These local mediators induce epithelial cell lipoxygenase to produce oxygen radicals which are important in allowing infiltration of the inflamed intestinal mucosa by myeloperoxidase containing activated neutrophils (Hibi *et al.* 1993). These neutrophils produce further superoxide radicals (nitric oxide) which, together with low molecular weight chelates derived from denatured haemoglobin and iron therapy, amplify the inflammatory response and subsequent mucosal damage (Babbs 1992; Rachmilewitz *et al.* 1995). Glycose aminoglycans contribute to the leak of protein and fluid, thrombosis and tissue remodelling (Murch *et al.* 1993). There are therefore self-perpetuating cycles of reactive oxygen metabolite formation, inflammation, and mucosal/vascular injury (Koizumi *et al.* 1992). An extension of the crypt abscesses, through direct membrane disruption, lipid peroxidation, generation of secondary toxic oxidants and uninhibited mucosal proliferation ensues (Babbs 1992). Chemotactic products of lipid peroxidation provide positive feedback to accelerate the inflammatory–oxidative process, leading to an acute exacerbation of the disease (Figure 5.1). Mucosal inflammation in ulcerative colitis is therefore related to an influx into the lamina propria of luminal macromolecules with toxic, antigenic, immune, and chemoattractive properties. Understanding of this pathway has recently opened up therapeutic possibilities (Babbs 1992).

Smoking

It is suggested that a history of current smoking offers protection against developing ulcerative colitis (Tysk and Jarnerot 1992,

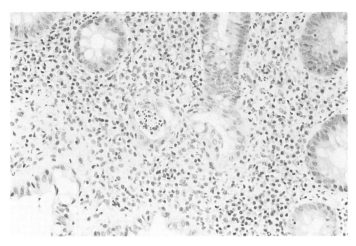

Figure 5.1 Active ulcerative colitis. There is inflammation of the colonic mucosa with crypt abscess formation. The mucosal glands are markedly distorted. H&E×100.

Koutroubakis *et al.* 1996). Only 27% of those with ulcerative colitis are current smokers, compared with 78% of those with Crohn's disease. The risk to a patient who has smoked of developing colitis relative to one who has never smoked is 0.5–0.8, the risk reducing progressively with increasing numbers of cigarettes smoked (Sandler *et al.* 1992). It is cessation of smoking that contributes to the development of colitis, the risk for ex-smokers being greater than for non-smokers (relative risk 2.0–4.4). Ex-smokers comprise 70% of those with ulcerative colitis, half of these developing symptoms within 3 years of stopping smoking. The clinical course of the disease also appears to be related to smoking habits, clinical improvement occurring within 6 weeks in half of the colitics who resume smoking.

Both maternal and passive smoking at birth are associated with an increased risk of developing inflammatory bowel disease, although this is greater for Crohn's disease than for ulcerative colitis (relative risk 2.0) (Silverstein *et al.* 1994). Childhood passive smoking appears to influence adult susceptibility to the development of colitis, although in adults passive smoking is associated with a reduced risk of colitis, which is unrelated to sex, education, or age at onset of symptoms (Sandler *et al.* 1992). These findings suggest that there is either a brief induction time before a protective effect of smoking develops or that patients selectively stop smoking due to their experiencing early symptoms of the disease (Pullan 1996). Doppler studies have shown a significantly increased rectal blood flow in those with ulcerative colitis, which is maximal in those who are non-smokers (Guslandi *et al.* 1995). The protective effects of smoking in ulcerative colitis may therefore be related to its ability to reduce rectal blood flow towards normal values.

Dietary factors

The possibility of an allergic reaction to foodstuffs initiating an immunological response in colitis has been long suggested (Koutroubakis *et al.* 1996); Mishkin 1997. Despite these earlier studies, strong support for a dietary aetiology of ulcerative colitis have remained elusive. Although not proven to be the case, an allergic response to milk continues to be suggested, colitics having higher levels of anti-casein antibodies than controls (Bernstein *et al.* 1994; Mishkin 1997). Elemental diets significantly improve the number of bowel movements in patients with colitis despite the

gross appearance of rectal mucosa remaining unaltered. Similarly, high-fibre diets produce a greater clinical improvement in those with quiescent colitis compared with controls (70% versus 25%). Low-alcohol consumption and regular consumption of fast foods have also been implicated with increasing the risk of developing colitis (Persson *et al.* 1993). The finding that a diet containing fish oil improves clinical symptoms is recognized to be due to its affect on eicosanoid synthesis (Aslan and Triadafilopoulos *et al.* 1992; Stenson *et al.* 1992). The interaction between dietary and immunological factors is suggested by the 15-fold risk of developing ulcerative colitis in patients with coeliac disease.

Bacteriological factors

Although cytomegalovirus has been implicated in some studies, viruses do not appear to be important in the aetiology of ulcerative colitis. The former belief that bacillary or amoebic dysentery can initiate ulcerative colitis no longer applies. However, in tropical countries these infections are still commonly associated with exacerbations of colitis (Macpherson *et al.* 1996). In contrast to Crohn's disease antibodies to *Mycobacterium paratuberculosis* are rarely found in ulcerative colitis. Although *Campylobacter jejuni* or *Clostridium difficile* may enter into the differential diagnosis they are rarely implicated in the development of ulcerative colitis.

Mucosal-associated flora are altered in active ulcerative colitis for both total flora, obligate anaerobes, micro-aerobes and facilitative organisms. The most common bacteria associated with ulcerative colitis are colonic commensals, particularly *Escherichia coli*. The colonic mucosa is invaded by bacteria in almost all cases of ulcerative colitis, while bacteria adherence is found in only 5% of normal colons (Ohkusa *et al.* 1995). The adhesive property of *E. coli* isolates in those with ulcerative colitis is similar to that of pathogenic intestinal *E. coli*, suggesting a possible pathogenic role for this organism (Olusanya *et al.* 1992). The aetiological role of bacteria is unknown. It has been suggested that in genetically susceptible individuals a bacterial metabolite of bile acid metabolism may contribute to the development of ulcerative colitis. It is also possible that bacteria may degrade colonic sulphomucins, which are known to be reduced in patients with ulcerative colitis.

Psychological aspects

Patients with ulcerative colitis tend to be highly strung and introspective. Although it is suggested that relapses occur at times of emotional stress only 10% of relapses occur when patients are under pressure. Claims of dramatic improvement from psychotherapy have not been substantiated by psychiatric tests, which reveal that patients have normal psychosomatic development. The psychogenic aetiology of ulcerative colitis in adults therefore remains unproven. It is suggested that perinatal health events and social class are important contributory factors to inflammatory bowel disease in a significant number of these cases (Rigas *et al.* 1993).

Drugs

Non-steroidal anti-inflammatory drugs, but not oral contraceptives, have been implicated in inducing ulcerative colitis and in activating quiescent colitis (Lashner *et al.* 1990; Sandler *et al.* 1992).

Genetic factors

Family members are at increased risk of developing inflammatory bowel disease relative to other members of the community (Thompson *et al.* 1996). A positive family history is found in

10–20% of those with ulcerative colitis, which is higher than is seen in Crohn's disease. However, the concordance among monozygotic twins is higher for Crohn's disease than ulcerative colitis, suggesting a polygenic inheritance. The genetic heterogeneity of the condition is also suggested by the finding of significantly increased levels of antineutrophil antibodies in relatives of patients with ulcerative colitis (Reumaux *et al.* 1993, Papo *et al.* 1996). Probert and colleagues (1993) investigated the prevalence and comparative risks of family history in 1254 patients with inflammatory bowel disease in England. The comparative risk of developing ulcerative colitis in first-degree relatives of patients with ulcerative colitis was increased by approximately 15, but the risk of Crohn's disease was not increased. The study supports the view that Crohn's disease and ulcerative colitis arise in people with a genetic predisposition and exposed to some, as yet unknown, environmental factor. There appears to be a single genotype with 10–15 genes which predispose to inflammatory bowel disease (Mazlam and Hodgson 1994).

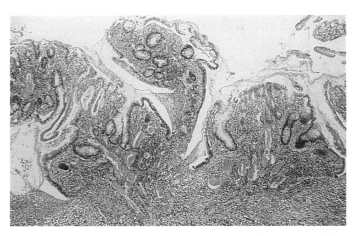

Figure 5.3 Active ulcerative colitis. There is inflammation of the mucosa with pseudopolyp formation and considerable distortion of mucosal glands. H&E×40.

Pathology

Macroscopic appearance

In ulcerative colitis the length and transverse diameter of the colon and rectum is reduced. The serosal surface is intact and retains its normal shiny appearance in all but the most fulminating cases, while the mucosal surface is granular and friable with marked venous congestion. Full thickness ulceration may be linear and related to the attachments of the taeniae coli. In ulcerative colitis the inflammatory changes are continuous even in the presence of a macroscopic appearance suggesting patchy involvement. The disease starts in the rectum and sigmoid and spreads proximally in continuity, but even in total colitis the mucosal changes remain greatest in the distal colon.

'Pseudo-polyps' represent areas of deep ulceration surrounding an area of less ulcerated mucosa giving the appearance of a relative protrusion into the lumen (Figures 5.2 and 5.3). Pseudo-polyps are more prominent in the colon than in the rectum and often remain after healing as evidence of past disease ('colitis polyposa'). The terminal ileum is involved for 5–20 cm in 10% of colectomy specimens and always in the presence of total colitis. Strictures in ulcerative colitis suggest the possibility of Crohn's disease or malignancy.

Microscopic appearance

Inflammation is most marked in the mucosa and to a lesser extent the submucosa. Cases with appendiceal involvement are unlikely to develop purulent appendicitis as inflammation is confined to the mucosa. Transmural inflammation is only seen in fulminant disease when mucosal loss can be extensive. Exposure of the muscle implies imminent perforation. In active disease there is infiltration of the lamina propria by plasma cells, eosinophils, and neutrophils (Figure 5.1). Histiocytes occur near disrupted crypt abscesses and, although foreign body giant cells are occasionally seen, the non-caseating granulomata of Crohn's disease do not occur. Infiltration of the crypts with neutrophils forms the characteristic crypt abscesses of acute disease. However, crypt abscesses are non-specific, being found also in appendicitis, infective colitis and Crohn's disease. There is prominent dilatation of the thin-walled vessels of the mucosa and submucosa with oedema. Mucin depletion of the goblet cells is an important finding, often being the only abnormality in mild disease (Figure 5.4). As the inflammation resolves, the goblet cell population is restored and the vascular congestion, crypt abscesses, and inflammatory cell response are reduced. There is reactive epithelial hyperplasia and restoration of epithelial continuity. Cases in remission show persistent histological changes despite sigmoidoscopic abnormalities. These include mucosal atrophy,

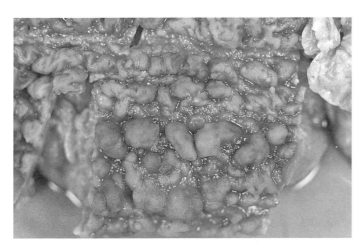

Figure 5.2 Pseudopolyp formation in ulcerative colitis.

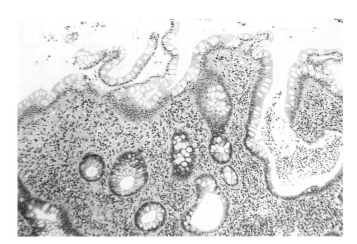

Figure 5.4 Active ulcerative colitis showing goblet cell depletion. H&E×100.

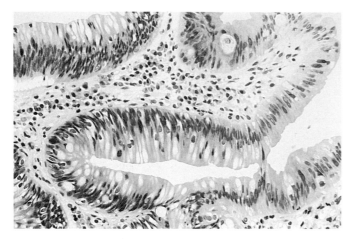

Figure 5.5 Low-grade dysplasia in ulcerative colitis. Note the stratification of nuclei and goblet cell depletion. H&E×250.

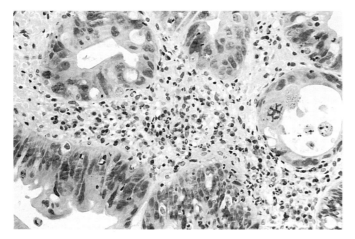

Figure 5.6 High-grade dysplasia in ulcerative colitis. There is marked cytological atypia with the mucosal glands. H&E×250.

branching of the crypts, thickening of the muscularis mucosae and fat in the lamina propria. These inflammatory and reparative changes may mimic neoplastic change (dysplasia) making assessment of premalignant change difficult in ulcerative colitis (Schneider and Stolte 1993) (Figures 5.5 and 5.6).

The assessment of dysplasia in ulcerative colitis is subjective. There is a disturbingly low level of agreement in diagnosing high-grade dysplasia among specialist pathologists, variation between observers often not differing from chance. In a review of cases at St Mark's Hospital, London, the overall agreement between the pathologists was poor; each pair agreeing on between 42% and 65% of the slides (Melville *et al.* 1989). The best agreement was for slides that were said to show no dysplasia. Comparison with clinical outcome indicated that the pathologists most likely to diagnose dysplasia in patients with carcinoma were also likely to diagnose dysplasia in patients who did not go on to develop carcinoma. Calculating an average grade of dysplasia did not significantly improve diagnostic accuracy (Melville *et al.* 1989).

In ulcerative colitis DNA analysis has been advocated as a useful predictor of the degree of dysplasia and hence of possible carcinoma. The percentage, however, of abnormal DNA (DNA aneuploidy) in dysplasia varies considerably, from 0 to 20% in mild dysplasia, 5–30% in moderate dysplasia and 10–45% in severe dysplasia (Melville *et al.* 1989). It may be that microspectrophotometric measurement of DNA content will prove a useful screening procedure in the assessment and diagnosis of dysplasia in ulcerative colitis (Suzuki *et al.* 1990; Paganelli *et al.* 1993; Hartmann *et al.* 1995).

Clinical presentation

Symptoms

Diarrhoea with passage of blood and mucus are the classical symptoms of colitis. Volume of stool is an important indicator of disease severity as large volumes indicate sufficient mucosal damage to affect sodium and water reabsorption. Nocturnal diarrhoea also suggests severe disease but frequency is less reliable as it may occur from large volume diarrhoea. Urgency of defecation and incontinence occur due to hypersensitivity and poor compliance of the rectum which with distension produces prolonged sphincter relaxation. The diarrhoea of ulcerative colitis has also been attributed to changes in gastrointestinal motility. A contribution to diarrhoea may also come from inhibition of the sodium potassium-ATPase and impaired carbohydrate absorption by actively inflamed mucosa. The presence of free oxygen radicals and inhibitory neurotransmitters result in inhibition of myosin light chain phosphorylation (Snape *et al.* 1991). The net effect is an electromechanical dissociation resulting in an increase in low amplitude propagation contractions and an overall decrease in the force of muscle contraction with variable colonic transit times. Consequently, constipation may occur, faecal studies revealing that 10% of attacks of distal colitis are associated with proximal faecal stasis. Those with proctosigmoiditis may therefore have overflow incontinence around a solid rectal stool while patients with left-sided disease may be constipated in the right colon while passing small amounts of diarrhoea from the affected segment.

In severe cases blood, often dark red with clots, is mixed with pus, mucus, and faecal material. In contrast, bleeding from proctitis is bright red on the surface of an often constipated stool. Colicky abdominal pain frequently accompanies the diarrhoea, especially in the more severe cases. Constant abdominal pain is more ominous implying peritoneal irritation. Pain may be the only feature of perforation in those on steroid therapy while shoulder tip pain implies perforation of toxic megacolon (Bitton and Peppercorn 1995).

Signs

Examination of patients with mild disease is unremarkable, but those with extensive disease are often anaemic and cachectic. The cachectic effects of alpha tumour necrosis factor may contribute to the inadequate growth that is seen (Murch *et al.* 1993). Mild pyrexia (less than 38°C) is seen in acute exacerbations irrespective of the extent of the disease. Higher temperatures imply fulminant disease or sepsis. Oral manifestations and finger clubbing are more typical of Crohn's disease. Abdominal examination is usually normal. Tenderness, localized or generalized, and distension suggest the possibility of a megacolon or imminent perforation. The perineum may show a perianal abscess, fistula, or fissure formation, although these are more suggestive of Crohn's disease. Rectal examination is usually normal or reveals blood on the glove. Very rarely palpable granularity, thickening, or fibrosis of the rectum is detected.

Investigations

Blood tests

The most powerful predictors of disease activity are volume and frequency of stool, temperature, pulse, anaemia, weight loss, and erythrocyte sedimentation rate (ESR). There is good observer agreement in the clinical assessment of disease activity using these parameters. Other markers of disease that correlate with endoscopic activity faecal alpha-1-antitrypsin and serum albumin (Moran *et al.* 1995; Oudkerk-Pool *et al.* 1995). Progressive alkalosis on blood gas analysis has been associated with increasing severity of disease, megacolon being indicated by a pH of over 7.5 (Fallingborg *et al.* 1993). Microalbuminuria is a useful disease activity marker for inflammatory bowel disease correlating strongly with ESR, C-reactive protein and the severity of colonic inflammation (Mahmud *et al.* 1996). Abnormal liver function tests occur in 10% of patients and are usually transient, reflecting acute relapse, malnutrition, or minor fatty infiltration (Broome *et al.* 1994). Persistently raised enzymes, particularly alkaline phosphatase is seen in 3% of patients, even in quiescent disease. Stools should be sent from all patients to exclude an infective cause such as *Salmonella*, *Campylobacter*, *Shigella*, or *C. difficile*.

Ulcerative colitis may be divided in severe, moderate and mild disease according to the classification of Truelove and Witts (1955). Severe disease is the passage of six or more bloody stools per day associated with fever, tachycardia, anaemia, and an ESR over 30 mm/h. About 15% of patients will fall into this category. Most patients (60%) have mild disease, defined as four or less stools per day with minimal blood loss and no systemic disturbance. The remaining patients have moderately severe disease. Depressed red blood cell folate is associated with an increased risk of dysplasia and cancer in patients with ulcerative colitis and may be a risk factor for neoplastic transformation (Lashner 1995).

Endoscopy

Sigmoidoscopy should be performed in all patients. Bowel preparation is not required, as it is dangerous in fulminant cases while in quiescent disease the hyperaemia resulting from enemas makes mucosal assessment difficult. Biopsies are safe provided they are taken carefully from below the peritoneal reflection. Biopsies should always be taken even if the mucosa looks normal as histologically there is almost always inflammation. True ulcerative colitis with a sigmoidoscopically and histologically normal mucosa only occurs in very mild cases in which the disease has completely regressed. The earliest sigmoidoscopic change is loss of the normal vascular pattern progressing to hyperaemic oedematous mucosa and contact bleeding. The mucosa then becomes granular and friable. In severe disease the lumen contains blood and pus. The mucosa is inflamed, oedematous, and ulcerated with contact bleeding. In long-standing disease the mucosa is pale and atrophic, the presence of pseudopolyps suggesting previous attacks of severe colitis.

The accuracy of colonoscopy in diagnosing ulcerative colitis is 90%; features suggesting Crohn's disease are discontinuity, cobblestone mucosa, linear ulcers, and perianal disease (Quinn *et al.* 1994). Despite this it is impossible to distinguish ulcerative colitis from Crohn's disease in 7% of cases, particularly in severe disease (Pera *et al.* 1987). The acute phase or severe disease is associated with deep ulceration, there is a significant risk of perforation and colonoscopy is best avoided or performed with great caution. In mild disease the colonoscopic appearances may be normal but histology reveals mucosal abnormalities. The underestimation of the extent of disease by barium enema relative to colonoscopy is therefore greatest in mild disease. Colonoscopy also has the advantage over barium enema of allowing biopsy of polyps, strictures and random biopsy for dysplasia. Random colonoscopic biopsies increase the sensitivity of cancer diagnosis in ulcerative colitis but areas of dysplasia are patchy and multiple repeated biopsies are necessary. Foci of dysplasia, which occur in 85% of colons removed for cancer in patients with ulcerative colitis, are often identified well away from the cancer itself. Biopsy of areas of macroscopic abnormality, such as strictures, flat nodular plaques, or polyps increases the chances of detecting dysplasia. However, a barium enema may be helpful in some patients in guiding endoscopists to biopsy abnormal areas.

Radiology

Abdominal radiographs

Plain abdominal X-rays are helpful in assessing the extent of ulcerative colitis, agreeing with colonoscopic or colectomy findings in 80% of cases. Abnormalities are detected in 90% in those with extensive colitis while 75% of patients with rectosigmoid disease have normal plain films (Gore and Ghahremani 1995). The features on a plain abdominal film that are most useful in assessing the extent of colitis are irregular mucosal profile, thickening of the colonic wall and flattening or swelling of the inter-haustral folds (Figure 5.7). Faeces rarely accumulate in an inflamed segment and is therefore a useful marker of the extent of disease. Failure to visualize the right colon and the presence of small bowel gas indicate extensive disease and a poor prognosis. Small bowel gas is apparent in 75% of patients who

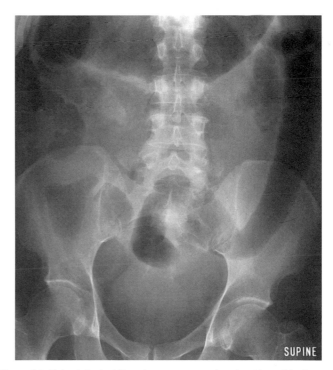

Figure 5.7 Plain abdominal X-ray in severe, extensive ulcerative colitis showing colonic wall thickening, loss of haustral folds and absence of faeces.

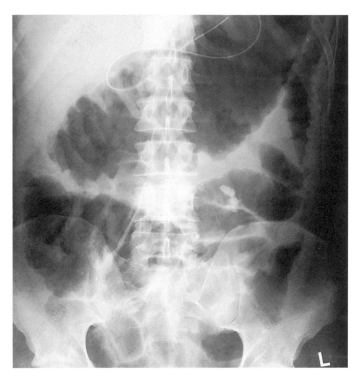

Figure 5.8 Toxic megacolon. Note mucosal oedema causing thumb-print indentation of left colon.

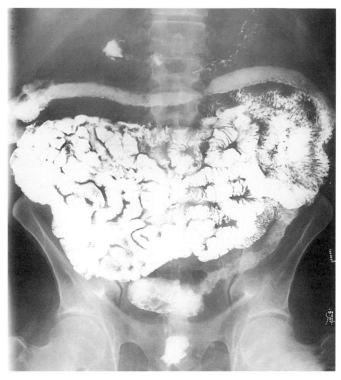

Figure 5.9 Barium follow through examination demonstrating total colitis.

will fail to respond to medical therapy and in over 20% of patients who subsequently develop toxic megacolon (Caprilli *et al.* 1987; Chew *et al.* 1991). In children the presence of small bowel gas and absence of stool in one or more colonic segments is also indicative of severe disease (Taylor *et al.* 1986; Kirschner 1996).

The normal transverse diameter of the colon does not exceed 5.5 cm. In toxic dilatation the diameter is greater than 6.5 cm, the normal haustral folds are lost and irregular mucosal contour with intraluminal projections representing deep ulcers is seen (Gore and Ghahremani 1995) (Figure 5.8). Intramural air implies impending perforation. Megacolon normally involves the transverse colon, although the sigmoid colon may be involved independently or as well. Moving the patient may distribute the gas and allow identification of more extensive segments of the colon. An increase in the presacral space on lateral X-ray to greater than 2 cm occurs in half of those with long standing colitis. This is related to peri-rectal inflammation and oedema but may also be seen in obese patients, radiation proctitis or in rectal or prostatic cancer. Air enema radiology is useful in assessing the extent of disease, particularly in those with severe colitis (Almer *et al.* 1995).

Barium enema

In the acute situation a contrast enema may be associated with bacteraemia in 12% of cases, while perforation or megacolon can be precipitated. If an urgent radiological diagnosis is required, a water soluble enema is safer. Alternatively, a per-oral antegrade barium enema gives good pictures of the rectosigmoid region in almost 100% of cases, the sigmoid colon in 77% and the rectum in 54% (Figure 5.9). A recent rectal biopsy is not a contraindication to barium enema provided it has been taken carefully from below the peritoneal reflection.

The earliest radiographic findings are fine mucosal granularity (Gore and Ghahremani 1995). This is usually maximal in the rectum, although rectal sparing may occur in 20% of cases especially if topical steroids have been used. As the disease becomes more severe, superficial ulcers are seen, deep ulcers suggesting Crohn's disease. The ulcers may coalesce, leaving only islands of intact mucosa. Pseudopolyps imply severe total colitis with mucosa loss (Figure 5.2). Severe ulceration and pseudopolyp formation results in a fluffy appearance with barium occasionally lying outside the bowel lumen. Post-inflammatory polyps may be of a 'filiform' type or be large and sessile (Figure 5.10). They are seen in up to 20% of patients. Distinction from neoplastic polyps is difficult and colonoscopic excision biopsy is advised (Pera *et al.* 1987). Strictures are not that uncommon but distinction from Crohn's disease or carcinoma is difficult. As most cancers in ulcerative colitis are annular, all strictures should be biopsied. Raised plaque-like areas on barium enema suggests epithelial dysplasia and points to the possibility of a malignant stricture. In long-standing disease there is widening of the pre-sacral space, loss of haustration, and shortening of the colon giving a hose-pipe appearance.

Double contrast barium enema is superior in diagnosing the extent of colitis than plain films or single contrast enemas and has better observer agreement (Lindstrom and Noren 1992). The specificity for distinguishing between ulcerative colitis and Crohn's disease is 93–98% for double contrast enema compared with 82% for single contrast studies. This is principally due to double contrast enemas being more sensitive (91% versus 70%) in detecting early disease, there being little difference between double and single contrast enemas in assessing advanced disease (Figures 5.11–5.13). Occasionally, an inflammatory carcinoma may have the appearances of colitis, while in 4% of those with colitis the barium enema may mimic the findings of ischaemic colitis.

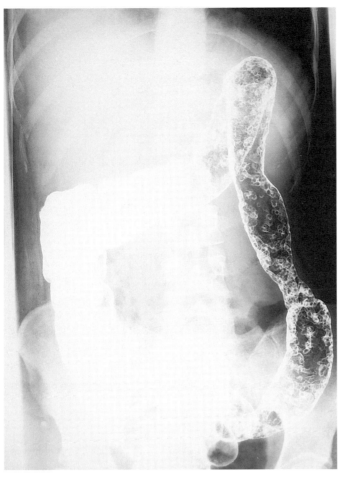

Figure 5.10 'Filiform' type post-inflammatory polyps.

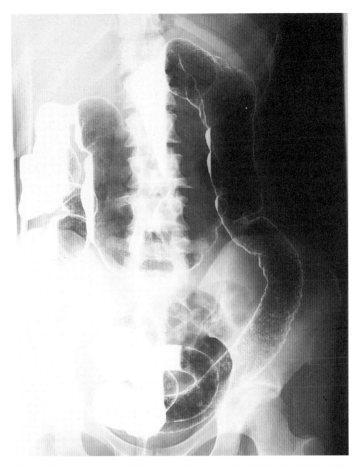

Figure 5.11 Double contrast barium enema in acute or chronic ulcerative colitis showing 'collar stud' ulcerations.

Ultrasound scanning

The thickness of the bowel wall is important in distinguishing ulcerative colitis from Crohn's disease and is related to disease activity. In ulcerative colitis, the bowel wall is less thickened than in Crohn's disease and tends to be located in the left, rather than the right lower quadrant. In severe acute colitis, the sensitivity of ultrasound scan for distinguishing colitis from Crohn's disease is 91%. Instilling water into the colon gives an overall sensitivity of 90% and correctly distinguishes between colitis and Crohn's disease in 86% of cases. In the future, colonoscopic ultrasound scan may prove valuable (Tamaki et al. 1994).

Bowel wall thickening can also be detected by computerized tomography (CT) or magnetic resonance imaging (MRI) scanning (Giovagnoni et al. 1993; Philpotts et al. 1994). Typical features are an inhomogeneous attenuation and targeted appearance in the rectum characterized by proliferation of perirectal fat. However, a prominent submucosal pattern may represent submucosal fat rather than inflammation. CT scanning is more sensitive than plain radiographs at assessing bony changes, pneumatosis coli in severe colitis, and in distinguishing benign from malignant intraluminal strictures. MRI is comparable with colonoscopy in differentiating ulcerative colitis from Crohn's disease and in gauging the severity of the disease (Shoenut et al. 1994). Transmural assessment, sagittal imaging, and the lack of invasiveness are potential advantages of MRI.

Radioisotope scanning (Figure 5.14)

Two principal radioisotopes, indium[111] and technetium[99] (Tcm) have been used to assess ulcerative colitis. (Arndt et al. 1997; Delgado et al. 1997). Indium[111] white cell scanning has a sensitivity of 90%, specificity of 90% and accuracy of 86% for detecting and assessing the extent of inflammatory bowel disease (Stahlberg et al. 1997). Correlation with barium studies is obtained in 80%, histology confirming the diagnosis in 70% of cases. Faecal excretion of indium[111] has a 97% sensitivity for detecting inflammatory bowel disease but lacks sensitivity for the extent of disease. Therefore, indium[111] is useful in evaluating recurrent disease and permits screening of active disease. It may be used as an adjunct to, or instead of barium enemas.

Technetium scanning in inflammatory bowel disease has a sensitivity of 95%, specificity of 97%, and 75% correlation with barium enema or colonoscopy, identifying more extensive disease than barium studies in 20% of cases (Papos et al. 1993, Almers et al. 1996). It is also claimed to be more reliable than barium enema at distinguishing ulcerative colitis from Crohn's disease (Li et al. 1994). However, technetium[99] sucralfate scintigraphy and technetium[99]-labelled IgG scanning underestimate the extent of disease and correlate poorly with colonoscopic assessment. In contrast, one study showed agreement between technetium HMPAO and colonoscopy in 68 of 70 cases (kappa = 0.94), technetium being superior to indium[111] scanning (Vilien et al. 1992). Technetium[99m]-colloid pelvic pouch emptying scans allow a useful assessment of those with stable pouch function or pouchitis (Thoeni et al. 1990;

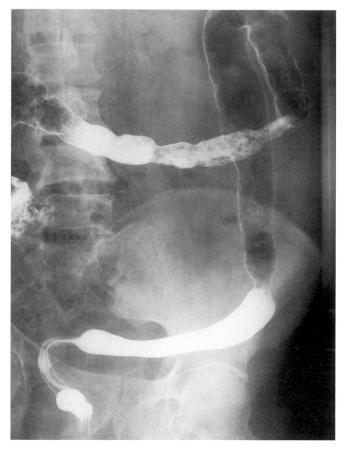

Figure 5.12 Barium enema showing typical 'hose-pipe' colon of chronic colitis.

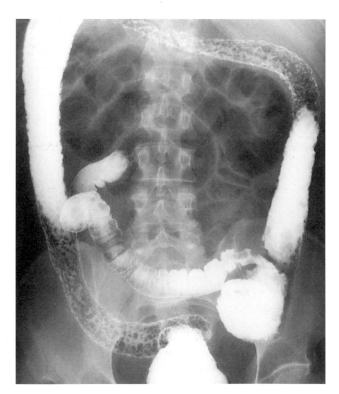

Figure 5.13 Barium enema showing total colonic involvement with pseudo-polyp formation and backwash ileitis.

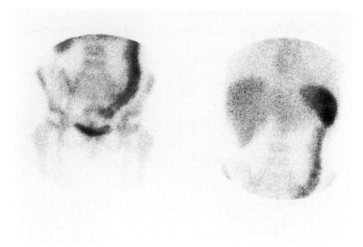

Figure 5.14 Technetium labelled white cell scan showing distal colitis.

Woolfson *et al.* 1991). Other isotopes that may be used to assess ulcerative colitis are chromium[51] EDTA enema excretion and selenium HCAT scanning. However, the correlation with pathology and hence the clinical usefulness of radio-isotope scanning remains to be determined.

Course of the disease

Patients presenting for the first time represent 40% of those experiencing acute attacks, the remainder representing episodes of relapse. The cumulative risk of remaining relapse free at 2, 5, and 10 years after diagnosis is 20%, 10%, and less than 5%, respectively (Hendriksen *et al.* 1985). About 75% of those presenting with colitis there is complete absence of symptoms between attacks, but relapses can be expected at variable frequencies. Only 5% of patients experience a single attack and have no further problems during their lifetime, even though histological abnormalities may persist. In the remainder the severe initial attack does not resolve necessitating surgical intervention. Risk of relapse is directly related to the length of remission between the first attack and the first relapse, and is unrelated to either the severity or extent of the disease. Approximately 40% of patients will relapse within 2 years of diagnosis. The relapse rate at 5 years in younger patients is 80%, compared with 40% in those presenting at an older age (Hendriksen *et al.* 1985).

The factors determining the outcome of ulcerative colitis are the prognosis of the first attack, the frequency of relapse and the incidence of complications such as colorectal cancer or liver disease. In the first year of presentation, 10% of cases will run a fulminant course requiring surgery while 70% will experience moderately severe and 20% a mild disease (Hendriksen *et al.* 1985). At any given time 50% of patients will be asymptomatic, 30% will have mild symptoms and 20% moderate or severe disease. Irrespective of race, the frequency of pancolitis is 1%, while 30% will have distal colitis and a further 30% proctitis (Probert *et al.* 1992). Resection rate depends upon management policy and ranges from 3% to 26% at 5 years. In specialized centres, over one-third of patients undergo colectomy during their first attack, the colectomy rate for total colitis, left-sided disease and distal disease on presentation being 36%, 38% and 25%, respectively (Leijonmarck 1990). The resection rate at 5 years for those with total colitis is 35% while at 25 years 65% of patients will have had their colon excised (Hendrikson *et al.* 1985).

Proctitis represents about 10% of those with ulcerative colitis and behaves as a less virulent disease. The risk of extension to the sigmoid colon is 20% at 10 years and 30% at 20 years, while that of involvement of the hepatic flexure is 6% and 7%, respectively. Total resolution occurs in 45% of cases, severe relapse occurring in only 10%. Consequently, the colectomy rate at 10 years is 5%, being similar at 20 years (6%). Overall life expectancy is no different in those with proctitis than in age–sex-matched controls, 80% of patients dying from causes unrelated to their colitis (Nordenholtz *et al.* 1995, Persson *et al.* 1996).

In a review by Langholz and colleagues (1992) no significant excess mortality was found after the first year, but in the year of diagnosis the relative risk of death was 2.4. The cumulative colectomy rate was 32.4% 25 years after diagnosis. The initial extent of disease significantly influenced the colectomy probability, being 35% in total colitis, 19% in colitis involving the transverse colon and 9% in distal colitis within the first 5 years after diagnosis. The relative risk of colorectal cancer for patients with ulcerative colitis was 0.9, the calculated lifetime risk being 3.5% compared with 3.7% for the general Danish population. It appears that with active medical treatment, patients who are left with their colon intact bear no significantly increased risk of colorectal malignancy (Rhodes 1996).

Colitis in children

About 14% of patients will develop symptoms before the age of 16 years and a third of these will have a positive family history (Hofley and Piccoli 1994). The disease is usually severe, two-thirds of children having total colonic involvement and 10% fulminant disease. Although the symptoms and signs are similar to those of adults, relapse and complications are more common with two-thirds of patients running a chronic, insidious course (Kirschner 1996). Extra-intestinal manifestations are also more frequent, while the risk of colon cancer is 3% at 10 years after the onset of symptoms. Growth retardation and delayed sexual maturity are particular features in children, there being an average 15% reduction in ideal body weight (Hofley and Piccoli 1994). This is related to chronic protein loss but is not as marked as in Crohn's disease. Growth retardation often responds to steroid therapy, failure to do so may be an indication for surgery (Kirschner 1996). Other indications for surgery are similar to those in adults.

Children often respond well to an ileal pouch procedure, although the frequency of defecation and possible septic complications can affect schooling (Orkin *et al.* 1990, Rintala and Lindahl 1996). Children cope with the ileostomy of traditional proctocolectomy remarkably well and it is not until adolescence that they appreciate the social, sexual, and psychological aspects of a stoma (Sedgwick *et al.* 1991). An ileorectal anastomosis provides excellent functional results without a stoma and with minimal risk to bladder or sexual function. However, the risk of recurrent proctitis or cancer is significant and requires to be explained to parents and later to the children.

Colitis in the elderly

Ulcerative colitis in elderly patients usually consists of inactive total colitis or incapacitating distal disease. Extra-intestinal manifestations such as erythema nodosum or pyoderma gangrenosum are relatively common. Relapse presenting as acute colitis in the over-60s is uncommon but is associated with a high mortality (20%) due to the insidious onset of dilatation and perforation in the absence of significant symptoms or signs. Mortality is further increased by the diagnostic difficulty in distinguishing symptoms from ischaemic colitis and the reluctance to operate on elderly, unfit patients. Although the risks of emergency surgery are considerable, elderly patients tolerate elective surgery well. Patients who therefore fail to respond to conventional medical therapy should be considered for elective surgery, rather than waiting for complications to arise.

Colitis in pregnancy

Infertility in women with colitis is no higher than that of the normal population (7%), although those with total colitis often voluntarily defer pregnancy until there is symptomatic improvement. Male fertility is uninfluenced by colitis or its treatment with the exception of sulphasalazine. Reversible abnormalities in semen analysis occur in 70% of men on this drug. Pelvic surgery for colitis may influence both male and female sexual function. Overall, patients with ulcerative colitis have the same incidence of abortion, congenital abnormality, and stillbirth as the general population. However, spontaneous abortion and stillbirths are higher than expected for those who develop a severe relapse or their first attack during pregnancy. The risk of relapse is no higher in pregnant patients and may in fact be less than that of the general population if patients are maintained on their medication during pregnancy. Despite this, almost half of patients will experience a mild deterioration in symptoms and only one-third will go into remission during pregnancy.

Most patients can be managed medically until the 33rd week when Caesarean section is generally safe. 5-ASA drugs should be continued as the risks to the fetus are greater from relapse than from the drugs. 5-ASA derivatives are generally safer than sulphasalazine. Although steroids cross the placenta they are generally safe during pregnancy and in the puerperium. If colectomy is required during pregnancy it is generally safe (Cooksey *et al.* 1985). Women who become pregnant after colectomy may be delivered vaginally, but Caesarean section is frequently performed, particularly in those with pouches (Scaglia *et al.* 1993). Intestinal obstruction occurs in 10% of pregnant patients with a pouch, but almost always settles with conservative treatment.

Complications

Toxic dilatation

This is defined as a diameter of the transverse colon greater than 5.5 cm. It often occurs during the first attack of colitis, and is more common in ulcerative colitis than Crohn's disease, although it may also occur with amoebic colitis, ischaemic colitis, pseudomembranous colitis, and bacillary dysentery (Heppell *et al.* 1986). The risk of perforation is related to the size of the colon and the depth of ulceration (Figure 5.15). Colonic dilatation still carries an overall mortality of 33%, being 3% in those without, and up to 40% in those with, perforation (Heppell *et al.* 1986; Bitton and Peppercorn 1995). Delay in operating, particularly in those on steroids who have developed silent perforation is the single most important factor affecting mortality. One-third of patients with toxic dilatation will respond to conservative treatment, although most of

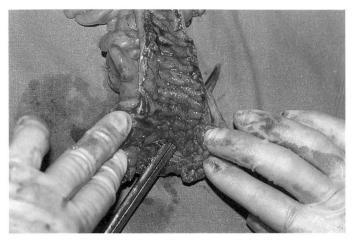

Figure 5.15 Colonic perforation (indicated by the scissors) in a case of severe colitis.

these will require colectomy for further dilatation or severe attacks. Therefore, if there is any deterioration or no improvement within

72 h with bowel rest, fluid replacement, steroids, and antibiotics, surgery is indicated. Other poor risk factors include free gas on radiology during admission. Opiates or anticholinergic drugs can precipitate megacolon.

A wide spectrum of hepatobiliary (Table 5.3), ocular, skin, arthritic, and other conditions (Table 5.4) occurs in ulcerative colitis (Figure 5.16). Oral lesions may also occur (Lisciandrano *et al.* 1996).

Mortality

Ulcerative colitis is usually not associated with an increased mortality relative to the normal population, with the exception of the first 2 years after diagnosis. This initial excess mortality is related to the severity of the first attack. The cumulative mortality at 2 years of those presenting with a severe first attack is up to 30%, while that of those presenting with extensive disease may be 20%. Older studies suggest that the mortality of those with severe or moderate disease is 40% and 20%, respectively at 5 years, compared with 10% at 15 years for mild disease. Modern results from specialized units report an overall mortality at 5 years of 5%. However, all studies confirm that after the first 2 years, overall mortality is similar to the rest of the population. Most deaths are associated with

Table 5.3 Hepatobiliary complications of ulcerative colitis

Complication	Features	Author
Sclerosing cholangitis	3% of all ulcerative colitics	Wiesner 1994
	25–45 years, males > females	Broome *et al.* 1995
	Unrelated to severity/extent of UC	Brentall *et al.* 1996
	Might increase risk of colorectal cancer	Kartheuser *et al.* 1996
	Gallstones common	Loftus *et al.* 1996
	Alkaline phosphatase markedly elevated	Penna *et al.* 1996
	ERCP: irregular strictures of bile ducts	
	Therapy	
	Cholestyramine, vitamin K	
	Steroids do not affect course of disease	
	Stenting, hepaticojejunostomy, liver transplant	Mikkola *et al.* 1995
Gallstones	Increased if sclerosing cholangitis or extensive ileal resection	Mikkola *et al.* 1995
Chronic active hepatitis	Incidence increased	Mikkola *et al.* 1995
Fatty infiltration	Usually confined to severe disease	Mikkola *et al.* 1995
	Related to protein malnutrition	
Peri-cholangitis	Unrelated to disease severity	Mikkola *et al*.1995
	Unaffected by colectomy	
Cirrhosis	1% of those with ulcerative colitis	Lever *et al.* 1993
	Associated with extensive disease	*Zins et al.* 1995
	Associated with high operative mortality if colectomy (20%)	Kartheuser *et al.* 1996
	Liver transplant effective	
Cholangiocarcinoma	Related to duration and extent of disease	Herzog and Goldblum 1996
	Up to 20-fold increase with extensive colitis	
	May occur in absence of other complications	
	Unaffected by colectomy	
	Diagnosis	
	ERCP: distinguish from sclerosing cholangitis	
	Treatment	
	Stenting or surgical resection	

Table 5.4 Other extra-intestinal complications of ulcerative colitis

Complication	Features	Author
Ocular lesions	*Uveitis* Up to 10% of those with colitis Associated with skin lesions, arthritis, stomatitis May resolve spontaneously or with colectomy Topical steroids effective *Episcleritis* Presents with pain and scleral injection Related to relapse of colitis May resolve spontaneously or with colectomy Topical steroids effective *Superficial keratitis* *Blepharitis* *Retinitis* Retrobulbar neuritis	Hofley *et al.* 1994 Soukiasian *et al.* 1994
Skin lesions	*Pyoderma gangrenosum* Affects 1–5% of those with ulcerative colitis Accounts for half of all skin conditions in colitics Usually confined to severe cases Progresses to necrotic ulcer Responds to colectomy May recur if severe disease in rectal stump *Erythema nodosum* 2–4% of colitics more common in females Associated with arthritis or iritis Usually associated with relapse of colitis Raised tender swelling on leg or arm (Figure 5.16) Responds to colectomy May recur with pouchitis *Exfoliative dermatitis* Associated with severe disease or sulphasalazine Responds to colectomy *Cutaneous vasculitis* Responds to steroid therapy	Graham *et al.* 1994 Tjandra and Hughes 1994 Dwarakanath *et al.* 1995
Arthritis	Migratory, asymmetrical arthropathy Occurs in 10% of colitics Affects knees, wrists, and elbows Associated with erythema nodosum and uveitis Resolves spontaneously or with colectomy May recur with pouchitis *Ankylosing spondylitis* Occurs in 10% of colitics Colitics account for 20% of all cases of spondylitis Represents 30-fold increase Equal sex incidence 'Bamboo spine' Salicylates and NSAIDs helpful Colectomy rarely affects progression	Burgos-Vargas 1993 Gran and Husby 1993 Mahoney 1993 Adachi Y *et al.* 1996 Andreyev *et al.* 1996
Oral	Stomatitis Candida Aphthoid ulceration	Lisciandrano *et al.* 1996
Other manifestations	Hypertrophic osteoarthropathy Stomatitis Amyloid Pericarditis Fibrosing alveolitis Extracolonic malignancy (connective tissue and brain tumours)	Lossos *et al.* 1995 Maeder 1996 Ekbom *et al.* 1991

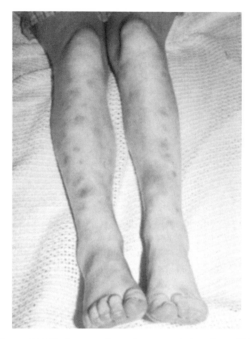

Figure 5.16 Erythema nodosum in a case of ulcerative colitis.

an acute attack, particularly if there has been perforation or delay in surgical intervention. Deaths from colorectal cancer are now recognized to be less important than was previously believed (Hendriksen *et al.* 1985). Recent suggestions that primary sclerosing cholangitis increases the risks of colorectal cancer in ulcerative colitis remain unproven (Brentnall *et al.* 1996; Loftus *et al.* 1996). Over the last three decades there has been a world-wide reduction in mortality from ulcerative colitis, irrespective of age or sex, which is most marked in younger patients (Probert *et al.* 1993). The overall mortality in children is about 5% with up to half of children presenting with colitis having a colectomy during their lifetime.

Medical management

After healing half of the patients will remain in remission without therapy. Although more than half of acute attacks improve without treatment, many relapse again within 2 months. Most patients therefore require medical treatment. The medical management of ulcerative colitis involves pharmacological agents, nutritional therapy, and psychological support. Trials of disease-modifying agents have employed a variety of 'end points' including symptoms, laboratory results, endoscopic findings or quality of life assessments (Irvine *et al.* 1994; Robinson *et al.* 1994; Kornbluth and Sachar 1997). Consequently, comparison of drug efficacy between trials is difficult. In an attempt to provide a baseline for therapeutic intervention in ulcerative colitis, assessment was made of the placebo arms of 11 trials of acute disease and six trials of remission follow-up (Meyers and Janowitz 1989).

Pharmacology

5-aminosalicylic acid preparations

Sulphasalazine is a chemical combination of 5-ASA and sulphapyridine joined by an azo bond. In the colon, bacteria break down the

azo bond releasing the individual moieties. 5-ASA is the active part of the combination (Azad Khan *et al.* 1977). Sulphasalazine and 5-ASA derivatives has been demonstrated to heal acute relapses and maintain remission of ulcerative colitis (Schroeder *et al.* 1987; Miner *et al.* 1995; Mesalamine Study Group 1996). Side-effects occur in up to 30% of patients, being sufficiently severe to require stopping the preparation in up to 15% (Taffet and Das 1983; Sviri *et al.* 1997). Because the side-effects are largely due to the sulphapyridine moiety, preparations containing only 5-ASA have been developed.

Plain 5-ASA is rapidly and completely absorbed in the upper gastrointestinal tract (Myers *et al.* 1987). This causes increased systemic levels with associated potential nephrotoxicity (Staerk Laursen*et al.* 1990). It also fails to deliver 5-ASA to the colon where it is poorly absorbed and believed to act locally (Ireland and Jewell 1990; Kamm and Senapati 1992). Three methods of enhanced colonic delivery have been devised. Asacol (mesalazine enteric coated) is a 5-ASA preparation coated with a pH-dependent resin which dissolves at pH 7 or above. Pentasa (mesalazine slow release) contains granules of 5-ASA coated in a resin which allows slow release throughout the bowel (Figure 5.17). Dipentum (olsalazine) contains two 5-ASA molecules joined by an azo bond similar to that used in sulphasalazine and released in a similar fashion. Of the newer 5-ASA preparations, olsalazine is the most colon specific with higher colonic concentrations and lower serum urinary levels than the other formulations (Staerk Laursen *et al.* 1990). Mesalazine slow release (Pentasa) is the least colon specific and this may be of benefit in treating small bowel Crohn's disease (Gendre *et al.* 1993). Side-effects are fewer with the newer 5-ASAs, but watery diarrhoea is commoner with olsalazine (Sandberg-Gertzen *et al.* 1986; Kruis *et al.* 1995). This diarrhoea should be distinguished from a flare-up of the colitis and can be improved by taking the medication with meals. Nephrotoxicity is a potential but rare problem with all 5-ASA preparations. The increased frequency of adverse renal events associated with Asacol may simply reflect prescribing habits.

Despite the differences in formulation, the majority of studies in ulcerative colitis have shown none of the four preparations to be

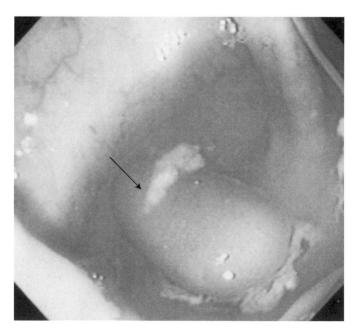

Figure 5.17 Colonoscopic picture of intact mesalazine capsule (arrowed) entering the caecum.

more effective than any other. One recent study in ulcerative colitis found olsalazine superior to mesalazine enteric coated and sulphasalazine in reducing the rate of relapse (Courtney et al. 1992). The results of this trial need to be confirmed by other studies. For the moment sulphasalazine remains the initial drug of choice in ulcerative colitis except for those males in whom oligospermia would be undesirable. There is little to choose between the other three preparations.

Steroids

In 1955 Truelove and Witts established the value of corticosteroids in the acute treatment of ulcerative colitis. The benefit of steroids has been repeatedly shown for acute attacks of both ulcerative colitis and Crohn's disease, but has little place in maintaining remission (Jarnerot et al. 1985; Modigliani et al. 1990). Corticosteroids act by modifying the inflammatory response. Side-effects include weight gain and acne in the short term and loss of bone density in the long term. Growth retardation may occur in children on long-term steroids. The ideal preparation should have high anti-inflammatory potency with low mineralocorticoid activity. Limiting systemic absorption by topical delivery or increasing hepatic metabolism are desirable.

At present, prednisolone is the oral corticosteroid of choice. When an intravenous alternative is required methylprednisolone at four-fifths the prednisolone dose or hydrocortisone at four times the prednisolone dose have the equivalent anti-inflammatory potency. Topical administration may be given by enema, suppository or rectal foam preparation. When only distal disease is present, these preparations reduce the systemic corticosteroid load, especially when prednisolone is attached to a carrier as in prednisolone metasulphobenzoate (McIntyre et al. 1986). Other preparations have used beclomethasone dipropionate (Bansky et al. 1987), tixocortol pivalate (Hanauer et al. 1986), and budesonide (Danielsson et al. 1987). All are as effective as prednisolone and with fewer systemic side-effects. Budesonide appears to be the one showing greatest promise, being significantly more effective than prednisolone without causing any significant depression of plasma cortisone levels. It is possible that in the future an oral preparation of budesonide may replace prednisolone in the treatment of inflammatory bowel disease (Gilvarry and O'Morain 1993).

Other immunosuppressants

Azathioprine is metabolized to 6-mercaptopurine (6-MP) in the liver. Both are purine analogues and affect DNA synthesis. In the treatment of inflammatory bowel disease they may be considered as equivalent. Seventy-three per cent of ulcerative colitis patients unresponsive to steroids or 5-ASAs respond to 6-MP allowing steroid dosage to be reduced (Present et al. 1988; Hawthorne et al. 1992, George et al. 1996). Side-effects are significant and must be fully discussed with patients. Common side-effects include leucopenia, anaemia, rash, and arthralgia. The leucopenia must be monitored by initially fortnightly and then monthly full blood counts. There is a recognized risk of malignancy when these drugs are used in renal transplant patients and to date two cases of patients with histiocytic lymphoma of the brain have been reported out of 1000 Crohn's disease patients on immunosuppression (Linn and Peppercorn 1992). Azathioprine and 6-MP should be stopped for 3 months prior to a patient planning to become pregnant, although the risk of birth defects is negligible if patients do become pregnant (Alstead et al. 1990). They may also be safely used in children with refractory disease (Verhave et al. 1990).

The optimal dosing schedule is unclear and there is debate as to whether or not mild neutropenia is needed for therapeutic effect (Hanauer 1993). One regimen suggests slowly increasing from 50 mg daily to 2 mg/kg per day (or until mild neutropenia occurs) over 1–2 months. The treatment should be continued for at least 1 year but not indefinitely without attempts at withdrawal (Linn and Peppercorn 1992).

Other immunosuppressants that have been tried in inflammatory bowel disease include cyclosporin which suppresses cell-mediated immunity and the folic acid antagonist methotrexate. Both may have a role in inflammatory bowel disease that has proven refractory to other medication (Brynskov et al. 1989; Lichtiger and Present 1990; Egan and Sandborn 1996). Cyclosporin enemas appear to be effective in 50% of patients with refractory ulcerative colitis and have the advantage of minimal systemic absorption (Ranzi et al. 1989). In children cyclosporin is effective in achieving clinical remission in 80% of cases with refractory fulminant colitis; however, within 1 year, most initial responders will require colectomy (Treem et al. 1995). In the majority of patients, the role of cyclosporin therapy is to ameliorate symptoms rapidly and prevent precipitous colectomy, improve nutrition and psychological adaptation, and reduce the steroid dose leading to surgery in a well-prepared patient. Unlike Crohn's disease, antibiotics are not of benefit in ulcerative colitis.

Lipo-oxygenase inhibitors

Arachidonic acid is the substrate in the production of leukotriene B_4 by one of the lipo-oxygenase pathways. Leukotriene B_4 is believed to have a key role in the inflammatory response of inflammatory bowel disease (Laursen et al. 1994). Inhibition of this pathway may be achieved by eicosapentaenoic acid (EPA, fish oil) or by a specific 5-lipo-oxygenase inhibitor (Zileuton). As additional therapy in ulcerative colitis, EFA is effective (Tobin et al. 1990; Cummings 1997). Use of Zileuton significantly reduces the leukotriene B_4 concentration in rectal dialysis fluid and was clinically beneficial in those not on 5-ASAs (Laursen et al. 1994). Other agents which have been reported to have beneficial effects include heparin, topical lignocaine, nicotine, immunotherapy and oxygen free radical scavengers (Gaffney et al. 1991; Pullan et al. 1993).

Nutritional therapy

This may be used to improve the nutrition status of the patient or to treat the disease (Wu and Craig 1995). Many patients with inflammatory bowel disease requiring hospitalization are undernourished and therefore may run into postoperative surgical complications. Most can be managed by oral or enteral supplementation with the occasional patient requiring parenteral nutrition (Wu and Craig 1995). The importance of adequate nutrition during an acute attack is demonstrated by high nitrogen losses occurring in patients on steroids who do not receive sufficient protein intake (O'Keefe et al. 1989). In patients with anaemia refractory to treatment with iron and vitamins, treatment with oral iron and recombinant erythropoietin can raise haemoglobin levels (Schreiber et al. 1996).

Medical treatment

Mild flare-up

In mild disease patients pass no more than four bowel motions per day which may or may not contain blood. The patient remains systemically well. This situation can usually be managed by increasing the dose of oral 5-ASA preparations to six or more tablets per day or the addition of topical preparations (Schroeder et al. 1987). When the disease is predominantly a proctitis or confined to the left side of the colon, topically administered preparations are effective. Enema formulations reach the splenic flexure and suppositories the sigmoid colon (Campieri et al. 1986). Foam preparations are preferred by patients over liquid formulations (Somerville et al. 1985). Some patients with left-sided disease develop constipation and faecal loading of the proximal colon. Treatment of this with an osmotic laxative or by a high-fibre diet may significantly improve the distal inflammation. Therapy should be continued until symptomatic remission is achieved and the patient then considered for maintenance therapy (Nilsson et al. 1995; Kornbluth and Sachar 1997).

Moderate flare-up

In moderate disease more than four motions per day are passed. In this situation or on failure of mild disease to respond to the above therapy, oral prednisolone should be added. Prednisolone 40 mg is given daily for 2 weeks and if the symptoms resolve, the daily dose reduced weekly by increments of 10 mg down to 20 mg/day and by 5–2.5 mg increments below this (Hanauer 1993).

Severe flare-up

In the presence of systemic symptoms such as pyrexia and tachycardia, evidence of anaemia or hypoalbuminaemia, the patient should be admitted to hospital. Initial management is by fluid, electrolyte, and blood replacement as required and intravenous hydrocortisone 400 mg daily. Malnourished patients may be started on parenteral nutrition. Temperature, pulse, and blood pressure should be monitored and an abdominal X-ray obtained to exclude dilatation or perforation. The abdominal X-ray should be repeated in patients who show no evidence of responding. Stool samples should be sent for culture to exclude an infective cause including C. difficile. In the absence of proven infection, antibiotics are of no value (Chapman et al. 1986). If colonic dilatation or ileus is present, a nasogastric tube should be inserted and the patient fasted. Oral food intake can be maintained if these findings are absent (McIntyre et al. 1986). Patients ill enough to require admission to hospital ought to be assessed by both a physician and a surgeon.

Seventy per cent of patients treated with intravenous steroids will respond within 5 days. Those who do improve may be changed to oral prednisolone 40 mg daily and a 5-ASA preparation. In such patients, steroids should only be reduced slowly. Patients who have not improved during the first 5 days and also those who deteriorate at any stage during their admission should be considered for urgent surgery. Factors predicting a poor response to medical therapy include the passage of more than 12 stools in the first 24 h, a temperature greater than 38°C or pulse greater than 100/min at any stage and a persistently low serum albumin (Lennard-Jones et al. 1975). One preliminary report suggests the benefit of cyclosporin given to patients who were refractory to 10 days intravenous steroids and in whom a colectomy would otherwise have been indicated. Eleven of 15 patients improved (Lichtiger and Present 1990).

Refractory colitis

One-quarter of patients will not respond to treatment for moderate colitis yet not become systemically ill and develop severe colitis. Several alternatives are available for these patients. Irrespective of the extent of disease, 5-ASA enemas should be added to maximum doses of oral 5-ASA preparations to alleviate the symptoms attribut-

able to rectal disease (Porro et al. 1995). High-dose intravenous steroids may induce remission in otherwise refractory patients (Jarnerot et al. 1985). The addition of an immunosuppressant (6-MP) can produce remission in 75% of patients who are unresponsive to steroids or 5-ASA preparations allowing steroid dosage to be reduced in almost all these cases (Present et al. 1988). Cyclosporin can also be used (Lichtiger and Present 1990). Those with refractory distal disease may respond to short chain fatty acid enemas (Patz et al. 1996; Cummings 1997). Care must be taken that the patient's general health and nutrition do not continue to deteriorate while trying these second line options. By delaying an operation in these cases, the patient comes to surgery in a poorer physical condition than might otherwise have been the case.

Maintenance therapy

For the majority of patients continuation of the 5-ASA preparation at half the dose that induced remission is sufficient (Kruis et al. 1995). This may be maintained indefinitely. One-quarter of patients requiring steroids to induce remission will continue to require them to prevent relapse (Hanauer 1993). For such patients, the introduction of azathioprine or 6-MP will allow reduction in the dose of steroid required or a complete cessation in the majority of cases. After maintaining remission for at least 1 year, consideration should be given to withdrawing the immunosuppressant therapy (Linn and Peppercorn 1992).

The management of ulcerative colitis in pregnancy and in children is the same as that for non-pregnant adults. When pregnancy is being planned, azathioprine or 6-MP should be stopped. However, unplanned pregnancies while on these drugs have shown negligible rates of birth defects. Of the adverse effects of drugs in children, a primary concern is the avoidance of growth retardation. If steroids are required, alternative day dosing may reduce their side-effects.

Surgical treatment

Absolute indications for surgery in patients with ulcerative colitis are (Farouk and Pembertan 1997):

1. Acute fulminating colitis which deteriorates with, or does not respond to, medical therapy.
2. Toxic dilatation or perforation.

Relative indications for surgery are:

1. Continued bleeding with persistent chronic diarrhoea or repeated relapse.
2. When symptomatic relief can only be achieved by continuous steroid therapy.

Emergency surgery

Emergency panproctocolectomy or subtotal colectomy with primary ileorectal anastomosis has been associated with an operative mortality of up to 35%. Most authors therefore recommend subtotal colectomy leaving a rectal stump as an effective life-saving procedure, being associated with an operative mortality of under 10%. However, many patients continue to complain of rectal bleeding and the extra-intestinal manifestations, especially skin and joint complications, often persist in the presence of residual disease. In addition, the risk of cancer developing is about 3% if the rectal stump is retained for over 10 years (Oakley *et al.* 1985). Two-thirds of patients therefore undergo excision of the rectal stump within 2 years of emergency subtotal colectomy, the overall life-time risk of rectal excision being 75% (Oakley *et al.* 1985). An ileorectal anastomosis or pouch procedure may then performed with an operative mortality similar to the corresponding elective procedure (1–5%) (Johnson *et al.* 1986). Emergency subtotal colectomy is inappropriate in the presence of massive bleeding from the rectum or if there is a perforation near the peritoneal reflection. In such circumstances the rectum should be mobilized and divided at the pelvic floor (proctocolectomy and anal mucosectomy).

Elective surgery

Panproctocolectomy and ileostomy

This is still the 'gold standard' surgical procedure having the advantage of removing all the diseased colon, and hence the risk of cancer, in one operation. Operative mortality for elective cases is acceptable at about 3% but rises to 10% for urgent cases. The procedure is not recommended in the emergency situation as operative mortality is over 20%. Recovery following proctocolectomy is generally good, most patients returning to normal activities within 2 months. The risk of sepsis (10–15%) is slightly less than following restorative proctocolectomy. The major disadvantage of the procedure is the need for a stoma and its associated problems. Many patients find an ileostomy distasteful, transient depression being seen in up to half of patients, although this is partly related to steroid withdrawal. Patients are also worried about the social and sexual effects of the stoma, which may be exacerbated by bladder or sexual dysfunction related to the pelvic surgery (Scaglia *et al.* 1993). One-third of patients complain of an impaired sex life, but in almost 60% sexual satisfaction is improved following proctocolectomy due to a general improvement in well-being. Up to 35% of patients have persistent urinary symptoms after proctocolectomy and 15% have autonomic denervation resulting in urinary retention (Kelly 1992).

Complications of the ileostomy include diarrhoea (up to 25% of patients), bleeding, stenosis, prolapse, herniation, intestinal obstruction (in 10%), and a 10% increase above normal in the incidence of urinary calculi (Figure 5.18). Despite these problems, 80% of patients are satisfied with their stoma. However, 80% of those who are converted to a restorative proctocolectomy state that they prefer

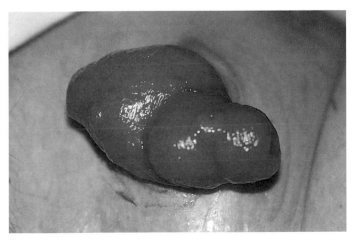

Figure 5.18 Prolapse of an ileostomy.

the greater freedom social and sexual freedom of the pouch (Moody 1993). Failure of the perineal wound to heal is not as major a problem as in Crohn's disease.

Ileorectal anastomosis

This associated with a low operative mortality (1–5%) and anastomotic leak rate (3–6%) (Oakley *et al.* 1985; Leijonmarck 1990). The risk of anastomotic breakdown is reduced if a stapling, rather than a hand-sewn technique is used (Kelly 1992). Stool frequency is usually four times per day, antidiarrhoeal medication being required by 20–30% of patients. Urgency occurs in up to one-third of patients and is related to intermittent relapses of proctitis, patients requiring medical treatment at some stage with 10–30% taking long-term medication to control symptoms related to the retained rectum (Oakley *et al.* 1985; Leijonmarck 1990). Modifying the technique to perform a caeco-anal anastomosis has no advantage, as severe colitis develops in the retained caecum.

The principal concern of ileorectal anastomosis is the associated risk of cancer in the residual rectum, which occurs in about 4% of cases overall, 2.5 times the risk of age–sex-matched controls (Oakley *et al.* 1985). The risk increases with time (Johnson *et al.* 1986). Consequently, at long-term follow-up, less than half of patients still retain their ileorectal anastomosis. Patients should therefore undergo annual sigmoidoscopy.

Mean hospital stay following ileorectal anastomosis is 20 days, being 60 days in the 6% who develop major complications. Mean stool frequency is four motions per day, patients being continent unless stools are very liquid. Nocturnal defecation occurs in less than 5% of cases (Oakley *et al.* 1985, Leijonmarck 1990).

A direct comparison between an ileorectal anastomosis and the pouch procedure revealed a mean stool frequency of 4.5 per day for ileorectal anastomosis compared with 3.7 per day for the W pouch. Half of those with an ileorectal anastomosis were on medication, compared with 20% of those with pouch procedures.

The indications for subtotal colectomy and ileorectal anastomosis have diminished since the introduction of the pelvic pouch procedure. The operation may still have a place in adolescents who do not wish their studies disrupted by the often long recovery and small risk of sexual dysfunction associated with a pelvic pouch. It may also be suitable for older patients with mild rectal disease and good anal tone or those troubled by severe ileostomy diarrhoea. Ileorectal anastomosis may be satisfactorily used as a palliative operation in those with advanced (Dukes' C and D) colorectal cancer complicating ulcerative colitis. In those without cancer, the risks of this complication developing in the rectal stump should always be borne in mind.

Continent reservoir ileostomy (Kock pouch)

This is now rarely employed as complications may occur in up to 70% of patients with 25% requiring reoperation. Complications include desusception of the nipple valve (10–40%), pouchitis (5–40%), intestinal obstruction (15%), and faecal fistula or peritonitis (15%), often related to necrosis of the conduit or nipple valve (5%).

Restorative proctocolectomy

Restorative proctocolectomy with pelvic pouch reservoir is intended to remove all the diseased mucosa and hence the risk of cancer, while avoiding the disadvantages of an ileostomy (Giebel and Sabiers 1996). However, even in cases where excision of the mucosa

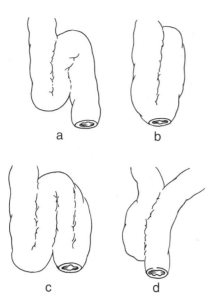

Figure 5.19 The different shapes of pouch in restorative proctocolectomy. A = 'S' pouch; B = 'J' pouch; C = 'W' pouch; D = 'Y' pouch).

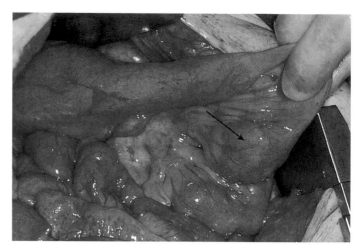

Figure 5.21 'J' pouch following completion (see colour plates).

was considered complete, histological studies reveal islands of residual mucosa within the rectal cuff or anal canal. Hence the risk of recurrent colitis, polyps, and cancer is not totally eliminated, and all have been reported to occur, although very rarely, within the pelvic pouch (Stern *et al.* 1990) (Figure 5.19).

Crohn's disease is a contraindication to performing a pelvic pouch procedure. However, colonoscopic biopsies and even careful pathological examination of a complete colectomy specimen cannot reliably distinguish between ulcerative colitis and Crohn's disease. Performing an initial colectomy and delaying the formation of the pouch until there is histological proof of ulcerative colitis is no guarantee, as 5–10% of resected colons will turn out to have Crohn's disease despite histological evidence suggesting ulcerative colitis (Poppen *et al.* 1992). Performing a frozen section during the operation also fails to detect cases of Crohn's disease. Similarly, if the pouch is fashioned as a one-stage procedure at the same time as removing the colon, 10% of cases will turn out to have Crohn's disease, despite radiological, endoscopic, and histological evidence to the contrary (Poppen *et al.* 1992). There therefore appears to be

little difference in complications and outcome in performing the pouch synchronously with the colectomy or as a later procedure (Figures 5.20 and 5.21). Consequently, most large series now report 5–10% of patients undergoing restorative proctocolectomy for presumed ulcerative colitis will turn out to have Crohn's disease (Foley *et al.* 1995). Complications, principally anal or vaginal fistula requiring ileostomy or pouch excision, occur in half of these patients, compared with only 3% of those who truly have ulcerative colitis (Grobler *et al.* 1993). If suspicion about the diagnosis exists, a preliminary colectomy should be performed for histological examination prior to completion of the pouch. However, patients should be warned that even if this policy is carried out, there is still a 5–10% risk that they will develop problems due to undetected Crohn's disease (Sagar *et al.* 1996).

Acute complications are fewer, functional pouches greater, stool control better, and overall hospitalization shorter than patients with a mucosectomy and handsewn ileoanal anastomosis. There is no evidence from controlled trials that performing a covering loop ileostomy provides any advantage and may in fact be associated with a higher incidence of intestinal obstruction (Grobler *et al.* 1993; Gorfine *et al.* 1995). However, in patients taking over 20 mg prednisolone daily, an ileostomy may be safer (Tjandra *et al.* 1993) (Figure 5.22). Preserving the omentum is associated with a lower

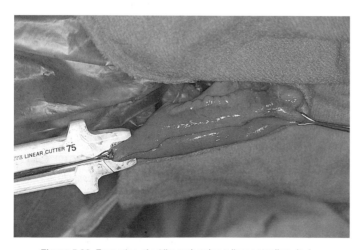

Figure 5.20 Formation of a 'J' pouch using a linear stapling device.

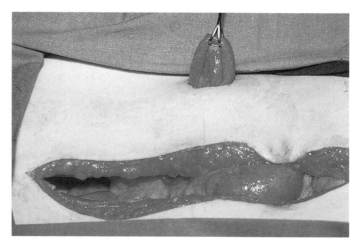

Figure 5.22 Formation of a loop ileostomy during restorative proctocolectomy.

incidence of postoperative complications, but does not alter the risk of small bowel obstruction (30%). Wexner and colleagues (1993) have performed 20 laparoscopically assisted pouch procedures for colitis, mean operating time being 3.9 (2.5–6.5) h with a median (range) length of hospitalization of 8.1 (4–19) days. The functional results are comparable with that of the open operation.

The complications of restorative proctocolectomy are shown in Table 5.5. Early postoperative complications occur in one-third of patients with 20% requiring reoperations, most often because of haemorrhage or pelvic sepsis (Jarvinen and Luukkonen 1993) (Figures 5.23 and 5.24). Late morbidity is seen in 30%. Failure of the operation is indicated by removal of the pouch or construction of a secondary loop ileostomy and ranges from 0 to 30%, usually being about 5% (Wexner *et al.* 1990; Kelly 1992; Jarvinen and Luukonen 1993, Koresen *et al.* 1996).

The incidence of small bowel obstruction (15–20%) after an ileo-rectal anastomosis is less than that following restorative procto-colectomy (up to 40% particularly if a covering ileostomy is preformed) (Kelly 1992) (Figure 5.25). Because of the cancer risk and generally comparable functional results, most authors now suggest that restorative proctocolectomy is preferable to ileorectal anastomosis (Kelly 1992, Giebel and Sabiers 1996).

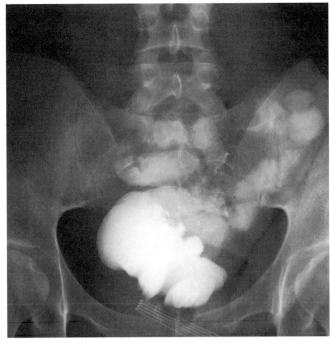

Figure 5.23 Normal 'pouchogram' in a case of suspected pelvic sepsis following pouch formation.

Table 5.5 The complications of restorative proctocolectomy

Complication	Feature	Author
Operative mortality	1% (Similar to proctocolectomy and ileostomy or ileorectal anastomosis) Closely related to surgeon's experience of pouch procedure	Johnston *et al.* 1996 Mikkola *et al.* 1996
Pelvic sepsis	3–33% depending on definition Due to infected haematoma or anastomotic leakage (cuff abscess) Unrelated to sutured or stapled anastomosis	Romanos *et al.* 1996 Ziv *et al.* 1996 Isbister and Prasad 1997
Anastomotic stricture	Occurs in 4–30% of cases Usually responds to a single dilatation Does not affect long-term functional results	Herbst *et al.* 1996 Paye *et al.* 1996 Senapati *et al.* 1996
Small bowel obstruction	Occurs in 6–40% of cases Higher in those with covering ileostomy or if colectomy and pouch performed at the same operation Bowel resection increases frequency of defecation and incontinence	Johnston *et al.* 1996 Romanos *et al.* 1996
Fistula	Occurs in 2–10% of cases Related to anastomotic leakage, Crohn's disease or trapping vagina in staple line Appears after ileostomy closure	Wexner *et al.* 1990
Pouchitis	Occurs in 33% within 5 years Aetiology unknown Extra-intestinal manifestations may develop or recur 90% responds to metronidazole	Oresland *et al.* 1990 Lohmuller *et al.* 1990 Luukkonen *et al.* 1994 Hurst *et al.* 1996 Keighley 1996 Penna *et al.* 1996 Stahlberg *et al.* 1996
Failure of operation	Usually 5–10% Related to Crohn's disease Recurrent colitis or tumour may occur	Wexner *et al.* 1990 Kelly 1992 Jarvinen and Luukkonen 1993 Korgsen *et al.* 1996 Sagar *et al.* 1996 Thompson-Fawcett and Mortensen 1996 MacRae *et al.* 1997

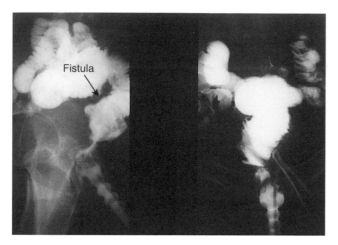

Figure 5.24 'Pouchogram' showing pouch-vaginal fistula (which settled spontaneously).

The functional results of restorative proctocolectomy improve for at least 2 years after operation and are best in children (Kelly 1992). Results from patients with indeterminate colitis are not quite as good as for proven ulcerative colitis (McIntyre *et al.* 1995, Stewenius *et al.* 1996). Complete continence occurs in over 85% of patients, about 5% experiencing faecal leakage during the day and 10% at night (Wexner *et al.* 1989). Over half of patients with a pouch take antidiarrhoeal medication. Although 90% of patients can discriminate between gas, liquid, and solid, 15–30% wear pads and one-third are incontinent of flatus. Frequency of defecation also improves with time being eight stools per day at 1 month, six at

6 months, and five after 9 months. The length of small bowel used to construct the pouch is the major determinant of stool frequency, although pouch volume, compliance and motor activity are also important. The capacity of J pouches and hence their functional results, increases for 2 years following the operation (Oresland *et al.* 1990). The triplicated S pouch increases the capacity of the reservoir and provided a short efferent limb is used, the initial functional results are better than with the J pouch (Wexner *et al.* 1989). A quadruple W pouch has the increased capacity of an S pouch without the problems of the efferent limb and greater compliance relative to the J pouch. However, with time, the functional results of most pouches, J, S, or W are generally comparable and there appears to be little to choose between pouch designs.

There is little disturbance of bladder function with restorative proctocolectomy and the incidence of impotence in males is under 10%, being more common in those over 50 years (Wexner *et al.* 1989). However, one-third of females will have sexual dysfunction, mainly dyspareunia or faecal leakage during intercourse. Pouch formation does not adversely affect ability to become pregnant and vaginal delivery is generally safe (Counihan *et al.* 1994; Juhasz *et al.* 1995). Almost all patients can return to work following restorative proctocolectomy and 90% are satisfied with the result (Wexner *et al.* 1989; Damgaard *et al.* 1995; Kohler and Troidl 1995). However, it is suggested that quality of life assessment is already satisfactory after 'cure' of the disease, and restitution of normal defecation by a pouch does not yield much further improvement (Weinryb *et al.* 1995).

Inflammation in the ileal reservoir (pouchitis) occurs in about one-third of patients within 5 years of operation (Luukkonen *et al.* 1994; Mignon *et al.* 1995, Stahlberg *et al.* 1996). Its aetiology is unknown. There is an alteration in the aerobe to anaerobe ratio resulting in a fall in luminal short chain fatty acids and change in bile acid metabolism (Chapman *et al.* 1994). The bacterial overgrowth is probably a result of stasis, although there is neither radiographic evidence of stasis or proof that treatment with fatty acids improve symptoms (Mignon *et al.* 1995). Alternative theories are that colonic metaplasia occurring in the ileum is subjected to the same inflammatory process responsible for the original colitis or that there is mucosal ischaemia supplemented by migration of endotoxins (Hosie *et al.* 1992; Luukonen *et al.* 1994). Crohn's disease and adhesive *E. coli* in the ileal pouch do not appear to be responsible (Subramani *et al.* 1993).

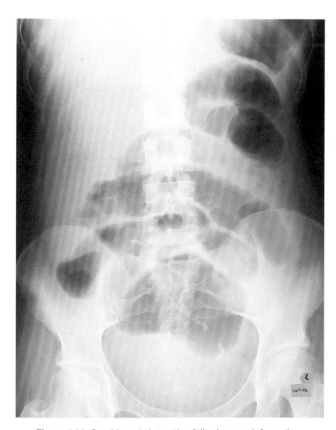

Figure 5.25 Small bowel obstruction following pouch formation.

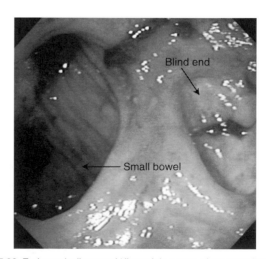

Figure 5.26 Endoscopically normal 'J' pouch in a case of suspected pouchitis.

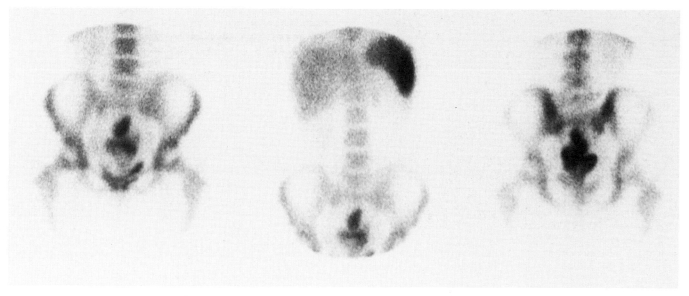

Figure 5.27 Technetium-labelled white cell scan showing an inflamed pouch.

The clinical features of pouchitis are bloody diarrhoea and pyrexia (Hurst *et al.* 1996). Extra-intestinal manifestations, particularly those which respond to colectomy (arthritis, skin and eye complications) may occur for the first time or relapse with an episode of pouchitis. Recurrent episodes of pouchitis are likely in up to two-thirds of those who develop the condition (Lohmuller *et al.* 1990). Sigmoidoscopy, preferably with a flexible instrument, reveals a haemorrhagic, oedematous mucosa with apthous ulceration (Figure 5.26). Biopsy reveals a characteristic neutrophil inflammatory infiltrate, the severity of which correlates with clinical and endoscopic features. Pouchitis is often associated with thrombocytosis, leucocytosis, hypoalbuminaemia, and raised alkaline phosphatase (Santavirta *et al.* 1991). Radio-isotope studies with indium have a specificity of 80% and sensitivity of 70% (Figure 5.27). Pouchitis responds to metronidazole therapy in 90% of cases, a response being almost diagnostic. 5-ASA and steroids may be used topically or orally, although oral steroids should be reserved for those with systemic or extra-intestinal symptoms who fail to respond to other treatments.

References

Adachi Y, *et al.* Rheumatoid arthritis associated with ulcerative colitis. *J. Gastroenterol.* 1996; 31: 590–5.

Almer S, *et al.* Air enema radiology compared with leukocyte scintigraphy for imaging inflammation in active ulcerative colitis. *Eur. J. Gastroenterol. Hepatol.* 1995; 7: 59–64.

Almer S, Granerus G, Franzen L, Strom M. Technetium-99m scintigraphy: more accurate assessment of ulcerative colitis with exametazime-labelled leucocytes than with antigranulocyte antibodies. *Eur. J. Nucl. Med.* 1996; 23: 247–55.

Alstead EM, *et al.* Safety of azathioprine in pregnancy in inflammatory bowel disease. *Gastroenterology* 1990; 99: 443–6.

Andreyev HJ, *et al.* Joint symptoms after restorative proctocolectomy in ulcerative colitis and familial polyposis coli. *J. Clin. Gastroenterol.* 1996; 23: 35–9.

Arndt JW, *et al.* Inflammatory bowel disease activity assessment using technetium-99m-HMPAO leukocytes. *Dig. Dis. Sci.* 1997; 42: 387–93.

Aslan A, Triadafilopoulos G. Fish oil fatty acid supplementation in active ulcerative colitis: a double blind, placebo controlled, crossover study. *Am. J. Gastroenterol.* 1992; 87: 432–7.

Azad Khan AK, Piris J, Truelove SC. An experiment to determine the active therapeutic moiety of sulphasalazine. *Lancet* 1977; ii: 892–5.

Babbs CF. Oxygen radicals in ulcerative colitis. *Free Radical Biol. Med.* 1992; 13: 169–81.

Bansky G, *et al.* Treatment of distal ulcerative colitis with beclomethasone enemas: high therapeutic efficacy without endocrine side effects. A prospective, randomized, double blind trial. *Dis. Colon Rectum* 1987; 30: 288–92.

Bernstein CN, *et al.* Milk tolerance in adults with ulcerative colitis. *Am. J. Gastroenterol.* 1994; 89: 872–7.

Bioque G, *et al.* Evidence of genetic heterogeneity in IBD: 1. The interleukin-1 receptor antagonist in the predisposition to suffer from ulcerative colitis. *Eur. J. Gastroenterol. Hepatol.* 1996; 8: 105–10.

Bischoff SC, Grabowsky J, Manns MP, Quantification of inflammatory mediators in stool samples of patients with inflammatory bowel disorders and controls. *Dig. Dis. Sci.* 1997; 42: 394–403.

Bitton A, Peppercorn MA. Emergencies in inflammatory bowel disease. *Crit. Care Clin.* 1995; 11: 513–29.

Brentnall TA, *et al.* Risk and natural history of colonic neoplasia in patients with primary sclerosing cholangitis and ulcerative colitis. *Gastroenterology* 1996; 110: 331–8.

Broome U, *et al.* Primary sclerosing cholangitis and ulcerative colitis: evidence for increased neoplastic potential. *Hepatology* 1995; 22: 1404–8.

Brynskov J, *et al.* A placebo controlled, double blind, randomized trial of cyclosporine therapy in active chronic Crohn's disease. *N. Engl. J. Med.* 1989; 321: 45–50.

Burgos-Vargas R. Spondyloarthropathies and psoriatic arthritis in children. *Cur. Opin. Rheumatol.* 1993; 5: 634–43.

Campieri M, *et al.* Retrograde spread of 5 aminosalicylic acid enemas in patients with active ulcerative colitis. *Dis. Colon Rectum* 1986; 29: 108–10.

Capobianchi MR, *et al.* Absence of circulating interferon in patients with inflammatory bowel disease. Suggestion against an autoimmune etiology. *Clin. Exp. Immunol.* 1992; 90: 85–7.

Chapman RW, Selby WS, Jewell DP. Controlled trial of intravenous metronidazole as an adjunct to corticosteroids in severe ulcerative colitis. *Gut* 1986; 27: 1210–2.

Colombel JF, *et al.* Antineutrophil cytoplasmic autoantibodies in inflammatory bowel diseases. *Gastroenterol. Clin. Biol.* 1992; 16: 656–60.

Counihan TC, *et al.* Fertility and sexual and gynecologic function after ileal pouch anal anastomosis. *Dis. Colon Rectum* 1994; 37: 1126–9.

Courtney MG, *et al*. Randomised comparison of olsalazine and mesalazine in prevention of relapses in ulcerative colitis. *Lancet* 1992; 339: 1279–81.

Cummings JH. Short-chain fatty acid enemas in the treatment of distal ulcerative colitis. *Eur. J. Gastroenterol. Hepatol.* 1997; 9: 149–533.

Damgaard B, Wettergren A, Kirkegaard P. Social and sexual function following ileal pouch anal anastomosis. *Dis. Colon Rectum* 1995; 38: 286–9.

Danielsson A, *et al*. A controlled randomized trial of budesonide versus prednisolone retention enemas in active distal ulcerative colitis. *Scand. J. Gastroenterol.* 1987; 22: 987–92.

Delgado Castro M, *et al*. The diagnostic value of Tc-99m human polyclonal immunoglobulin imaging compared to Tc-99m HMPAO labeled leukocytes in inflammatory bowel disease. *Clin. Nucl. Med.* 1997; 22: 17–20.

Dwarakanath AD, *et al*. 'Sticky' neutrophils, pathergic arthritis, and response to heparin in pyoderma gangrenosum complicating ulcerative colitis. *Gut* 1995; 37: 585–8.

Ekbom A, *et al*. Extracolonic malignancies in inflammatory bowel disease. *Cancer* 1991; 67: 2015–9.

Egan LJ, Sandborn WJ. Methotrexate for inflammatory bowel disease: pharmacology and preliminary results. *Mayo Clin. Proc.* 1996; 71: 69–80.

Farouk R, Pemberton JH. Surgical options in ulcerative colitis. *Surg. Clin. North Am.* 1997; 77: 85–94.

Foley EF, *et al*. Rediversion after ileal pouch anal anastomosis. Causes of failures and predictors of subsequent pouch salvage. *Dis. Colon Rectum* 1995; 38: 793–8.

Gaffney PR, *et al*. Response to heparin in patients with ulcerative colitis. *Lancet* 1991; 337: 238–9.

Gendre JP, *et al*. Oral mesalamine (Pentasa) as maintenance treatment in Crohn's disease: a multicenter placebo controlled study. The Groupe d'Etudes Therapeutiques des Affections Inflammatoires Digestives (GETAID). *Gastroenterology* 1993; 104: 435–9.

George J, *et al*. The long-term outcome of ulcerative colitis treated with 6-mercaptopurine. *Am. J. Gastroenterol.* 1996; 91: 1711–4.

Giebel GD, Sabiers H. Ileal pouch-anal anastomosis for ulcerative colitis and polyposis coli: is the risk of carcinoma formation conclusively averted? *Eur. J. Surg. Oncol.* 1996; 22: 372–6.

Gilvarry JM, O'Morain CA. New treatments in inflammatory bowel disease. Eur. J. Gastroenterol. Hepatol. 1993; 5: 893–902.

Giovagnoni A, *et al*. MR imaging of ulcerative colitis. *Abdom. Imaging* 1993; 18: 371–5.

Gore RM, Ghahremani GG. Radiologic investigation of acute inflammatory and infectious bowel disease. *Gastroenterol. Clin. North Am.* 1995; 24: 353–84.

Gorfine SR, *et al*. Restorative proctocolectomy without diverting ileostomy. *Dis. Colon Rectum* 1995; 3: 188–94.

Graham JA, *et al*. Pyoderma gangrenosum in infants and children. *Pediat. Dermatol.* 1994; 11: 10–7.

Gran JT, Husby G. The epidemiology of ankylosing spondylitis. *Semin. Arthrit. Rheumat.* 1993; 22: 319–34.

Grobler SP, *et al*. Outcome of restorative proctocolectomy when the diagnosis is suggestive of Crohn's disease. *Gut* 1993; 34: 1384–8.

Grzybowska K, Kozlowski W. The level of immunoglobulins in the small and large intestinal mucosa from children with ulcerative colitis. *Patologia Polska* 1993; 44: 217–20.

Guslandi M, Polli D, Sorghi M, Tittobello A. Rectal blood flow in ulcerative colitis. *Am. J. Gastroenterol.* 1995; 90: 579–80.

Hanauer SB. Medical therapy of ulcerative colitis. *Lancet* 1993; 342: 412–7.

Hanauer SB. Inflammatory bowel disease. N. Engl. J. Med. 1996; 334: 841–8.

Hanauer SB, Kirsner JB, Barrett WE. The treatment of left sided ulcerative colitis with tixocortol pivalate. *Gastroenterology* 1986; 90: A1449.

Hartmann DP, *et al*. Flow cytometric DNA analysis of ulcerative colitis using paraffin embedded biopsy specimens: comparison with morphology and DNA analysis of fresh samples. *Am. J. Gastroenterol.* 1995; 90: 590–6.

Haruta J, *et al*. Phenotypic and functional analysis of lamina propria mononuclear cells from colonoscopic biopsy specimens in patients with ulcerative colitis. *Am. J. Gastroenterol.* 1992; 87: 448–54.

Hawthorne AB, *et al*. Randomised controlled trial of azathioprine withdrawal in ulcerative colitis. *Br. Med. J.* 1992; 305: 20–2.

Hendriksen C, Kreiner S, Binder V. Long term prognosis in ulcerative colitis—based on results from a regional patient group from the county of Copenhagen. *Gut* 1985; 26: 158–63.

Heppell J, *et al*. Toxic megacolon. An analysis of 70 cases. *Dis. Colon Rectum* 1986; 29: 789–92.

Herbst F, Sielezneff I, Nicholls RJ. Salvage surgery for ileal pouch outlet obstruction. *Br. J. Surg.* 1996; 83: 368–71.

Herzog K, Goldblum JR. Gallbladder adenocarcinoma, acalculous chronic lymphoplasmacytic cholecystitis, ulcerative colitis. *Mod. Pathol.* 1996; 9: 194–8.

Hiatt RA, Kaufman L. Epidemiology of inflammatory bowel disease in a defined northern California population. *Western J. Med.* 1988; 149: 541–6.

Hibi T, *et al*. Interleukin 2 and interferon gamma augment anticolon antibody dependent cellular cytotoxicity in ulcerative colitis. *Gut* 1993; 34: 788–93.

Hofley P, *et al*. Asymptomatic uveitis in children with chronic inflammatory bowel diseases. *J. Ped. Gastroenterol. Nutrit.* 1993; 17: 397–400.

Hofley PM, Piccoli DA. Inflammatory bowel disease in children. Med. Clin. North Am. 1994; 78: 1281–302.

Hosie KB, *et al*. Ileal mucosal absorption of bile acid in man: validation of a miniature flux chamber technique. *Gut* 1992; 33: 490–6.

Hurst RD, *et al*. Prospective study of the incidence, timing and treatment of pouchitis in104 consecutive patients after restorative proctocolectomy. *Arch. Surg.* 1996; 131: 497–506.

Isbister WH, Prasad J. The surgical management of nonspecific inflammatory bowel disease: a small personal experience. *N. Z. Med. J.* 1997; 110: 56–8.

Ireland A, Jewell DP. Mechanism of action of 5 aminosalicylic acid and its derivatives. *Clin. Sci.* 1990; 78: 119–25.

Irvine EJ, *et al*. Quality of life: a valid and reliable measure of therapeutic efficacy in the treatment of inflammatory bowel disease. *Gastroenterology* 1994; 106: 287–96.

Izzo RS, *et al*. Interleukin-8 and neutrophil markers in colonic mucosa from patients with ulcerative colitis. *Am. J. Gastroenterol.* 1992; 87: 1447–52.

Jarnerot G, Rolny P, Sandberg-Gertzen H. Intensive intravenous treatment of ulcerative colitis. Gastroenterology 1985; 89: 1005–13.

Jarvinen HJ, Luukkonen P. Experience with restorative proctocolectomy in 201 patients. *Ann. Chir. Gynaecol.* 1993; 82: 159–64.

Jayanthi V, *et al*. Low incidence of ulcerative colitis and proctitis in Bangladeshi migrants in Britain. *Digestion* 1992; 52: 34–42.

Johnson WR, *et al*. The outcome of patients with ulcerative colitis managed by subtotal colectomy. *Surg. Gynecol. Obstet.* 1986; 162: 421–5.

Johnston D, *et al*. Prospective controlled trial of duplicated (J) versus quadruplicated (W) pelvic ileal reservoirs in restorative proctocolectomy for ulcerative colitis. *Gut* 1996; 39: 242–7.

Juhasz ES, *et al*. Ileal pouch anal anastomosis function following childbirth. An extended evaluation. *Dis. Colon Rectum* 1995; 38: 159–65.

Kamm MA, Senapati A. Drug management of ulcerative colitis. Br. Med. J. 1992; 305: 35–8.

Kartheuser AH, *et al*. Comparison of surgical treatment of ulcerative colitis associated with primary sclerosing cholangitis: ileal pouch-anal anastomosis versus Brooke ileostomy. *Mayo Clinic Proceed.* 1996; 71: 748–56.

Keighley MR. Review article: the management of pouchitis. *Aliment. Pharmacol. Therapeut.* 1996; 10: 449–57.

Kelly KA. Anal sphincter saving operations for chronic ulcerative colitis. *Am. J. Surg.* 1992; 163: 5–11.

Kirschner BS. Ulcerative colitis in children. Pediatr. Clin. North Am. 1996; 43: 235–54.

Kohler L, Troidl H. The ileoanal pouch: a risk benefit analysis. *Br. J. Surg.* 1995; 82: 443–7.

Koizumi M, *et al*. Expression of vascular adhesion molecules in inflammatory bowel disease. *Gastroenterology* 1992; 103: 840–7.

Korsgen S, *et al*. Results from pouch salvage. *Brit. J. Surg.* 1996; 83: 372.

Koutroubakis I, *et al*. Environmental risk factors in inflammatory bowel disease. Hepato-Gastroenterol. 1996; 43: 381–93.

Kruis W, *et al*. Double blind dose finding study of olsalazine versus sulphasalazine as maintenance therapy for ulcerative colitis. *Eur. J. Gastroenterol. Hepatol.* 1995; 7: 391–6.

Kvist N, *et al*. Malignancy in ulcerative colitis. Surgical Dept., Rigshospitalet, Copenhagen, Denmark. *Scand. J. Gastroenterol.* 1989; 24: 497–506.

Langholz E, Munkholm P, Davidsen M, Binder V. Colorectal cancer risk and mortality in patients with ulcerative colitis. *Gastroenterology* 1992; 103: 1444–51.

Langholz E, *et al*. Incidence and prevalence of ulcerative colitis in Copenhagen county from 1962 to 1987. *Scand. J. Gastroenterol.* 1992; 26: 1247–56.

Lashner BA. Prediction rules for ulcerative colitis. *Am. J. Gastroenterol.* 1995; 90: 1737–8.

Lashner BA, Kane SV, Hanauer SB. Colon cancer surveillance in chronic ulcerative colitis: historical cohort study. *Am. J. Gastroenterol.* 1990; 85: 1083–7.

Laursen LS, *et al*. Selective 5 lipoxygenase inhibition by Zileuton in the treatment of relapsing ulcerative colitis: a randomised double blind placebo controlled multicentre trial. *Eur. J. Gastroenterol. Hepatol.* 1994; 6: 209–15.

Lee FI, Jewell DP, Mani V, *et al*. A randomised trial comparing mesalazine and prednisolone foam enemas in patients with acute distal ulcerative colitis. *Gut.* 1996; 38: 229–33.

Leijonmarck CE. Surgical treatment of ulcerative colitis in Stockholm county. *Acta Chir. Scand. Suppl.* 1990; 554: 1–56.

Lennard-Jones JE, Ritchie JK, Hilder W, Spicer CC. Assessment of severity in colitis: a preliminary study. *Gut* 1975; 16: 579–84.

Lever E, *et al*. Primary biliary cirrhosis associated with uclerative colitis. *Am. J. Gastroenterol.* 1993; 88: 945 7.

Li DJ, Freeman A, Miles KA, Wraight EP. Can 99Tcm HMPAO leucocyte scintigraphy distinguish between Crohn's disease and ulcerative colitis? *Br. J. Radiol.* 1994; 67: 472–7.

Lichtiger S, Present DH. Preliminary report: cyclosporin in treatment of severe active ulcerative colitis. *Lancet* 1990; 336: 16–9.

Lindstrom E, Noren B. Air enema revisited in assessment of colitis. *Acta Radiol.* 1992; 33: 360–4.

Linn FV, Peppercorn MA. Drug therapy for inflammatory bowel disease: Part II. *Am. J. Surg.* 1992; 164: 178–85.

Lisciandrano D, *et al*. Prevalence of oral lesions in inflammatory bowel disease. *Am. J. Gastroenterol.* 1996; 91: 7–10.

Loftus EV Jr, *et al*. Risk of colorectal neoplasia in patients with primary sclerosing cholangitis. *Gastroenterology* 1996; 110: 432–40.

Lohmuller JL, *et al*. Pouchitis and extraintestinal manifestations of inflammatory bowel disease after ileal pouch anal anastomosis. *Ann. Surg.* 1990; 211: 622–7.

Lossos A, *et al*. Neurologic aspects of inflammatory bowel disease. *Neurology* 1995; 45: 416–21.

Luukkonen P, Jarvinen H, Tanskanen M, Kahri A. Pouchitis—recurrence of the inflammatory bowel disease? *Gut* 1994; 35: 243–6.

Macpherson A, Khoo UY, Forgacs I, Philpott-Howeard J, Bjarnason I. Mucosal antibodies in inflammatory bowel disease are directed against intestinal bacteria. *Gut.* 1996; 38: 365–75.

MacRae HM, *et al*. Risk factors for pelvic pouch failure. *Dis. Colon Rectum.* 1997; 40: 257–62.

Maeder UH. The complete heart-block—an extraintestinal manifestation of ulcerative colitis. *Zeitschrift fur Gastroenterol.* 1996; 34: 27–9.

Mahoney BP. Rheumatologic disease and associated ocular manifestations. *J. Am. Optometric. Assoc.* 1993; 64: 403–15.

Mahmud N, McDonald GS, Kelleher D, Weir DG. Microalbuminuria correlates with intestinal histopathological grading in patients with inflammatory bowel disease. *Gut* 1996; 38: 99–103.

Mayberry JF, Ballantyne KC, Hardcastle JD, Mangham C, Pye GAD. Epidemiological study of asymptomatic inflammatory bowel disease: the identification of cases during a screening programme for colorectal cancer. *Gut* 1989; 30: 481–3.

McIntyre PB, *et al*. Therapeutic benefits from a poorly absorbed prednisolone enema in distal colitis. *Gut* 1985; 26: 822–4.

McIntyre PB, *et al*. Controlled trial of bowel rest in the treatment of severe acute colitis. *Gut* 1986; 27: 481–5.

McIntyre PB, *et al*. Indeterminate colitis. Long term outcome in patients after ileal pouch anal anastomosis. *Dis. Colon Rectum.* 1995; 38: 51–4.

Melville DM, *et al*. Observer study of the grading of dysplasia in ulcerative colitis: comparison with clinical outcome. *Hum. Pathol.* 1989; 20: 1008–14.

Mesalamine Study Group. An oral preparation of mesalamine as long term maintenance therapy for ulcerative colitis. A randomized, placebo controlled trial. *Ann. Intern. Med.* 1996; 124: 204–11.

Meyers S, Janowitz HD. The 'natural history' of ulcerative colitis: an analysis of the placebo response. *J. Clin. Gastroenterol.* 1989; 11: 33–7.

Mignon M, Stettler C, Phillips SF. Pouchitis—a poorly understood entity. *Dis. Colon Rectum* 1995; 38: 100–3.

Mikkola K, *et al*. Liver involvement and its course in patients operated on for ulcerative colitis. *Hepato-gastroenterol.* 1995; 42: 68–72.

Mikkola K, Luukkonen P, Jarvinen HJ. Restorative compared with conventional proctocolectomy for the treatment of ulcerative colitis. *Eur. J. Surg.* 1996; 162: 315–9.

Miner P, Hanauer S, Robinson M, Schwartz J, Arora S. Safety and efficacy of controlled release mesalamine for maintenance of remission in ulcerative colitis. Pentasa UC Maintenance Study Group. *Dig. Dis. Sci.* 1995; 40: 296–304.

Mishkin S. Dairy sensitivity, lactose malabsorption, and elimination diets in inflammatory bowel disease. *Am. J. Clin. Nutrit.* 1997; 65: 564–7.

Modigliani R, *et al*. Clinical, biological, and endoscopic picture of attacks of Crohn's disease. Evolution on prednisolone. Groupe d'Etude Therapeutique des Affections Inflammatoires Digestives. *Gastroenterology* 1990; 98: 811–8.

Moody GA, Bhakta P, Mayberry JF. Disinterest in local self help groups amongst patients with inflammatory bowel disease in Leicester. *Int. J. Colorectal Dis.* 1993; 8: 181–3.

Moran A, Jones A, Asquith P. Laboratory markers of colonoscopic activity in ulcerative colitis and Crohn's colitis. *Scand. J. Gastroenterol.* 1995; 30: 356–60.

Morita N, *et al*. Incidence and prevalence of inflammatory bowel disease in Japan: nationwide epidemiological survey during the year 1991. *J. Gastroenterol.* 1995; 30 Suppl 8: 1–4.

Moum B, Aadland E, Ekbom A, Vatn MH. Seasonal variations in the onset of ulcerative colitis. *Gut.* 1996; 38: 376–8.

Moum B, *et al*. Incidence of ulcerative colitis and indeterminate colitis in four counties of southeastern Norway, 1990–93. A prospective population-based study. The Inflammatory Bowel South-Eastern Norway (IBSEN) Study Group of Gastroenterologists. *Scand. J. Gastroenterol* 1996; 31: 362–6.

Murch SH, Braegger CP, Walker Smith JA, MacDonald TT. Location of tumour necrosis factor alpha by immunohistochemistry in chronic inflammatory bowel disease. *Gut* 1993; 34: 1705–9.

Myers B, *et al*. Metabolism and urinary excretion of 5 amino salicylic acid in healthy volunteers when given intravenously or released for absorption at different sites in the gastrointestinal tract. *Gut* 1987; 28: 196–200.

Nilsson A, *et al*. Olsalazine versus sulphasalazine for relapse prevention in ulcerative colitis: a multicenter study. *Am. J. Gastroenterol.* 1995; 90: 381–7.

Niv Y, Abukasis G. Prevalence of ulcerative colitis in the Israeli kibbutz population. *J. Clin. Gastroenterol.* 1991; 13: 98–101.

Nordenholtz KE, *et al*. The cause of death in inflammatory bowel disease: a comparison of death certificates and hospital charts in Rochester, New York. *Am. J. Gastroenterol.* 1995; 90: 927–32.

O'Keefe SJ, Ogden J, Rund J, Potter P. Steroids and bowel rest versus elemental diet in the treatment of patients with Crohn's disease: the effects on protein metabolism and immune function. *Jpn. J. Parenter. Enteral. Nutr.* 1989; 13: 455–60.

Oakley JR, *et al*. Management of the perineal wound after rectal excision for ulcerative colitis. *Dis. Colon Rectum* 1985; 28: 885–8.

Odes HS, Fraser D, Krawiec J. Inflammatory bowel disease in migrant and native Jewish populations of southern Israel. *Scand. J. Gastroenterol.* Suppl 1989; 170: 36–8.

Ohkusa T, Okayasu I, Tokoi S, Araki A, Ozaki Y. Changes in bacterial phagocytosis of macrophages in experimental ulcerative colitis. *Digestion* 1995; 56: 159–64.

Olusanya O, *et al.* Surface properties, connective tissue protein binding and *Shiga* like toxin production of *Escherichia coli* isolated from patients with ulcerative colitis. *Int. J. Med. Microbiol. Virol. Parasitol. Infect. Dis.* 1992; 276: 254–63.

Oresland T, Fasth S, Nordgren S, Akervall S, Hulten L. Pouch size: the important functional determinant after restorative proctocolectomy. *Br. J. Surg.* 1990; 77: 265–9.

Orkin BA, Telander RL, Wolff BG, Perrault J, Ilstrup DM. The surgical management of children with ulcerative colitis. The old vs. the new. *Dis. Colon Rectum* 1990; 33: 947–55.

Oudkerk-Pool M, *et al.* Serological markers to differentiate between ulcerative colitis and Crohn's disease. *J. Clin. Pathol.* 1995; 48: 346–50.

Paganelli GM, *et al.* Abnormal rectal cell proliferation and p52/p35 protein expression in patients with ulcerative colitis. *Cancer Lett.* 1993; 73: 23–8.

Papos M, Nagy F, Lang J, Csernay L. Technetium-99m hexamethyl-propylene-amine-oxime labelled leucocyte scintigraphy in ulcerative colitis and Crohn's disease. *Eur. J. Nuclear Med.* 1993; 20: 766–9.

Papos M, *et al.* Antineutrophil cytoplasmic antibodies in relatives of patients with inflammatory bowel disease. *Am. J. Gastroenterol.* 1996; 91: 1512–5.

Patz J, Jacobsohn WZ, Gottschalk-Sabag S, Zeides S, Braverman DZ. Treatment of refractory distal ulcerative colitis with short chain fatty acid enemas. *Am. J. Gastroenterol.* 1996; 91: 731–4.

Paye F, *et al.* Pouch-related fistula following restorative proctocolectomy. *Br. J. Surg.* 1996; 83: 1574–7.

Pera A, *et al.* Colonoscopy in inflammatory bowel disease. Diagnostic accuracy and proposal of an endoscopic score. *Gastroenterology* 1987; 92: 181–5.

Penna C, *et al.* Pouchitis after ileal pouch-anal anastomosis for ulcerative colitis occurs with increased frequency in patients with associated primary sclerosing cholangitis. *Gut* 1996; 38: 234–9.

Persson PG, Leijonmarck CE, Bernell O, Hellers G, Ahlbom A. Risk indicators for inflammatory bowel disease. *Int. J. Epidemiol.* 1993; 22: 268–72.

Persson PG, *et al.* Survival and cause-specific mortality in inflammatory bowel disease: a population-based cohort study. *Gastroenterol.* 1996; 110: 1339–45.

Philpotts LE, Heiken JP, Westcott MA, Gore RM. Colitis: use of CT findings in differential diagnosis. *Radiology* 1994; 190: 445–9.

Poppen B, *et al.* Colectomy proctomucosectomy with S pouch: operative procedures, complications, and functional outcome in 69 consecutive patients. *Dis. Colon Rectum.* 1992; 35: 40–7.

Porro GB, *et al.* Pentasa dosage versus hydrocortisone in the topical treatment of active ulcerative colitis: a randomized, double blind study. *Am. J. Gastroenterol.* 1995; 90: 736–9.

Present DH, Chapman ML, Rubin PH. Efficacy of 6 mercaptopurine in refractory ulcerative colitis. *Gastroenterology* 1988; 94: A359.

Primatesta P, Goldacre MJ. Crohn's disease and ulcerative colitis in England and the Oxford record linkage study area: a profile of hospitalized morbidity. *Int. J. Epidemiol.* 1995; 24: 922–8.

Probert CS, Mayberry JF, Mann R. Inflammatory bowel disease in the rural Indian subcontinent: a survey of patients attending mission hospitals. *Digestion* 1990; 47: 42–639.

Probert CS, Jayanthi V, Pinder D, Wicks AC, Mayberry JF. Epidemiological study of ulcerative proctocolitis in Indian migrants and the indigenous population of Leicestershire. *Gut* 1992; 33: 687–93.

Probert CS, *et al.* Prevalence and family risk of ulcerative colitis and Crohn's disease: an epidemiological study among Europeans and South Asians in Leicestershire. *Gut* 1993; 34: 1547–51.

Pullan RD, *et al.* Transdermal nicotine treatment for ulcerative colitis: a controlled trial. *Gastroenterology* 1993; 104: A765.

Pullan RD. Colonic mucus, smoking and ulcerative colitis. *Ann. Roy. Coll. Surg. Eng.* 1996; 78: 85–91.

Quinn PG, Binion DG, Connors PJ. The role of endoscopy in inflammatory bowel disease. *Med. Clin. North Am.* 1994; 78: 1331–52.

Rachmilewitz D, *et al.* Enhanced colonic nitric oxide generation and nitric oxide synthase activity in ulcerative colitis and Crohn's disease. *Gut* 1995; 36: 718–23.

Rajput HI, Seebaran AR, Desai Y. Ulcerative colitis in the Indian population of Durban. *S. Afric. Med. J.* 1992; 81: 245–8.

Ranzi T, *et al.* Treatment of chronic proctosigmoiditis with cyclosporin enemas. *Lancet* 1989; ii: 97.

Reumaux D, *et al.* Antineutrophil cytoplasmic auto antibodies in sera from patients with ulcerative colitis after proctocolectomy with ileo anal anastomosis. *Adv. Exp. Med. Biol.* 1993; 336: 523–5.

Rhodes JM. Unifying hypothesis for inflammatory bowel disease and associated colon cancer: sticking the pieces together with sugar. *Lancet* 1996; 347: 40–4.

Rigas A, *et al.* Breast feeding and maternal smoking in the etiology of Crohn's disease and ulcerative colitis in childhood. *Ann. Epidemiol.* 1993; 3: 387–92.

Rintala RJ, Lindahl H. Restorative proctocolectomy for ulcerative colitis inchildren—is the J-pouch better than straight pull-through? *J. Pediat. Surg.* 1996; 31: 530–3.

Robinson M, Hanauer S, Hoop S, Zbrozek A, Wilkinson C. Mesalamine capsules enhance the quality of life for patients with ulcerative colitis. *Aliment. Pharmacol. Ther.* 1994; 8: 27–34.

Romanos J, *et al.* Restorative proctocolectomy in children and adolescents. *J. Pediat. Surg.* 1996; 31: 1655–8.

Sagar PM, Dozois RR, Wolff BG. Long-term results of ileal pouch-anal anastomosis in patients with Crohn's disease. *Dis. Colon. Rectum* 1996; 39: 893–8.

Sandberg-Gertzen H, Jarnerot G, Kraaz W. Azodisal sodium in the treatment of ulcerative colitis. A study of tolerance and relapse prevention properties. *Gastroenterology* 1986; 90: 1024–30.

Sandler RS, Sandler DP, McDonnell CW, Wurzelmann JI. Childhood exposure to environmental tobacco smoke and the risk of ulcerative colitis. *Am. J. Epidemiol.* 1992; 35(6): 603–8.

Santavirta J, Mattila J, Kokki M, Matikainen M. Mucosal morphology and faecal bacteriology after ileoanal anastomosis. *Int. J. Colorectal Dis.* 1991; 6: 38–41.

Scaglia M, Bronsino E, Canino V, Hulten L. The impact of conventional proctocolectomy on sexual function. *Minerva Chir.* 1993; 48: 903–10.

Schneider A, Stolte M. Differential diagnosis of adenomas and dys-plastic lesions in patients with ulcerative colitis. *Z. Gastroenterol.* 1993; 31: 653–6.

Schreiber S, *et al.* Recombinant erythropoietin for the treatment of anemia in inflammatory bowel disease. *N. Engl. J. Med.* 1996; 334: 619–23.

Schroeder KW, Tremaine WJ, Ilstrup DM. Coated oral 5 aminosalicylic acid therapy for mildly to moderately active ulcerative colitis. A randomized study. *N. Engl. J. Med.* 1987; 317: 1625–9.

Sedgwick DM, *et al.* Population based study of surgery in juvenile onset ulcerative colitis. *Br. J. Surg.* 1991; 78: 176–8.

Senapati A, *et al.* Stenosis of the pouch anal anastomosis following restorative proctocolectomy. *Int. J. Colorect. Dis.* 1996; 11: 57–9.

Shivananda S, *et al.* Incidence of inflammatory bowel disease across Europe: is there a difference between north and south? Results of the European Collaborative Study on Inflammatory Bowel Disease (EC-IBD). *Gut* 1996; 39: 690–7.

Shoenut JP, *et al.* Comparison of magnetic resonance imaging and endoscopy in distinguishing the type and severity of inflammatory bowel disease. *J. Clin. Gastroenterol.* 1994; 19: 31–5.

Silverstein MD, Lashner BA, Hanauer SB. Cigarette smoking and ulcerative colitis: a case control study. *Mayo Clinic Proc.* 1994; 69: 425–9.

Snape WJ Jr, Williams R, Hyman PE. Defect in colonic smooth muscle contraction in patients with ulcerative colitis. *Am. J. Physiol.* 1991; 261: G987–91.

Sola Lamoglia R, *et al.* Chronic inflammatory intestinal disease in Catalonia (Barcelona and Gerona). *Revista Espanola de Enfermedades Digestivas* 1992; 81: 7–14.

Somerville KW, *et al.* Effect of treatment on symptoms and quality of life in patients with ulcerative colitis: comparative trial of hydrocortisone acetate foam and prednisolone 21 phosphate enemas. *Br. Med. J.* 1985; 291: 866.

Soukiasian SH, Foster CS, Raizman MB. Treatment strategies for scleritis and uveitis associated with inflammatory bowel disease. *Am. J. Ophthalmol.* 1994; 118: 601–11.

Srivastava ED, *et al.* Incidence of ulcerative colitis in Cardiff over 20 years: 1968–87. *Gut* 1992; 33: 256–8.

Staerk Laursen L, *et al.* Disposition of 5 aminosalicylic acid by olsalazine and three mesalazine preparations in patients with ulcerative colitis: comparison of intraluminal colonic concentrations, serum values, and urinary excretion. *Gut* 1990; 31: 1271–6.

Stahlberg D, *et al.* Pouchitis following pelvic pouch operation for ulcerative colitis. Incidence, cumulative risk, and risk factors. *Dis. Colon Rectum* 1996; 39: 1012–8.

Stahlberg D, *et al.* Leukocyte migration in acute colonic inflammatory bowel disease: comparison of histological assessment and Tc-99m-HMPAO labeled leukocyte scan. *Am. J. Gastroenterol.* 1997; 92: 283–8.

Stenson WF, *et al.* Dietary supplementation with fish oil in ulcerative colitis. *Ann. Intern. Med.* 1992; 151: 609–14.

Stern H, Walfisch S, Mullen B, McLeod R, Cohen Z. Cancer in an ileoanal reservoir: a new late complication? *Gut* 1990; 31: 473–5.

Stewenius J, *et al.* Ulcerative colitis and indeterminate colitis in the city of Malmo, Sweden. A 25 year incidence study. *Scand. J. Gastroenterol.* 1995; 30: 38–43.

Stewenius L, *et al.* Operations in unselected patients with ulcerative colitis and indeterminate colitis. A long-term follow-up study. *Eur. J. Surg.* 1996; 162: 131–7.

Stowe SP, *et al.* An epidemiologic study of inflammatory bowel disease in Rochester, New York. Hospital incidence. *Gastroenterol.* 1990; 98: 104–10.

Subramani K, *et al.* Refractory pouchitis: does it reflect underlying Crohn's disease? *Gut* 1993; 34: 1539–42.

Suzuki K, Muto T, Masaki T, Morioka Y. Microspectrophotometric DNA analysis in ulcerative colitis with special reference to its application in diagnosis of carcinoma and dysplasia. *Gut* 1990; 31: 1266–70.

Sviri S, *et al.* Mesalamine-induced hypersensitivity pneumonitis. A case report and review of the literature. *J. Clin. Gastroenterol.* 1997; 24: 34–6.

Taffet SL, Das KM. Sulfasalazine. Adverse effects and desensitization. *Dig. Dis. Sci.* 1983; 28: 833–42.

Tamaki Y, *et al.* Evaluation of colon diseases by using new method of extracorporeal ultrasonic examination during usual colon endoscopy. *Nippon Shokakibyo Gakkai Zasshi.* 1994; 91: 36–41.

Tartter PI, Heimann TM, Aufses AH Jr. Blood transfusion, skin test reactivity, and lymphocytes in inflammatory bowel disease. *Am. J. Surg.* 1986; 151: 358–61.

Taylor GA, *et al.* Plain abdominal radiographs in children with inflammatory bowel disease. *Pediatr. Radiol.* 1986; 16: 206–9.

Thoeni RF, Fell SC, Engelstad B, Schrock TB. Ileoanal pouches: comparison of CT, scintigraphy, and contrast enemas for diagnosing postsurgical complications. *Am. J. Roentgenol.* 1990; 154: 73–8.

Thompson NP, Driscoll R, Pounder RE, Wakefield AJ. Genetics versus environment in inflammatory bowel disease: results of a British twin study. *Br. Med. J.* 1996; 312: 95–6.

Thompson-Fawcett MW, Mortensen NJ. Anal transitional zone and columnar cuff in restorative proctocolectomy. *Br. J. Surg.* 1996; 83: 1047–55.

Tjandra JJ, *et al.* Omission of temporary diversion in restorative proctocolectomy—is it safe? *Dis. Colon Rectum* 1993; 36: 1007–14.

Tjandra JJ, Hughes LE. Parastomal pyoderma gangrenosum in inflammatory bowel disease. *Dis. Colon Rectum* 1994; 37: 938–42.

Tobin A, Suzuki Y, O'Morain C. A controlled double blind crossover study of eicosapentanoic acid (EPA) in chronic ulcerative colitis (UC). *Gastroenterology* 1990; 98: A207.

Tragnone A, *et al.* Incidence of inflammatory bowel disease in Italy: a nationwide population-based study. Gruppo Italiano per lo Studio del Colon e del Retto (GISC). *Int. J. Epidemiol.* 1996; 25: 1044–52.

Treem WR, Cohen J, Davis PM, Justinich CJ, Hyams JS. Cyclosporine for the treatment of fulminant ulcerative colitis in children. Immediate response, long term results, and impact on surgery. *Dis. Colon Rectum* 1995; 38: 474–9.

Truelove SC, Witts LJ. Cortisone in ulcerative colitis. Final reports on a therapeutic trial. *Br. Med. J.* 1955; ii: 1041–8.

Tysk C, Jarnerot G. Seasonal variation in exacerbations of ulcerative colitis. *Scand. J. Gastroenterol.* 1993; 28: 95–6.

Verhave M, Winter HS, Grand RJ. Azathioprine in the treatment of children with inflammatory bowel disease. *J. Pediatr.* 1990; 117: 809–14.

Vilien M, *et al.* Leucocyte scintigraphy to localize inflammatory activity ulcerative colitis and Crohn's disease. *Scand. J. Gastroenterol.* 1992; 27(7): 582–6.

Wardle TD, Hall L, Turnberg LA. Platelet activating factor: release from colonic mucosa in patients with ulcerative colitis and its effect on colonic secretion. *Gut* 1996; 38: 355–61.

Weinryb RM, *et al.* A prospective study of the quality of life after pelvic pouch operation. *J. Am. Coll. Surg.* 1995; 180: 589–95.

Wexner SD, *et al.* Long term functional anal. Results after restorative procto colectomy *Dis. Colon Rectum* 1989; 32: 275–81.

Wexner SD, *et al.* The ileoanal reservoir. *Am. J. Surg.* 1990; 159: 178–83.

Wexner SD, *et al.* Laparoscopic colorectal surgery: a prospective assessment and current perspective. *Br. J. Surg.* 1993; 80: 1602–5.

Wiesner RH. Current concepts in primary sclerosing cholangitis. *Mayo Clin. Proceed.* 1994; 69: 969–82.

Woolfson K, *et al.* Pelvic pouch emptying scan: an evaluation of scintigraphic assessment of the neorectum. *Int. J. Colorectal Dis.* 1991; 6: 29–32.

Wu S, Craig RM. Intense nutritional support in inflammatory bowel disease. *Dig. Dis. Sci.* 1995; 40: 843–52.

Vucelic B, *et al.* Ulcerative colitis in Zagreb, Yugoslavia: incidence and prevalence 1980–1989. *Int. J. Epidemiol.* 1991; 20: 1043–7.

Yoshida Y, Murata Y. Inflammatory bowel disease in Japan: studies of epidemiology and etiopathogenesis. *Med. Clin. North Am.* 1990; 74: 67–90.

Zins BJ, *et al.* Pouchitis disease course after orthotopic liver transplantation in patients with primary sclerosing cholangitis and an ileal pouch-anal anastomosis. *Am. J. Gastroenterol.* 1995; 90: 2177–81.

Ziv Y, *et al.* Stapled ileal pouch anal anastomoses are safer than handsewn anastomoses in patients with ulcerative colitis. *Am. J. Surg.* 1996; 171: 320–3.

6 Crohn's disease

Incidence

Crohn's disease is named after Burrill Bernard Crohn who described the condition of terminal ileitis in 1932. It may affect any part of the gastrointestinal tract, although it has a propensity to occur in the small bowel, especially the terminal ileum and colon (Hanauer 1996; Oberhuber *et al.* 1997) (Figure 6.1). Crohn's disease occurs throughout the world with incidence rates of between one and four cases per 100 000 population per year and prevalence rates up to 10 times this figure (de Dombal 1985). However, exact incidence figures are compounded by difficulty in establishing the correct diagnosis. In about 15% of patients it is difficult to distinguish Crohn's disease from ulcerative colitis and the clinical features may also be mimicked by enterocolonic infections (see Chapters 3 and 5).

Crohn's disease is most commonly found in Europe and North America, with a slight excess in females over males and a preponderance in young persons whose disease begins in early adult life. About two-thirds of patients develop symptoms between 10 and 30 years of age and 10% after the age of 50 years (Lind *et al.* 1985). However, as symptoms may not be marked, the diagnosis of Crohn's disease may be delayed for up to 10 years in almost 10% of patients.

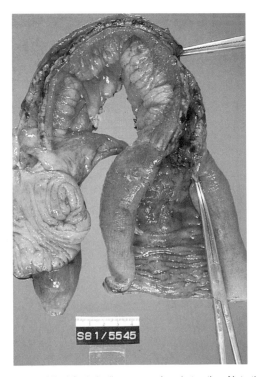

Figure 6.1 Terminal ileal Crohn's disease causing obstruction. Note the proximally dilated small bowel.

Time trend studies suggest an overall increase in incidence with a tendency towards a plateau in recent years in some areas. The number of patients in complete remission for 10 years after the initial attack is practically zero. Despite this, 80% of patients with the disease have full work capacity.

Aetiology

The precise aetiological mechanisms of Crohn's disease remain obscure, although environmental, microbial, and immunological factors are involved (Kirsner 1991; Colombel and Gower-Rousseau 1994, Mishina *et al.* 1996). The hypothesis of genetic susceptibility is based on the frequency of familial forms (6–33%) and higher relative risk in first-degree relatives (between 10 and 21 times) (Thompson *et al.* 1996; Cottone *et al.* 1997). To date, no genetic marker has been found for Crohn's disease, although molecular biology techniques have revealed a significant association with HLA-DR1, DQW5 genotypes and chromosome 16 (Hugot *et al.* 1996). Epidemiological evidence in favour of an environmental cause includes an increased incidence since the Second World War, a north–south incidence gradient (established in the USA and probably in Europe), and a predominance in urban areas. Smoking has also been shown to have a detrimental effect, perhaps via modification in the microcirculation of the intestinal wall and smoking may be a risk factor for surgical recurrence of the disease (Cottone *et al.* 1994; Cosnes *et al.* 1996). Despite some contradictory results, there is no convincing evidence that either the contraceptive pill or any particular foodstuffs increase the risk of Crohn's disease. Similarly, there is no reliable evidence showing that psychiatric factors have an effect on the appearance or aggravation of the disease.

Perinatal infection has, however, been shown to affect incidence and subjects born during periods of flu epidemics have a higher relative risk. Morphological and epidemiological studies have implicated the measles virus as a potential component cause, particularly when exposure occurs *in utero* or early in life. There appears to be an increased incidence of Crohn's disease among people born during measles epidemics (Ekbom *et al.* 1994).

Similarities between Crohn's disease and intestinal mycobacterial infection, particularly Johne's disease in ruminants, have been widely recognized. After demonstration of the transmission of granulomata from Crohn's disease by injecting intestinal homogenates into the footpads of mice there followed many studies attempting to identify infective agents within the bowel of patients with the disease (Smith and Wakefield 1993). Although *Mycobacterium paratuberculosis* has been identified in intestinal tissue from a proportion of patients with Crohn's disease a convincing role for this agent in its aetiology has not been established (Walmsley *et al.*

1996). Likewise, extensive studies into bacterial and viral agents potentially associated with Crohn's disease have been inconclusive.

Based on current knowledge, the sequence leading Crohn's disease would include one or more perinatal events such as viral infection acting on a genetically susceptible subject and resulting in a modified immune response (Hanauer 1996). Later in life an as yet unknown environmental factor, perhaps cell-wall deficient mycobacteria or viral infection of the bowel or vascular endothelium, leads to an inappropriate immune response. This results in chronic T-lymphocyte activation, with tissue damage induced by secondary macrophage activation (MacDonald and Murch 1994; Mingrone *et al.* 1996). Crohn's disease may well represent a chronic granulomatous vasculitis in reaction to a persistent infection with the measles virus within the vascular endothelium. This granulomatous inflammation, perhaps aggravated by either a hypercoagulable state or mechanical stress may result in the clinical features of Crohn's disease (Wakefield *et al.* 1995). In ulcerative colitis, by contrast, there is no strong evidence for T-cell activation, and humoral mechanisms predominate. Despite the fundamental differences in initiating mechanisms, the two conditions have many 'downstream' inflammatory processes in common.

Pathology

Macroscopic appearance

The gross pathology of Crohn's disease is the same at all levels of the gastrointestinal tract. The disease is segmental and discontinous and is characterized by sharply outlined foci separated by normal bowel (skip lesions). In the early stages the mucosa is red and may show pin-point haemorrhagic lesions and aphthous ulcers, the cause of which is unknown (Sankey *et al.* 1993). The classical fissures are narrow deep ulcers which may be transmural and form fistulas (Figure 6.2). When fissuring is extensive the elevated mucosa produces a 'cobble-stone' appearance which is seen in approximately 25% of patients (Figures 6.3 and 6.4). During the course of the disease the bowel wall becomes fibrotic leading to an increase in thickness and stricture formation. These can be single or multiple, and short or long and produce the classical 'hose-pipe' appearance of the affected segment.

In areas of gross stricturing the muscularis mucosae comprises almost 10% of the total wall thickness (Lee *et al.* 1991) (Figure 6.5).

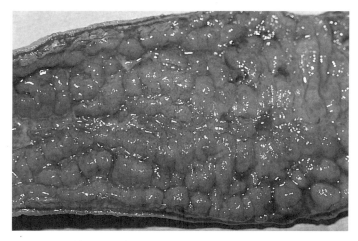

Figure 6.3 Cobble-stone appearance in the colon.

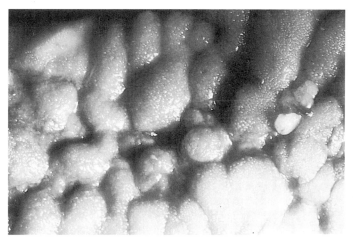

Figure 6.4 Close-up view of cobble-stone appearance.

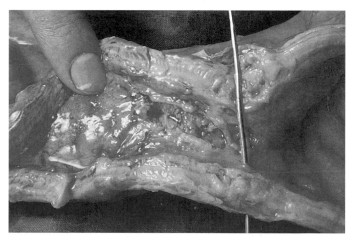

Figure 6.5 Crohn's disease showing marked thickening of the wall. A perforation is also present (indicated by the probe).

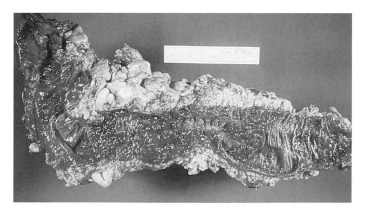

Figure 6.2 Resected Crohn's specimen showing mucosal ulceration, thickening, and mesenteric encroachment (see colour plates).

The increased mass of muscularis mucosae smooth muscle may be responsible in part for the commonly observed stricture formation. As extreme muscularis mucosae hyperplasia appears to be peculiar to Crohn's disease, it may serve as an additional marker differentiating it from other diseases.

There is often an associated serositis and involvement of the peri-intestinal fat (mesenteric encroachment) which can lead to adhesion formation between adjacent structures. Multiple white nodules or 'tubercules' may be present on the serosal surface and are composed of granulomata and lymphoid aggregates. Regional lymph nodes are usually enlarged.

Microscopic appearance

The microscopic features are those of a chronic granulomatous inflammatory disorder (Figure 6.6). There is a spectrum of appearances ranging from an acute inflammatory reaction to a fibrotic picture. The characteristic diagnostic feature are epithelioid granulomata which are found in 50–70% of cases. The presence of granulomata depends on the severity of the inflammatory process. Fewer are found in the terminal ileum than in the colon, and they are most numerous in the rectum. The incidence of granulomata decreases with age, duration of illness and under conservative therapy and they may be absent in fulminant acute onset disease (Schmitz-Mooremann *et al.* 1984). Granulomata in Crohn's disease are found in the seemingly uninvolved intestinal mucosa as well as in the affected mucosa so that biopsy of macroscopically normal mucosa can be useful (Kuramoto *et al.* 1987).

As well as epithelioid macrophages the granulomata typically contain Langhan's-type giant cells in which Schaumann bodies may be present along with lymphocytes and plasma cells.

In the absence of granulomata other features can suggest a diagnosis of Crohn's disease. Immunostaining for macrophages, vessel wall, and blood constituents has allowed identification of small mucosal capillaries which are not otherwise apparent. In Crohn's disease damage and rupture of these small capillaries occurs before infiltration of the lamina propria by inflammatory cells. Loss of the overlying epithelium seems to follow this vascular damage. Later superficial well defined ulcers form; these result from mural oedema, and proliferation of mucosal and submucosal lymphoid tissue. In addition, the inflammation in Crohn's disease is transmural and includes serosal fat but tends to be focal and consist of aggregates of lymphocytes and plasma cells. At ulcer margins there are crypt abscesses. Fissures are very suggestive of Crohn's but may be seen in fulminant ulcerative colitis and lymphomatous infiltration. They contain polymorphs and are lined by granulation tissue, epithelioid and giant cells. They extend deep into the bowel wall and are the basis of fistulas seen grossly. Less specific features are submucosal oedema, fibrosis, lymphangiectasia, pyloric gland metaplasia in crypts, Paneth cell metaplasia, and occasionally arteritis.

If the histological changes are non-specific, cases are labelled 'indeterminate colitis' or terminal ileitis. Other diagnosis such as ulcerative colitis and an infective or ischaemic aetiology need to be considered. The diagnosis can also be difficult in the burnt out phase of the disease if fibrosis, vascular changes, and neuronal hypertrophy are the only findings.

The inflammatory changes in Crohn's disease are not usually associated with the glandular distortion, goblet cell depletion, crypt abscess formation or cryptitis seen in ulcerative colitis. The inflammation tends to be more severe in the submucosa and may be peri-lymphatic. Eosinophils are more prominent in ulcerative colitis but can be seen in both conditions.

Diagnosis

This is based on a correlation of symptoms, physical signs, endoscopic, radiological, and histological assessments. A simple clinical activity index has been devised based on the history and physical findings (Table 6.1). Laboratory investigations (full blood count, erythrocyte sedimentation rate, electrolytes, and serum proteins) help establish the nutritional state of the patient and are an index of disease activity. Decreased serum iron and albumin are frequently found and patients may have vitamin B_{12} and folic acid deficiency. Microalbuminuria is a useful disease activity marker for inflammatory bowel disease correlating strongly with erythrocyte sedimentation rate, C-reactive protein and the severity of colonic inflammation (Mahmud *et al.* 1996). Some patients with long-standing active disease will exhibit the anaemia of chronic disease due to suppression of erythropoiesis (Schreiber *et al.* 1996). Low levels of zinc and vitamin A reflect decreased absorption or reduced intake. Frank malabsorption with steatorrhoea can be present in patients with extensive small bowel disease or bacterial overgrowth.

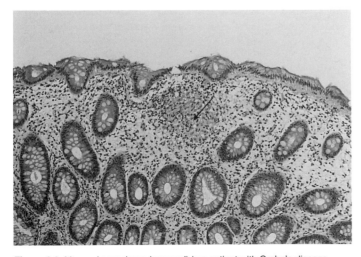

Figure 6.6 Mucosal granuloma (arrowed) in a patient with Crohn's disease H&E×100.

Table 6.1 Crohn's disease activity index based on clinical features

Clinical feature	Scoring
General well-being	0 = Very well
	1 = Well
	2 = All right
	3 = Poor
	4 = Terrible
Abdominal pain	0 = Rare or none
	1 = Mild
	2 = Moderate
	3 = Severe
Liquid stools	Number per day
Abdominal mass	0 = Absent
	1 = Possible and non-tender
	2 = Probable and minimal tenderness
	3 = Definite and tender
Complications	e.g. arthralgia, apthous ulceration (See Table 6.2)
	Score 1 point for each complication

Endoscopy

Rectal examination may reveal the characteristic changes of perianal disease with inflammation, skin tags and fistulae (Platell *et al.* 1996) (Figure 6.7). The affected rectum shows a spectrum of disease ranging from 2 to 3 mm aphthous ulcers to gross inflammation (Figure 6.8). Oedema and thickened mucosal folds are common. Rectal strictures or symmetrical narrowing may also be seen but pseudopolyps are less common than in ulcerative colitis. Rectal biopsy should be performed even if the rectum appears normal as rectal inflammation will be found in 60% of those with Crohn's colitis, 30% of those with ileitis, and 20% of those with ileocolitis. Granulomata are present in 4% and microgranulomas in 8% of those with macroscopically normal rectal mucosa. Deep circumscribed ulcers are sometimes seen along the longitudinal plane of

the bowel. The characteristic cobble-stone appearance is more common in the colon than the rectum. It is the patchy nature of the mucosal abnormality with intervening areas of apparently normal tissue that is the most useful endoscopic aid distinguishing Crohn's disease from ulcerative colitis.

In a multicentre trial of 130 patients with Crohn's disease who underwent colonoscopy the most common lesions were ulceration and aphthous ulcers, followed by pseudopolyps, cobble-stone lesions and stenosis (Lorenz-Meyer *et al.* 1985). Patients with Crohn's colitis alone had more serious inflammation than those with involvement of both the small and large intestine. In those with previous resections, inflammation near the anastomosis was frequently accompanied by stenosis.

Colonoscopy with multiple biopsies is superior to either colonoscopy alone or barium studies in assessing the extent of disease (Holdstock *et al.* 1984). In one study of patients undergoing both radiological and endoscopic investigation 15% of patients were considered to have extensive colitis on barium enema, 34% on the colonoscopic appearance alone compared with 62% on colonoscopic biopsy (Coremans *et al.* 1984). Cannulation and biopsy of the terminal ileum at colonoscopy provides further information about the extent of inflammation (Coremans *et al.* 1984).

Radiology

The small bowel follow-through or enema have become the procedure of choice for the diagnosis of small bowel disease (Carlson

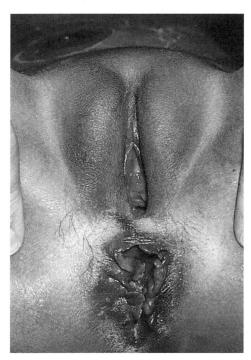

Figure 6.7 Typical Crohn's disease perineum showing skin tags and longitudinal ulceration.

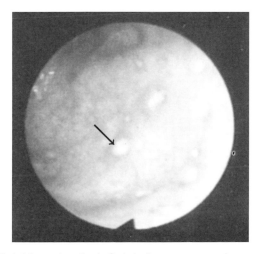

Figure 6.8 Aphthous ulceration in Crohn's disease seen on colonoscopy (see colour plates).

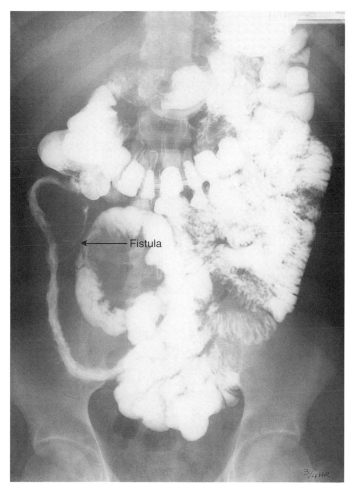

Figure 6.9 Barium follow-through showing severe Crohn's disease with long stricture and fistula formation.

1986) (Figure 6.9). Commonest appearances are thickening of the valvulae conniventes, oedema of the wall, and fissure ulceration. Scattered aphthoid ulcers throughout the small intestine are not uncommon but will not be seen with a barium meal and follow through. Stricturing may result in dilatation of the proximal bowel.

Double contrast barium enema visualizes both the colon and the terminal ileum if there is reflux of barium into the small intestine (Figure 6.10). The characteristic cobble-stone appearance is due to a combination of deep longitudinal ulceration, narrow transverse slit ulceration and oedema of the bowel wall (Figure 6.11). The radiological incidence of longitudinal ulcers in the small intestine is significantly higher than in the colon (Yao *et al.* 1989). Cobble-stoning is positively correlated and longitudinal ulceration negatively correlated with disease activity, reflecting the fact that colonic involvement often indicates more severe disease than small intestinal involvement alone. Barium studies may also reveal fine mucosal detail, aphthoid ulcers, and spiculation (rosethorn appearance), especially in the left colon (Figures 6.12 and 6.13). Longitudinal submucosal tracts (Marshak's sign) are highly suggestive of Crohn's disease. Contraction of the colonic lumen may be symmetrical or isolated (stricture). Typically there is less contraction of the colon and less evidence of descent of the splenic flexure than in ulcerative colitis, and pseudopolyps are less frequent (Figure 6.14). Nevertheless, differentiation from ulcerative colitis can be extremely difficult

If a retrograde barium enema is considered contraindicated in acute colonic inflammation, antegrade evaluation is a safe and effective alternative (Figure 6.9). The right and left colon are well seen in almost all cases to the junction of the descending and sigmoid colon, the sigmoid in 75% and the rectum in 55% of patients (Cohen *et al.* 1986). There is also excellent correlation between the extent of disease seen on antegrade study and retrograde enema, endoscopy, and surgery.

Relative to computerized tomography (CT) barium studies are better at demonstrating mucosal disease, sinus tracts, postsurgical

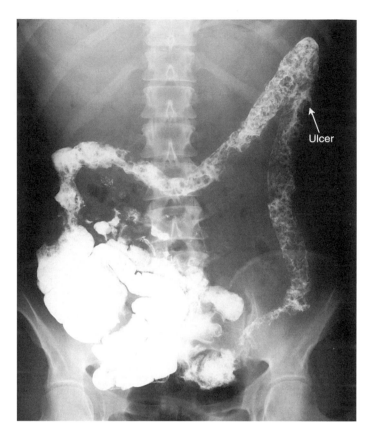

Figure 6.11 Barium study showing severe Crohn's disease with cobble-stoning and linear ulceration (arrow).

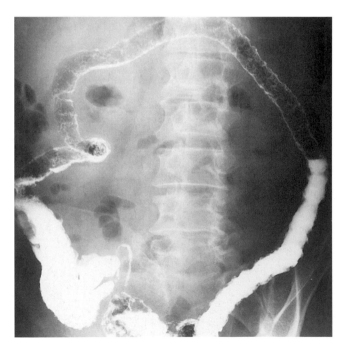

Figure 6.10 Barium enema showing severe Crohn's disease affecting the entire colon and terminal ileum.

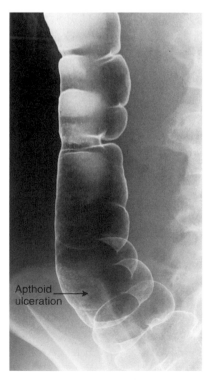

Figure 6.12 Barium enema showing the multiple white dots of aphthoid ulceration (arrowed).

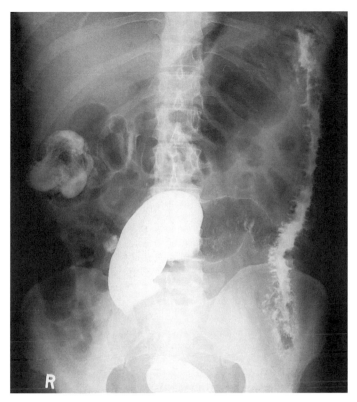

Figure 6.13 Barium enema in severe disease showing rosethorn ulceration and longitudinal ulceration.

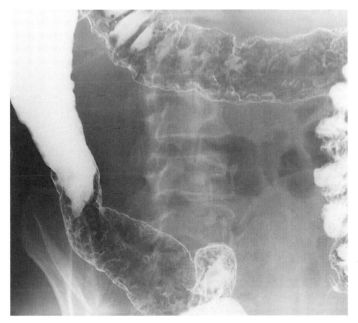

Figure 6.14 Case of Crohn's disease showing pseudopolyps.

anatomy, and relation of recurrence to an anastomosis. CT, however, is superior in demonstrating mesenteric inflammation, abscesses, enterovesical and enterocutaneous fistulas or fistulas to the iliopsoas muscle and sacrum (Orel *et al.* 1987; Sahat *et al.* 1997). In many clinical circumstances both CT and contrast studies can be

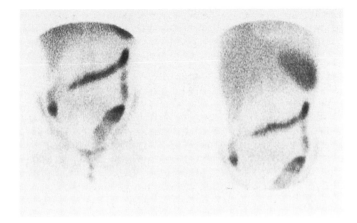

Figure 6.15 Technetium-labelled white cell scan in Crohn's colitis showing the classical skip lesions.

performed as they are complementary. Doppler sonography is also correlated with disease activity (Van Oostayen *et al.* 1997).

Scintiscanning with indium-labelled 111 leucocytes is reported to be as accurate as barium enema in localizing the site of inflammatory involvement in the colon and can aid decision-making in patients with fistulas and sinus tracts (Even Sapir *et al.* 1994; Arndt *et al.* 1997; Stahlberg *et al.* 1997) (Figure 6.15).

Clinical features

The clinical features of Crohn's disease depend not only on the location and extent of the disease but also on the onset of specific complications which are often the presenting features. The disease is localized to the ileocolic region in 60% of patients, the small bowel in 20%, and the large bowel in 20% (Lind *et al.* 1985). Crohn's disease isolated to the appendix has also been described and appears to run a less aggressive course (see Chapter 14) (Figure 6.16).

Patients with Crohn's disease most often seek medical attention because of chronic intermittent diarrhoea with colicky abdominal pain and general malaise. Diarrhoea occurs in 70–80% of patients

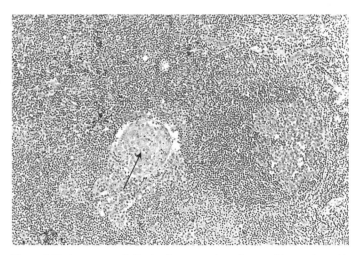

Figure 6.16 Acute appendicitis showing a granuloma (arrowed) in a patient with Crohn's disease. H&E×250.

while in 15% of cases Crohn's disease of the terminal ileum presents with acute abdominal pain mimicking acute appendicitis (McCue *et al.* 1988). Recurrent abdominal pain occurs in two-thirds of patients with ileal or ileocolic disease and is the indication for laparotomy in 15% of those undergoing surgery. Rectal bleeding is a feature of colorectal disease and is not usually found with small bowel involvement only. As associated peptic ulcer disease is also common in Crohn's disease it may be difficult to distinguish the source of bleeding (Yardley and Hendrix 1997).

Patients may also present with small bowel obstruction (usually subacute), perforation, abscess formation, fistula formation, haemorrhage, toxic dilatation of the colon, or peritonitis. About 10% of patients first come to medical attention because of perianal disease. Manifestations of malabsorption including steatorrhoea, protein wasting, and deficiencies of vitamin B_{12}, folic acid, and iron, usually occur only when the disease is extensive.

Signs

Examination may reveal anaemia, weight loss, dehydration, extra-intestinal manifestations, abdominal distension from small or large bowel obstruction, and abdominal tenderness. Free perforation is rare. An enterocutaneous fistula may present through an old appendix scar while flexion deformity of the hip indicates a psoas abscess. Perianal complications are seen in one-quarter of those with small bowel disease, 40% of those with combined small and large bowel, and one-half of those with large bowel involvement (Platell *et al.* 1996). Perianal lesions may be the sole manifestation of Crohn's disease in 5% of patients. Fistulas are often multiple and can be associated with extensive tracking into the groin, scrotum, labia, vagina, urethra, prostate, or seminal vesicles. Tissue destruction by sepsis may produce sphincter impairment and incontinence. Alternatively, an anorectal stricture may result with transient resolution of the sepsis. Fissures in Crohn's disease are characteristically large indolent, laterally sited, and relatively painless. If it affects an entire quadrant the resultant anal canal ulcer extends into the rectum producing an exquisitely painful lesion that frequently requires faecal diversion for symptomatic relief. Oral aphthous ulceration is common and precedes intestinal symptoms by up to 1 year in one-third of patients (Lisciandrano *et al.* 1996) (Figure 6.17).

Complications

Most of the complications of Crohn's disease are so common that they are considered as integral features of the disease. These include abscess, fistula formation, intestinal obstruction, and malnutrition. Severe life-threatening gastrointestinal haemorrhage is rare but generally requires removal of diseased bowel at the time of the first episode of massive haemorrhage (Robert *et al.* 1991) (Figure 6.18). Although the majority of abscesses associated with Crohn's disease require surgical treatment, radiologically assisted percutaneous drainage may be helpful (Weismayr *et al.* 1994).

Most fistulas derive from transmural penetration of the bowel wall by a fissure with escape of enteric content and formation of an abscess that penetrates into an adjacent viscous or through a wound. Enterocutaneous fistulas may be single or multiple and usually arise from the affected segment of bowel (Figure 6.19). Spontaneous fistulas are uncommon and arise from external drainage of an abscess usually secondary to perforated ileocaecal Crohn's disease. More usual is the occurrence of fistulas through an abdominal incision site, the source being an area of recurrent disease at an ileocolic anastomosis. Frequently, there are associated problems such as enteroenteric or enterovesical fistulas. A further variety is the fistula that occurs early in the postoperative period. Enteroenteric fistulas most commonly occur between two loops of small bowel. Ileosigmoid fistulas are frequently associated with severe nutritional depletion and in fewer than 20% will the fistulous track be apparent on the barium enema examination. In contrast to diverticulitis the small bowel is the source of the fistula and invariably the sigmoid colon is free of Crohn's disease.

About 80% of fistulas arise in the ileum, 15% in the ileocaecal valve, and 5% in the colon (Kelly and Preshaw 1989). The majority

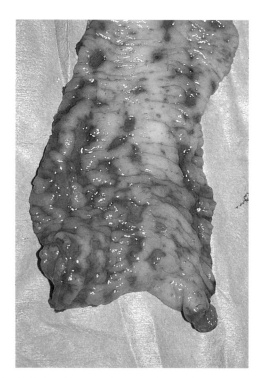

Figure 6.18 Crohn's colitis necessitating a colectomy for acute, severe haemorrhage.

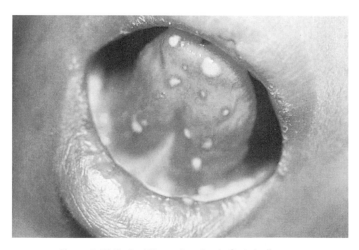

Figure 6.17 Oral aphthous ulceration in Crohn's disease.

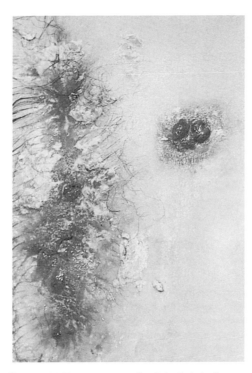

Figure 6.19 Enterocutaneous fistula in Crohn's disease.

Table 6.2 Extra-intestinal manifestations of Crohn's disease

Complication	Feature
Hepatobiliary	Fatty infiltration
	Cholelithiasis
	Sclerosing cholangitis
	Chronic active hepatitis
	Granulomatous hepatitis
	Cirrhosis
	Amyloid
	Liver abscess
	Cholangiocarcinoma
Ocular	Uveitis
	Episcleritis
Arthritis	Migratory, asymmetrical arthropathy
	Sacro-ileitis
	Ankylosing spondylitis
Skin	Pyoderma gangrenosum
	Erythema nodosum
	Aphthous stomatitis
Oral	Stomatitis
	Aphthoid ulcers
	Candida
Renal	Calculi
	Pyelonephritis
	Amyloid
	Obstructive uropathy
Cardiovascular	Vasculitis
	Pericarditis
	Systemic thrombosis
	Takayasu's disease
Pulmonary	Pleural effusion
	Fibrosing alveolitis

are located either at the proximal end of a stricture (60%) or within a stricture (30%), 10% are not associated with strictures. About 75% of fistulas in those with previous bowel resection for Crohn's disease arise from the anastomosis and almost all the remainder in association with strictures (Kelly and Preshaw 1989).

The incidence of enterovesical fistulas in Crohn's disease is 2.5% (Heyen *et al.* 1989). Three-quarters of these patients present with urinary symptoms (pneumaturia, haematuria, or urinary tract infection). Persistent symptomatic fistulas should be treated by resection of the affected segment of bowel with primary anastomosis if appropriate. In enterovesical fistula the defect in the bladder should be closed over an indwelling catheter which should not be removed until there is radiological confirmation that the bladder defect has healed satisfactorily. Managing the fistula by bypass or defunctioning may result in persistent sepsis which may be fatal (Glass *et al.* 1985).

About 30% of all Crohn's disease patients will have extra-intestinal manifestations (Williams and Harned 1987; Danzi 1988) (Table 6.2). These systemic manifestations are probably the result of increased mucosal permeability to dietary and bacterial antigens stimulating B lymphocytes to produce excessive amounts of antibody. In one study extra-intestinal diseases were seen in 55% of patients with Crohn's disease, most frequently related to colonic involvement (joint disease 21%, eye 12%, liver pathology 12%, skin 8%, amyloid 6%) (Lind *et al.* 1985) (Figures 6.20–6.23).

Almost one-half of patients undergoing operation for abdominal mass related to Crohn's disease will have a fistula (Figures 6.24 and 6.25). Although a fistula is present in 35% of all patients undergoing surgery for complicated Crohn's disease, it is the primary indication for operation in only 7% (Michelassi *et al.* 1993). About 70% of fistulas are diagnosed pre-operatively, 27% intraoperatively, and the remaining 3% only after examination of the resected specimen (Michelassi *et al.* 1993).

A multicentre study of 225 patients with perianal disease followed up over a median of 6 years found an anal fistula in 85%, an

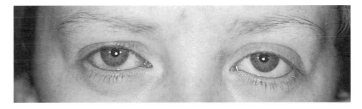

Figure 6.20 Conjunctivitis associated with Crohn's disease (see colour plates).

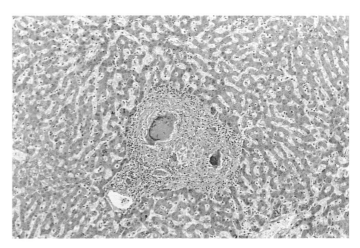

Figure 6.21 Granulomatous hepatitis in a patient with Crohn's disease H&E×250.

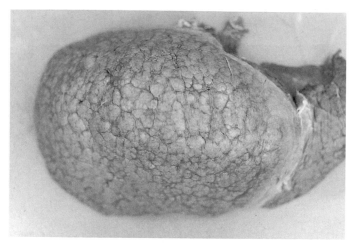

Figure 6.22 Cirrhosis of the liver associated with Crohn's disease.

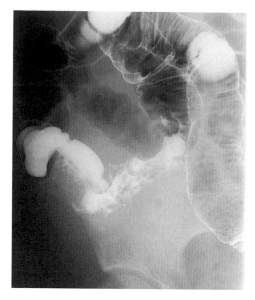

Figure 6.24 Barium enema showing abnormality of the sigmoid colon with gas inthe adjacent small bowel suggesting a fistula.

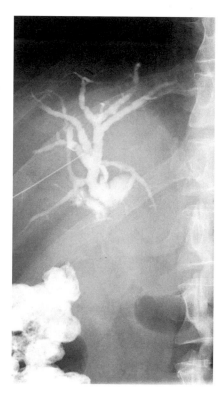

Figure 6.23 Percutaneous transhepatic cholangiogram showing sclerosing cholangitis

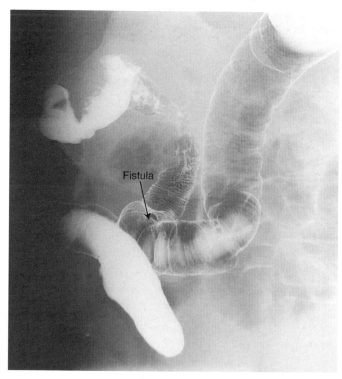

Figure 6.25 Barium enema of same patient as Figure 6.24 showing fistulous connection between large and small bowel (arrowed).

abscess in 45%, and fissures in 25% of patients (Pescatori *et al.* 1995). Diarrhoea and anal pain were the most common symptoms. Anal lesions preceded the onset of intestinal symptoms in 20% of cases. In perianal Crohn's disease, both anal fissures and abscesses can be relatively asymptomatic and overlooked. Consequently, patients may not present until extensive tissue destruction has occurred (Figure 6.26). The large anal skin tags of Crohn's disease may make perianal hygiene difficult, leading to perianal dermatitis (Figure 6.27). Superficial infection which undermines the skin may coalesce to leave large areas of ulceration with intervening skin bridges. Extensive maceration may also occur in the presence of acute proctitis. Despite this, half of all perianal disease in children and over two-thirds of fissures in adults may heal spontaneously

(Hyams 1996, Tolia 1996). One-third of asymptomatic fistulas may also heal spontaneously, although a quarter of patients may develop further fistulas within 10 years (Figure 6.28). Healing of abscesses and fistulas in Crohn's disease takes on average 4 weeks longer to occur than in other patients. Amyloid may supervene in long-standing cases, while carcinoma of the vulva, perianal area, and lymphomas occur with increased frequency in patients with Crohn's disease. Bowen's disease and squamous cell carcinoma have also been reported in the perineal sinuses of patients with Crohn's

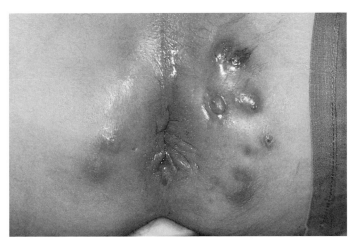

Figure 6.26 Perianal Crohn's disease showing extensive abscess and fistula formation.

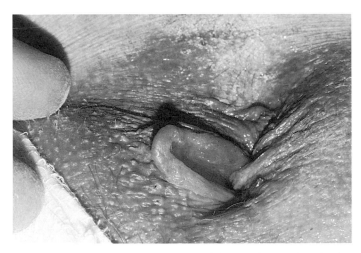

Figure 6.27 Large anal skin tag with characteristic deep ulceration in perianal Crohn's disease.

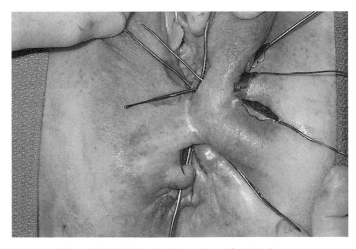

Figure 6.28 Multiple fistulas in perianal Crohn's disease.

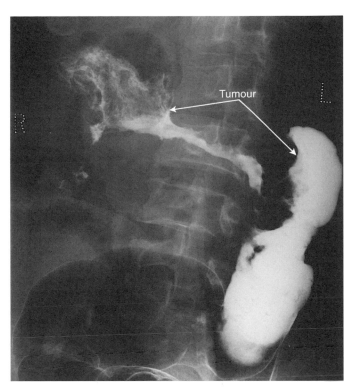

Figure 6.29 Malignant stricture in a patient with long-standing Crohn's disease. Note the soft tissue mass and the dilated transverse colon. Ultrasound scan identified liver metastases.

disease. In addition, female patients may develop sexual problems related to a combination of abdominal pain and fear of faecal leaks.

There are varying reports as to an increased risk of cancer in long-standing Crohn's disease (Bernstein and Rogers 1996, Rhodes 1996) (Figure 6.29). The relative risk of colorectal cancer in a series of 281 patients followed for at least 12 years was 3.4 (Gillen *et al.* 1994). As in ulcerative colitis the age of onset and extent of colonic involvement are important (Bansal and Sonnenberg 1996; Ribeiro *et al.* 1996). Patients with extensive colitis showed an 18-fold increase in risk. The relative risk for colonic disease was fivefold, while patients with just rectal involvement had no greater risk of colonic cancer than the normal population. Against this, another study failed to show an increase in the lifetime risk of cancer in patients with Crohn's disease, although the risk of rare small bowel cancer was significantly increased (Munkholm *et al.* 1993).

Medical treatment

Details concerning the drugs used in the medical management of Crohn's disease are discussed in detail in the medical management section of the section on ulcerative colitis (see Chapter 5). Treatment regimens for the various aspects of Crohn's disease are outlined below.

Mild/moderate disease

Patients not already on a 5-aminosalicylic acid (5-ASA) preparation should be started on one, rapidly increasing to therapeutic doses (up to 4 g/day or more). Because of its delivery to the small bowel as well as the colon, an oral mesalazine preparation (Asacol or Pentasa) may be preferable (Gendre *et al.* 1993). The use of metronidazole has been shown to be as effective as sulphasalazine in the treatment of acute Crohn's disease (Ursing *et al.* 1982). Other broad-spectrum antibiotics such as ciprofloxacin are also being tried.

If there is no response, the addition of a short course of steroids is indicated beginning with 40 mg/day prednisolone and gradually tapering down as remission is achieved (Summers *et al.* 1979; Malchow *et al.* 1984). Newer steroids that act topically (budesonide) and are either poorly absorbed or have a high first pass metabolism are effective and may well be preferable in view of their reduced side-effects (de Kaski *et al.* 1991; Löfberg *et al.* 1991; Greenberg *et al.* 1996). If a response to steroids is not forthcoming, a 4-week trial of an elemental diet should be considered. This is as effective as steroids in inducing remission and can work in cases that have been refractory to steroids (O'Morain *et al.* 1984; O'Morain 1990). Although not scientifically proven, it would appear that many gastroenterologists now use steroids and an elemental diet in combination rather than as alternatives (Payne-James and Silk 1990).

When a mild/moderate flare-up of symptoms has not responded to the above therapy, consideration should be given to two specific situations: bacterial overgrowth and an irritable bowel syndrome-type picture. Bacterial overgrowth may occur in Crohn's disease and is responsive to treatment with metronidazole. Irritable bowel syndrome symptoms are not uncommon in Crohn's disease and relate more to a sensory-motor upset of the gut wall than mucosal inflammation. Such symptoms may respond to antispasmodics and antidiarrhoeal agents (Kornbluth *et al.* 1993).

Severe disease

The onset of systemic symptoms such as fever and tachycardia or the failure of moderate disease to respond to treatment warrant the patient's admission to hospital. In the case of severe acute disease it is important to exclude toxic dilatation or perforation. Close observation of temperature, pulse, and blood pressure is necessary and an abdominal X-ray should be performed. Patients should be started on intravenous fluid replacement and intravenous administration of hydrocortisone 400 mg daily.

In such cases the colon is often the predominant site of Crohn's involvement and management of colonic dilatation should be the same as for toxic megacolon due to ulcerative colitis (Figure 6.30). Failure to respond to 5 days of intravenous steroid therapy or deterioration while on steroids are relative indications for surgery.

Refractory disease

Without deteriorating or developing signs of systemic illness, some patients will remain refractory to treatment with steroids and 5-ASA preparations. In such patients the immunosuppressant 6-mercaptopurine/azathioprine is of proven benefit (Bouhnik *et al.* 1996). In one study, two-thirds of patients treated with 6-mercaptopurine improved compared with only 8% in the placebo group (Present *et al.*, 1980). There was an associated reduction or cessation of steroid therapy in three-quarters of those on 6-mercaptopurine compared with 36% of the placebo group. Patients failing to respond steroids or azathioprine/6-mercaptopurine may respond to methotrexate (Kozarek *et al.* 1991; Egan and Sandborn 1996) or cyclosporin (Brynskov *et al.* 1985; Sandborn *et al.* 1996).

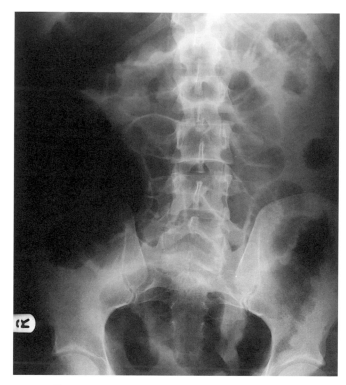

Figure 6.30 Toxic megacolon in severe Crohn's disease.

Distal disease

When disease activity is confined to the rectum and sigmoid colon, topical applications may be all that are required. Steroid and 5-ASA preparations are both effective. Perianal disease is often a problem in Crohn's disease. Associated proctitis must be treated aggressively with topical therapy as well as oral medication. The same principles of treatment apply to perianal fistulas as to fistulas at other sites. Other forms of perianal disease may also respond to metronidazole. Fissures and areas of ulceration benefit from topical application of steroids or 5-ASA preparations. Surgery should be avoided where possible because of poor postoperative healing. This is especially applicable to haemorrhoid surgery.

Complications

Obstruction

Intestinal obstruction in Crohn's disease typically occurs in the ileocaecal area. It may be due to the oedema of acute inflammation, stricture formation, or adhesive bands in those with previous surgery or bad fistulous disease. When the obstruction is due to inflammation, treatment with steroids may provide relief. However, the relief is often temporary and returns on stopping the steroids. Regardless of the specific cause, most cases of obstruction in Crohn's disease settle over the course of a few days on conservative therapy. Although this allows a period of time to plan elective surgery, it does not obviate the need for surgical intervention.

Fistulas and abscess formation

Fistulas may occur between loops of bowel, to other organs such as the bladder or vagina, or to the skin. Many are asymptomatic and even those that discharge large volumes on to the skin surface may be surprisingly painless. The initial management is medical unless an abscess is present or a distal obstruction is the cause of the fistula. Metronidazole is the initial drug of choice. Its value is limited by side-effects in the long term and the fact that the fistula often recurs on cessation of therapy. 6-mercaptopurine has been reported to close fistulas in one-third of cases and to reduce the output from a further third (Present *et al.* 1980; Korelitz and Present 1985). Cyclosporin has also been reported to heal fistulas, including those refractory to other forms of therapy (Present and Lichtiger 1992).

Maintenance therapy

Although debated for many years, recent studies have confirmed that maintenance therapy with 5-ASA preparations does prevent relapse (Anonymous 1990; Prantera *et al.*, 1992; Bayless 1996). Generally, mesalazine has been used because it is released in the small bowel. Doses have tended to be higher than the maintenance doses for ulcerative colitis, e.g. 2–4 g mesalazine daily. Such treatment should probably be maintained indefinitely. In the specific case of maintaining remission after surgical resection, 5-ASAs have also proven beneficial, mesalazine reducing the 2-year relapse rate from 41% to 18% (Caprilli *et al.* 1994).

Low-dose steroids do not prevent relapse in patients with inactive disease (Summers *et al.* 1979). However, some patients relapse rapidly on stopping steroids and they may be regarded as having chronically active disease. Such patients do benefit from continuation of low doses of steroids.

Azathioprine or 6-mercaptopurine are indicated for maintaining remission and reducing the dosage of steroid required. Azathioprine prevents a relapse in 95% of patients over a 1-year period compared with a 41% relapse rate when the drug was withdrawn (O'Donoghue *et al.* 1978).

Indications for surgery

Surgery is generally performed for complications of Crohn's disease and less commonly for failure of medical management (Fazio and Wu 1997) (Table 6.3). The operation rate 10 years from diagnosis for patients with ileocolitis is 90% and for Crohn's colitis 66%. Perianal disease assumes a significant role as an indication for operation in ileitis, ileocolitis, and colitis. Sepsis and obstruction are also indications. Intestinal obstruction and internal fistulas associated with sepsis are the main indications for surgery in patients with ileocolitis. For Crohn's colitis the major reasons for surgery include toxicity, poor response to medical therapy, debility, bleeding, and extra-intestinal manifestations. Many fistulas may be treated conservatively with parenteral nutrition. Toxic megacolon may be treated similarly to that of ulcerative colitis. Subtotal colectomy with ileostomy is the most widely used procedure for toxic dilatation and it is the procedure of choice in the presence of free perforation.

Surgical principles in Crohn's disease are:

(1) deal only with the specific complication that is the indication for the operation;
(2) do not remove bowel just because it is affected by the disease;
(3) the worst affected portion of bowel causing obstruction or fistula should be resected and do not remove more bowel than is necessary;
(4) do not leave stenosed bowel even in a defunctioned segment;
(5) in the small bowel it is preferable to avoid a bypass.

Table 6.3 Indications for surgery in colonic Crohn's disease

Complication	Feature
Absolute	Free perforation
	Impending perforation (toxic megacolon)
	Undrained intra-abdominal abscess
	Uncontrollable intestinal haemorrhage
Relative	Fistula
	Enteroenteric
	Enterovesical
	Enterovaginal
	Enterocutaneous
	Perianal disease
	Fistula
	Fissure
	Abscess
	Persistent symptoms
	Pain
	Obstruction
	Diarrhoea (uncontrollable)
	Malnutrition
	Growth retardation
	Medical
	Need for long-term steroids
	Side-effects of steroids or other drugs

Laparoscopic surgery does not compromise these principles (Ludwig *et al.* 1996; Reissman *et al.* 1996). The risk of recurrent disease is no greater if there is residual disease at the site of the anastomosis, but is related to the presence of granulomata in the resected specimen (Anseline *et al.* 1997). However, patients undergoing operation for radiologically proven Crohn's disease in whom no macro-

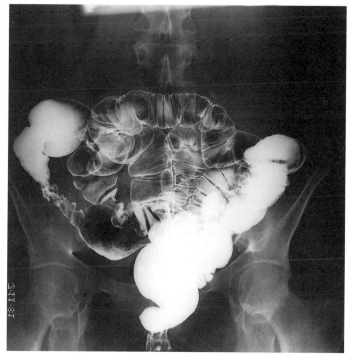

Figure 6.31 Recurrent Crohn's disease at the anastomotic site following a right hemicolectomy.

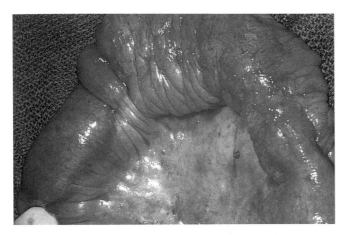

Figure 6.32 Mesenteric environment typical of Crohn's disease.

scopically abnormal small bowel can be detected at laparotomy should not have a resection deferred as almost all cases so treated will subsequently deteriorate and require further surgery (Butterworth *et al.* 1992) (Figure 6.31). In these cases, histology reveals an unusually superficial distribution of inflammation. Such minor abnormalities can be detected from the slight resistance to the passage of a partly inflated urinary catheter balloon along the small bowel. In such cases stricturoplasty is effective (Ozuner *et al.* 1996). However, mesenteric encroachment and narrowing are usually clinically obvious (Figure 6.32).

In a review of perianal Crohn's disease, medical treatment alone cured only 15% of cases, while combined medical and surgical treatment either cured or improved 62% of patients (Pescatori *et al.* 1995). Fifty per cent had an intestinal resection. Rectovaginal fistulas required intestinal surgery in 36% and anal surgery in 20% of the cases, half of these with good results. Of the patients who had anal surgery, 58% had a positive outcome. Recurrence of anal disease requiring further surgery occurred in 25% of the cases. Therefore limited surgery appears to achieve satisfactory results in more than one-half of the patients affected by perianal Crohn's lesions, whereas medical treatment alone cured only one in six patients.

Many surgeons have cautioned against radical operations for perianal Crohn's disease as the results of treatment are often more disabling than the original problem (Sangwan *et al.* 1996). Others advocate active if not aggressive surgical intervention. Early aggressive surgical management of suppurative complications of perianal Crohn's disease before complex management problems arise result in a high incidence of healing and a low risk of subsequent proctectomy (Williamson *et al.* 1995). In general, perianal lesions are not treated unless they are producing significant symptoms. Abscesses are treated by simple incision and drainage, although if recurrent they may be treated by the long-term use of loosely applied seton sutures (Faucheron *et al.* 1996). Should this fail to be effective and a course of metronidazole produce minimal response, fistulotomy can be performed if the rectum appears normal and the fistula does not affect the sphincter mechanism. The outcome of high fistulas is less satisfactory, and proctectomy is ultimately required in a number of patients; therefore, for high fistulas a conservative approach is primarily recommended (Halme and Sainio 1995). In selected cases where an internal opening is easily seen and when there is concern regarding the amount of sphincter muscle that would be divided by

performing a fistulotomy, an advancement rectal mucosal flap with or without a covering stoma is advised, provided the rectum appears normal (Makowiec *et al.* 1995). The ileostomy can be closed approximately 2–3 months later. If extensive perianal disease or rectovaginal fistulas are associated with rectal Crohn's disease, simple deroofing of abscesses or insertion of a seton is recommended (McCourtney and Finlay 1995). If these measures and conventional therapy such as metronidazole fail to keep the patient reasonably comfortable faecal diversion is usually necessary (Hull and Faazio 1997; Tsang and Rothernberger 1997). Subsequently, proctocolectomy may be required.

Anal fissures are not treated unless associated with pain. In this situation Crohn's disease of the rectum is usually absent. Dilatation using anaesthesia or in selected cases conservative sphincterotomy may be used. In patients requiring extensive colonic resection, ileorectal anastomosis may be considered when the rectum is spared of disease, if it distends well with air insufflation and sphincter tone is adequate. The presence of perianal sepsis, fistula and ileal disease are also contraindications to ileorectal anastomosis. A covering loop ileostomy may be performed. Revisional surgery is required in 10–15% of cases. Sexual dysfunction in males under 50 years occurs in 5% of those undergoing proctocolectomy and bladder dysfunction in 15%. This is largely preventable by conservative resection techniques.

References

Anonymous. Coated oral 5 aminosalicylic acid versus placebo in maintaining remission of inactive Crohn's disease. International Mesalazine Study Group. *Aliment. Pharmacol. Ther.* 1990; 4: 55–64.

Anseline PF, Wlodarczyk J, Murugasu R. Presence of granulomas is associated with recurrence after surgery for Crohn's disease: experience of a surgical unit. *Br. J. Surg.* 1997; 84: 78–82.

Arndit JW, Grootscholten MI, van Hogezand RA Griffioen G, Lamers CB, Pauwels EK. Inflammatory bowel disease activity assessment using technetium-99m-HMPAO leukocytes. *Dig. Dis. Sci.* 1997; 42: 387–93.

Bansal P, Sonnenberg A. Risk factors of colorectal cancer in inflammatory bowel disease. *Am. J. Gastroenterol.* 1996; 91: 44–8.

Bayless TM. Maintenance therapy for Crohn's disease. *Gastroenterology* 1996; 110: 299–302.

Bernstein D, Rogers A. Malignancy in Crohn's disease. *Am. J. Gastroenterol.* 1996; 91: 434–40.

Bouhnik Y, Lemann M, Mary JY, Scemama G, Tai R, Matuchansky C, *et al.* Long term follow-up of patients with Crohn's disease treated with azathioprine or 6 mercaptopurine. *Lancet* 1996; 347: 215–9.

Brynskov J, Freund L, Rasmussen SN, Lauritsen K, de Muckadell OS, Williams N, *et al.* A placebo controlled, double blind, randomized trial of cyclosporine therapy in active chronic Crohn's disease. *N. Engl. J. Med.* 1989; 321: 845–50.

Butterworth RJ, Williams GT, Hughes LE. Can Crohn's disease be diagnosed at laparotomy? *Gut* 1992; 33: 140–2.

Caprilli R, Andreoli A, Capurso L, Corrao G, D'Albasio G, Gioieni A, *et al.* Oral mesalazine (5 aminosalicylic acid; Asacol) for the prevention of post operative recurrence of Crohn's disease. *Aliment. Pharmacol. Ther.* 1994; 8: 35–43.

Carlson HC. Perspective: the small bowel examination in the diagnosis of Crohn's disease. *Am. J. Roentgenol.* 1986; 147: 63–5.

Cohen AJ, Rowen SJ, Pelot D, Dana ER. The role of antegrade barium studies in the evaluation of colitis. *Am. J. Gastroenterol.* 1986; 81: 656–61.

Colombel JF, Gower-Rousseau C. Etiology of Crohn disease. Current data. *Presse Med.* 1994; 23: 558–60.

Coremans G, Rutgeerts P, Geboes K, Van den Oord J, Ponette E, Vantrappen G. The value of ileoscopy with biopsy in the diagnosis of intestinal Crohn's disease. *Gastrointest. Endoscopy* 1984; 30: 167–72.

Cosnes J, Carbonnel F, Beaugerie L, Le Q uintrec Y, Gendre JP. Effects of cigarette smoking on the long term course of Crohn's disease. *Gastroenterology* 1996; 110: 424–31.

Cottone M, Rosselli M, Orlando A, Oliva L, Puleo A, Cappello M, *et al.* Smoking habits and recurrence in Crohn's disease. *Gastroenterology* 1994; 106: 643–8.

Cottone M, Brignola C, Rosselli M, Oliva L, Belloli C, Cipolla C, Orlando A, De Simone G, Aiala MR, Di Mitri R, Gatto G, Buccellato A. Relationship between site of disease and familial occurence in Crohn's disease. *Dig. Dis. Sci.* 1997; 42: 129–32.

Danzi JT. Extra-intestinal manifestations of idiopathic inflammatory bowel disease. *Arch. Intern. Med.* 1988; 148: 297–302.

de Dombal FT. Epidemiology of Crohn's disease of the colon. *Ann. Gastroenterol. Hepatol.* 1985; 21: 191–200.

de Kaski MC, Peters AM, Lavender JP, Hodgson HJ. Fluticasone propionate in Crohn's disease. *Gut* 1991; 32: 657–61.

Egan LJ, Sandborn WJ. Methotrexate for inflammatory bowel disease: pharmacology and preliminary results. *Mayo Clin. Proc.* 1996; 71: 69–80.

Ekbom A, Wakefield AJ, Zack M, Adami HO. Perinatal measles infection and subsequent Crohn's disease. *Lancet* 1994; 344: 508–10.

Even Sapir E, Barnes DC, Martin RH, LeBrun GP. Indium-111 white blood cell scintigraphy in Crohn's patients with fistulas and sinus tracts. *J. Nuclear Med.* 1994; 35: 245–50.

Faucheron, JL, Saint-Marc O, Guibert L, Parc R. Long-term seton drainage for high anal fistulas in Crohn's disease—a sphincter-saving operation? *Dis. Colon Rectum* 1996; 39: 208–11.

Fazio VW, Wu JS. Surgical therapy for Crohn's disease of the colon and rectum. *Surg. Clin. North Am.* 1997; 77: 197–210.

Gendre JP, Mary JY, Florent C, Modigliani R, Colombel JF, Soule JC, *et al.* Oral mesalamine (Pentasa) as maintenance treatment in Crohn's disease: a multicenter placebo controlled study. The Groupe d'Etudes Therapeutiques des Affections Inflammatoires Digestives (GETAID). *Gastroenterology* 1993; 104: 435–9.

Gillen CD, Andrews HA, Prior P, Allan RN Crohn's disease and colorectal cancer. *Gut* 1994; 35: 651–5.

Glass RE, Ritchie JK, Lennard Jones JE, Hawley PR, Todd IP. Internal fistulas in Crohn's disease. *Dis. Colon Rectum* 1985; 28: 557–61.

Greenberg GR, Feagan BG, Martin F, Sutherland LR, Thomson AB, Williams CN, *et al.* Oral budesonide as maintenance treatment for Crohn's disease: a placebo controlled, dose ranging study. Canadian Inflammatory Bowel Disease Study Group. *Gastroenterology* 1996; 110: 45–51.

Halme L, Sainio AP. Factors related to frequency, type, and outcome of anal fistulas in Crohn's disease. *Dis. Colon Rectum* 1995; 38: 55–9.

Hanauer SB. Inflammatory bowel disease. *N. Engl. J. Med.* 1996; 334: 841–8.

Heyen F, Ambrose NS, Allan RN, Dykes PW, Alexander Williams J, Keighley MR. Enterovesical fistulas in Crohn's disease. *Ann. R. Coll. Surg. Engl.* 1989; 71: 101–4.

Holdstock G, DuBoulay CE, Smith CL. Survey of the use of colonoscopy in inflammatory bowel disease. *Dig. Dis. Sci.* 1984; 29: 731–4.

Hugot JP, Laurent Puig P, Gower Rousseau C, Olson JM, Lee JC, Beaugerie L, *et al.* Mapping of a susceptibility locus for Crohn's disease on chromosome 16. *Nature* 1996; 379: 821–3.

Hull TL, Faxio VW. Surgical approaches to low anovaginal fistula in Crohn's disease. *Am. J. Surg.* 1997; 173: 95–8.

Hyams JS. Crohn's disease in children. *Pediatr. Clin. North Am.* 1996; 43: 255–77.

Kelly JK, Preshaw RM. Origin of fistulas in Crohn's disease. *J. Clin. Gastroenterol.* 1989; 11: 193–6.

Kirman I, Nielsen OH. Expression of common gamma chain on peripheral blood mononuclear cells in Crohn's disease. *Dig. Dis. Sci.* 1997; 42: 372–7.

Kirsner JB. Inflammatory bowel disease. Part I: Nature and pathogenesis. *Disease-A-Month* 1991; 37: 605–66.

Kirsner JB. Crohn's disease: yesterday, today, and tomorrow. *Gastroenterol.* 1997; 112: 1028–30.

Korelitz BI, Present DH. Favorable effect of 6 mercaptopurine on fistulas of Crohn's disease. *Dig. Dis. Sci.* 1985; 30: 58–64.

Kornbluth A, Salomon P, Sachar DB. Crohn's disease. In: Sleisenger MH, Fordtran JS, eds. *Gastrointestinal disease. pathophysiology/diagnosis/management*, 5th edn. Philadelphia: WB Saunders, 1993: 1270–304.

Kozarek RA, Patterson DJ, Botoman VA, Ball TJ, Gelfand MD. Methotrexate use in inflammatory bowel disease patients who have failed azathioprine or 6 mercaptopurine. *Gastroenterology* 1991; 100: A222.

Kuramoto S, Oohara T, Ihara O, Shimazu R, Kondo Y. Granulomas of the gut in Crohn's disease. A step sectioning study. *Dis. Colon Rectum* 1987; 30: 6–11.

Lee EY, Stenson WF, DeSchryver Kecskemeti K. Thickening of muscularis mucosae in Crohn's disease. *Mod. Pathol.* 1991; 4: 87–90.

Lind E, Fausa O, Elgjo K, Gjone E. Crohn's disease. Clinical manifestations. *Scand. J. Gastroenterol.* 1985; 20: 665–70.

Lisciandrano D, Ranzi T, Carrassi A, Sardella A, Campanini MC, Velio P, Bianchi PA. Prevalence of oral lesions in inflammatory bowel disease. *Am. J. Gastroenterol.* 1996; 91: 7–10.

Löfberg R, Danielsson A, Salde L. Oral budesonide in active ileocecal Crohn's disease—a pilot trial with a topically acting steroid. *Gastroenterology* 1991; 100: A226.

Lorenz Meyer H, Malchow H, Miller B, Stock H, Brandes JW. European Cooperative Crohn's Disease Study (ECCDS): colonoscopy. *Digestion* 1985; 31: 109–19.

Ludwig KA, Milsom JW, Church JM, Fazio VW. Preliminary experience with laparoscopic intestinal surgery for Crohn's disease. *Am. J. Surg.* 1996; 171: 52–5.

MacDonald TT, Murch SH. Aetiology and pathogenesis of chronic inflammatory bowel disease. *Baillières Clin. Gastroenterol.* 1994; 8: 1–34.

Mahmud N, McDonald GS, Kelleher D, Weir DG. Microalbuminuria correlates with intestinal histopathological grading in patients with inflammatory bowel disease. *Gut* 1996; 38: 99–103.

Makowiec F, Jehle EC, Becker HD, Starlinger M. Clinical course after transanal advancement flap repair of perianal fistula in patients with Crohn's disease. *Br. J. Surg.* 1995; 82: 603–6.

Malchow H, Ewe K, Brandes JW, Goebell H, Ehms H, Sommer H, *et al.* European Cooperative Crohn's Disease Study (ECCDS): results of drug treatment. *Gastroenterology* 1984; 86: 249–66.

McCourtney JS, Finlay IG. Setons in the surgical management of fistula in ano. *Br. J. Surg.* 1995; 82: 448–52.

McCue J, Coppen MJ, Rasbridge SA, Lock MR. Crohn's disease of the appendix. *Ann. R. Coll. Surg. Engl.* 1988; 70: 300–3.

Michelassi F, Stella M, Balestracci T, Giuliante F, Marogna P, Block GE. Incidence, diagnosis, and treatment of enteric and colorectal fistulas in patients with Crohn's disease. *Ann. Surg.* 1993; 218: 660–6.

Mingrone G, Greco AV, Benedetti G, Capristo E, Semeraro R, Zoli G, Gasbarrini G. Increased resting lipid oxidation in Crohn's disease. *Dig. Dis. Sci.*. 1996; 41: 72–6.

Mishina D, Katsel P, Brown ST, Gilberts EC, Greenstein RJ. On the etiology of Crohn disease. *Proc. Nat. Acad. Science USA.* 1996; 93: 9816–20.

Moum B, Ekbom A, Vatn M, Aadland E, Sauar J, Lygren I, Schulz T, Stray N, Fausa O. Inflammatory bowel disease: re-evaluation of the diagnosis in a prospective population based study in south eastern Norway. *Gut* 1997; 40: 328–32.

Munkholm P, Langholz E, Davidsen M, Binder V. Intestinal cancer risk and mortality in patients with Crohn's disease. *Gastroenterology* 1993; 105: 1716–23.

Oberhuber G, Puspok A, Oesterreicher C, Novacek G, Zauner C, Burghuber M, Vogelsang H, Potzi R, Stolte M, Wrba F. Focally enhanced gastritis: a frequent type of gastritis in patients with Crohn's disease. *Gastroenterol.* 1997; 112: 698–706.

O'Donoghue DP, Dawson AM, Powell Tuck J, Bown RL., Lennard Jones JE. Double blind withdrawal trial of azathioprine as maintenance treatment for Crohn's disease. *Lancet* 1978; ii: 955–7.

O'Morain CA. Does nutritional therapy in inflammatory bowel disease have a primary or an adjunctive role? *Scand. J. Gastroenterol.* Suppl 1990; 172: 29–34.

O'Morain CA, Segal AW, Levi AJ. Elemental diet as primary treatment of acute Crohn's disease: a controlled trial. *Br. Med. J.* 1984; 288: 1859–62.

Orel SG, Rubesin SE, Jones B, Fishman EK, Bayless TM, Siegelman SS. Computed tomography vs barium studies in the acutely symptomatic patient with Crohn disease. *J. Comput. Assist. Tomography* 1987; 11: 1009–16.

Ozuner G, Fazio VW, Lavery IC, Church JM, Hull TL. How safe is strictureplasty in the management of Crohn's disease? *Am. J. Surg.* 1996; 171: 57–60.

Payne-James JJ, Silk DB. Gastroenterologists and nutritional support. *Gut* 1990; 31: 483.

Pescatori M, Interisano A, Basso L, Arcana F, Buffatti P, Di Bella F, *et al.* Management of perianal Crohn's disease. Results of a multicenter study in Italy. *Dis. Colon Rectum* 1995; 38: 121–4.

Platell C, Mackay J, Collopy B, Fink R, Ryan P, Woods R. Anal pathology in patients with Crohn's disease. *Aust. NZ. J. Surg.* 1996; 66: 5–9.

Prantera C, Pallone F, Brunetti G, Cottone M, Miglioli M. Oral 5 amino-salicylic acid (Asacol) in the maintenance treatment of Crohn's disease. The Italian IBD Study Group. *Gastroenterology* 1992; 103: 363–8.

Present DH, Lichtiger S. The efficacy of cyclosporine in the treatment of the fistula of Crohn's disease. *Gastroenterology* 1992; 102: A680.

Present DH, Korelitz BI, Wisch N, Glass JL, Sachar DB, Pasternack BS. Treatment of Crohn's disease with 6 mercaptopurine. A long term, randomized, double blind study. *N. Engl. J. Med.* 1980; 302: 981–7.

Reissman P, Salky BA, Pfeifer J, Edye M, Jagelman DG, Wexner SD. Laparoscopic surgery in the management of inflammatory bowel disease. *Am. J. Surg.* 1996; 171: 47–50.

Rhodes JM. Unifying hypothesis for inflammatory bowel disease and associated colon cancer: sticking the pieces together with sugar. *Lancet* 1996; 347: 40–4.

Ribeiro MB, Greenstein AJ, Sachar DB, Barth J, Balasubramanian S, Harpaz N, *et al.* Colorectal adenocarcinoma in Crohn's disease. *Ann. Surg.* 1996; 223: 186–93.

Robert JR, Sachar DB, Greenstein AJ. Severe gastrointestinal hemorrhage in Crohn's disease. *Ann. Surg.* 1991; 213: 207–11.

Sahai A, Belair M, Gianfelice D, Cote S, Gratton J, Lahaie R. Percutaneous drainage of intra-abdominal abscesses in Crohn's disease: short and long-term outcome. *Am. J. Gastroenterol.* 1997; 92: 275–81.

Sandborn WJ, Tremaine WJ, Lawson GM. Clinical response does not correlate with intestinal or blood cyclosporine concentrations in patients with Crohn's disease treated with high dose oral cyclosporine. *Am. J. Gastroenterol.* 1996; 91: 37–43.

Sangwan YP, Schoetz DR Jr, Murray JJ, Roberts PL, Coller JA. Perianal Crohn's disease. Results of local surgical treatment. *Dis. Colon Rectum* 1996; 39: 529–35.

Sankey EA, Dhillon AP, Anthony A, Wakefield AJ, Sim R, More L, *et al.* Early mucosal changes in Crohn's disease. *Gut* 1993; 34: 375–81.

Schmitz Moormann P, Pittner PM, Malchow H, Brandes JW. The granuloma in Crohn's disease. A bioptical study. *Pathol. Res. Pract.* 1984; 178: 467–76.

Schreiber S, Howaldt S, Schnoor M, Nikolaus S, Bauditz J, Gasche C, *et al.* Recombinant erythropoietin for the treatment of anemia in inflammatory bowel disease. *N. Engl. J. Med.* 1996; 334: 619–23.

Smith MS, Wakefield AJ. Viral association with Crohn's disease. *Ann. Med.* 1993; 25: 557–61.

Stahlberg D, Veress B, Mare K, Granqvist S, Agren B, Richter S, Lofberg R. Leukocyte migration in acute colonic inflammatory bowel disease: comparison of histological assessment and Tc-99m-HMPAO labeled leukocyte scan. *Am. J. Gastroenterol.* 1997; 92: 283–8.

Summers RW, Switz DM, Sessions JT Jr, Becktel JM, Best WR, Kern F Jr, *et al.* National Cooperative Crohn's Disease Study: results of drug treatment. *Gastroenterology* 1979; 77: 847–69.

Thompson NP, Driscoll R, Pounder RE, Wakefield AJ. Genetics versus environment in inflammatory bowel disease: results of a British twin study. *Br. Med. J.* 1996; 312: 95–6.

Tolia V. Perianal Crohn's disease in children and adolescents. *Am. J. Gastroenterol.* 1996; 91: 922–6.

Tsang CB, Rothenberger DA. Rectovaginal fistulas. Therapeutic options. *Surg. Clin. North Am.* 1997; 77: 95–114.

Ursing B, Alm T, Barany F, Bergelin I, Ganrot Norlin K, Hoevels J, *et al.* A comparative study of metronidazole and sulfasalazine for active Crohn's disease: the cooperative Crohn's disease study in Sweden. II. Result. *Gastroenterology* 1982; 83: 550–62.

van Oostayen JA, Wassser MN, van Hogezand RA Griffioen G, Biemond I, Lamers CB de Ross A. Doppler sonography evaluation of superior mesenteric artery flow to assess Crohn's disease activity: correlation with clinical evaluation, Crohn's disease activity index, and alpha l-antitrypsin clearance in feces. *Am. J. Roentgenol.* 1997; 168: 429–33.

Wakefield AJ, Ekbom A, Dhillon AP, Pittilo RM, Pounder RE. Crohn's disease: pathogenesis and persistent measles virus infection. *Gastroenterology* 1995; 108: 911–6.

Walmsley RS, Ibbotson JP, Chahal H, Allan RN. Antibodies against Mycobacterium paratuberculosis in Crohn's disease. *QJM.* 1996; 89: 217–21.

Wiesmayr M, Bankier A, Fleischmann D, Karnel F. Percutaneous drainage of intra abdominal abscesses in Crohn disease. *Aktuelle Radiol.* 1994; 4: 184–7.

Williams SM, Harned RK. Hepatobiliary complications of inflammatory bowel disease. *Radiol. Clin. North Am.* 1987; 25: 175–88.

Williamson PR, Hellinger MD, Larach SW, Ferrara A. Twenty year review of the surgical management of perianal Crohn's disease. *Dis. Colon Rectum* 1995; 38: 389–92.

Yao T, Okada M, Fuchigami T, Iida M, Takenaka K, Date H, Fujita K. The relationship between the radiological and clinical features in patients with Crohn's disease. *Clin. Radiol.* 1989; 40: 389–92.

Yardley JH, Hendrix TR. Gastroduodenal Crohn's disease: the focus is on focality. *Gastroenterol.* 1997; 112: 1031–2.

7 Diverticular disease

Incidence

Diverticular disease is predominantly a disease of the twentieth century. At the beginning of the century, only 25 cases had been reported, yet it is now the commonest condition with identifiable pathology affecting the large intestine in Western countries. It is difficult to estimate the incidence of diverticular disease in the general population, most reports having resorted to radiological or autopsy studies. Early large studies reported colonic diverticula to occur in 6% of all barium enemas and 5% of autopsies (Rankin and Brown 1930), figures very similar to a more recent autopsy study (Richter *et al.* 1991). However, other barium enema or autopsy studies report the prevalence of diverticulosis to range between 15% and 40%, depending on age (Parks 1969; Levy *et al.* 1985; Chia *et al.* 1991), while in those over 50 years, 25% of colonoscopies will show evidence of diverticula (De Reuck *et al.* 1990). The exact prevalence of diverticulitis is also unknown. Between 15% and 30% of patients with diverticula on radiology or autopsy are thought to have evidence of active inflammation (Kubo *et al.* 1985; Dozle and Daiss 1992). Less than 20% of those with diverticulitis will require hospital admission. Subsequent progression of radiologically proven diverticulosis to diverticulitis occurs in up to 20% of cases (Sugihara *et al.* 1984; Rege and Nahrwold 1989). Acute diverticulitis is said to account for 4% of all hospital admissions in Western countries and 2% of emergency laparotomies for acute abdominal pain. Over the past 30 years, operations for diverticulitis have remained constant, despite a reduction in hospital admissions for the condition, suggesting an increase in the severity and septic complications of the disease (Chia *et al.* 1991). Diverticular disease accounts for 11% of colon resections in those over 70 years.

There is a striking correlation in the incidence of diverticular disease with age (Cheskin *et al.* 1990; Ozick *et al.* 1994). Approximately 5% of patients are under 40 years of age, but thereafter the condition rises steadily such that diverticula occur in 30% of 50 year olds and 50% of 80 year olds (Parks 1969; Acosta *et al.* 1992). The mean age at diagnosis is 65 years, 25% of patients being over 75 years at presentation (Vayre 1990). Diverticular disease presenting in those less than 40 years is rare but tends to run an aggressive course, often requiring operation (Acosta *et al.* 1992). The sex distribution is variable; some studies showing a slight male, and others a slight female, predominance (Parks 1969).

There is considerable geographical and racial variation in diverticular disease. The prevalence in developing countries is 2%, compared with 15–20% seen in Europe or America (Ogunbiyi 1989; Chia *et al.* 1991; Ibrarullah *et al.* 1991). In Western and African countries the condition is predominantly left sided, 66% of diverticula occurring solely in the sigmoid colon (Segal and Leibowitz 1989; Walker and Seeal 1997). In contrast, 70% of diverticular disease in Orientals is confined to the right colon and occurs in a younger age group (Sugihara *et al.* 1984; Chia *et al.* 1991; Nakada *et al.* 1995). Total colonic involvement occurs in 10% of Western and 20% of Oriental patients with diverticular disease (Parks 1969; Sugihara *et al.* 1984).

Aetiology

There is no association between diverticula in the duodenum and colon so that colonic diverticular disease is unlikely to represent part of a generalized gastrointestinal diverticular tendency (De Koster *et al.* 1991). It has long been recognized that colonic diverticula represent acquired herniation of the mucosa at points of maximum weakness of the colonic wall, where the blood vessels enter between the mesenteric and antimesenteric taenia and to a lesser extent between the antimesenteric taenia (Slack 1962, McCarthy *et al.* 1996) (Figure 7.1). Muscular spasm and irregular uncoordinated contraction of the affected colon increase the intraluminal pressure and precipitate the herniation, explaining the muscular hypertrophy seen pathologically and the radiological features of spasm (Condon 1985; Ozick *et al.* 1994). This muscular thickening is due to a 200% increase in the elastin content of the taenia, leading to contraction and corrugation of the circular muscle in the presence of normal muscle cells (Whiteway and Morson 1985). As a consequence, the tensile strength decreases distally as the colonic wall thickness increases (Watters *et al.* 1985). The increase in diverticular disease with age is related to this progressive elastosis and shortening of the taeniae coli with time (Watters *et al.* 1985; Whiteway and Morson 1985). This is related to changes in cross-linking of collagen with age (Wess *et al.* 1995). The age-related changes in elastosis and tensile strength are maximal in the left side

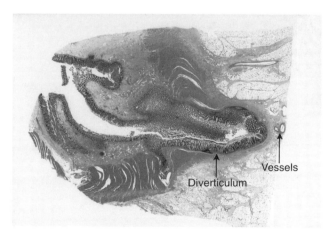

Figure 7.1 Tissue section mount from a colonic diverticulum (H&E). Note the full thickness herniation through the muscle in close conjunction with the blood vessels (arrowed).

which is the narrowest and thickest part of the colon (Watters and Smith 1990).

Colonic pressure measurements are significantly higher in both the resting and postprandial states in those with diverticular disease relative to controls and in symptomatic compared with asymptomatic patients (Cortesini and Pantalone 1991). The intraluminal pressure reverts to normal levels following sigmoid colectomy. Although slow wave rhythms are not responsible, disturbances in the amount of vasoactive intestinal peptide in the bowel wall may contribute to the obstructive motility patterns (Katschinski *et al.* 1990; Milner *et al.* 1990). A combination of the higher intraluminal pressure and smaller calibre of the left colon predisposes to the characteristic distribution of the diverticula. The excessive segmentation causes intermittent colonic obstruction resulting in severe pain which can occur without the presence of inflammation (Painter 1985).

Numerous epidemiological studies imply that lack of fibre in the diet is a major aetiological factor for diverticular disease (Segal and Leibowitz 1989; Ihekwaba 1992). The segmentation required to propel the viscous faeces produced by a low-fibre diet creates the higher intracolonic pressures seen in this condition. Most authors now agree that diverticular disease represents an interaction between racial and environmental factors, of which dietary fibre and ageing are the most important (Burkitt *et al.* 1985; Segal and Leibowitz 1989). In Western countries, early weaning and the small stools associated with a low-fibre diet that only intermittently distend the colon may initiate the elastosis associate with diverticular disease (Whiteway and Morson 1985). Such changes explain the time lag between alteration in diet and the incidence of diverticular disease.

Lack of physical exercise and chronic renal failure, especially adult autosomal dominant polycystic disease, have been associated with diverticular disease (Abramson *et al.* 1991; Aldoori *et al.* 1995). Over 40% of patients on chronic ambulatory peritoneal dialysis have colonic diverticula accounting for a quarter of episodes of peritonitis in this group (Tranaeus *et al.* 1990). In contrast, the previously reported relationship between pelvic phleboliths and diverticular disease remains unproven (de Vries *et al.* 1992). Non-steroidal anti-inflammatory drugs (NSAIDs) have recently been implicated in the aetiology of complicated diverticular disease (Wilson *et al.* 1990; Campbell and Steele 1991; Riddell *et al.* 1992; Bjarnason *et al.* 1993). Other studies have emphasized the risk of perforated diverticular disease for patients on corticosteroids (Weiner *et al.* 1993).

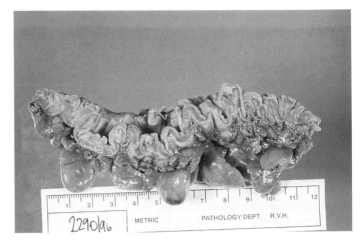

Figure 7.2 Diverticular disease of the sigmoid colon in longitudinal section. Note the sacculation and the thickening of the bowel wall.

of cases, followed by the descending, transverse, ascending colon and caecum, in decreasing order of frequency. On sectioning the gross specimen, there is thickening of the muscle layers, with sacculation of the bowel (Figure 7.2).

Microscopic appearance

Diverticula contain only two layers, an inner mucosal and outer serosal layer. Even though hypertrophy of both the longitudinal and circular muscle coat may be present even in the absence of inflammation, it is now recognized that there is a marked increase in the elastin content of the taeniae (Whiteway and Morson 1985) (Figure 7.3). Variable degrees of inflammation are usually seen, often with foci of foreign-body reaction to vegetable material from the faeces or to barium. Inflammation begins in a narrow-necked diverticulum which becomes obstructed. Bacterial proliferation, mucosal transgression and inflammatory exudate with raised intraluminal pressure precipitate necrosis of the thin-walled sac with micro-perforation. The inflammatory process may spread to involve the adjacent colonic wall and, depending on the site of the diverticulum, may be contained in the mesocolon (Hackford and Veidenheimer 1985). Rupture into the peritoneum without direct communication with the bowel lumen results in peritoneal contamination with pus. Direct communication with the lumen results in faecal peritonitis and is

Pathology

Macroscopic appearances

Colonic diverticula are acquired pulsion diverticula of herniated mucosa and submucosa. The diverticula occur between the mesenteric taenia and the two antimesenteric taeniae at the site of entry of the blood vessels (Figure 7.1). Antimesenteric diverticula are usually only 2–3 mm in size and usually occur in advanced or long-standing cases. The diverticula penetrate the bowel wall and appear on the outside of the intestine covered by serosa or fat according to their location. Their appearance is globular and they communicate with the bowel lumen by a narrow neck. Small diverticula in fat patients may be relatively inapparent, as they often project into the appendices epiploicae. The sigmoid colon is the site of disease in 80%

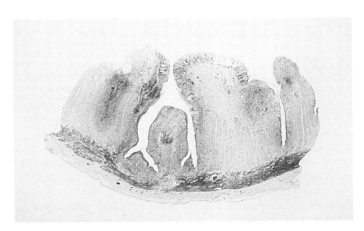

Figure 7.3 Tissue section mount through wall of the sigmoid colon showing diverticuli extending deeply into the hypertrophic muscularis propria.

associated with the greatest mortality. The speed of onset of perforation determines the extent of containment of the contamination by fibrin, omentum, or adjacent viscera. However, initially contained infection may rupture to become widespread, whereas free perforation with subdiaphragmatic gas may become contained. With each attack the pericolonic fibrosis increases until the wall becomes encased by a fibrous reaction, leading to obstruction (Whiteway and Morson 1985). In contrast to carcinoma, the mucosa of diverticular disease is always intact and never ulcerated.

Clinical presentation

Symptoms

Diverticular disease may be associated with pain, varying in site, severity and duration; alteration of bowel habit from diarrhoea, constipation or a combination of both, and bleeding (Ogunbiyi 1989, Metcalf *et al.* 1996). These symptoms are non-specific, only 20% of patients with such complaints being found to have diverticulitis (Bertschinger 1993). In diverticular disease, recurrent symptoms are uncommon, only 20% of patients admitting to repeated pain, the majority of these being over 50 years old (Bertschinger 1993). In contrast, severe diverticulitis is the first manifestation of the disease in 50% of cases, and 80% of those with perforated diverticular disease will deny previous symptoms (Hackford and Vedenheimer 1985). Consequently, there is a poor correlation between pre-operative symptoms and operative findings (Moreaux 1991). Uncomplicated diverticulosis was formerly believed to be asymptomatic, representing an incidental finding during investigation for other conditions. It is now recognized that diverticulosis and diverticulitis represent a disease spectrum with a similar aetiology. The excessive segmentation responsible for both conditions produces pain, flatulence, and alteration in bowel habit, inflammation being a secondary, rather than a primary, phenomenon (Painter 1985). Half of patients with diverticulosis will have symptoms, of which alteration in bowel habit is the most common (25%) (Sugihara *et al.* 1984). It is suggested that two clinical types of diverticular disease exist. One is associated with pain, bowel symptoms or fistula, resection identifying only a few diverticula with histological evidence of perforation (Ryan 1991). The less common variety presents with bleeding, associated with densely packed extensive diverticula with no histological evidence of perforation (Ryan 1991).

Signs

Diverticulosis is associated with no clinical signs. Diverticulitis may be evident as tenderness, usually in the left iliac fossa, with or without a palpable mass, which may be detectable rectally. Such findings are entirely non-specific. Occasionally, there may be signs and symptoms of bowel obstruction. This is usually due to small bowel adherent to an inflamed diverticular segment, or, much less commonly, dilated large bowel from a tight diverticular stricture. Psoas spasm, associated with leg or thigh pain and occasionally emphysema of the left thigh is suggestive of retroperitoneal perforation (Haiart *et al.* 1989). This presentation is more common in the elderly, females and those with delayed diagnosis and is associated with a considerable mortality (Ravo *et al.* 1985).

Diagnosis

Although an elevated white cell count is seen in 75% of patients with diverticulitis, blood tests are of little benefit in making the diagnosis (Morris *et al.* 1986). Perforation should be considered in the absence of clinical signs if patients on steroids have an elevated temperature or white cell count (Weiner *et al.* 1993). Sigmoidoscopy is frequently abnormal, but has a low specificity and sensitivity as spasm often prevents an adequate view and the presence of diverticula does not exclude a neoplasm higher in the colon (Morris *et al.* 1986). Colonoscopy or barium enema is therefore preferable (Figure 7.4).

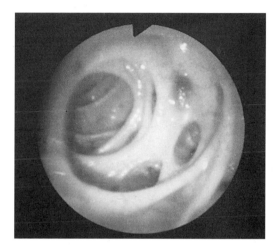

Figure 7.4 Colonoscopic view of diverticular disease.

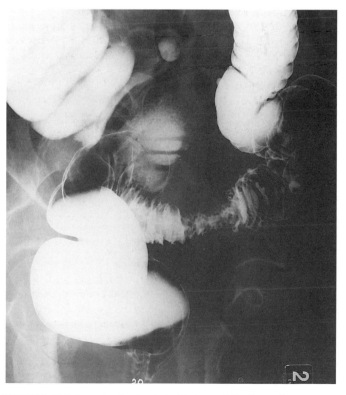

Figure 7.5 Barium enema showing typical features of diverticular disease including spasm.

In only 60% of patients clinically felt to have complicated diverticular disease is the diagnosis confirmed on barium enema by radiological evidence of spasm or perforation (Morris *et al.* 1986) (Figure 7.5). An accurate distinction between diverticular disease and polyps or neoplasm may be difficult on barium enema (Figures 7.6 and 7.7). Consequently, 5% of operations for diverticular disease are because carcinoma cannot be excluded radiologically (Moreaux and Vons 1990; Gravie *et al.* 1991). Features which favour the diagnosis of diverticular disease are a long affected segment, gradual transition to abnormal bowel without shouldering, a bizarre, fringed contour, an intact mucosa, and the presence of diverticula in other parts of the colon. Even when these features are present, the distinction may be difficult (Figure 7.8). Early reports suggested that it was impossible to distinguish radiologically diverticular disease from carcinoma in up to 20% of cases. More recent reports comparing barium enema with colonoscopy reveal that barium enema reporting of sigmoid diverticular disease is inaccurate in 35–43% of cases (Aldridge and Sim 1986). This is because in up to 25% of those with diverticular disease a colonic polyp may also be present, about 5% of the polyps being malignant. In addition, diverticulosis occurs in almost 20% of those with colon cancer (Morosi *et al.* 1991). Nevertheless, in patients over 60 years presenting with rectal bleeding from supposed diverticular disease, colonoscopy should be performed (Metcalf *et al.* 1996). If colonoscopy reveals crescenteric mucosal folds close to diverticula, the bleeding is likely to be due to diverticular disease. These mucosal folds are found in 2% of colonoscopies, 80% being due to diverticular disease. They are formed by venous congestion and mucosal redundancy secondary to spastic contraction of the muscle coat (Kelly 1991; Gore *et al.* 1992).

There has been concern that performing a barium enema during an attack of acute diverticulitis may potentiate perforation or complications. There is little evidence for this, many feeling that, if per-

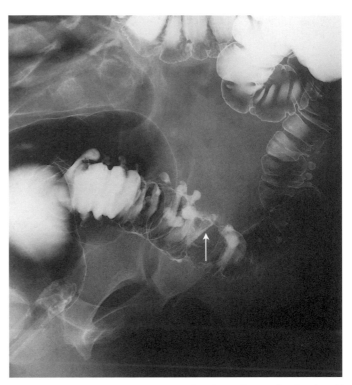

Figure 7.7 Barium enema in a patient with diverticular disease showing sigmoid polyp (arrowed).

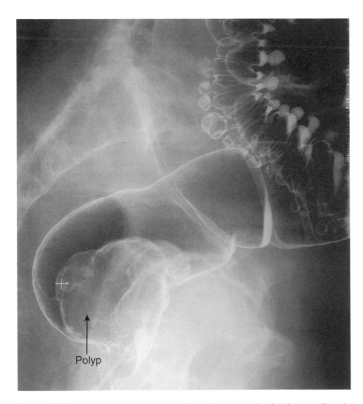

Figure 7.6 Barium enema showing coexistent large rectal polyp (arrowed) and diverticular disease.

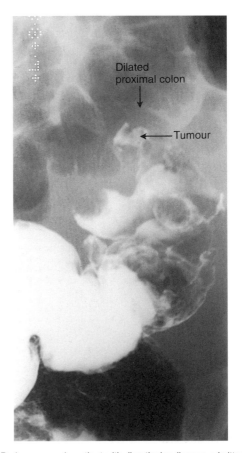

Figure 7.8 Barium enema in patient with diverticular disease admitted with large bowel obstruction. The obstructing lesion turned out to be carcinoma.

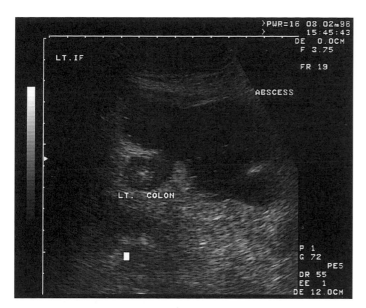

Figure 7.9 Ultrasound scan showing peri-colic collection in perforated diverticular disease.

formed carefully with water-soluble contrast media, it is the investigation of choice for both confirming the diagnosis and planning treatment (Moreaux 1991; Bazzocchi *et al.* 1992). Radiological features suggesting diverticular disease are intramural thickening, localized extravasation, thickened folds with distortion and spasticity, and mucosal tethering. If barium enema is delayed until inflammation settles, these features are absent and the main benefit is to exclude coexistent carcinoma. Patients who cannot tolerate a barium enema may be given barium orally (Papadaki *et al.* 1993).

In the acute phase, ultrasound or computerized tomography (CT) scanning can non-invasively detect the gross and subtle changes of diverticular disease (Schwerk *et al.* 1992; Jacobs and Birnbaum 1995) (Figure 7.9). The sensitivity, specificity and accuracy of ultra-

sound are all about 98% (Schwerk *et al.* 1992; Zielke *et al.* 1997). Hypoechoic areas with target lesions support the diagnosis, while hyperechogenicity suggests peridiverticulitis (Wilson and Toi 1990; Schwerk *et al.* 1992). The CT findings of diverticular disease consist of mixed attenuation areas often containing gas, extracolonic masses and bowel wall thickening or oedema (Pillari *et al.* 1984, Hachigian *et al.* 1992; Ambrosetti *et al.* 1997) (Figure 7.10). CT abnormalities are detected in over 60% of patients with acute diverticular disease, abscesses being detected, and potentially drained, in one-third (Morris *et al.* 1986; Hachigian *et al.* 1992; McLoughlin *et al.* 1995, Shuler *et al.* 1996).

Complications

Inflammatory or bleeding complications occur in 15–20% of patients. Diverticular disease or its complications accounts for up to 20% of all colectomies performed in Western countries (Walsh *et al.* 1990). Over the past 30 years, the presentation of diverticular disease has tended to become more severe, septic complications in particular becoming more common. Currently, emergency procedures account for two-thirds of surgical operations performed for diverticular disease. Factors increasing the risk of developing complications are age under 50 years, a short history of left-sided abdominal pain (18–36 months), and a short diverticular segment (7 cm or less) (Cortesini and Pantalone 1991). Younger patients are more likely to present with perforation and seven times more likely to present with fistulation than older patients and therefore frequently require operation early during their first hospital admission (Freischlag *et al.* 1986; Acosta *et al.* 1992; Schauer *et al.* 1992; Mader *et al.* 1994).

Complicated diverticular disease is associated with a 6–15% mortality (Berry *et al.* 1989; Hold *et al.* 1990; Elliott *et al.* 1997). Whereas the mortality from elective surgery is 2%, that of urgent operations is 10%, while emergency operation is associated with mortality of up to 40%, largely related to faecal peritonitis (Vayre 1990; Scholefield *et al.* 1991). Mortality is related to prolonged symptom duration, pre-operative hypotension, coexisting illness, increasing age, faecal peritonitis, and persistent postoperative sepsis (Corder and Williams 1990; Rothenberger and Wiltz 1993). Mortality is significantly higher in patients over 70 years, being related to the presence of two or more pre-operative diseases, the requirement for emergency surgery, and the development of post-operative complications, particularly infection (Letoquart *et al.* 1992). The morbidity of operations for diverticular disease is 20–30%. The wound infection rate is up to 30% while leakage from both primary anastomosis and colostomy closure can be about 10%.

Patients with diverticular disease do not appear to be at increased risk of developing colon cancer, despite a low-fibre diet being implicated in both conditions. In a follow-up study of over 7000 patients with diverticular disease, there was no significant increased risk for the development of carcinoma of the colon or rectum (Stefansson *et al.* 1993).

Obstruction

Diverticular disease may be complicated by stenosis (Kurgansky and Foxwell 1993). Although complete obstruction is uncommon in diverticular disease, 10% of surgical procedures in diverticular disease are for obstructive symptoms (Rodkey and Welch 1984) (Figure 7.11). Approximately 15% of large bowel obstructions are

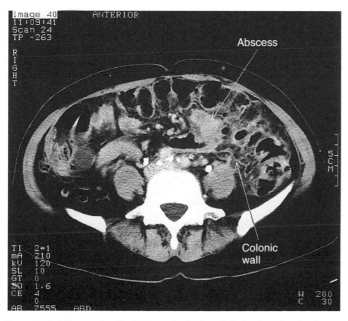

Figure 7.10 CT scan showing thickened colonic wall (1.4 cm) and peri-colic collection in perforated diverticular disease.

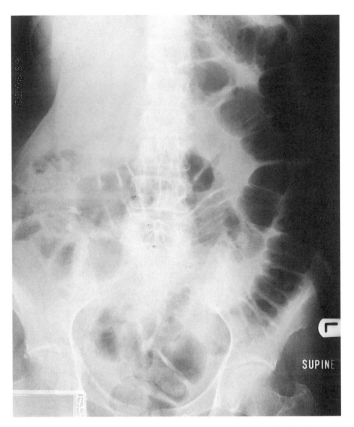

Figure 7.11 Plain abdominal X-ray in a patient with stenosing diverticular disease. Note the obstruction is incomplete, with gas present in the rectum.

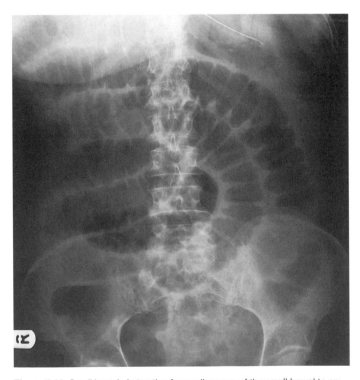

Figure 7.12 Small bowel obstruction from adherence of the small bowel to an area of inflamed diverticular disease.

caused by diverticular disease. Small bowel obstruction may also occur from adherence to an inflamed diverticular segment (Figure 7.12). Inflammatory oedema in an incompletely obstructed colon may result in complete obstruction, which often resolves as the inflammation settles. Stricture of the sigmoid colon is seen in 2% of colonoscopies, 75% of these being due to diverticular disease, the remaining 25% to carcinoma (King *et al.* 1990). However, even with colonoscopic biopsies, distinction between the two conditions can be difficult and operation may be required. Alternatively, balloon dilatation may be performed in conjunction with regular colonoscopic biopsies.

Perforation

Perforation accounts for almost half of those requiring operation for complicated diverticular disease and is the most frequent cause of death in those dying from diverticular disease (Moreaux 1991; Richter *et al.* 1991). Even patients undergoing elective surgery may have histological evidence of micro-perforation, the risk being particularly high (1 in 4) in those on ambulatory peritoneal dialysis (Tranaeus *et al.* 1990). Aspirin ingestion may be another aetiological factor (Lanas *et al.* 1997).

At operation free pus is found in 60% of those with clinical perforation and a phlegmonous mass in the remainder (Huber *et al.* 1991; Sarin and Boulos 1991). If perforated diverticular disease is suspected clinically, operation will reveal an inflammatory mass or localized abscess in 10%, free pus without detectable perforation in 10% and an obvious perforation in 25% (Lambert *et al.* 1986; Medina *et al.* 1991; Letoquart *et al.* 1992).

Haemorrhage

Bleeding is common in diverticular disease, but accounts for only 5% of operations performed for this condition (Gravie *et al.* 1991). Early literature reviews comprising several thousand patients found between 11% and 17% of patients had experienced haemorrhage. More recent studies suggest that bleeding occurs in 20% of patients admitted with left-sided and 5% of right-sided diverticular disease (Boulos *et al.* 1984). Diverticular disease accounts for 25% of gastrointestinal bleeding investigated by colonoscopy (Canedo-Acosia and Jalazar-Mendola 1990). In patients with renal disease, 10% of all gastrointestinal bleeds and one-third of colonic bleeds are due to diverticular disease (Gheissari *et al.* 1990). Diverticular disease was formerly believed to be the commonest cause of lower intestinal bleeding, although some cases may have been due to angiodysplasia. Although bleeding may occasionally be mild, minor rectal bleeding is uncommon in uncomplicated diverticular disease. Mild rectal bleeding is much more likely to be due to colonic polyps or carcinoma than diverticular disease, which represents only 2% of obscure intestinal bleeding (Thompson *et al.* 1987). In one study of diverticular disease, one-third of patients also had polyps (Boulos *et al.* 1984). Bleeding occurred in 65% of those with polyps compared with 20% of those with purely diverticular disease (Boulos *et al.* 1984). Consequently, patients with diverticular disease experiencing mild rectal bleeding should be investigated for polyps or tumour, rather than attributing the symptoms to the diverticular disease. In the few cases in which diverticular disease is responsible, colonoscopy may reveal bleeding from inflamed mucosal crescents at the opening of the diverticula (Kelly 1991; Gore *et al.* 1992). The bleeding from diverticular disease is often brisk (Bokhari *et al.* 1996). In a study of 50 patients with massive intestinal bleeding, 38% of cases were due to diverticular disease (Browder *et al.* 1986). Such torrential bleeding is normally associated with diverticulosis

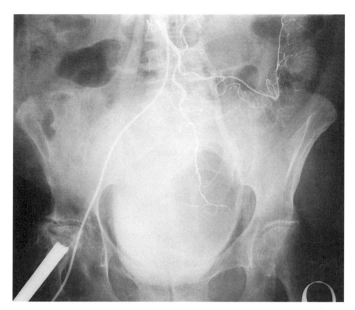

Figure 7.13 Inferior mesenteric arteriogram in a patient with bleeding diverticular disease.

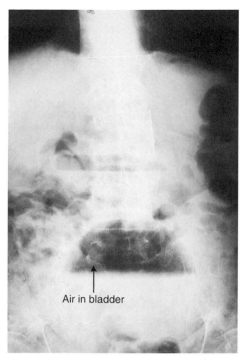

Figure 7.14 Plain abdominal X-ray in a case of vesicocolic fistula secondary to diverticular disease. Note the presence of large amounts of air in the bladder.

rather than diverticulitis. Angiography is particularly useful for investigating heavy intestinal bleeding (over 0.5 ml/min), locating the bleeding source, excluding angiodysplasia, and allowing the correct operation to be chosen (Browder *et al.* 1986; Uden *et al.* 1986; McGuire 1994) (Figure 7.13). Radionucleotide scanning can also provide valuable information in the presence of active bleeding (more than 0.1 ml/min), although some suggest that colonoscopy, particularly after gentle, rapid preparation, is the most beneficial investigation. It is important to exclude a rectal cause of the bleeding by proctosigmoidoscopy, as the extraperitoneal rectum is almost impossible to evaluate intra-operatively and it is the area to be left *in situ* should 'blind' resection (subtotal resection) be necessary. However, this is rarely necessary as bleeding stops spontaneously in 75% of cases and 99% of patients requiring less than four units of transfusion per day (McGuire 1994). When a bleeding diverticulum is removed, rebleeding is rare (Bokhari *et al.* 1996).

Fistula

Fistula formation is caused by rupture of a diverticular abscess into a neighbouring viscus or through the skin. Fistulation accounts for 10–20% of those operated on for complicated diverticular disease (Moreaux and Vons 1990; Huber *et al.* 1991). Fistulas are found in 3% of gastrograffin enemas performed for diverticular disease (Raymond and Gibler 1989). However, in centres with specialist referral patterns, up to 20% of patients with diverticulitis will be found to have fistulas (Raymond and Gibler 1989). Three-quarters of large bowel fistulas are caused by diverticular disease, although a distinction from other causes of fistulation, such as Crohn's disease or carcinoma may occasionally be difficult (Finkelstein and Jamieson 1987). The commonest fistula is a colovesical fistula, for which diverticular disease is the most frequent cause (Puyol *et al.* 1990).

Approximately half of the fistulas from diverticular disease are into the bladder, colovesical fistula accounting for 15% of those undergoing surgery for diverticular disease. Colovesical fistulas are uncommon in women, due to protection from the interposed uterus. Terminal pneumaturia with recurrent urinary tract infections is pathognomic, but often absent (Puyol *et al.* 1990). Similarly, faecal

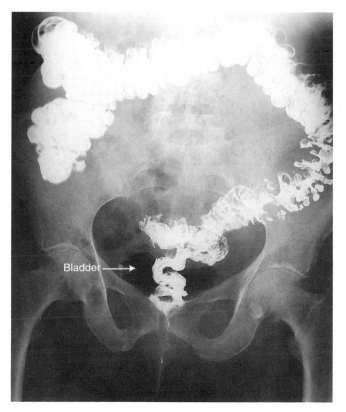

Figure 7.15 Barium enema in vesicocolic fistula. Note the free gas and flecks of barium in the bladder.

material is rarely present in the urine. The finding of air in the bladder on plain radiographs is nearly always due to a fistula and the presence of a conical elevation of the bladder is also highly suggestive (Figure 7.14). The radiological investigations available are intravenous and retrograde urography, serial voiding cystourethography and barium enema (Puyol *et al.* 1990; Grissom and Snyder 1991) (Figure 7.15). However, these tests are rarely positive. X-raying the urine for barium following a barium enema may be helpful (Bach *et al.* 1981). CT scan may reveal thickening and adherence of the colonic and bladder walls. The finding of posterior cystitis on cystoscopy is highly suggestive of a fistula, although an actual opening is identified in less than half of the cases. Colovaginal fistula occurs almost exclusively in women who have had a previous hysterectomy. Presentation is with a foul-smelling vaginal discharge, vaginitis, dyspareunia, and the passage of flatus or faeces per vagina.

Treatment

Conservative treatment

The majority (85%) of patients with uncomplicated diverticulitis are satisfactorily treated by a high-fibre diet (Roberts *et al.* 1995). Such a diet often prevents further attacks and tends to be associated with fewer symptoms, fewer complications, and fewer operations (Sarin and Boulos 1991; Ozick *et al.* 1994). However, 20% of patients will fail to take the diet regularly. Both a high roughage diet and lactulose increase bowel frequency and stool consistency, alleviating symptoms in 70% of those with pain and 66% of those with alteration in bowel habit (Smits *et al.* 1990; Thorburn *et al.* 1992). In uncomplicated diverticular disease antispasmodics or a poorly absorbed antibiotic (rifaximin) can produce significant symptomatic relief (Papi *et al.* 1992; Bertschinger 1993; Papi *et al.* 1995). Mortality from non-surgical treatment of uncomplicated cases is less than 1% (Hackford and Vedenheimer 1985). Patients with suspected localized sepsis secondary to diverticular disease should be treated conservatively in the first instance with systemic antibiotics (Krukowski *et al.* 1985). Many cases, even with abscess formation, will resolve with appropriate antibiotic therapy. Cases complicated by abscess formation which do not settle can be successfully treated with CT-guided drainage provided the patient is stable (Rothenberger and Wiltz 1993). This overcomes the immediate sepsis, allowing bowel preparation and planned excision to be performed. Mortality of resection is then about 2%, clinically apparent anastomotic leakage occurring in about 3% of cases (Gravie *et al.* 1991).

Surgical treatment

Traditional indications for operation are a failure to respond to conservative therapy and the development of complications (Krukowski *et al.* 1985; Roberts *et al.* 1995; Wedell 1997). However, patients with localized peritonitis can often be managed without operation and large abscesses may spontaneously resolve or be drained percutaneously under radiological control (McLoughlin *et al.* 1995). Even the presence of generalized contamination, as shown by free gas under the diaphragm, may not require surgery. Repeated clinical examination and early radiological investigation are often necessary before deciding surgical intervention should be performed. As such, clinical or radiological evidence of perforation or localized sepsis is not necessarily an indication for surgery, as large abscesses may

resolve with appropriate antibiotic therapy. Persistence of peritoneal irritation, pyrexia, tachycardia, and an elevated white cell count indicate failure to respond to conservative therapy and the necessity for surgery (Figure 7). When the indications for operation are more critically defined, the frequency of surgical intervention falls. With such a policy, Krukowski *et al.* (1985) found the proportion of operations performed as an emergency fell during the periods 1977–79, 1980–83, and 1984–86 from 43% to 28% to 15%, repectively. Despite this, mortality and morbidity were both steadily reduced during this time. Although radiological studies aid the decision-making, the decision to operate is essentially based on clinical findings. Those with strictures often require surgery unless carcinoma can be confidently excluded. Patients under the age of 40 years or who are immunosuppressed require early surgical intervention, as their disease frequently runs an aggressive course (Freischlag *et al.* 1986). In some series the indications for surgery are recurrent acute diverticulitis (40%), perforation/abscess (46%), fistula (7%), bleeding (5%), and stricture/possible carcinoma (2%) (Moreau and Vows 1990; Gravie *et al.* 1991). Two attacks of acute diverticulitis may warrant elective surgical intervention to reduce the risk of having to perform emergency surgery during a subsequent acute attack (Gravie *et al.* 1991; Bottingelli *et al.* 1990). In those under 55 years the initial attack of diverticulitis tends to be severe, while recurrent acute diverticulitis can be expected in over 50% of cases. Surgery has therefore been suggested after the first admission for severe acute diverticulitis in this age group (Hackford and Vedenheimer 1985). Consequently, some centres have recently increased the proportion of elective cases from 45% to 57% in an attempt to pre-empt emergency surgery and reduce morbidity and mortality (Karavias *et al.* 1993).

In elective cases, resection and primary anastomosis is the procedure of choice, even if an unsuspected abscess is encountered (Weder *et al.* 1997). Myotomy is of little benefit (Cagliani and Ross 1989). Excellent long-term results are claimed in 85% of all those undergoing elective surgery and in 82% of those operated on for chronic pain (Moreau and Vows 1990). Sigmoid colectomy reduces colonic motility to normal values and effectively relieves symptoms (Cortesini *et al.* 1989). Following sigmoid colectomy, 85% of patients will remain symptom-free, while 11% will experience recurrent symptoms and 3% recurrent infection (Moreaux 1991). Completely excising the sigmoid colon reduces the likelihood of recurrent symptoms (Moreaux 1991). In a series of over 500 cases from the Mayo clinic, symptoms recurred in 12% of those undergoing limited sigmoid resection compared with 7% if the entire sigmoid colon was removed (Benn *et al.* 1986).

Progression of diverticulosis into colon proximal to the sigmoid occurs in only 15% of cases, diverticulitis developing in about one in 10 (Wolff *et al.* 1984). Therefore, if the sigmoid colon only is involved, there is little advantage in resecting more proximal bowel as the risk of subsequent recurrent diverticular disease is slight. Mortality from elective colectomy is about 2% and morbidity about 10% (Levien *et al.* 1989; Walsh *et al.* 1990).

Recently, there have reports of both uncomplicated diverticular disease and diverticular fistulas treated by laparoscopic sigmoid colectomy, but further studies are required before the value of this technique can be fully assessed (Senagore *et al.* 1993; Hewett and Stitz 1995, O'Sullivan *et al.* 1996).

In diverticular disease complicated by bleeding, segmental resection is the treatment of choice, if sigmoid diverticular disease is confidently diagnosed as the source of colonic bleeding. Otherwise subtotal colectomy should be considered, as 'blind' hemicolectomy fails in 30% of cases, with considerable morbidity and mortality. There is no advantage in preserving the caecum during subtotal colectomy, as the bleeding source may be caecal angiodysplasia, while the functional results are no different from direct ileorectal anastomosis (Fasth et al. 1983). In a study of 20 patients with massive bleeding from diverticular disease, 45% were located in the right colon (Egger et al. 1992). Over half the patients stopped bleeding after transfusion of three units of blood, but 45% required emergency surgery with a 22% mortality (Egger et al. 1992). After 5 years follow up, only 10% of the conservatively treated group had required surgery for rebleeding. Patients bleeding from the right colon or requiring a transfusion of more than six units should be considered for surgery.

Patients with fistulation may be treated conservatively in the first instance followed by elective surgery. The optimal operation for fistulation is elective resection of the offending diverticular segment with primary anastomosis and interposition of omentum between colon and bladder (Puyol et al. 1990; Grissom and Snyder 1991; Moquet et al. 1991). Complete correction of the fistula can thereby be achieved with the low morbidity and mortality associated with elective resection of diverticular disease (Karamchandani and West 1984). Excision of the thickened bladder wall is rarely necessary, although a urinary catheter should remain in place for at least 7 days postoperatively. If primary anastomosis cannot be performed, a proximal colostomy will be required. Colovaginal fistulas are treated in a manner similar to colovesical fistulas. Colocutaneous fistulas are usually secondary to previous surgery and are best treated by parenteral nutrition and staged surgical resection.

The treatment of diverticular disease complicated by perforation remains controversial, as no randomized trials have been performed. Complications secondary to perforation were formerly treated by drainage alone or defunctioning transverse colostomy, drainage and antibiotics. Patients were then placed on a high-fibre diet and admitted several months later for colostomy closure and possible colonic resection. Many now consider a transverse colostomy to be aesthetically and theoretically unattractive, being ineffective in the most severe forms of disease and unnecessary in the less severe. The mortality, morbidity, and combined hospital stay for this three-stage procedure is significant (14%, 24%, and 52 days, respectively) (Hackford et al. 1985). Several studies have now shown a significant advantage in operations involving excision, compared with defunctioning, of the affected segment. Compared with colostomy alone, primary resection is associated with a lower number of procedures per patient (1.5 versus 2.1), reduced combined hospital stay (32 days versus 50 days), and decreased wound infection (16% versus 32%) (Hackford et al. 1985; Sarin and Bouls 1991). Patients undergoing resection and exteriorization (Hartmann's procedure) also have a significantly reduced overall mortality (7%) relative to those undergoing defunctioning colostomy and drainage (26%) (Peoples et al. 1990; Khan et al. 1995). The highest mortality is from drainage alone (odds ratio 4 relative to Hartmann's procedure). In addition, faecal fistula complicates 20% of drainage procedures alone. Even in the presence of obvious perforation there is no survival advantage from transverse colostomy and drainage over resection of the affected segment. There is no evidence that simple suture closure of the perforation reduces the risk of further bacterial contamination (Krukowski et al. 1985). It is therefore recommended that Hartmann's procedure should be performed in most cases of septic complications from diverticular disease (Pain and Cahill 1991, Belmonte et al. 1996). However, in poor risk patients, the mortality from a Hartmann's procedure can rise to over 20% and morbidity

to almost 70%, while 33–50% of patients will be left with a permanent stoma (Khan et al. 1995).

A major disadvantage of Hartmann's procedure is the morbidity associated by the colostomy and its closure. Complications can be expected in up to 35% of patients having their Hartmann's procedure reversed. One study suggests that the optimum time for closure of the stoma to minimize the risk of complications is within 4 months of the original surgery.

Recently, there has been a trend to performing resection and primary anastomosis, wherever possible (Wedell et al. 1997). This was originally suggested only in the most favourable circumstances, if necessary using on table lavage (Hold et al. 1990). In some specialized centres, primary anastomosis is performed for 95% of elective cases, even in the presence of an unsuspected abscess (Moreaux and Vons 1990). In complicated diverticular disease, primary anastomosis is advocated for all cases without free perforation; in one series the proportion of patients undergoing primary anastomosis, Hartmann's procedure and transverse colostomy/drainage being 60%, 35%, and 5% (Huber et al. 1991). In such circumstances, mortality is 2% and morbidity about 20%, hospital stay being 20 days (Corder and Williams 1990; Huber et al. 1991; Medina et al. 1991). The addition of a covering colostomy to protect the primary anastomosis is of no benefit as overall morbidity actually increases to 20–40% (Hackford et al. 1985; Hold et al. 1990).

It is probable that morbidity and mortality depend less on the actual operative procedure than on associated co-morbid conditions, immune and nutritional status, severity of disease, and faecal or purulent peritonitis. With a high index of suspicion, early diagnosis, adequate resuscitation and early operation, good immediate and long-term morbidity, and mortality figures can be expected (Gravie et al. 1991; Rothenberger and Wiltz 1993). In the absence of concomitant disease, with good pre- and postoperative management and an experienced colonic surgeon primary anastomosis should be considered, even in the presence of faecal peritonitis. In other circumstances, a Hartmann's procedure should probably be performed (Elliott et al. 1997).

Right-sided diverticular disease

In the right colon, two histologically distinct types of diverticula exist. In addition to the false diverticula similar to that of the left colon, a true, congenital, and often single caecal diverticulum occurs. The entire colon is involved in 10–20% of patients from Western countries with diverticular disease, while in 5% the changes are confined to the right colon (Parks 1969; Sugihara et al. 1984). However, in Orientals 70% of diverticular disease is confined to the right colon (Segal and Leibowitz 1989; Chia et al. 1991; Nakada et al. 1995, Lo and Chu 1996).

Right-sided diverticular disease is often asymptomatic, only 3–15% of patients developing inflammation (Kubo et al. 1985; Nakada et al. 1995) (Figure 7.16). Clinical presentation is similar to that of appendicitis. However, the average age at presentation is 45 years, being older than that of appendicitis but younger than most patients with left-sided diverticulitis (Gouge et al. 1983). The history if often longer than that of appendicitis and the pain is located solely in the right iliac fossa (Lo and Chu 1996). Despite these differences, pre-operative diagnosis is of 'appendicitis' in 70% of cases, caecal diverticulitis being suspected in only 7% (Sardi

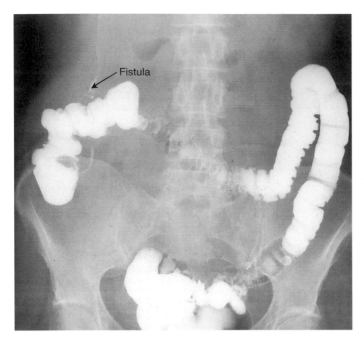

Figure 7.16 Barium enema in a patient with scattered diverticulae and a liver abscess showing a fistula into the liver (arrowed). At operation the source was found to be a diverticulum at the hepatic flexure.

et al. 1987). A faecolith is present in almost 50% of cases, while CT scanning may help in the distinction from acute appendicitis. Even at operation, the correct diagnosis is made in only 60% of patients, carcinoma being incorrectly diagnosed in about one-third of cases (Sardi *et al.* 1987). Four types of right-sided diverticular disease are described.

1. The true, congenital caecal diverticulum, which is very rare.
2. A solitary false diverticulum, the presentation of which mimics acute appendicitis and is found at operation to have an inflamed caecal mass.
3. A diverticulum resulting from defects in the muscularis propria. This accounts for 4% of right-sided diverticular disease, virtually all presenting with rectal haemorrhage. Although this is often clinically felt to represent angiodysplasia, the mean age at presentation is younger, being 30 years (Kubo *et al.* 1985). The macroscopic appearances at operation are normal.
4. Single or multiple diverticula with similar aetiology and complications as left colonic diverticular disease.

Right-sided diverticular disease runs a less aggressive course than left-sided disease, with only 0.3% of patients requiring surgery (Nakada *et al.* 1995). If caecal diverticulitis presents as a mass, conservative treatment with antibiotics is best, allowing time to investigate the differential diagnoses of appendix mass, caecal carcinoma, or Crohn's disease (Sugihara *et al.* 1984). Operative cases with purely local inflammation and a confident diagnosis may be treated by simple inversion (approximately 5% of cases) or excision of the diverticulum (30% of cases) (Sardi *et al.* 1987). Appendicectomy should also be done to avoid future diagnostic confusion. Right hemicolectomy should be performed for extensive inflammation, severe bleeding, when carcinoma cannot be confidently excluded or when closure would compromise the ileocaecal valve (Gouge *et al.* 1983; Sugihara *et al.* 1984; Sardi *et al.* 1987). The overall mortality from right-sided diverticular disease is 2% (Sardi *et al.* 1987).

Giant colonic diverticulum

This is a rare complication of colonic diverticular disease, representing a large (over 5 cm) air-filled cystic structure attached to the antimesenteric border of the colon. Adjacent diverticular disease is almost invariable, the majority of giant diverticula being located in the sigmoid colon. It is thought to arise from inflammation narrowing the neck of the diverticulum and trapping bowel gas by a ball-valve mechanism. Clinical presentation is variable, the diagnosis often being made incidentally during investigation for another purpose or of an asymptomatic abdominal mass. Occasionally, vague symptoms of fullness, abdominal pain, or diarrhoea occur, while torsion or perforation is associated with signs of peritonitis. Plain radiographs often reveal an elliptical air-filled structure in relation to the sigmoid colon. However, a communication with the bowel lumen, which is always present pathologically, is identified in only two-thirds of barium enemas. CT scan identifies the diverticulum to have a wall which is smooth on the inside and rough on the outside, varying in thickness from 0.5 to 2 cm (Figure 7). Pathologically, there is an outer coat of fibrous tissue surrounding an inner lining of chronic granulation tissue. The condition is not malignant. The presence of muscle fibres suggests a duplication cyst rather than a giant diverticulum. Other diagnoses which should be considered are sigmoid volvulus, mesenteric cysts, emphysematous cystitis, an air-filled abscess cavity, or an enterovesical fistula. As this represents a complication of diverticular disease, excision of the diverticular segment containing the giant diverticulum with primary anastomosis is usually recommended.

References

Abramson SJ, Berdon WE, Laffey K, Ruzal Shapiro C, Nash M, Baer J. Colonic diverticulitis in young patients with chronic renal failure and transplantation. *Pediatr. Radiol.* 1991; 21: 352–4.

Acosta JA, Grebenc ML, Doberneck RC, McCarthy JD, Fry DE. Colonic diverticular disease in patients 40 years old or younger. *Am. J. Surg.* 1992; 58: 605–7.

Aldoori WH, Giovannucci EL, Rimm EB, Ascherio A, Stampfer MJ, Colditz GA, *et al.* Prospective study of physical activity and the risk of symptomatic diverticular disease in men. *Gut* 1995; 36: 276–82.

Aldridge MC, Sim AJW. Colonoscopy findings in symptomatic patients without X ray evidence of colonic neoplasms. *Lancet* 1986; ii: 833–4.

Ambrosetti P, Grossholz M, Becker C, Terrier F, Morel P. Computed tomography in acute left colonic diverticulitis. *Br. J. Surg.* 1997; 84: 532–4.

Bach CD, Resnik B, Flammenbaum W, *et al.* Colovesical fistula diagnosed by an unconventional procedure. *Br. Med. J.* 1981; 283: 1154.

Bazzocchi R, Grazia M, Bini A. Diagnostic timing in complicated and uncomplicated diverticular disease. *Minerva Chir.* 1992; 47: 261–7.

Belmonte C, Klas JV, Perez JJ, Wong WD, Rothenberger DA, Goldberg SM, Madoff RD. The Hartmann procedure. First choice or last resort in diverticular disease? *Arch. Surg.* 1996; 131: 612–5.

Benn PL, Wolff BG, Ilstrup DM. Level of anastomosis and recurrent colonic diverticulitis. *Am. J. Surg.* 1986; 151: 269–71.

Berry AR, Turner WH, Mortensen NJ, Kettlewell MG. Emergency surgery for complicated diverticular disease. A five year experience. *Dis. Colon Rectum* 1989; 32: 849–54.

Bertschinger P. Diverticulosis. *Schweiz. Rundsch. Med. Prax.* 1993; 82: 487–9.

Bjarnason I, Hayllar J, MacPherson AJ, Russell AS. Side effects of non-steroidal anti inflammatory drugs on the small and large intestine in humans. *Gastroenterology* 1993; 104: 1832–47.

Bokhari M, Vernava AM, Ure T, Longo WE. Diverticular hemorrhage in the elderly—is it well tolerated? *Dis. Colon Rectum* 1996; 39: 191–5.

Boulos PB, Karamanolis DG, Salmon PR, Clark CG. Is colonoscopy necessary in diverticular disease? *Lancet* 1984; i: 95–6.

Browder W, Cerise EJ, Litwin MS. Impact of emergency angiography in massive lower gastrointestinal bleeding. *Ann. Surg.* 1986; 204: 530–6.

Burkitt DP, Clements JL Jr, Eaton SB. Prevalence of diverticular disease, hiatus hernia, and pelvic phleboliths in black and white Americans. *Lancet* 1985; ii: 880–1.

Cagliani P, Rossi R. Our experience in diverticular disease of the colon. Resection and myotomy intervention. *Minerva. Chir.* 1989; 44: 613–8.

Campbell K, Steele RJ. Non steroidal anti inflammatory drugs and complicated diverticular disease: a case control study. *Br. J. Surg.* 1991; 78: 190–1.

Canedo Acosta J, Salazar Mendoza R. Colonoscopy in hemorrhagic lesions of the colon. *Rev. Gastroenterol. Mex.* 1990; 55: 185–90.

Cheskin LJ, Bohlman M, Schuster MM. Diverticular disease in the elderly. *Gastroenterol. Clin. North Am.* 1990; 19: 391–403.

Chia JG, Wilde CC, Ngoi SS, Goh PM, Ong CL. Trends of diverticular disease of the large bowel in a newly developed country. *Dis. Colon Rectum* 1991; 34: 498–501.

Condon RE. Diverticular disease of the left colon. *Helv. Chir. Acta.* 1985; 52: 409.

Corder AP, Williams JD. Optimal operative treatment in acute septic complications of diverticular disease. *Ann. R. Coll. Surg. Engl.* 1990; 72: 82–6.

Cortesini C, Pantalone D. Usefulness of colonic motility study in identifying patients at risk for complicated diverticular disease. *Dis. Colon Rectum* 1991; 34: 339 42.

De Koster E, Mante M, Denis P, Nyst JF, Otero J, Van Geel J, et al. Juxtapapillary duodenal diverticula and diverticula of the colon: is there a general 'gastrointestinal diverticular disease'? *Acta Gastroenterol. Belg.* 1991; 54: 191–4.

De Reuck M, Nyst JF, Jonas C, De Koster E, Deltenre M. Endoscopic findings compared with clinical findings in diverticular disease of the colon. *Acta Gastroenterol. Belg.* 1990; 53: 354–8.

de Vries EH, Ginai AZ, Robben SG, Hop WC. Pelvic phleboliths: is there an association with diverticulitis? *Br. J. Radiol.* 1992; 65: 868–70.

Dolle W, Daiss W. Internistic therapy of acute diverticulitis. *Schweiz. Rundsch. Med. Prax.* 1992; 81: 861–2.

Egger B, Gertsch P, Wagner HE. Anemia inducing colonic diverticular hemorrhages. *Schweiz. Med. Wochenschr.* 1992; 122: 936–9.

Elliott T, Yego S, Irwin T. Five-year audit of the acute complications of diverticular disease. *Br. J. Surg.* 1997; 84: 534–8.

Fasth S, Hedlund H, Svaninger G, et al. Functional results after subtotal colectomy and caecortical anastomosis. *Acta Chir. Scand.* 1983; 149: 623–7.

Finkelstein JA, Jamieson CG. An association between anti inflammatory medication and internal pelvic fistulas. *Dis. Colon Rectum* 1987; 30: 168–70.

Freischlag J, Bennion RS, Thompson JE Jr. Complications of diverticular disease of the colon in young people. *Dis. Colon Rectum* 1986; 29: 639–43.

Gheissari A, Rajyaguru V, Kumashiro R, Matsumoto T. Gastrointestinal hemorrhage in end stage renal disease patients. *Int. J. Surg.* 1990; 75: 93–5.

Gore S, Shepherd NA, Wilkinson SP. Endoscopic crescentic fold disease of the sigmoid colon: the clinical and histopathological spectrum of a distinctive endoscopic appearance. *Int. J. Colorectal Dis.* 1992; 7: 76–81.

Gouge TH, Coppa CF, Eng K, et al. Management of diverticulitis of the ascending colon: 10 years' experience. *Am. J. Surg.* 1983; 145: 387.

Gravie JF, Quinaux D, Sezeur A, Gallot D, Malafosse M. Elective surgical treatment of colonic diverticulosis. *Ann. Gastroenterol. Hepatol.* 1991; 27: 65–8.

Grissom R, Snyder TE. Colovaginal fistula secondary to diverticular disease. *Dis. Colon Rectum* 1991; 34: 1043–9.

Hachigian MP, Honickman S, Eisenstat TE, Rubin RJ, Salvati EP. Computed tomography in the initial management of acute left sided diverticulitis. *Dis. Colon Rectum* 1992; 35: 1123–9.

Hackford AW, Veidenheimer MC. Diverticular disease of the colon: current concepts and management. *Surg. Clin. North Am.* 1985; 65: 347–63.

Hackford AW, Schoetz DJ Jr, Coller JA, Veidenheimer MC. Surgical management of complicated diverticulitis. The Lahey Clinic experience, 1967 to 1982. *Dis. Colon Rectum* 1985; 28: 317–21.

Haiart DC, Stevenson P, Hartley RC. Leg pain: an uncommon presentation of perforated diverticular disease. *J. R. Coll. Surg. Edinburgh* 1989; 34: 17–20.

Hewett PJ, Stitz R. The treatment of internal fistulae that complicate diverticular disease of the sigmoid colon by laparoscopically assisted colectomy. *Surg. Endosc.* 1995; 9: 411–3.

Hold M, Denck H, Bull P. Surgical management of perforating diverticular disease in Austria. *Int. J. Colorectal. Dis.* 1990; 5: 195–9.

Huber MA, Woisetschlager R, Sulzbacher H, Wayand W. Surgical therapy of complicated diverticular disease. *Zentralbl Chir.* 1991; 116: 999–1007.

Ibrarullah M, Sikora SS, Saxena R, Kapoor VK, Kackcer L, Awasthi S. Diverticular disease of colon, Indian variant. *Trop. Gastroenterol.* 1991; 12: 87–90.

Ihekwaba FN. Diverticular disease of the colon in black Africa. *J. R. Coll. Surg. Edinburgh* 1992; 37: 107–9.

Jacobs JE, Birnbaum BA. CT of inflammatory disease of the colon. *Semin. Ultrasound CT MR* 1995; 16: 91–101.

Karamchandani MC, West CF Jr. Vesicoenteric fistulas. *Am. J. Surg.* 1984; 147: 681–3.

Karavias T, Hager K, Ernst M, Dollinger U. Changes in surgery of diverticulitis. *Zentralbl. Chir.* 1993; 118: 76–80.

Katschinski M, Lederer P, Ellermann A, Ganzleben R, Lux G, Arnold R. Myoelectric and manometric patterns of human rectosigmoid colon in irritable bowel syndrome and diverticulosis. *Scand. J. Gastroenterol.* 1990; 25: 761–8.

Kelly JK. Polypoid prolapsing mucosal folds in diverticular disease. *Am. J. Surg. Pathol.* 1991; 15: 871–8.

Khan AL, Ah See AK, Crofts TJ, Heys SD, Eremin O. Surgical management of the septic complications of diverticular disease. *Ann. R. Coll. Surg Engl.* 1995; 77: 16–20.

King DW, Lubowski DZ, Armstrong AS. Sigmoid stricture at colonoscopy—an indication for surgery. *Int. J. Colorectal Dis.* 1990; 5: 161–3.

Krukowski ZH, Koruth NM, Matheson NA. Evolving practice in acute diverticulitis. *Br. J. Surg.* 1985; 72: 684–6.

Kubo A, Kagaya T, Nakagawa H. Studies on complications of diverticular disease of the colon. *Jpn. J. Med.* 1985; 24: 39–43.

Kurgansky D, Foxwell MM Jr. Pyoderma gangrenosum as a cutaneous manifestation of diverticular disease. *South Med. J.* 1993; 86: 581–4.

Lambert ME, Knox RA, Schofield PF, Hancock BD. Management of the septic complications of diverticular disease. *Br. J. Surg.* 1986; 73: 576–9.

Lanas A, Serrano P, Bajador E, Esteva F, Benito R, Sainz R. Evidence of aspirin use in both upper and lower gastrointestinal perforation. *Gastroenterol.* 1997; 112: 683–9.

Letoquart JP, Bansard JY, Kunin N, La Gamma A, Podeur L, Aussel D, et al. Surgical treatment of colonic diverticulosis: results of a series of 70 cases. *J. Chir.* 1992; 129: 345–51.

Levien DH, Mazier WP, Surrell JA, Raiman PJ. Safe resection for diverticular disease of the colon. *Dis. Colon Rectum* 1989; 32: 30–2.

Levy N, Stermer E, Simon J. The changing epidemiology of diverticular disease in Israel. *Dis. Colon Rectum* 1985; 28: 416–18.

Lo CY, Chu KW. Acute diverticulitis of the right colon. *Am. J. Surg.* 1996; 171: 244–6.

Mader TJ. Acute diverticulitis in young adults. *J. Emerg. Med.* 1994; 12: 779–82.

McCarthy DW, Bumpers HL, Hoover EL. Etiology of diverticular disease with classic illustrations. *J. Nat. Med. Assoc.* 1996; 88: 389–90.

McGuire HH Jr. **Bleeding colonic diverticula. A reappraisal of natural history and management.** *Ann. Surg.* **1994; 220: 653–6.**

McLoughlin RF, Mathieson JR, Cooperberg PL, Atkinson KG, Christensen RM, MacFarlane JK. Peritoneal abscesses due to bowel perforation: effect of extent on outcome after percutaneous drainage. *J. Vasc. Interv. Radiol.* 1995; 6: 185–9.

Medina VA, Papanicolaou GK, Tadros RR, Fielding LP. Acute perforated diverticulitis: primary resection and anastomosis? *Conn. Med.* 1991; 55: 258–61.

Metcalf JV, Smith J, Jones R, Record CO. Incidence and causes of rectal bleeding in general practice as detected by colonoscopy. *Brit. J. Gen. Pract.* 1996; 46: 161–4.

Milner P, Crowe R, Kamm MA, Lennard Jones JE, Burnstock G. Vasoactive intestinal polypeptide levels in sigmoid colon in idiopathic constipation and diverticular disease. *Gastroenterology* 1990; 99: 666–75.

Moquet PY, Letoquart JP, Pompilio M, Kunin N, La Gamma A, Mambrini A. Sigmoido-uterine fistula of diverticular origin. Review of the literature apropos of a case. *J. Chir.* 1991; 128: 419–23.

Moreaux J, Vons C. Elective resection for diverticular disease of the sigmoid colon. *Br. J. Surg.* 1990; 77: 1036–8.

Moreaux J. **Diverticular sigmoiditis: surgical treatment.** *Bull. Acad. Natl Med.* **1991; 175: 1285–91.**

Morosi C, Ballardini G, Pisani P, Bellomi M, Cozzi G, Vidale M, et al. Diagnostic accuracy of the double contrast enema for colonic polyps in patients with or without diverticular disease. *Gastrointest. Radiol.* 1991; 16: 345–7.

Morris J, Stellato TA, Lieberman J, Haaga JR. The utility of computed tomography in colonic diverticulitis. *Ann. Surg.* 1986; 204: 128–32.

Nakada I, Ubukata H, Goto Y, Watanabe Y, Sato S, Tabuchi T, et al. Diverticular disease of the colon at a regional general hospital in Japan. *Dis. Colon Rectum* 1995; 38: 755–9.

Ogunbiyi OA. Diverticular disease of the colon in Ibadan, Nigeria. *Afr. J. Med. Sci.* 1989; 18: 241–4.

O'Sullivan GC, Murphy D, O'Brien MG, Ireland A. Laparoscopic management of generalized peritonitis due to perforated colonic diverticula. *Amer. J. Surg.* 1996; 171: 432–4.

Ozick LA, Salazar CO, Donelson SS. Pathogenesis, diagnosis, and treatment of diverticular disease of the colon. *Gastroenterologist* 1994; 2: 299–310.

Pain J, Cahill J. **Surgical options for left sided large bowel emergencies.** *Ann. R. Coll. Surg. Engl.* **1991; 73: 394–6.**

Painter NS. **The cause of diverticular disease of the colon, its symptoms and its complications. Review and hypothesis.** *J. R. Coll. Surg. Edinburgh* **1985; 30: 118–22.**

Papadaki PJ, Vassiliou PM, Zavras GM, Kounis NG, Hadjioannou N, Fezoulidis IB, et al. A modified per os double contrast examination of the colon in the elderly. *Rofo. Fortschr. Geb. Rontgenstr. Neuen. Bildgeb. Verfahr.* 1993; 158: 320–4.

Papi C, Ciaco A, Koch M, Capurso L. Efficacy of rifaximin on symptoms of uncomplicated diverticular disease of the colon. A pilot multicentre open trial. Diverticular Disease Study Group. *Ital. J. Gastroenterol.* 1992; 24: 452–6.

Papi C, Ciaco A, Koch M, Capurso L. Efficacy of rifaximin in the treatment of symptomatic diverticular disease of the colon. A multicentre double blind placebo controlled trial. *Aliment. Pharmacol. Ther.* 1995; 9: 33–9.

Parks TG. Natural history of diverticular disease of the colon. A review of 521 cases. *Br. Med. J.* 1969; 4: 639–42.

Peoples JB, Vilk DR, Maguire JP, Elliott DW. Reassessment of primary resection of the perforated segment for severe colonic diverticulitis. *Am. J. Surg.* 1990; 159: 291–3.

Pillari G, Greenspan B, Vernace FM, Rosenblum G. Computed tomography of diverticulitis. *Gastrointest. Radiol.* 1984; 9: 263–8.

Puyol M, Alcaraz A, Romero JA, Vargas C, Gonzalez S, Barrera M, et al. Entero-urinary fistula. A study of 22 cases. *Arch. Esp. Urol.* 1990; 43: 457–60.

Rankin FW, Brown PW. Diverticulitis of the colon. *Surg. Gynecol. Obstet.* 1930; 50: 836–39.

Ravo B, Khan SA, Ger R, et al. Unusual extraperitoneal presentations of diverticulitis. *Am. J. Gastroenterol.* 1985; 80: 346–51.

Raymond PL, Gibler WB. Detection of colovesical fistula in the emergency department: report of a case. *Am. J. Emerg. Med.* 1989; 7: 191–5.

Rege RV, Nahrwold DL. **Diverticular disease.** *Curr. Probl. Surg.* **1989; 26: 133–89.**

Richter S, v.d. Linde J, Dominok GW. Diverticular disease. Pathology and clinical aspects based on 368 autopsy cases. Chirurgische Klinik, Krankenhauses Cottbus. *Zentralbl. Chir.* 1991; 116: 991–8.

Riddell RH, Tanaka M, Mazzoleni G. Non steroidal anti inflammatory drugs as a possible cause of collagenous colitis: a case control study. *Gut* 1992; 33: 683–6.

Roberts P, Abel M, Rosen L, Cirocco W, Fleshman J, Leff E, et al. Practice parameters for sigmoid diverticulitis. The Standards Task Force American Society of Colon and Rectal Surgeons. *Dis. Colon Rectum* 1995; 38: 125–32.

Rodkey GV, Welch CE. Changing patterns in the surgical treatment of diverticular disease. *Ann. Surg.* 1984; 200: 466–78.

Rothenberger DA, Wiltz O. **Surgery for complicated diverticulitis.** *Surg. Clin. North Am.* **1993; 73: 975–92.**

Ryan P. Two kinds of diverticular disease. *Ann. R. Coll. Surg. Engl.* 1991; 73: 73–9.

Sardi A, Gokli A, Singer JA. Diverticular disease of the cecum and ascending colon. A review of 881 cases. *Am. Surg.* 1987; 53: 41–5.

Sarin S, Boulos PB. Evaluation of current surgical management of acute inflammatory diverticular disease. *Ann. R. Coll. Surg. Engl.* 1991; 73: 278–82.

Schauer PR, Ramos R, Ghiatas AA, Sirinek KR. Virulent diverticular disease in young obese men. *Am. J. Surg.* 1992; 164: 443–6.

Scholefield JH, Wyman A, Rogers K. Management of generalized faecal peritonitis—can we do better? *J. R. Soc. Med.* 1991; 84: 664–6.

Schwerk WB, Schwarz S, Rothmund M. Sonography in acute colonic diverticulitis. A prospective study. *Dis. Colon Rectum* 1992; 35: 1077–84.

Segal I, Leibowitz B. The distributional pattern of diverticular disease. *Dis. Colon Rectum* 1989; 32: 227–9.

Senagore AJ, Luchtefeld MA, Mackeigan JM, Mazier WP. Open colectomy versus laparoscopic colectomy: are there differences? *Am. J. Surg.* 1993; 59: 549–53.

Shuler FW, Newman CN, Angood PB, Tucker JG, Lucas GW. Nonoperative management for intra-abdominal abscesses. *Amer. Surg.* 1996; 62: 218–22.

Slack WW. The anatomy, pathology and some clinical features of diverticulitis of the colon. *Br. J. Surg.* 1962; 50: 185–90.

Smits BJ, Whitehead AM, Prescott P. Lactulose in the treatment of symptomatic diverticular disease: a comparative study with high fibre diet. *Br. J. Clin. Pract.* 1990; 44: 314–8.

Stefansson T, Ekbom A, Sparen P, Pahlman L. Increased risk of left sided colon cancer in patients with diverticular disease. *Gut* 1993; 34: 499–502.

Sugihara K, Muto T, Morioka Y, et al. Diverticular disease of the colon in Japan. A review of 615 cases. *Dis. Colon Rectum* 1984; 27: 531–7.

Tancer ML, Veridiano NP. Genital fistulas secondary to diverticular disease of the colon: a review. *Obst. Gynecol. Survey* 1996; 51: 67–73.

Thompson JN, Salem RR, Hemingway AP, et al. Specialist investigation of obscure gastrointestinal bleeding. *Gut* 1987; 28: 47–51.

Thorburn HA, Carter KB, Goldberg JA, Finlay IG. Does ispaghula husk stimulate the entire colon in diverticular disease? *Gut* 1992; 33: 352–6.

Tranaeus A, Heimburger O, Granqvist S. Diverticular disease of the colon: a risk factor for peritonitis in continuous peritoneal dialysis. *Nephrol. Dial. Transplant.* 1990; 5: 141–7.

Uden P, Jiborn H, Jonsson K. Influence of selective mesenteric arteriography on the outcome of emergency surgery for massive, lower gastrointestinal hemorrhage. A 15-year experience. *Dis. Colon Rectum* 1986; 29: 561–6.

Vayre P. Surgical treatment of sigmoid diverticulitis. *J. Chir.* 1990; 127: 547–51.

Walker AR, Segal I. Effects of transition on bowel diseases in sub-Saharan Africans. *Eur. J. Gastroenterol. Hepatol.* 1997; 9: 207–10.

Walsh RM, Aranha GV, Freeark RJ. Mortality and quality of life after total abdominal colectomy. *Arch. Surg.* 1990; 125: 1564–6.

Watters DA, Smith AN. Strength of the colon wall in diverticular disease. *Br. J. Surg.* 1990; 77: 257–9.

Watters DA, Smith AN, Eastwood MA, *et al.* Mechanical properties of the colon: comparison of the features of the African and European colon *in vitro. Gut* 1985; 26: 384–92.

Wedell J, Banzhaf G, Chaoui R, Fischer R, Reichmann J. Surgical management of complicated colonic diverticulitis. *Br. J. Surg.* 1997; 84: 380–3.

Weiner HL, Rezai AR, Cooper PR. Sigmoid diverticular perforation in neurosurgical patients receiving high dose corticosteroids. *Neurosurgery* 1993; 33: 40–3.

Wess L, Eastwood MA, Wess TJ, Busuttil A, Miller A. Cross linking of collagen is increased in colonic diverticulosis. *Gut* 1995; 37: 91–4.

Whiteway J, Morson BC. Pathology of ageing—diverticular disease. *Clin. Gastroenterol.* 1985; 14: 829–46.

Wilson RG, Smith AN, Macintyre IM. Complications of diverticular disease and non steroidal anti inflammatory drugs: a prospective study. *Br. J. Surg.* 1990; 77: 1103–4.

Wilson SR, Toi A. The value of sonography in the diagnosis of acute diverticulitis of the colon. *Am. J. Roentgenol.* 1990; 154: 1199–202.

Wolff BG, Ready RL, MacCarty RL, *et al.* Influence of sigmoid resection on progression of diverticular disease of the colon. *Dis. Colon Rectum* 1984; 27: 646–7.

Zielke A, Hasse C, Nies C, Kisker O, Voss M, Sitter H, Rothmund M. Prospective evaluation of ultrasonography in acute colonic diverticulitis. *Br. J. Surg.* 1997; 84: 385–8.

8 Polypoid disease and polyposis syndromes

Colorectal polyps may be classified as neoplastic or non-neoplastic. Neoplastic polyps arise from a particular parent cell type, normally columnar epithelium, and are of tubular, villous, and tubulovillous varieties. Non-neoplastic polyps include hyperplastic (metaplastic), hamartomatous, and inflammatory lesions. About three-quarters of all colorectal polyps are adenomas, 20% are hyperplastic with 5% being inflammatory polyps (Pines *et al.* 1992; Pennazio *et al.* 1993; Vamosi-Nagy *et al.* 1993; Fucci *et al.* 1994) (Figure 8.1).

Incidence and aetiology (Table 8.1)

Autopsy studies suggest that neoplastic and hyperplastic polyps both occur in 15–25% of the population (Johannsen *et al.* 1989; Pines *et al.* 1992). Similar figures are found in those without symptoms

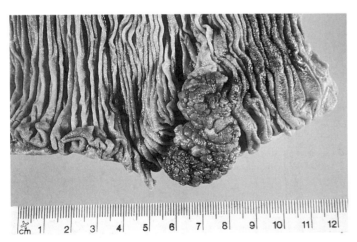

Figure 8.1 Tubulovillous adenoma of the colon.

Table 8.1 The incidence and aetiology of polyps

Polyp type	Features
Neoplastic	More common in Western countries
	Prevalence 20% of the population
	Incidence increases with age
	Over 65 years males < females
	'Left-to-right' shift in incidence in time trend studies
	Multiple in 30% of cases
	Aetiology similar to colorectal cancer
Hyperplastic	Prevalence 20% of the population
	Incidence increases with age
	Male/female ratio 4 : 1
	Aetiology: dyskinesis of the proliferative compartment

undergoing colonoscopic screening, but up to half of symptomatic patients undergoing screening will be found to have a polyp of some description (Vamosi-Nagy *et al.* 1993; Rex 1994). However, the incidence varies with geographic location and race (Offerhaus *et al.* 1991). It is estimated that 725 000 Americans harbour at least one adenomatous polyp, the overall incidence of these polyps in Western countries being about 45/100 000 for men and 30/100 000 for women (Johannsen *et al.* 1989; Koretz 1993). This incidence has remained relatively stable for men but has increased for women over the last 20 years (Johannsen *et al.* 1989; Offerhaus *et al.* 1991). The incidence of hyperplastic polyps is about 20/100 000 in males and 8/100 000 in females and is increasing in both men and women (Chatrenet *et al.* 1991).

Neoplastic polyps are single in 70% of cases, two to four polyps occurring in 25% of patients with five or more polyps being noted in 5% (Nguyen *et al.* 1991). If multiple polyps are present the risk of colon cancer is doubled. It is stated that over two-thirds of all polyps occur in the rectosigmoid region with fewer than 10% in the caecum (Pines *et al.* 1992). However, autopsy and endoscopic studies suggest that about one-third of adenomas are now located proximal to the splenic flexure (Offerhaus *et al.* 1991; Nguyen *et al.* 1991; Levi *et al.* 1993). There, therefore, appears to be a 'left to right' shift in the distribution of colorectal polyps, similar to that seen in colorectal cancer (Bondonio *et al.* 1992). One study revealed the ratio of right-sided to left-sided adenomas to have increased from 0.55 in the 1970s to 0.8 in the 1980s (Offerhaus *et al.* 1991). Another study noted the proportion of colorectal polyps situated in the ascending colon to have significantly increased from 8% to 17% over this period, with similar, but less extensive, changes in the transverse colon (8–11%) (Levi *et al.* 1993). Over this time period, the incidence of ascending colon polyps rose from 1/100 000 to 5/100 000, while there was a marked decrease in the prevalence of left-sided adenomas (12/1000 compared with 7/1000) (Offerhaus *et al.* 1991; Levi *et al.* 1993). Over 80% of these adenomas of the right colon are under 5 mm in diameter, 90% are sessile and 95% are tubular displaying no, or only slight, dysplasia. They are therefore small, rarely dysplastic and unlikely to evolve into malignancy. This shift from distal to proximal sites may be due to greater detection of multiple polyps, the incidence of which is strongly age and site-related (Johannsen *et al.* 1989; DiSario *et al.* 1991). Multiple adenomatous polyps tend to occur in the right side of the bowel, being most frequent in the transverse colon, then the ascending colon and then, in decreasing frequency, the sigmoid, descending colon, and rectum. Almost 60% of hyperplastic polyps arise in the rectum and a further 30% in left colon (Chatrenet *et al.* 1991; DiSario *et al.* 1991).

Tubular adenomas are the most common neoplastic polyps of the mucosa of the colon and rectum, accounting for 80% of adenomatous polyps and 50% of all colorectal polyps (Griffioen *et al.* 1989;

DiSario *et al.* 1991; Nguyen *et al.* 1991). They occur eight to 10 times more commonly than villous adenomas, which therefore comprise about 5–10% of all polyps.

Age and sex distribution

The prevalence of adenomatous polyps increases markedly with age. The average age at diagnosis of all polyps is about 50 years, which is 10 years earlier than that of colorectal cancer (Cajucom *et al.* 1992). Villous adenomas tend to occur in a slightly older population, with a mean age at diagnosis of 62 years. Adenomas become more prevalent with age, a screening colonoscopy study of asymptomatic elderly men revealing 40% had adenomas and 34% hyperplastic polyps (often multiple) (DiSario *et al.* 1991). As for colon cancer, the sex ratio of adenomas changes with age, from being slightly more frequent in females in those under 65 years, to a male predominance in the over-65s. The prevalence of hyperplastic polyps is also markedly age-dependent and the male to female ratio is 4:1 (Chatrenet *et al.* 1991).

Geographical and racial distribution

The incidence of colorectal polyps reflects that of colorectal cancer, being more common in countries with a Western life-style. Variations within races also exist, Ashkenazi (European-American-born) Jews having a 2.5-fold risk of colorectal polyps compared with African-Asian-born Jews (Bat *et al.* 1986). In America, the overall prevalence of adenomas in blacks is lower than in whites (Offerhaus *et al.* 1991). As with colorectal cancer, blacks have a higher prevalence of right-sided adenomas (six per 1000) than left-sided adenomas (four per 1000) (Offerhaus *et al.* 1991).

Aetiology

The environmental and genetic factors that are thought to be responsible for causing neoplastic polyps are similar to those for colorectal cancer (Cole *et al.* 1996). They are described in the aetiology of malignant colorectal conditions (see Chapter 10).

In hyperplastic polyps the underlying defect is a form of dyskinesis in which the proliferative compartment of the crypt becomes elongated and hyperplastic. Migration of cells above the proliferative zone is slowed because cells are retained longer than their normal counterparts so that the cells become excessively mature (Risio *et al.* 1995). These changes are more marked in smokers than non-smokers (Zahm *et al.* 1991).

Pathology (Table 8.2)

Macroscopic appearance

Almost three-quarters of adenomatous polyps are pedunculated, although small adenomas are typically sessile. With screening the average size of most polyps removed is now about 5 mm, with 90% measuring under 1 cm (DiSario *et al.* 1991). Villous adenomas are generally larger (average size over 2 cm) than the other types. Tubulovillous or villous adenomas comprise 70% of polyps over 1 cm, while in lesions larger than 2 cm, 60% are villous adenomas and 30% tubulovillous adenomas (Nguyen *et al.* 1991). The larger the villous adenoma the more likely it is to be in the rectum—60% of lesions larger than 4 cm occur in the rectum while only 15% of villous adenomas originate in the proximal colon.

Villous adenomas have a cauliflower appearance with frond-like projections (Figure 8.2). No appreciable extension of the muscularis mucosa into the villous process is detectable and a sparse core of delicate connective tissue is apparent. They are usually solitary, only

Table 8.2 Pathological features of colorectal polyps

Polyp type	Feature
Neoplastic polyps	80% of neoplastic polyps
Tubular	Usually < 1 cm and pedunculated
Villous and tubulovillous	20% of neoplastic polyps
	Often > 1 cm and pedunculated
	Tend to occur near rectum
	Usually solitary
	Risk of synchronous cancer—10%
	Greater malignant potential than tubular adenoma
Hyperplastic	90% under 5 mm
	90% occur in rectum and left colon
	Usually sessile
	Synchronous adenomas in 20% of cases
	May occur as giant or inverted polyps
Other types of polyp	Inflammatory myoglandular polyps
	Filiform polyposis
	Serrated adenoma

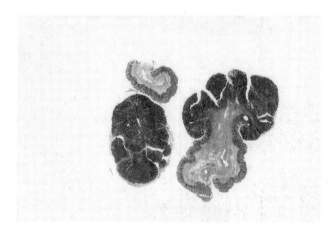

Figure 8.2 Tissue section mount of a tubulovillous adenoma in longitudinal and transverse section.

4% being multiple. Synchronous cancers occur with 10% of villous adenomas and synchronous tubular adenomas with 30%.

Hyperplastic polyps appear as small, sessile nodules arising on the mucosal folds (DiSario *et al.* 1991; Isbister *et al.* 1993) (Figure 8.3). Over 90% are less than 5 mm (average size 3 mm) and 90% are located in the left colon or rectum (Chatrenet *et al.* 1991; DiSario *et al.* 1991). Irrespective of size, pedunculated tumours are most commonly adenomas, whereas sessile tumours in the rectum and sigmoid colon are usually hyperplastic (Isbister 1993). Large hyperplastic polyps may become pedunculated and mistaken for adenomas but they usually retain the same colour as normal mucous membrane.

Microscopic appearance

In the normal colonic crypt, the proliferative compartment is restricted to the lower three-quarters of the crypt, with the majority of mitoses being found in the lower one-third. Expansion of the proliferative fraction of the crypt occurs in polyps and in the mucosa of those patients at high risk of developing colonic cancer. Large bowel adenomas appear to be derived from a single altered

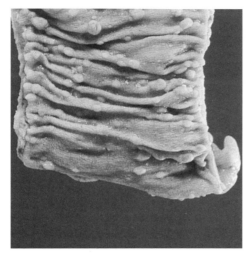

Figure 8.3 Hyperplastic polyps.

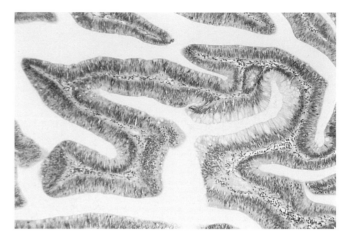

Figure 8.6 Tubulovillous adenoma showing focal low-grade dysplasia. H&E×100.

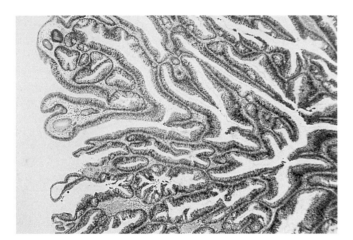

Figure 8.4 Tubulovillous adenoma of the colon. H&E×40.

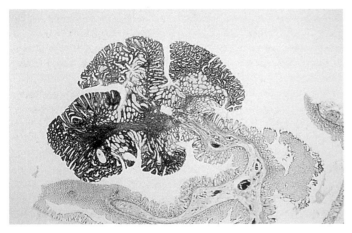

Figure 8.5 Low power view of tubulovillous adenoma of the colon. H&E×25.

large-bowel mucosa that includes an uninterrupted projection of the muscularis mucosa (Figure 8.5). Blood vessels, lymphatics, and connective tissue provide the nutrient supply and support to the head of the polyp which occupies the submucosal position and is in direct continuity with the submucosa of the contiguous bowel. Villous adenomas display slender villi with the intervillous epithelium lying directly above the muscularis mucosae. Severe dysplasia is more commonly associated with villous growth and positive mucin staining (Griffioen *et al.* 1989). Mucinous carcinomas show a significant association with villous adenomas, which is not surprising in view of their similar cytology. Tubulovillous adenomas are intermediate in terms of their architectural configuration, size and malignant potential between tubular and villous adenomas (Figure 8.6).

Hyperplastic polyps are distinguished from neoplastic polyps (adenomas) by the fact that the proliferative zone is restricted to the lower one-half of the crypt and that the individual epithelial cells differentiate as the cells migrate towards the mucosal surface—hyperplastic polyps do not progress to carcinomas (Figures 8.7). However, in one-fifth of cases they are found in association with adenomas (Chatrenet *et al.* 1991; Isbister 1993). In hyperplastic polyps, although the cells at the base of the crypt are hyperplastic, maturation and differentiation are maintained. The mucosa is thickened with enlarged vesicular cells and prominent nucleoli. Above the proliferative zone, the crypts are serrated and lined by mucin-laden

crypt cell with the progeny of that cell progressing as a clone to cancer.

Histological examination of tubular adenomas reveals closely packed epithelial tubules with little papillary infolding (Figure 8.4). The pedunculated tubular adenoma has a stalk bridged with normal

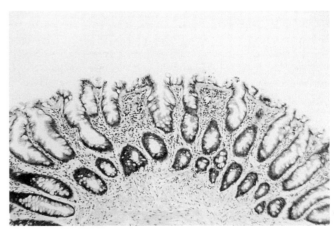

Figure 8.7 Hyperplastic polyp of the colon. H&E×100.

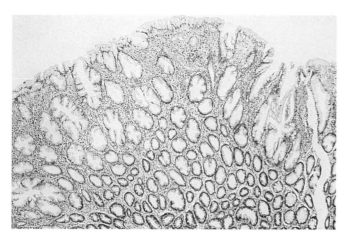

Figure 8.8 Large hyperplastic polyp of the colon. There is no evidence of dysplasia H&E×100.

columnar cells. Multiple large hyperplastic polyps (>1 cm) occasionally occur and may be distinct from the more common diminutive polyps (Warner 1994; Tsai and Lu 1995; Weston and Campbell 1995) (Figure 8.8). About 20 cases of diffuse hyperplastic polyposis of the colon have been reported, with a slightly increased risk of colorectal cancer (Kusunoki *et al*. 1991). Inverted hyperplastic polyps are an unusual but distinctive polyp of the proximal colon which may be multiple and share the phenotypic changes of regular hyperplastic polyps. The pathogenesis of this epithelial inversion probably relates to misplacement of epithelium through anatomical defects in the muscularis mucosae due to mechanical forces. The polyps may mimic both adenomas and carcinomas but the neoplastic potential of inverted hyperplastic polyposis is likely to be very low (Shepherd 1993). The number of argyrophilic nucleolar organizer regions (AgNORs) per cell is claimed to distinguish hyperplastic polyps from adenomas with high-grade dysplasia and from all the adenocarcinomas. (Bufo *et al*. 1992).

A small numbers of polyps cannot be classified into the above categories. Inflammatory myoglandular polyps are distinct clinico-pathologically from other types of colorectal polyps (Nakamura *et al*. 1992). They are believed to be caused by chronic trauma from the faecal stream and peristalsis of the bowel. Endoscopic examination reveals solitary pedunculated, red polyps with a smooth surface. They are found especially in the sigmoid colon and occasionally distal rectum (Nakamura *et al*. 1992; Gomez-Navarro *et al*. 1994). Histologically, the characteristic features are inflammatory granulation tissue in the lamina propria mucosae, proliferation of smooth muscle, and hyperplastic glands with occasional cystic dilatation (Nakamura *et al*. 1992; Gomez Navarro *et al*. 1994). They can be differentiated from juvenile and inflammatory polyps by the presence of abundant smooth-muscle cells in the inflamed lamina propria mucosae. Their locations and macroscopic appearance distinguish these polyps from mucosal prolapse syndrome and polyps developed after colostomy and from inflammatory polyps, in that they lack a fibrin cap (Nakamura *et al*. 1992; Gomez Navarro *et al*. 1994).

Filiform polyposis is a rare condition which is usually found in association with chronic inflammatory bowel disease (Rozenbajgier *et al*. 1992) (see Chapter 1, Figure 1.14). The condition is characterized by the presence of numerous, densely packed, filiform polyps in the colon, which may resemble villous adenomas on endoscopy. Microscopy reveals inflammatory pseudopolyps covered by largely normal and non-dysplastic colonic epithelium. The condition

alone is not an indication for bowel resection but complications, such as massive haemorrhage or intestinal obstruction from the underlying inflammatory bowel disease, may necessitate surgical intervention (Rozenbajgier *et al*. 1992). Giant inflammatory polyps may also be associated with idiopathic inflammatory bowel disease. They may produce intestinal obstruction or intestinal bleeding, requiring endoscopic polypectomy or surgery. Electron microscopy shows fibroblasts, myofibroblasts, mast cells, lymphocytes, collagen fibres, capillaries, and venules. They may have an important role in the excessive granulation, angiogenesis, and fibrotic process in giant inflammatory polyps (Balazs 1990).

The serrated adenoma is a rare but distinct entity described in recent years (Balazs *et al*. 1994). Although the tumours contain hyperplastic and adenomatous areas, the tendency for malignant transformation is similar to that of pure adenomas (Balazs *et al*. 1994). Inflammatory fibroid polyps are uncommon lesions that may occur throughout the gastrointestinal tract and may present with intestinal blood loss (Harned *et al*. 1992). Most appear as large, intramural masses at radiological examination. Some are pedunculated and all are solitary (Harned *et al*. 1992). The lesions originate in the submucosa and are composed of fibroblasts, inflammatory cells, and a network of blood vessels.

Dysplasia and malignant transformation

The risk of colorectal carcinoma in patients with adenomatous polyps is between three and six times that of the general population (Meagher and Stuart 1994). However, the risk of malignancy in a given individual is relatively small; over 85% of those with adenomas are unlikely to develop malignancy within their lifetime. The risk of malignant transformation is related to the degree of cellular atypia, 5–10% of polyps showing evidence of severe dysplasia, carcinoma *in situ*, or invasive carcinoma (Pennazio *et al*. 1993; Matsumoto *et al*. 1994; Shiri *et al*. 1994). Adenoma size and the extent of the villous component are major independent polyp risk factors associated with high-grade dysplasia and malignancy. Relative to small adenomas, medium-sized adenomas are three times and large adenomas, eight times, more likely to display high-grade dysplasia, while the risk for villous adenomas is between three and 11 times that of tubular adenomas (O'Brien *et al*. 1990). The number of adenomas affects the risk for high-grade dysplasia, patients with five or more adenomas showing a high risk (15%) of having colon cancer that is particularly prone to arise from the right side of the colon (O'Brien 1990; Schuman *et al*. 1990).

In mild dysplasia both goblet cells and columnar cells are recognized. Nuclei are slightly enlarged and crowded with numerous mitoses (Figure 8.9). With loss of differentiation these cell types are replaced by a single population of immature columnar cells secreting little mucus. As dysplasia increases, the nuclei enlarge, becoming elongated, hyperchromic and pseudo-stratified. In severe or high-grade dysplasia, nucleoli are prominent, there is architectural branching and a haphazard arrangement of endocrine and Paneth cells. Moderate to high-grade dysplasia occurs in one-third of adenomas and is significantly associated with larger size and villous architecture (8% of villous adenomas have high-grade dysplasia) (DiSario *et al*. 1991; Nguyen *et al*. 1991). Observer variation studies indicate a high level of agreement between pathologists in distinguishing hyperplastic from adenomatous polyps (Demers *et al*. 1990). However, assessment of the degree of dysplasia, particularly between moderate or severe atypia, is poor (Demers *et al*. 1990).

The adenomatous epithelium is superficial to the muscularis mucosa in all tubular adenomas, invasion of the muscularis being a

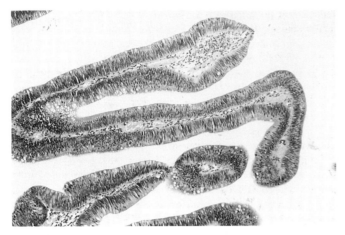

Figure 8.9 Tubulovillous adenoma showing low-grade dysplasia. H&E×100.

feature of malignancy. The incidence of malignant transformation in colorectal polyps varies with the indication for colonoscopy. It is about 1% for screening of asymptomatic patients but up to 15% for polyps removed from symptomatic individuals (Vamosi-Nagy *et al.* 1993). The risk of malignancy is closely related to polyp size and type. Almost half of villous adenomas over 2 cm are malignant compared with 5% of smaller lesions. This represents a 10-fold increased risk of malignancy over tubular adenomas. The risk of carcinoma in tubular adenomas under 1 cm is 1%, 1–2 cm 10%, and over 2 cm 34% (Muto *et al.* 1975). The corresponding figures for tubulovillous adenomas are 4%, 7%, and 45%, while those for villous adenomas are 9%, 10%, and 53% (Muto *et al.* 1975) (Table 8.3). However, tumours are occasionally reported in polyps under 5 mm in size (Cosgrove *et al.* 1991). Sessile polyps, especially if found in the rectum or sigmoid, have a higher incidence (20%) of cancer than the more common polypoid lesions (7%) (Matsumoto *et al.* 1994). Although the risk of malignancy in any given polyp is independent of the number of polyps present, the cumulative risk of malignancy is proportional to the total number of polyps, so that in patients with more than eight polyps, the risk is over 10%

Table 8.3 The risk of malignant transformation (%) related to polyp type and size

Polyp type	< 1 cm	1–2 cm	> 2 cm
Tubular	1	10	34
Tubulovillous	4	7	45
Villous	9	10	53

Taken from Muto *et al.* (1975)

Table 8.4 The risk of further adenomas and cancer (%) related to time

	Adenoma			Carcinoma		
Years of observation	5	10	15	5	10	15
Single adenomas	14%	33%	50%	1%	2%	5%
Multiple adenomas	33%	67%	80%	7%	12%	12%

(Ottenjann and Wormann 1985). Studies of polyps which have not been removed suggest that the incidence of malignancy increases with time, the cumulative risk of cancer in polyps greater than 1 cm at 5, 10, and 20 years being 2.5%, 8%, and 24% respectively (Stryker *et al.* 1987). This relationship with time is also related to the number of polyps present (Table 8.4).

Several pathological techniques have been investigated to identify polyps which are likely to undergo malignant transformation. In one study severe dysplasia in the index adenoma was significantly but weakly associated with size (>1 cm), peduncular shape and villous architecture on univariate, but only villous architecture on multivariate analysis (Chapuis *et al.* 1993). This suggests that it is unlikely that strong predictors of a patient developing a metachronous adenoma or colorectal cancer can be identified on the basis of an index adenoma found at initial colonoscopy. (Chapuis *et al.* 1993). Almost half of colorectal polyps will stain positive for CEA or CA19-9, but this is not related to either the degree of dysplasia or risk of malignancy (Afdhal *et al.* 1987). Similarly, although a high c-*myc* protein or p53 tissue level correlates with dysplasia, immunohistochemical staining is of little benefit in predicting malignant transformation (Allen *et al.* 1987; Imaseki *et al.* 1989; Pavelic *et al.* 1992; Darmon *et al.* 1994). DNA aneuploidy is found in 15–35% of adenomatous polyps and is also generally unhelpful in identifying patients with polyps at high risk of developing cancer (Sciallero *et al.* 1988). Neither is DNA ploidy useful in predicting the development of a metachronous adenoma (Griffioen *et al.* 1992). Morphometric image analysis is also of little benefit in determining dysplasia and malignant potential within adenomatous polyps (Tsuno *et al.* 1993; Meijer *et al.* 1994).

In polyps that are malignant, an adequate margin is the most important factor in predicting the prognosis of endoscopically resected colorectal adenomas containing well-differentiated adenocarcinomas (Cunningham *et al.* 1994). In a study of well-differentiated adenocarcinomas arising in polyps that were thought to be completely excised endoscopically, the only factor that had an adverse effect on outcome was the distance of the cancer to the cautery mark (<1 mm). Although rectal location was associated with the residual cancer, poor prognosis could have been predicted by the inadequate margins. Venous and/or lymphatic invasion occurs in 15% of malignant polyps, with a significant association with recurrent or Dukes' C carcinoma in polyps otherwise regarded as completely excised (Muller *et al.* 1989). A combination of haematoxylin and eosin and elastic van Gieson stains will usually identify the presence of vascular invasion (Muller *et al.* 1989).

Hyperplastic polyps

Hyperplastic colonic polyps are generally regarded as being of little clinical significance. There is no firm evidence that they progress to dysplasia or neoplasia and any association was felt to be coincidental in conditions that are progressively common with age (Marshall 1992). However, several case reports and a clustering phenomenon suggest that they may arise in abnormal colonic mucosa that is predisposed to develop neoplastic lesions (Isbister 1993; Warner 1994).

Clinical presentation of adenomatous polyps

Most patients with colorectal polyps are asymptomatic. Rectal bleeding is the most important symptom and is relatively more common in villous adenomas. In occult bleeding, tumour size correlates with the presence of faecal occult bloods (Uno and Munakata 1995). However, neither the frequency nor duration of bleeding or the total blood loss correlate with polyp size. Villous adenomas may produce

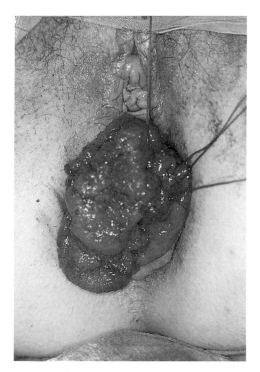

Figure 8.10 Large rectal polyp prolapsing through the anus (see colour plates).

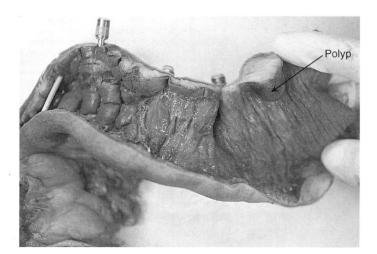

Figure 8.11 Polyp (arrowed) causing an ileocolic intussusception with infarction of the colon.

a mucous discharge. Occasionally, this may take the form of a profuse mucous diarrhoea, with water and electrolyte depletion resulting in a hypokalaemic, hypochloraemic metabolic acidosis, and circulatory collapse. Large polyps in the rectum may produce tenesmus and prolapse through the rectum (Figure 8.10). Adenomas in the colon may give rise to colicky central abdominal pain from intussusception (Figure 8.11). A large pedunculated polyp arising proximal to the dentate line may prolapse through the anus and be mistaken for a prolapsed haemorrhoid. Despite original suggestions, there is no evidence that skin tags are associated with a higher than usual risk of colonic polyps (Brendler *et al.* 1989; Ochsendorf *et al.* 1990). In one study age was a more important predictor of colorectal polyps than symptoms or history (Steine *et al.* 1994). Significant

predictors of polyps were age 40–79 years (odds ratio 2.5–5.0) and rectal bleeding (odds ratio 1.8).

Diagnosis of adenomatous polyps

The majority of cases, being asymptomatic, are identified coincidentally on sigmoidoscopy, colonoscopy, or barium enema. Investigation of the entire colon is necessary as 40% of those with colorectal polyps will have synchronous polyps elsewhere in the colon (Griffioen *et al.* 1989) (Figure 8.12). Colonoscopy is the most sensitive investigation for detecting colorectal polyps, not only detecting all small polyps found on flexible sigmoidoscopy but also identifying several other polyps missed by the sigmoidoscopy (Norfleet and Mitchell 1993). It is also reproducible, interobserver agreement being almost 100% for lesions over 1 cm and 85% for lesions smaller than this (Hixson *et al.* 1994). There is a good correlation between colonoscopic appearances and histological findings, the sensitivity of colonoscopy in assessing pathological type being 92% and specificity 72% (Kilche *et al.* 1994). As villous elements become more prominent in the histology, finely granular and/or villous surface patterns, adherent mucus, and a characteristic colour (slightly reddish with white spots) becomes more frequent endoscopically (Iida *et al.* 1990). Endoscopy using the sprayed dye technique is useful for visualizing the finely granular and/or villous surface pattern, while endoscopic ultrasound has been used to decrease the risk of haemorrhage or perforation before resection of large polyps (Iida *et al.* 1990; Souquet *et al.* 1993). An endoscope compatible, optical fibre system that produces laser-induced fluorescence spectra is claimed to differentiate adenomas correctly from normal colonic mucosa and hyperplastic polyps, with a sensitivity of 100% and specificity of 97% (Cothren *et al.* 1990; Romer *et al.* 1995). Five per cent of adenomas are pale and can be mistaken for hyperplastic polyps (Kilche *et al.* 1994). Histologically, they show mucus hypersecretion and low-grade dysplasia (Kilche *et al.* 1994).

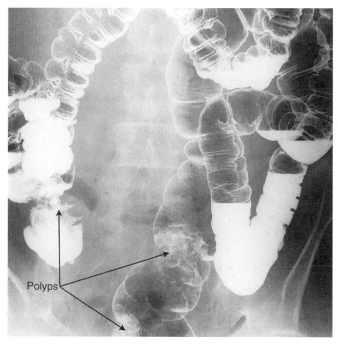

Figure 8.12 Double contrast barium enema showing synchronous villous adenomas in the rectum, sigmoid colon and caecum (arrowed). The mucus covering an adenoma prevents barium from coating the polyp, so aiding identification.

technique for colorectal polyps is 66–71% and 32–41%, respectively (Okada *et al.* 1994). CT colography is claimed to be accurate at detecting polyps over 5 mm diameter (Hara *et al.* 1996).

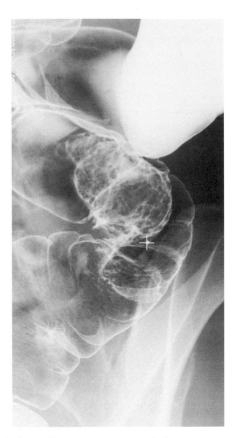

Figure 8.13 Large villous adenoma seen on barium enema examination.

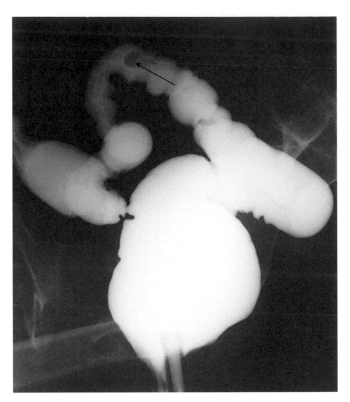

(a)

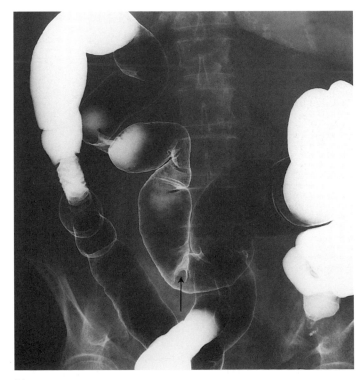

(b)

Figure 8.14 Polyps seen more readily on single contrast (a) than on double contrast barium enema (b). This is unusual—the double contrast study normally gives better mucosal detail.

Relative to colonoscopy the sensitivity of barium enema is 70% (Griffioen *et al.* 1989) (Figure 8.13). Double contrast barium enema has a sensitivity approaching 100% for the detection of polyps over 1 cm in diameter and 80% in those 6–9 mm in size, but is less sensitive (55%) in detecting polyps 4–5 mm and 2–3 mm (20%) in size (Rex *et al.* 1992) (Figure 8.14a,b). Factors contributing to false-negative interpretation on barium enema are the presence of air bubbles, overlap of bowel loops, and luminal faecal debris. In addition there is substantial inaccuracy in the measurement of colonic polyps on barium enema examination, with a 15–30% variation in the cross-sectional anatomical size (Ott *et al.* 1989) (Figure 8.15). However, barium enema is more sensitive than colonoscopy in detecting polyps in patients with diverticular disease (Figure 8.16). In severe diverticulosis (over 15 diverticula) barium enema detects one in four polyps found by sigmoidoscopy, compared with 70% in mild diverticulosis (Stefansson *et al.* 1994). The bowler-hat and carpenter's signs can distinguish colonic polyps from diverticula. If the bowler hat points toward the centre of the long axis of the bowel, it represents an intraluminal structure (i.e. a polyp). If, however, it points away from the centre of the long axis of the bowel, it represents an extraluminal structure (i.e. a diverticulum). At radiography, hyperplastic polyps classically appear as smooth, sessile elevations less than 5 mm in diameter. The radiological criteria for an atypical hyperplastic polyp at double-contrast barium enema examination include size greater than 5 mm, lobulation, and/or pedunculation. However, in one study half of hyperplastic polyps fitted the criteria for being atypical, the average size being 7 mm (Levine *et al.* 1990). The combination of double contrast barium enema and CT scanning is reproducible and reduces the radiation dose by 50%. Relative to colonoscopy, the sensitivity and positive predictive value of this

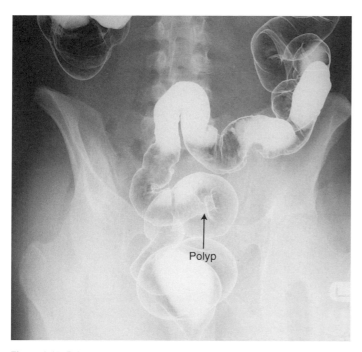

Figure 8.15 Polyp in the sigmoid colon (arrowed) that was initially not recognized on barium enema examination. The patient had a Dukes' C tumour excised from this site 1 year later.

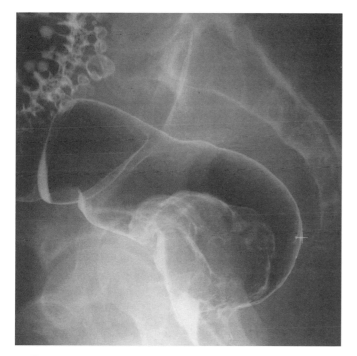

Figure 8.16 Large rectal polyp in association with diverticular disease.

Treatment

As the risk factors for adenomatous polyps are similar to those for colorectal cancer, it is hoped that prevention of colorectal polyps, and hence colorectal cancer, may be possible with dietary intervention (Greenberg *et al.* 1994; Nelson 1994). However, any appreciable effect of such trials will take many years to become apparent. In the meantime it is agreed that the best method of reducing the

risk of malignant transformation is to remove all colorectal polyps. Using the recommendations of the American Cancer Society (serial endoscopies a year apart) the incidence of adenomatous polyps is 10% for the first examination, 5% for the second, and 2% for the third (Riff 1990). The National Polyp Study found a significant reduction in the number of cancers subsequently detected in patients undergoing polypectomy relative to both adenoma-bearing and average-risk reference groups (Winawer *et al.* 1993).

Colonoscopic polypectomy reduces the risk of colorectal cancer by 70% and colorectal cancer death by 60% (Jorgensen *et al.* 1993; Meagher and Stuart 1994; Muller and Sonnenberg 1995) (Figure 8.17). In the National Polyp Study, five asymptomatic early-stage colorectal cancers were detected by follow-up colonoscopy (three at 3 years, one at 6 years, and one at 7 years) in over 1400 patients followed for 5–9 years after polypectomy (Winawer *et al.* 1993). No symptomatic cancers were detected. This represented a reduction in the incidence of colorectal cancer of 90% over those who did not have polyps removed and 75% over the general population (Winawer *et al.* 1993). Following polypectomy, most rectal cancers develop in patients whose adenomas have been inadequately removed; the risk being very low after complete removal (Atkin *et al.* 1992). The risk of subsequent colon cancer depends on the histological type, size, and number of adenomas in the rectosigmoid. In one study, cancer developed in 3.5% of those who had a rectosigmoid adenoma that was tubulovillous, villous, or greater than 1 cm (Atkin *et al.* 1992). In contrast, colorectal cancers developed in only 0.5% of those with small tubular adenomas (whether single or multiple) (Atkin *et al.* 1992). If not removed, polyps less than 5 mm grow at a rate of 1–2 mm over 2 years (Hoff *et al.* 1986).

It is accepted that an adenomatous polyp found during proctosigmoidoscopy warrants total colonoscopy with polypectomy, because of a 40% chance of a synchronous adenoma or cancer (Marshall 1992; Opelka *et al.* 1992). However, it is unclear whether this policy should apply to hyperplastic polyps (Fraser and Niv 1993; Warner 1994). Some reports suggest that the finding of a hyperplastic polyp on sigmoidoscopy is associated with adenomas in the more proximal colon in between one-third and one-half of cases (Ansher *et al.* 1989; Foutch *et al.* 1991; Opelka *et al.* 1992; Isbister 1993; Arrigoni *et al.* 1995). In one study, proximal neoplasms were found in 10% of those with no distal polyps, 33% of those with only small distal and 60% of those with at least one polyp >5 mm

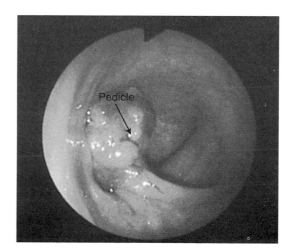

Figure 8.17 Pedunculated polyp highly amenable to total excision via colonoscopic polypectomy.

in diameter (Pennazio *et al.* 1993). The proximal neoplasm percentage was the same in patients with at least one adenomatous small polyp and those with only hyperplastic small polyps so that the authors felt that total colonoscopy is justified in all patients with distal polyps, regardless of their size and histotype (Pennazio *et al.* 1993; Read *et al.* 1997). However, other studies indicate that distal hyperplastic polyps are not strong predictors of the risk of proximal adenomas (Achord 1991; Rex *et al.* 1992; Fraser and Niv 1993; Rex 1994; Warner 1994). It is, however, suggested that small polyps seen during sigmoidoscopy should always be biopsied to determine their type, as small adenomas and hyperplastic polyps are often endoscopically indistinguishable, (DiSario *et al.* 1991; Marshall 1992; Fraser and Niv 1993). Follow-up of patients with hyperplastic polyps may also be indicated as there is an association with metachronous adenomatous polyps and colorectal cancer (Isbister 1993, Warner 1994).

Follow-up (Table 8.5)

Patients who have had adenomatous polyps are at increased risk of developing further polyps or colorectal cancer and so should undergo follow-up colonoscopy. The risk of further polyps is 25% at 2 years, while the incidence of metachronous carcinoma in those who have had a polyp excised is 6%, an incidence rate of 4.6 per 1000 person-years of follow-up (Lofti *et al.* 1986; Griffioen *et al.* 1989). Risk factors for developing further polyps include polyp size, male sex, the presence of multiple lesions at the initial examination and a recurrent polyp at previous colonoscopy (Hofstad *et al.* 1994). The overall recurrence rate is 70% in patients with multiple polyps compared with 50% in those with a single polyp. Approximately one-half of patients with multiple polyps, particularly older males, will demonstrate further neoplastic polyps within 2 years (Hixson *et al.* 1994). In one-third to one-half of cases, these appear to be new lesions developing *de novo* at a site different from the index polyp and are unlikely to have been missed at the initial colonoscopy (Hixson *et al.* 1994). Patients with atypia in initial polyps develop new polyps after a mean time of 12 months compared with 24 months in patients without atypia. In one study the mean time from a colon with no polyps to the diagnosis of a new adenomatous polyp less than 5 mm in size was 12 months, compared with 20 months for the development of polyps over 5 mm (Nava *et al.* 1987).

Patients with large colorectal polyps (more than 1 cm in diameter) should be closely followed up after treatment of the initial polyp, regardless of the site, or histological type, the age or sex of the patient, or the type of initial treatment (excision or fulguration) (Lofti *et al.* 1986). Follow-up not only reduces the risk of subsequent colorectal cancer to that of the general population but appears to reduce the incidence of colorectal cancer deaths to below that of the normal population (Jorgensen *et al.* 1993). There is considerable debate concerning the optimum follow-up regimen. Most agree that follow-up colonoscopic examinations are particularly warranted in patients with tubulovillous, villous, or large adenomas in the rectosigmoid, particularly if the adenomas are also multiple (Atkin *et al.* 1992). Some feel that patients with a single, small tubular adenoma which is only mildly dysplastic may not require regular surveillance as the risk of cancer is very low.(Atkin *et al.* 1992; Koretz 1996).

If the initial colonoscopy does not identify any adenomas, no further follow-up is required. If more than two adenomas are found, repeat colonoscopy should be performed 1 year later as endoscopists may overlook 10% of small polyps at first colonoscopy (Beck *et al.* 1995). Some suggest that if the only risk factor was a single small tubular adenoma, techniques less costly and less invasive than colonoscopy should be employed for follow-up (Grossman *et al.* 1989). In one study those with a single tubular adenoma less than 10 mm and who had no first-degree relatives with colorectal cancer had only a 3% prevalence of advanced colonic neoplasms (tubular adenomas greater than or equal to 10 mm in diameter; tubulovillous, villous, or severely dysplastic adenomas; or invasive cancers) found on colonoscopy; no greater than would be expected in the general population (Grossman *et al.* 1989). However, if the adenoma was over 2 cm in size, was incompletely excised or revealed either severe dysplasia or carcinoma *in situ*, then colonoscopy should be performed 3–6 monthly for 1 year. The management of patients with invasive carcinoma removed by colonoscopic polypectomy remains controversial. Subsequent surgery is indicated when the removed invasive carcinoma shows at least one of the following findings: (i) carcinoma near the surgical margin; (ii) vessel invasion; (iii) extensive invasion; and (iv) poorly differentiated adenocarcinoma (Sugihara *et al.* 1989). Once repeat colonoscopy has identified a 'clean colon' further colonoscopy can be performed 2 yearly if multiple polyps were present initially and 4 yearly in the presence of a single polyp (Leicester 1993; Beck *et al.* 1995). Follow-up beyond this time depends on the age of the patient. In those over 70 years, further examination should only be performed in those who are likely to survive into their eighth decade (Winawer *et al.* 1993; Achord 1994; Reinus 1994).

Table 8.5 Metachronous formation of adenomatous polyps	
Depends on:	Polyp size Multiple polyps Recurrence after previous polypectomy Male sex
Risk of metachronous polyp	25% at 2 years 50% lifetime risk if single polyp 70% lifetime risk if multiple polyps
FOLLOW UP POLICY	
Adenoma < 1 cm	Repeat colonoscopy in 12 months
Adenoma > 2 cm	Repeat colonoscopy in 6 months
Colon clear but previous polyps	Repeat colonoscopy in 2 years if multiple polyps Repeat colonoscopy in 4 years if single polyp
Age over 70 years	No follow up

Hamartomatous polyps (Table 8.6)

These represent non-neoplastic epithelial polyps composed of tissues indigenous to the site of origin but arranged in a haphazard manner. Its growth is linked to that of the surrounding tissue and normally stops after puberty. There is no malignant potential.

Juvenile (mucus retention) polyps

Over 300 cases of juvenile polyposis have been reported (Desai *et al.* 1995). In 20–50% of the cases, juvenile polyposis occurs as a familial condition (Hofting *et al.* 1993; Sharma *et al.* 1995). They

Table 8.6 Syndromes associated with hamartomatous polyps

Syndrome	Location	Associated features
Juvenile polyposis	Colon, small bowel, stomach	Family history in 20–50% Colon cancer in some families Hamartomatous ± adenomatous component Usually single 90% within 20 cm of the anus Possibly pre-malignant
Peutz–Jeghers'	Small intestine (75%) stomach (25%) colon (30%)	Autosomal dominant Hamartomas with bands of smooth muscle in lamina propria Pigmented lesions of mouth, hands and feet Ovarian and sex cord tumours (5% of females) Hepatobiliary, breast and lung cancers
Neurofibromatosis	Stomach, small intestine	Generalized neurofibromatosis
Cowden's syndrome	Stomach, colon, skin	Autosomal dominant Tricholemmomas and papillomas in 80% Breast, ovarian, and thyroid cancer Multiple other hamartomas and lipomas/neuromas
Basal cell naevus syndrome	Colon	Multiple basal cell carcinomas

normally arise in children under 10 years old (median age 5 years) but may occasionally develop in adults (Latt *et al*. 1993). They are rarely seen in the first year of life. The sex incidence is equal. In up to two-thirds of cases, the polyp is single, most of the remaining cases having fewer than 10 polyps (Latt *et al*. 1993; Muthuphei 1994).

Pathologically, the underlying polyps are of the hamartomatous type, but it is known that juvenile polyps may contain adenomatous tissue, or may be accompanied by adenomas. They are 1–2 cm in diameter with a smooth surface, spherical head, narrow stalk, and a coarsely lobulated appearance. They have a bright red surface interspersed with patches of cysts filled with mucin. Three-quarters are slightly pedunculated. Microscopically there are dilated cystic spaces lined with normal colonic epithelium, which is often ulcerated, embedded in an excess of lamina propria containing inflammatory cells (Figure 8.18). Their hamartomatous origin is suggested by the predominance of lamina propria over the glandular component. They are composed of essentially normal tissues that are abnormally arranged and may have superimposed infection, ulceration, or infarction that modifies the histological picture.

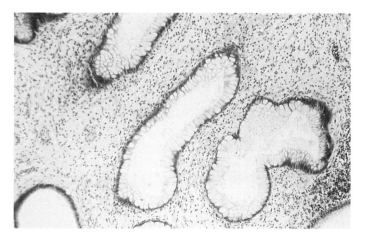

Figure 8.18 Juvenile polyp. Distended glands without dysplasia in stroma containing large numbers of eosinophils. H&E×100.

Clinically, about 90% arise within 20 cm of the anus, the remainder being evenly distributed throughout the colon so that total colonoscopy is advisable (Latt *et al*. 1993). Juvenile polyps may also develop in the stomach, duodenum, jejunum, or ileum (Hofting *et al*. 1993). Extra-intestinal anomalies are found in approximately 11% of patients (Hofting *et al*. 1993). A particular clinical feature is anaemia caused by chronic gastrointestinal bleeding and massive diarrhoea which may become life-threatening (Hofting *et al*. 1993). Prolapse through the anus is also common, while torsion, possibly with auto-amputation, occurs in 10% (Latt *et al*. 1993). Intussusception with intestinal obstruction is rare. Polyps in the rectum can be removed trans-anally or via a sigmoidoscopic snare. More proximal polyps can be removed colonoscopically. Recurrence may occur in up to 10% of cases.

Traditionally, juvenile polyps have been considered a benign, self-limiting process which resolves with age. The dictum that these polyps were usually solitary, were found predominantly in the rectosigmoid area, and were without malignant potential has been reconsidered in recent years with the increased use of colonoscopy (Heiss *et al*. 1993). There are now several case reports in both adults and children documenting the presence of adenomatous changes in this syndrome (Heiss *et al*. 1993). A reported malignant transformation rate of almost 20% justifies their classification as a precancerous condition, and has both therapeutic and, in particular, prophylactic consequences (Hofting *et al*. 1993). A more aggressive approach to patients found to have multiple juvenile polyps on barium enema, including colonoscopic biopsies at several sites to determine the presence of adenomatous changes, with colectomy and endorectal pull-through has therefore been advocated (Heiss *et al*. 1993; Hofting *et al*. 1993).

Cowden's disease

This is an autosomal dominant condition associated with multiple hamartomas affecting the skin and mucous membranes (Hizawa *et al*. 1994). It is probably a variant of juvenile polyposis. One-third of patients harbour gastrointestinal hamartomas anywhere from the oesophagus to the rectum. Multiple colonic polyps 1–4 mm in diameter with a rectosigmoid distribution and a hamartomatous microscopical appearance is characteristic. Facial papules (trichil-emmomas) and oral papillomas occur in over 80% of patients. Other extra-intestinal lesions include keratosis, lipomas, haemangiomas, neuromas, and lesions of the breast, ovary, and thyroid. There is no convincing evidence that colorectal cancer develops but patients may acquire breast or thyroid tumours (Visvanathan *et al.* 1992). Microscopical examination shows distinctive hamartomatous lesions characterized by disorganization and proliferation of the muscularis mucosae with minimally abnormal overlying mucosa (Hizawa *et al.* 1994).

Juvenile polyposis syndromes

These are rare conditions of infancy and early childhood (average age 7 years). They comprise of three clinical conditions: juvenile polyposis of infancy, familial juvenile polyposis coli, and generalized gastrointestinal polyposis. The principal presentations are haemorrhage, anaemia, hypoproteinaemia, and failure to thrive. Overall, associated congenital abnormalities (malrotation, cardiac defects, undescended testes, maldevelopment of the skull, and Meckel's diverticulum) occur in 30% of cases, being more common in the familial variant. Polyps may arise throughout the gastrointestinal tract but are principally located in the colon and rectum. They may therefore present with upper or lower intestinal haemorrhage obstruction or intussusception. In the familial variant, two-thirds of patients have a family history of colorectal cancer and 10% will develop colorectal cancer themselves. The development of cancer is probably related to adenomatous epithelium arising within the polyp. Consequently, careful screening is necessary for those with a strong family history of colon cancer.

Peutz–Jeghers' syndrome

The inheritance of this condition is autosomal dominant with variable penetrance. Sporadic mutation is not infrequent. It consists of gastrointestinal polyposis associated with mucocutaneous melanin pigmentation of the mouth, pharynx, lips, palms, soles, genitalia and

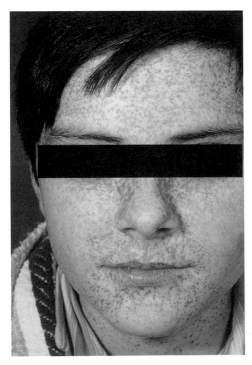

Figure 8.19 Facial pigmentation in Peutz–Jegher syndrome.

perineum (Buck *et al.* 1992; De Facq *et al.* 1995). All but the buccal freckles tend to fade after puberty while cutaneous pigmentation may not develop until after the polyps have formed (Figure 8.19). Careful examination of the buccal mucosa is therefore important in identifying those likely to develop this condition. Hamartomatous polyps, occurring in the small bowel (75%), colon (30%), and stomach (25%), are uniformly distributed throughout the affected segments.

Patients commonly present with recurrent colicky abdominal pain due to intermittent intussusception. Intestinal bleeding, anaemia and extrusion of the polyps may also occur. The risk of colorectal cancer is 5–13% (Giardiello *et al.* 1987). Tumours of the hepatobiliary system, breast, and lung have also been reported (Gardiello *et al.* 1987). About 5% of females develop ovarian cancers, half of which are hormonally active granulosa cell tumours (Easton *et al.* 1996). Symptomatic patients therefore require thorough investigation followed by careful surveillance, while some have advocated a combined surgical and endoscopic approach to clear as many polyps as possible. However, most would suggest that patients should be carefully followed, local resection being performed only for polyps which cause symptoms such as intussusception.

Neurofibromatosis (von Recklinghausen's disease)

The gastrointestinal tract may occasionally be involved in neurofibromatosis (Figure 8.20a, b). In such cases, the intestinal neurofibromata are derived from the submucosal primitive mesenchyme. The polyps are composed of a mixture of neurofibromata and juvenile polyps. The diagnosis is often not immediately apparent on barium enema or colonoscopy and biopsy is therefore frequently necessary (Hassell 1982).

Cronkhite–Canada syndrome

This is a rare form of adenomatous gastrointestinal polyposis which does not show a familial tendency. The disease presents with alopecia, skin pigmentation, nail dystrophy, protein-losing enteropathy, and electrolyte disturbances. Patients usually present in their 60s and it is equally common in both sexes (Daniel *et al.* 1982). Patients usually present with anorexia, copious diarrhoea with abdominal pain and distension. The nail, hair, and skin changes usually develop after the abdominal symptoms. Investigation reveals marked anaemia and a low serum potassium, calcium, phosphate, magnesium, and protein. Polyps are invariably present in the stomach and colon followed in frequency by the terminal ileum, duodenum, and remaining small bowel (Daniel *et al.* 1982). The oesophagus is spared (Daniel *et al.* 1982). The polyps are hamartomas with no malignant tendency. Although aggressive nutritional support is needed, surgery is only required for complications such as bleeding.

Inflammatory polyps (pseudo-polyps)

These represent non-neoplastic proliferations of either mucosa or granulation tissue in response to injury to the colorectal epithelium. Following full-thickness ulceration a regenerative process begins which results in bizarre configurations in the residual mucosa (Figure 8.21). These range from filiform tags to rounded masses. They are usually multiple, mucosal bridges often joining adjacent polyps. They are associated with chronic inflammatory conditions such as ulcerative colitis, Crohn's disease, amoebiasis, and schistosomiasis. Less commonly, inflammatory polyps are seen following diverticulitis and ischaemic colitis. Histologically, there is ulceration

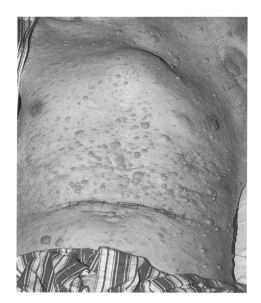

(a)

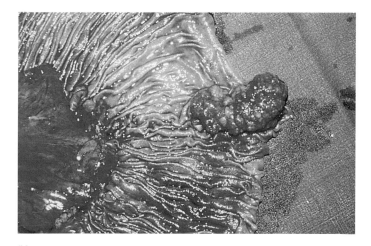

(b)

Figure 8.20 (a) Patient with neurofibromatosis. Investigation of intestinal bleeding revealed a small bowel neurofibroma (b).

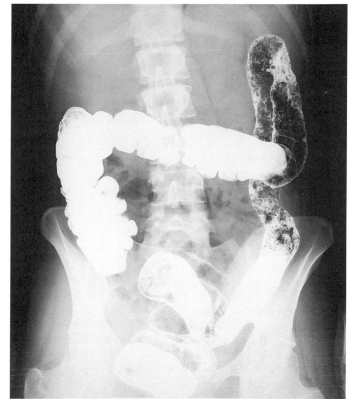

Figure 8.21 Pseudo-polyposis in a patient with chronic ulcerative colitis.

of the surrounding mucosa with a mild to moderate inflammatory response and granulation tissue. They are not pre-malignant.

Non-epithelial tumours (Table 8.7)

Familial adenomatous polyposis (FAP)

Incidence

This condition has an autosomal dominant non-sex-linked inheritance with a high degree of penetrance. Sporadic mutation accounts for a very small percentage of patients, tends to occur in males, and has a later clinical onset. Consequently, nearly half of affected offspring are at risk of developing the disease. FAP is estimated to affect between 1 in 8000 and 1 in 29 000 live births (Northover and Murday 1989). Over the last 30 years the incidence of FAP in Finland has increased from 0.6 to 2.4 per million (Jarvinen 1992). FAP is responsible for 0.5% of all colorectal cancers (Jarvinen 1992). Gardner's syndrome was originally thought to be distinct from FAP but mutation analysis suggests that it comprises part of the FAP disease phenotype (Williams and Peller 1994; Perniciaro 1995). The onset of polyposis is normally in the second and third decade, being rare before puberty. Polyp formation is usually initiated in puberty and increases dramatically with age. Over 80% of patients with the condition will have developed polyposis by the age of 25 years.

Aetiology

The gene for this condition is located on chromosome 5 (5q21). A mutation in one gene (adenomatous polyposis coli, APC gene) on this chromosome was identified as being transmitted to affected offspring in FAP families (Petersen 1994). This mutation has the features of a tumour suppressor gene, with 80% of the mutations being identified in exon 15 of chromosome 5 (Beroud and Soussi 1996). Most mutations are small deletions or single base substitutions which result in a premature stop codon and consequently truncation of the protein. Up to 20% of all APC mutations are accounted for by two specific exon 15 mutations (Spirio et al. 1993). The number of colorectal polyps which develop is probably determined by the exact position of the mutation (Horii et al. 1992). The most common is the 1309 mutation which leads to development of colonic polyps at a younger age, thus giving rise to an

Table 8.7 Non-epithelial syndromes

Syndrome	Inheritance and symptom onset	Gastrointestinal involvement	Associated abnormalities
Familial polyposis coli/ Gardner's syndrome	Autosomal dominant 10–40 years (85% before 25 years)	Colon (100%) Rectum 100% (rectal sparing if non-familial) Duodenum (90%) Stomach (50%)	Retinal pigmentation Osteomas of skull, mandible, long bones Exostoses, epidermal cysts, mesenteric fibromatosis, desmoid tumours, periampullary malignancy
Turcot's syndrome	Autosomal recessive 20–30 years	Colon Polyps fewer and larger than in FAP	Malignant CNS tumours Colorectal cancer common
Torre's syndrome	Autosomal dominant 20–30 years	Colon and rectum	Multiple skin tumours Low-grade visceral malignancy Colorectal cancer common
Oldfield's syndrome	40–50 years	Diffuse	Sebaceous cysts
Cronkite-Canada syndrome	Non-familial 50–60 years	Diffuse Non-malignant	Hyperpigmentation, alopecia, protein losing enteropathy, disaccharide deficiency, anaemia, electrolyte disturbances

earlier malignant transformation (Caspari *et al.* 1994; Beroud and Soussi 1996). In patients with the 5 base pair deletion at codon 1309, gastrointestinal symptoms and death from colorectal cancer occur about 10 years earlier than in patients with other mutations (Caspari *et al.* 1994). The APC gene probably acts by affecting colon cell maturation, although other factors, such as bile acid metabolism, may be important (Barker *et al.* 1994).

Pathology

In many cases the entire colorectum is involved with polyps being most frequent in the rectum and sigmoid colon (Figure 8.22). Non-familial variants often have rectal sparing and in such cases rectal cancer is very rare. The majority of polyps are pedunculated tubular adenomas measuring less than 1 cm. However, size may vary from a few millimetres to several centimetres and lesions may be sessile with the occasional villous component. Over half of patients form polyps in the stomach, particularly the antrum, while 90% of gene carriers develop polyps in the second and third parts of the duodenum. There is often clustering of polyps in the periampullary region, suggesting that bile acids play a part in their formation (Scates *et al.* 1993). The majority of gastric polyps are hamar-

tomatous lesions consisting of dilatation of the fundal glands. Patients have a 100–200-fold increase in the risk of periampullary tumours, which also occur 10–15 years earlier than in the general population Colectomy does not affect the natural history of periampullary tumours.

Colorectal cancer develops in almost 100% of cases unless prophylactic surgery is performed. Formerly over two-thirds of patients did develop carcinoma but screening has reduced this figure to about 3% (Petersen 1994, Debinski *et al.* 1996). The onset of carcinoma follows the onset of polyposis by 5–15 years. The distribution of colorectal cancer is similar to the normal population, most cases occurring in the rectosigmoid region. Tumours normally develop before age 40 years and have the same malignant potential as sporadic cancers. In about half of cancer cases multiple tumours are present, representing a 12-fold increase in multiple tumours over sporadic colorectal cancer. DNA analysis reveals the proliferative index and incidence of aneuploidy are similar to that seen in sporadic adenomas (Matthews *et al.* 1987). However, abnormal DNA content occurs at a smaller polyp size in FAP cases while a higher proliferative index is found in large FAP polyps.

Clinical presentation

Most patients have between 1000 and 2000 polyps, but occasionally over 5000 polyps may be present. Clinical symptoms normally follow the development of polyposis by 10–15 years. Rectal bleeding is the most common presenting symptom, occurring in 75% of affected individuals. Diarrhoea may develop in up to half of patients, while abdominal pain and mucus discharge are also common. Patients who present with colorectal cancer may also have symptoms of weight loss, anaemia, obstruction, or perforation secondary to the tumour.

In addition to polyps throughout the intestinal tract, a multitude of extra-colonic manifestations may occur (Figure 8.23). These include multiple osteomas particularly in the mandible, skull, and femur, and these may precede the development of polyps. These and the development of soft tissue tumours of the skin raise the suspicion that the patient may carry a new mutation of the APC gene. Less common associations include neoplasms of the duodenum, liver, gall-bladder, pancreas, brain, and, in women, thyroid and

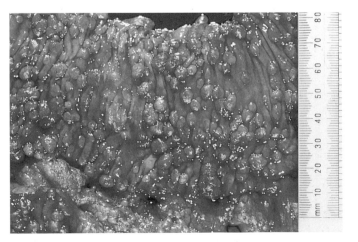

Figure 8.22 Familial polyposis coli.

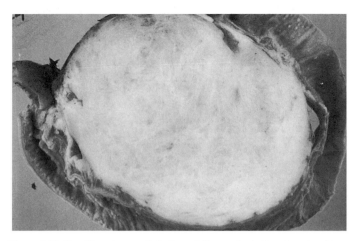

Figure 8.23 Small bowel mesenteric desmoid in a patient with polyposis coli.

breast cancer. Other associations are dental abnormalities (unerupted or supernummary teeth), postoperative fibromatosis, ocular lesions, and lymphoid hyperplasia of the terminal ileum.

Diagnosis

This is discussed in Chapter 9 on screening for colorectal cancer (Figure 8.24).

Treatment

In the future, DNA analysis techniques may make pre-symptomatic or even pre-natal diagnosis possible. In the meantime, care of FAP families will continue to depend on careful registration of family

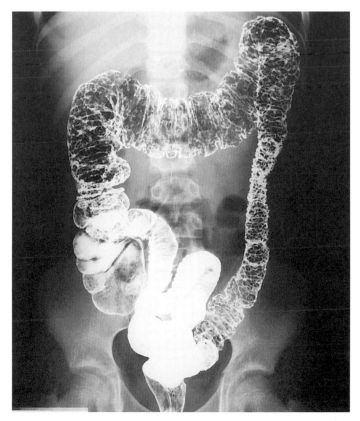

Figure 8.24 Barium enema showing polyposis coli.

information. If sufficient individuals within a family are affected, linkage studies with DNA markers mapping close to the gene is 99% reliable at identifying those inheriting the disease (Cunningham and Dunlop 1993). Mutation analysis is 100% accurate in identifying those carrying the APC gene who will therefore require careful follow-up. Those who do not carry the gene need no further surveillance (Mills *et al.* 1997).

Patients who carry the gene require prophylactic colectomy (Luk 1995). Proctocolectomy and ileostomy are reserved for patients with very low rectal tumours. Restorative proctocolectomy aims to preserve continence while abolishing the risk of malignancy (Ziv *et al.* 1995). However, patients with residual rectal mucosa from stapled anastomoses still require surveillance as a small risk of malignancy remains (Bertoni *et al.* 1995). In addition there is often considerable postoperative morbidity and bowel function is comparable (six motions per day) with that following ileorectal anastomosis. Subtotal colectomy with ileostomy is still a useful and successful mode of treatment for select patients with familial polyposis if they are followed up frequently and aggressively and if the surgeon maintains a low threshold for recommending completion proctectomy (Skinner *et al.* 1990). Total colectomy with ileorectal anastomosis requires vigorous surveillance of the rectal remnant. The risk of rectal cancer is highest in patients who had a colorectal cancer at the time of their original operation. Such a finding is therefore a contraindication to ileorectal anastomosis. However, regular surveillance lowers the incidence of cancer in the retained rectum (Sarre *et al.* 1987; Koretz 1996). About one-quarter subsequently will undergo definitive resection of the rectum over a follow-up of 10 years because of intractable benign polyps, with malignancy developing in 5% (Skinner *et al.* 1990).

The cumulative risk of rectal cancer is 3% at 5 years, 13% at 10 years, and 15% at 25 years after surgery (DeCosse and Cennerazzo 1992). In another study 97% of patients with less than 20 rectal polyps at their initial surgery were free of rectal cancer at 20 years (Sarre *et al.* 1987). In this study almost one-quarter of rectal polyps regressed after surgery, probably due to alterations in faecal pH from the ileorectal anastomosis (Sarre *et al.* 1987). Following colectomy and ileorectal anastomosis, it is more likely that patients will die of upper gastrointestinal malignancy than cancer in the retained stump. Subtotal colectomy with ileostomy is a valuable procedure if patients are followed up frequently and aggressively and if the surgeon maintains a low threshold for recommending completion proctectomy (Skinner *et al.* 1990). Total colectomy, rectal mucosectomy, and ileo-anal anastomosis eliminates the risk of malignancy, preserves anal sphincter function, and is readily adapted by children and young adults. Sulindac and NSAIDs show promise in reducing duodenal epithelial proliferation and polyp formation.

Upper gastrointestinal malignancies and desmoid tumours have overtaken colorectal cancer as the leading causes of death in these patients in some centres. However, the management of such polyps is difficult. Endoscopic or open polypectomy of the duodenal polyps is only temporary as new polyps will develop (Nugent *et al.* 1994). Similarly, prophylactic pancreaticoduodenectomy is a major undertaking which does not entirely remove the risk of duodenal cancer as further polyps may develop at the new site of bile entry. Careful endoscopic surveillance of the upper gastrointestinal polyps is therefore required, even after colectomy, to identify premalignant change in the stomach or duodenum.

Osteomas only require excision if they cause functional or cosmetic problems, while epidermoid cysts usually require excision only for cosmetic reasons. Desmoid tumours are benign (but potentially locally invasive), fibrous tumours which arise from musculoaponeurotic sheaths, most commonly the rectus abdominus muscle. They occur in 15% of patients with FAP, with a female predominance. The mean age of developing desmoid tumours is 30 years and over 80% arise after laparotomy and colectomy. CT scanning may help in the diagnosis (Doi *et al.* 1993). Surgical excision with insertion of a prosthetic mesh is indicated for symptoms such as pain. The intra-abdominal variant is difficult to manage because of compression of ureters, small bowel, and mesentery. Medical therapy is generally unsuccessful. Palliative surgical resection is indicated as radical resection results in unacceptable morbidity and mortality with the likely recurrence of the growth. They tend to recur and may arise in the scar following excision.

The hereditary flat adenoma syndrome

This is characterized by an autosomal dominant inherited predisposition to multiple colonic adenomas (usually less than 100) with proximal predominance and flat as opposed to polypoid growth (Rubio *et al.* 1996). Patients with the syndrome experience colorectal cancers in excess, and the lesions are distributed randomly in the colon. The prevalence is about 12% of polyps seen in referral centres (Lanspa *et al.* 1992). The polyps occur at a later age (median, 55 years) compared with age of onset of polyps in patients with FAP and patients with the Lynch syndromes. The syndrome and familial polyposis coli are linked to the same locus on chromosome 5q21–q22. The association between flat adenoma occurrence and various predictors (sex, race, prior colonic neoplasms, family history of cancer, synchronous adenomas) are similar to those seen with other adenomas (Lanspa *et al.* 1992). Gastric and duodenal polyps occur in about one-third of cases and there is also an associaion with periampullary carcinoma (Lynch *et al.* 1993). Histologically, flat adenomas consist of adenomatous change near the luminal surface of colonic tubules. The flat adenoma may represent an early stage of adenoma development that is manifested in a subset of patients from the general population and that, as an isolated event, does not provide a marker for a hereditary colon cancer-prone syndrome (Lanspa *et al.* 1992, Rubio *et al.* 1996).

Turcot's syndrome

This is a rare, probably autosomal recessive, disorder characterized by development of primary neuroepithelial tumours of the central nervous system and numerous adenomatous colorectal polyps (Mori *et al.* 1994; Scribano *et al.* 1995). The polyps, but not the neurological lesions, are related to the APC gene (Mori *et al.* 1994). Polyps are fewer in number and larger (>3 cm) than in FAP and the exact mode of inheritance is uncertain. It often presents with colorectal cancer in the second or third decade. The finding of polyposis in this condition should initiate CT scanning in a search for tumours of the nervous system (Tithecott *et al.* 1989; Scribano *et al.* 1995).

Torre's syndrome

This is a rare autosomal dominant disorder characterized by gastrointestinal polyps, colon cancer, multiple skin tumours, and multiple low-grade visceral malignancies (Schwartz *et al.* 1989). Associated skin tumours include basal cell carcinoma, squamous cell carcinoma and keratoacanthoma. Polyps are often confined to the colon and rectum with tumours arising in the sixth decade. Although an unusual disease, the syndrome requires recognition because these patients are at risk of multiple primary malignancies and may have family members also at risk (Schwartz *et al.* 1989).

References

Achord JL. Hyperplastic colon polyps do not predict adenomata. *Gastroenterology* 1991; 100: 1142–3.

Achord JL. Polyp guideline. *Am. J. Gastroenterol.* 1994; 89: 660–1.

Afdhal NH, Long A, Tobbia I, *et al.* Immunohistochemical Cal9-9 in primary colonic polyps and polyps synchronous with colorectal cancer. *Gut* 1987; 28: 594–600.

Allen DC, Foster H, Orchin JC, Biggart JD. Immunohistochemical staining of colorectal tissues with monoclonal antibodies to ras oncogene p21 product and carbohydrate determinant antigen 19-9. *J. Clin. Pathol.* 1987; 40: 157–62.

Ansher AF, Lewis JH, Fleischer DE, Cattau EL Jr, Collen MJ, O'Kieffe DA, *et al.* Hyperplastic colonic polyps as a marker for adenomatous colonic polyps. *Am. J. Gastroenterol.* 1989; 84: 113–7.

Arrigoni A, Pennazio M, Rossini FP. Rectosigmoid polyps as markers of proximal colonic neoplasms: a cost benefit analysis of different diagnostic protocols. *AntiCancer Res.* 1995; 15: 563–7.

Atkin WS, Morson BC, Cuzick J. Long term risk of colorectal cancer after excision of rectosigmoid adenomas. *N. Engl. J. Med.* 1992; 326: 658–62.

Balazs M. Giant inflammatory polyps associated with idiopathic inflammatory bowel disease. An ultrastructural study of five cases. *Dis. Colon Rectum* 1990; 33: 773–7.

Balazs M, Rigler A, Faller J. 'Serrated' adenoma—a little known type of colorectal tumors. *Orv. Hetil.* 1994; 135: 21–4.

Barker GM, Radley S, Bain I, Davis A, Lawson AM, Keighley MR, Neoptolemos JP. Biliary bile acid profiles in patients with familial adenomatous polyposis before and after colectomy. *Br. J. Surg.* 1994; 81: 441–4.

Bat L, Pines A, Ron E, *et al.* Colorectal adenomatous polyps and carcinoma in Ashkenazi and non Ashkenazi Jews in Israel. *Cancer* 1986; 58: 1167–71.

Beck DE, Opelka FG, Hicks TC, Timmcke AE, Khoury DA, Gathright JB Jr. Colonoscopic follow up of adenomas and colorectal cancer. *South Med J.* 1995; 88: 567–70.

Beroud C, Soussi T. APC gene: database of germline and somatic mutations in human tumors and cell lines. *Nucleic Acids Res.* 1996; 24: 121–4.

Bertoni G, Sassatelli R, Nigrisoli E, Tansini P, Roncucci L, Ponz de Leon M, Bedogni G. First observation of microadenomas in the ileal mucosa of patients with familial adenomatous polyposis and colectomies. *Gastroenterology* 1995; 109: 374–80.

Bondonio A, Picardi D, Sanesi A. Polyps of the proximal colon: rightward shift, malignancy potential and symptomatology. *Minerva Gastroenterol. Dietol.* 1992; 38: 21–5.

Brendler SJ, Watson RD, Katon RM, Parsons ME, Howatt JL. Skin tags are not a risk factor for colorectal polyps. *J. Clin. Gastroenterol.* 1989; 11: 299–302.

Buck JL, Harned RK, Lichtenstein JE, Sobin LH. Jeghers syndrome. *Radiographics* 1992; 12: 365–78.

Bufo P, Frassanito F, Maiorano E. Colorectal carcinoma and its precursors: role of argyrophilic nucleolar organizer regions (AgNORs). *Boll. Soc. Ital. Biol. Sper.* 1992; 68: 129–36.

Cajucom CC, Barrios GG, Cruz L, Varin C, Herrera L. Prevalence of colorectal polyps in Filipinos. An autopsy study. *Dis. Colon Rectum* 1992; 35: 676–80.

Caspari R, Friedl W, Mandl M, Moslein G, Kadmon M, Knapp M, *et al.* Familial adenomatous polyposis: mutation at codon 1309 and early onset of colon cancer. *Lancet* 1994; 343: 629–32.

Chapuis PH, Dent OF, Bokey EL, McDonald CA, Newland RC. Patient characteristics and pathology in colorectal adenomata removed by colonoscopic polypectomy. *Aust. N.Z. J. Surg.* 1993; 63: 100–4.

Chatrenet P, Milan C, Arveux P, Piard F, Dusserre Guion L, Faivre J. Colorectal hyperplasic polyps in the population of Cote d'Or, between 1976 and 1985. *Bull. Cancer* 1991; 78: 229–35.

Cole DE, Gallinger S, McCready DR, Rosen B, Engel, Malkin D. Genetic counselling and testing for susceptibility to breast, ovarian and colon cancer: where are we today? *Can. Med. Assoc. J.* 1996; 154: 149–55.

Cosgrove JM, Wolff WI, Tenenbaum N, Margolis IB. An appraisal of small and diminutive colonic polyps. *Surg. Endosc.* 1991; 5: 143–5.

Cothren RM, Richards Kortum R, Sivak MV Jr, Fitzmaurice M, Rava RP, Boyce GA, *et al.* Gastrointestinal tissue diagnosis by laser induced fluorescence spectroscopy at endoscopy. *Gastrointest. Endosc.* 1990; 36: 105–11.

Cunningham E, Dunlop M. Familial polyposis coli. *Curr. Pract. Surg.* 1993; 5: 181–5.

Cunningham KN, Mills LR, Schuman BM, Mwakyusa DH. Long term prognosis of well differentiated adenocarcinoma in endoscopically removed colorectal adenomata. *Dig. Dis. Sci.* 1994; 39: 2034–7.

Daniel ES, Ludwig SL, Lewin KJ, Ruprecht RM, Rajacich GM, Schwabe AD. The Cronkhite Canada syndrome. An analysis of clinical and pathologic features and therapy in 55 patients. *Med. Baltimore* 1982; 61: 293–309.

Darmon E, Cleary KR, Wargovich MJ. Immunohistochemical analysis of p53 overexpression in human colonic tumors. *Cancer Detect. Prev.* 1994; 18: 187–95.

De Facq L, De Sutter J, De Man M, Van der Spek P, Lepoutre L. A case of Peutz Jeghers syndrome with nasal polyposis, extreme iron deficiency anemia, and hamartoma-adenoma transformation: management by combined surgical and endoscopic approach. *Am. J. Gastroenterol.* 1995; 90: 1330–2.

DeCosse JJ, Cennerazzo W. Treatment options for the patient with colorectal cancer. *Cancer* 1992; 70 (Suppl.): 1342–5.

Debinski HS, Love S, Spigelman AD, Phillips RK. Colorectal polyp counts and cancer risk in familial adenomatous polyposis. *Gastroenterol.* 1996; 110: 1028–30.

Demers RY, Neale AV, Budev H, Schade WJ. Pathologist agreement in the interpretation of colorectal polyps. *Am. J. Gastroenterol.* 1990; 85: 417–21.

Desai DC, Neale KF, Talbot IC, Hodgson SV, Phillips RK. Juvenile polyposis. *Br. J. Surg.* 1995; 82: 14–7.

DiSario JA, Foutch PG, Mai HD, Pardy K, Manne RK Prevalence and malignant potential of colorectal polyps in asymptomatic, average risk men. *Am. J. Gastroenterol.* 1991; 86: 941–5.

Doi K, Iida M, Kohrogi N, Mibu R, Onitsuka H, Yao T, Fujishima M. Large intra abdominal desmoid tumors in a patient with familial adenomatosis coli: their rapid growth detected by computerized tomography. *Am. J. Gastroenterol.* 1993; 88: 595–8.

Easton DF, Matthews FE, Ford D, Swerdlow AJ, Peto J. Cancer mortality in relatives of women with ovarian cancer: the OPCS Study. Office of Population Censuses and Surveys. *Int. J. Cancer* 1996; 65: 284–94.

Foutch PG, DiSario JA, Pardy K, Mai HD, Manne RK. The sentinel hyperplastic polyp: a marker for synchronous neoplasia in the proximal colon. *Am. J. Gastroenterol.* 1991; 86: 1482–5.

Fraser GM, Niv Y. Hyperplastic polyp and colonic neoplasia. Is there an association? *J. Clin. Gastroenterol.* 1993; 16: 278–80.

Fucci L, Pirrelli M, Caruso ML. Carcinoma and synchronous hyperplastic polyps of the large bowel. *Pathologica* 1994; 86: 371–5.

Giardiello FM, Welsh SB, Hamilton SR, Offerhaus GJ, Gittelsohn AM, Booker SV, *et al.* Increased risk of cancer in the Peutz Jeghers syndrome. *N. Engl. J. Med.* 1987; 316: 1511–4.

Gomez Navarro E, del Rio Martin JV, Sarasa Corral JL, Melero Calleja E. Myoglandular inflammatory polyp located in the distal end of the rectum. *Rev. Esp. Enferm. Dig.* 1994; 85: 45–6.

Greenberg ER, Baron JA, Tosteson TD, Freeman DH Jr, Beck GJ, Bond JH, *et al.* A clinical trial of antioxidant vitamins to prevent colorectal adenoma. Polyp Prevention Study Group. *N. Engl. J. Med.* 1994; 331: 141–7.

Griffioen G, Bosman FT, Verspaget HW, de Bruin PA, Biemond I, Lamers CB. Mucin profiles and potential for malignancy of human colorectal adenomatous polyps. *Cancer* 1989; 63: 1587–91.

Griffioen G, Cornelisse CJ, Verspaget HW, Sier CF, Eulderink F, Bosman FT, Lamers CB. Association of aneuploidy in index adenomata with metachronous colorectal adenoma development and a comparison. *Cancer* 1992; 70: 2035–43.

Grossman S, Milos ML, Tekawa IS, Jewell NP. Colonoscopic screening of persons with suspected risk factors for colon cancer: II. Past history of colorectal neoplasms. *Gastroenterology* 1989; 96: 299–306.

Hara AK, Johnson CD, Reed JE, Ahlquist DA, Nelson H, Ehman RL, *et al.* Detection of colorectal polyps by computed tomographic colography: feasibility of a novel technique. *Gastroenterology* 1996; 110: 284–90.

Harned RK, Buck JL, Shekitka KM. Inflammatory fibroid polyps of the gastrointestinal tract: radiologic evaluation. *Radiology* 1992; 182: 863–6.

Hassell P. Gastrointestinal manifestations of neurofibromatosis in children. A report of two cases. *J. Can. Assoc. Radiol.* 1982; 33: 202–4.

Heiss KF, Schaffner D, Ricketts RR, Winn K. Malignant risk in juvenile polyposis coli: increasing documentation in the pediatric age group. *J. Pediatr. Surg.* 1993; 28: 1188–93.

Hirakata K, Nakata H, Nakayama T, Kajiwara Y, Kuroda Y. Primary malignant lymphoma of the rectum. *Pediatr Radiol.* 1989; 19: 474–6.

Hixson LJ, Fennerty MB, Sampliner RE, McGee DL, Garewal H. Two year incidence of colon adenomata developing after tandem colonoscopy. *Am. J. Gastroenterol.* 1994; 89: 687–91.

Hizawa K, Iida M, Matsumoto T, Kohrogi N, Suekane H, Yao T, Fujishima M. Gastrointestinal manifestations of Cowden's disease. Report of four cases. *J. Clin. Gastroenterol.* 1994; 18: 13–8.

Hoff G, Bjorneklett A, Moen IE, Jenssen E. Epidemiology of polyps in the rectum and sigmoid colon. Evaluation of breath methane and predisposition for colorectal neoplasia. *Scand. J. Gastroenterol.* 1986; 21: 193–8.

Hofstad B, Vatn M, Larsen S, Osnes M. Growth of colorectal polyps: recovery and evaluation of unresected polyps of less than 10 mm, 1 year after detection. *Scand. J. Gastroenterol.* 1994; 29: 640–5.

Hofting I, Pott G, Stolte M. The syndrome of juvenile polyposis. *Leber. Magen. Darm.* 1993; 23: 107–8.

Horii A, Nakatsuru S, Miyoshi Y, Ichii S, Nagase H, Kato Y, *et al.* The APC gene, responsible for familial adenomatous polyposis, is mutated in human gastric cancer. *Cancer Res.* 1992; 52: 3231–3.

Iida M, Iwashita A, Yao T, Kitagawa S, Sakamoto K, Fujishima M. Endoscopic features of villous tumors of the colon: correlation with histological findings. *HepatoGastroenterology* 1990; 37: 342–4.

Imaseki H, Hayashi H, Taira M, Ito Y, Tabata Y, Onoda S, *et al.* Expression of c myc oncogene in colorectal polyps as a biological marker for monitoring malignant potential. *Cancer* 1989; 64: 704–9.

Isbister WH. Hyperplastic polyps. *Aust. N.Z. J. Surg.* 1993; 63: 175–80.

Jarvinen HJ. Epidemiology of familial adenomatous polyposis in Finland: impact of family screening on the colorectal cancer rate and survival. *Gut* 1992; 33: 357–60.

Johannsen LG, Momsen O, Jacobsen NO. Polyps of the large intestine in Aarhus, Denmark. An autopsy study. *Scand. J. Gastroenterol.* 1989; 24: 799–806.

Jorgensen OD, Kronborg O, Fenger C. The Funen Adenoma Follow up Study. Incidence and death from colorectal carcinoma in an adenoma surveillance program. *Scand. J. Gastroenterol.* 1993; 28: 869–74.

Kilche I, Ardao G, Fosman E, Velazquez MS, Gualco G, Ribeiro M, Reissenweber N. Endoscopic pathologic correlation of rectocolonic lesions less than 10 mm. *Rev. Esp. Enferm. Dig.* 1994; 86: 510–4.

Koretz RL. Malignant polyps: are they sheep in wolves' clothing? *Ann. Intern. Med.* 1993; 118: 63–8.

Koretz RL. Polyp surveillance in patients with limited life expectancy. *JAMA* 1996; 275: 327.

Kusunoki M, Fujita S, Sakanoue Y, Shoji Y, Yanagi H, Yamamura T, Utsunomiya J. Disappearance of hyperplastic polyposis after resection of rectal cancer. Report of two cases. *Dis. Colon Rectum* 1991; 34: 829–32.

Lanspa SJ, Rouse J, Smyrk T, Watson P, Jenkins JX, Lynch HT. Epidemiologic characteristics of the flat adenoma of Muto. A prospective study. *Dis. Colon Rectum* 1992; 35: 543–6.

Latt TT, Nicholl R, Domizio P, Walker Smith JA, Williams CB. Rectal bleeding and polyps. *Arch. Dis. Child.* 1993; 69: 144–7.

Leicester R. Colorectal cancer: investigation. *Curr. Pract. Surg.* 1993; 5: 186–90.

Levi F, Randimbison L, La Vecchia C. Trends in subsite distribution of colorectal cancers and polyps from the Vaud Cancer Registry. *Cancer* 1993; 72: 46–50.

Levine MS, Barnes MJ, Bronner MP, Rubesin SE, Saul SH. Atypical hyperplastic polyps at double contrast barium enema examination. *Radiology* 1990; 175: 691–4.

Lotfi AM, Spencer RJ, Ilstrup DM, Melton LJ III. Colorectal polyps and the risk of subsequent carcinoma. *Mayo Clin. Proc.* 1986; 61: 337–43.

Luk GD. Diagnosis and therapy of hereditary polyposis syndromes. *Gastroenterologist* 1995; 3: 153–67.

Lynch HT, Smyrk TC, Lanspa SJ, Jenkins JX, Lynch PM, Cavalieri J, Lynch JF. Upper gastrointestinal manifestations in families with hereditary flat adenoma syndrome. *Cancer* 1993; 71: 2709–14.

Marshall JB. Polyps in the colon. Answers to key questions. *Postgrad. Med.* 1992; 92: 53–4, 57–60, 65.

Matsumoto T, Iida M, Yao T, Fujishima M. Role of nonpolypoid neoplastic lesions in the pathogenesis of colorectal cancer. *Dis. Colon Rectum* 1994; 37: 450–5.

Matthews JL, Glynn M, Parkins A, Cooke T. Alteration in colonic epithelial cell DNA associated with intestinal neoplasia: selection of high risk patients. *Br. J. Surg.* 1987; 74: 23–25.

Meagher AP, Stuart M. Does colonoscopic polypectomy reduce the incidence of colorectal carcinoma? *Aust. N.Z. J. Surg.* 1994; 64: 400–4.

Meijer GA, Fleege JC, Baak JP. Stereological assessment of architectural changes in dysplastic epithelium of colorectal adenomata. *Pathol. Res. Pract.* 1994; 190: 333–41.

Mills SJ Chapman PD, Burn J, Gunn A. Endoscopic screening and surgery for familial adenomatous polyposis: dangerous delays. *Br. J. Surg.* 1997; 84: 74–7.

Mori T, Nagase H, Horii A, Miyoshi Y, Shimano T, Nakatsuru S, *et al.* Germ line and somatic mutations of the APC gene in patients with Turcot syndrome and analysis of APC mutations in brain tumors. *Genes Chromosomes Cancer* 1994; 9: 168–72.

Muller AD, Sonnenberg A. Protection by endoscopy against death from colorectal cancer. A case control study among veterans. *Arch. Intern. Med.* 1995; 155: 1741–8.

Muller S, Chesner IM, Egan MJ, Rowlands DC, Collard MJ, Swarbrick ET, Newman J. Significance of venous and lymphatic invasion in malignant polyps of the colon and rectum. *Gut* 1989; 30(10): 1385–91.

Muthuphei MN. Multiple juvenile polyposis. A report of 2 cases. *S. Afr. J. Surg.* 1994; 32: 97–8.

Muto T, Bussey HJ, Morson BC. The evolution of cancer of the colon and rectum. *Cancer* 1975; 36: 2251–70.

Nakamura S, Kino I, Akagi T. Inflammatory myoglandular polyps of the colon and rectum. A clinicopathological study of 32 pedunculated polyps, distinct from other types of polyps. *Am. J. Surg. Pathol.* 1992; 16: 772–9.

Nava H, Carlsson G, Petrelli NJ, *et al.* Follow up colonoscopy in patients with colorectal adenomatous polyps. *Dis. Colon Rectum* 1987; 30: 465–8.

Nelson RL. Diet and adenomatous polyp risk. *Semin. Surg. Oncol.* 1994; 10: 165–75.

Nguyen HN, Walker S, Fritz P, Kreichgauer HP, Baum KD, Bode JC. The localization of colorectal polyps and carcinomas in relation to their size and the histological findings. *Dtsch. Med. Wochenschr.* 1991; 116: 1041–6.

Norfleet RG, Mitchell PD. *Streptococcus bovis* does not selectively colonize colorectal cancer and polyps. *J. Clin. Gastroenterol.* 1993; 17: 25–8.

Northover JM, Murday V. Familial colorectal cancer and familial adenomatous polyposis. *Baillières Clin. Gastroenterol.* 1989; 3: 593–613.

Nugent KP, Spigelman AD, Williams CB, Talbot IC, Phillips RK. Surveillance of duodenal polyps in familial adenomatous polyposis: progress report. *J. R. Soc Med.* 1994; 87: 704–6.

O'Brien MJ, Winawer SJ, Zauber AG, Gottlieb LS, Sternberg SS, Diaz B, *et al.* The National Polyp Study. Patient and polyp

characteristics associated with high grade dysplasia in colorectal adenomata. *Gastroenterology* 1990; 98: 371–9.

Ochsendorf FR, Leopolder Ochsendorf A, Holtermuller KH, Milbradt R. Soft skin fibromas: study of their importance and diagnostic significance for colonic neoplasms. *Hautarzt* 1990; 41: 207–11.

Offerhaus GJ, Giardiello FM, Tersmette KW, Mulder JW, Tersmette AC, Moore GW, Hamilton SR. Ethnic differences in the anatomical location of colorectal adenomatous polyps. *Int. J. Cancer* 1991; 49: 641–4.

Okada Y, Kusano S, Endo T. Double contrast barium enema study with computed radiography: assessment in detection of colorectal polyps. *J. Digit. Imaging* 1994; 7: 154–9.

Opelka FG, Timmcke AE, Gathright JB Jr, Ray JE, Hicks TC. Diminutive colonic polyps: an indication for colonoscopy. *Dis. Colon Rectum* 1992; 35: 178–81.

Ott DJ, Scharling ES, Chen YM, Gelfand DW, Wu WC. Positive predictive value and posttest probability of diagnosis of colonic polyp on single and double contrast barium enema. *Am. J. Roentgenol.* 1989; 153: 735–9.

Ottenjann R, Wormann B. Multiple colorectal polyps and carcinoma risk. *Dtsch. Med. Wochenschr.* 1985; 110: 1879–1882.

Pavelic ZP, Pavelic L, Kuvelkar R, Gapany SR. High c myc protein expression in benign colorectal lesions correlates with the degree of dysplasia. *AntiCancer Res.* 1992; 12: 171–5.

Pennazio M, Arrigoni A, Risio M, Spandre M, Rossini FP. Small rectosigmoid polyps as markers of proximal neoplasms. *Dis. Colon Rectum* 1993; 36: 1121–5.

Perniciaro C. Gardner's syndrome. *Dermatol. Clin.* 1995; 13: 51–6.

Petersen GM. Knowledge of the adenomatous polyposis coli gene and its clinical application. *Ann. Med.* 1994; 26: 205–8.

Pines A, Bat L, Rosenbaum J, Levo Y, Shemesh E. Are tiny polyps important when found on sigmoidoscopy in asymptomatic people? *J. Clin. Gastroenterol.* 1992; 15: 113–6.

Read TE, Read JD, Butterly LF. Importance of adenomas 5 mm or less in diameter that are detected by sigmoidoscopy. *N. Eng. J. Med.* 1997; 336: 8–12.

Reinus JF. Guidelines for clinical practice. Management of colorectal polyps. *Dig. Dis. Sci.* 1994; 39: 2282–4.

Rex DK. Endoscopic screening for colorectal cancer: recent studies from Indiana University. *Indiana Med.* 1994; 87: 68–73.

Rex DK, Smith JJ, Ulbright TM, Lehman GA. Distal colonic hyperplastic polyps do not predict proximal adenomata in asymptomatic average risk subjects. *Gastroenterology* 1992; 102: 317–9.

Riff ER, Dehaan K, Garewal GS. The role of sigmoidoscopy for asymptomatic patients. Results of three annual screening sigmoidoscopies, polypectomy, and subsequent surveillance colonoscopy in a primary care setting. *Cleve. Clin. J. Med.* 1990; 57: 131–6.

Risio M, Arrigoni A, Pennazio M, Agostinucci A, Spandre M, Rossini FP. Mucosal cell proliferation in patients with hyperplastic colorectal polyps. *Scand. J. Gastroenterol.* 1995; 30: 344–8.

Romer TJ, Fitzmaurice M, Cothren RM, Richards Kortum R, Petras R, Sivak MV Jr, Kramer JR Jr. Laser induced fluorescence microscopy of normal colon and dysplasia in colonic adenomas: implications for spectroscopic diagnosis. *Am. J. Gastroenterol.* 1995; 90: 81–7.

Rubio CA, Kato Y, Hirota T, Muto T. Histologic classification of endoscopically removed flat colorectal polyps: a multicentric study. *Japanese J. Cancer Res.* 1996; 87: 849–55.

Rozenbajgier C, Ruck P, Jenss H, Kaiserling E. Filiform polyposis: a case report describing clinical, morphological, and immunohistochemical findings. *Clin. Invest.* 1992; 70: 520–8.

Sarre RG, Jagelman DG, Beck GJ, *et al.* Colectomy with ileorectal anastomosis for familial adenomatous polyposis: the risk of rectal cancer. *Surgery* 1987; 101: 20–6.

Scates DK, Spigelman AD, Phillips RK, Venitt S. 32P postlabelling studies of target tissues and bile from patients with familial adenomatous polyposis and from unaffected controls. *IARC Sci Publ.* 1993; 124: 357–64.

Schuman BM, Simsek H, Lyons RC. The association of multiple colonic adenomatous polyps with cancer of the colon. *Am. J. Gastroenterol.* 1990; 85: 846–9.

Schwartz RA, Goldberg DJ, Mahmood F, DeJager RL, Lambert WC, Najem AZ, Cohen PJ. The Muir Torre syndrome: a disease of sebaceous and colonic neoplasms. *Dermatologica* 1989; 178: 23–8.

Sciallero S, Bruno S, Di Vinci A, Geido E, Aste H, Giaretti W. Flow cytometric DNA ploidy in colorectal adenomas and family history of colorectal cancer. *Cancer* 1988; 61: 114–20.

Scribano E, Loria G, Ascenti G, Cardia E, Molina D, Gaeta M. Turcot's syndrome: a new case in the first decade of life. *Abdom. Imaging* 1995; 20: 155–6.

Sharma AK, Sharma SS, Mathur P. Familial juvenile polyposis with adenomatous carcinomatous change. *J. Gastroenterol. Hepatol.* 1995; 10: 131–4.

Shepherd NA. Inverted hyperplastic polyposis of the colon. *J. Clin. Pathol.* 1993; 46: 56–60.

Shirai M, Nakamura T, Matsuura A, Ito Y, Kobayashi S. Safer colonoscopic polypectomy with local submucosal injection of hypertonic saline epinephrine solution. *Am. J. Gastroenterol.* 1994; 89: 334–8.

Skinner MA, Tyler D, Branum GD, Cucchiaro G, Branum MA, Meyers WC. Subtotal colectomy for familial polyposis. A clinical series and review of the literature. *Arch. Surg.* 1990; 125: 621–4.

Souquet JC, Napoleon B, Pujol B, Ponchon T, Keriven O, Lambert R. Echoendoscopy prior to endoscopic tumor therapy—more safety? *Endoscopy* 1993; 25: 475–8.

Spirio L, Olschwang S, Groden J, Robertson M, Samowitz W, Joslyn G, et al. Alleles of the APC gene: an attenuated form of familial polyposis. *Cell* 1993; 75: 951–7.

Stefansson T, Bergman A, Ekbom A, Nyman R, Pahlman L. Accuracy of double contrast barium enema and sigmoidoscopy in the detection of polyps in patients with diverticulosis. *Acta Radiol.* 1994; 35: 442–6.

Steine S, Stordahl A, Laerum F, Laerum E. Referrals for double contrast barium examination. Factors influencing the probability of finding polyps or cancer. *Scand. J. Gastroenterol.* 1994; 29: 260–4.

Stryker SJ, Wolff BG, Culp CE, Libbe SD, Ilstrup DM, MacCarty RL. Natural history of untreated colonic polyps. *Gastroenterology* 1987; 93: 1009–13.

Sugihara K, Muto T, Morioka Y. Management of patients with invasive carcinoma removed by colonoscopic polypectomy. *Dis. Colon Rectum* 1989; 32: 829–34.

Tithecott GA, Filler R, Sherman PM. Turcot's syndrome: a diagnostic consideration in a child with primary adenocarcinoma of the colon. *J. Pediatr. Surg.* 1989; 24: 1189–91.

Tsai CJ, Lu DK. Small colorectal polyps: histopathology and clinical significance. *Am. J. Gastroenterol.* 1995; 90: 988–94.

Tsuno N, Muto T, Kubota Y, Sawada T, Nagawa H. Morphometric analysis of colonic adenomatous polyps. *Jpn. J. Cancer Res.* 1993; 84: 310–4.

Uno Y, Munakata A. Endoscopic and histologic correlates of colorectal polyp bleeding. *Gastrointest. Endosc.* 1995; 41: 460–7.

Vamosi Nagy I, Koves I. Correlation between colon adenoma and cancer. *Eur. J. Surg. Oncol.* 1993; 19: 619–24.

Visvanathan R, Thambidorai CR, Myint H. Do dysplastic and adenomatous changes in large bowel hamartomas predispose to malignancy?—A report of two cases. *Ann. Acad. Med. Singapore* 1992; 21: 830–2.

Warner AS, Glick ME, Fogt F. Multiple large hyperplastic polyps of the colon coincident with adenocarcinoma. *Am. J. Gastroenterol.* 1994; 89: 123–5.

Weston AP, Campbell DR. Diminutive colonic polyps: histopathology, spatial distribution, concomitant significant lesions, and treatment of complications. *Am. J. Gastroenterol.* 1995, 90: 24–8.

Williams SC, Peller PJ. Gardner's syndrome. Case report and discussion of the manifestations of the disorder. *Clin. Nuclear Med.* 1994; 19: 668–70.

Winawer SJ, Zauber AG, Ho MN, O'Brien MJ, Gottlieb LS, Sternberg SS, et al. Prevention of colorectal cancer by colonoscopic polypectomy. The National Polyp Study Workgroup. *N. Engl. J. Med.* 1993; 329: 1977–81.

Zahm SH, Cocco P, Blair A. Tobacco smoking as a risk factor for colon polyps. *Am J Public Health* 1991; 81: 846–9.

Ziv Y, Church JM, Oakley JR, McGannon E, Fazio VW. Surgery for the teenager with familial adenomatous polyposis: ileo rectal anastomosis or restorative proctocolectomy? *Int. J. Colorectal Dis.* 1995; 10: 6–9.

9 Screening for colorectal cancer

An improvement in the overall survival of colorectal cancer requires both primary prevention and the eradication of potentially malignant lesions (Winawer *et al.* 1997). As many colorectal cancers develop from pre-existing benign adenomatous polyps it is hoped that removal of these polyps in asymptomatic individuals will reduce the subsequent incidence of colorectal cancer or increase the proportion of Dukes' A tumours (Lieberman 1992). It is hoped that detection and removal of adenomatous polyps may ultimately reduce cancer incidence; 8% of adenomas over 1 cm are malignant and severe dysplasia occurs in 20% of adenomas over 2 cm. Screening programmes for colorectal cancer therefore aim to detect early, asymptomatic cancers and adenomatous polyps which are 1 cm or more in diameter or that have a villous component histologically (Andrews *et al.* 1994; Ferrante 1996, Marshall 1996).

It is estimated that screening those from 50 to 75 years of age will reduce the chance of developing or dying from colorectal cancer by 10–75%, depending on which screening tests are used and how often screening is done (Eddy 1990). The success of a screening programme depends on both patient compliance, and its effectiveness (Bond 1997). Effectiveness is related to the sensitivity, specificity, and predictive value of the test together with its influence on cancer stage distribution, survival, and cost-effectiveness. An ideal screening programme should screen the entire population with highly sensitive tests but this is rarely practical or cost-effective (Ferrucci 1993, Nelson 1996). Such strategies are therefore often restricted to screening high-risk groups. Investigation of average-risk populations is feasible with cheap, reasonably sensitive tests (faecal occult bloods), but secondary investigation of those with positive results is then necessary and can be expensive (Lieberman 1994; Centers for Disease Control and Prevention 1996).

Methods of screening

Endoscopy (Table 9.1)

Colonoscopy is not an ideal screening tool for entire populations as it is labour-intensive, expensive, and associated with a complication rate of 0.2% (Rogge 1994; Ferrante 1996, Kewenter and Bervinge 1996). In the UK, it is estimated that screening for colorectal cancer would require 160 colonoscopies per 100 000 population per year, a figure which exceeds resources (Bennett 1987). The ability of colonoscopy to perform polypectomy does make it suitable as the secondary investigation of choice in patients with positive faecal occult bloods (FOBs) (Lieberman 1990). In those with positive FOBs, colonoscopy has a higher sensitivity (80% versus 57%), a higher specificity (95% versus 80%), lower cost per treatable lesion and lower cost per neoplasm detected, but higher cost per cancer detected than barium enema (Lashner and Silverstein 1990). The higher cost of colonoscopy is therefore offset by its greater sensitivity and its capacity for biopsy

Table 9.1 Comparison of endoscopic techniques in screening

Technique	Features
Rigid sigmoidoscopy	Unsuitable as sole screening procedure as: average distance of insertion is 17 cm visualizes at most 40% of colorectal cancers Uncomfortable May reduce incidence of rectal tumours
Flexible sigmoidoscopy	Detects over 50% of all colorectal cancers and polyps (but this may decrease as result of 'left-to-right' shift in colorectal cancer incidence) Significantly reduces colorectal cancer mortality Well tolerated (compliance 75–95%) Easy to learn (may be taught to nurse practitioners)
Colonoscopy	Not suitable for mass screening as: expensive labour intensive complication rate 0.2% Suitable secondary procedure if FOBs positive as: sensitivity 90% specificity 95% potentially therapeutic

and therapy. Alternatively, those with positive FOBs may be investigated by a combination of double contrast barium enema, flexible sigmoidoscopy, or both (Jensen 1990; Kewenter *et al.* 1995; Mendelson *et al.* 1995). The sensitivity for neoplasms greater than or equal to 1 cm in diameter is 70% for double contrast barium enema and 85% for flexible sigmoidoscopy. By combining the two techniques, sensitivity rises to 95% and specificity to 99% (Jensen 1990).

Rigid sigmoidoscopy is poorly suited to mass cancer screening of asymptomatic subjects as the average distance that a rigid sigmoidoscope is inserted is 17 cm, allowing potential visualization of at most, 40% of all colorectal cancers (Wilking *et al.* 1986) (Figure 9.1). In addition to being unpleasant, inconvenient, and accompanied by a small risk of perforation (0.01%), its effect in reducing cancer incidence is uncertain (Robinson *et al.* 1996).

Flexible sigmoidoscopic screening may potentially reduce the risk of colorectal cancer mortality by up to 70% (Ransohoff 1994). In one study, the risk for death from rectal and distal colon cancer was reduced among individuals having had a single flexible sigmoidoscopy (odds ratio = 0.2), compared with those who were not investigated (Newcomb *et al.* 1992). Flexible sigmoidoscopy has the potential for an effective screening test as it allows examination of the distal 30–60 cm of colon, where more than half of cancers and large adenomas can be found (Lush 1994; Vipon and Moshakis 1996) (Figure 9.2). The technique is simple to learn, 15–20 proce-

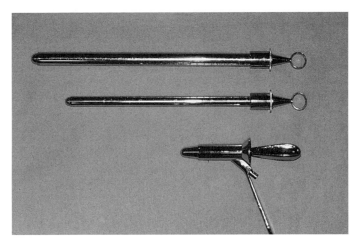

Figure 9.1 Comparison of the rigid adult sigmoidoscope, paediatric sigmoidoscope, and proctoscope. Their short length means that they are of limited value in screening the asymptomatic population.

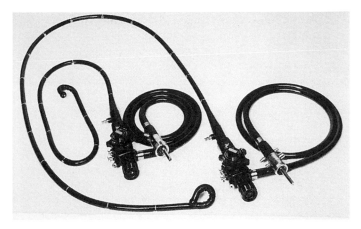

Figure 9.3 Comparison of the lengths of the 65-cm flexible sigmoidoscope and 160 cm colonoscope (Olympus Co).

dures being required for surgical trainees to become competent (Rodriguez-Bicas *et al.* 1993).

The 35 cm flexible sigmoidoscope appears preferable to the rigid sigmoidoscope, taking little longer (2 min versus 1 min) to introduce twice as far (mean of 33 cm versus 16 cm) and providing 20% additional information (Classen *et al.* 1985; Ackermann 1997). The flexible instrument also causes no or only slight discomfort in 80% of patients. In a study comparing the 35 and 60 cm flexible sigmoidoscope the mean time required to complete the examination was significantly less with the 35 cm instrument (2 min versus 5 min) (Dubow *et al.* 1985). Moderate to severe discomfort was experienced by 70% of patients with the 60 cm instrument compared with 30% with the 35 cm sigmoidoscope (Dubow *et al.* 1985). However, screening sigmoidoscopy examinations using colonoscopes suggest that 60 cm scopes have the optimal length for flexible endoscopy in unsedated patients undergoing standard sigmoidoscopy bowel preparation (Rex 1994, Vipon and Mushakis 1996). In such circumstances the 60 cm flexible sigmoidoscope detects 95% of polyps identified by a colonoscope so that the use of instruments longer than 60 cm gives little additional yield (Rex *et al.* 1990).

Careful explanation limits the degree of pain and embarrassment so that only 1% of patients would not have the test again (Kelly and Shank 1992; McCarthy and Moskowitz 1993). Compliance is, therefore, 75–95% being higher among those with a positive family history of colon cancer (McCarthy and Moskowitz 1993; Cauffmann *et al.* 1994; Wherry and Thomas 1994).

Some (including the American Cancer Society) recommend periodic flexible sigmoidoscopy screening for all adults aged 50 years and over, whereas others do not recommend screening at all (Centers for Disease Control and Prevention 1996). A selective screening policy for adults with a personal history of colon polyps or cancer, or a family history of colon, female genital, or breast cancer has also been advocated (Hahn 1990). Polyps detected by the 65 cm sigmoidoscope are an indication for full colonoscopy as there is concern that, with the left to right shift seen recently in colon cancer, flexible sigmoidoscopy will miss the one-third of colon tumours that are situated in the proximal colon (Morris *et al.* 1991). Flexible sigmoidoscopy will also fail to identify neoplasia in the 25–50% of patients with proximal colon cancers that are not associated with sentinel polyps in the distal colon (Dinning *et al.* 1994; Rex 1994) (Figure 9.3). However, in asymptomatic subjects (50–65 years) offered flexible sigmoidoscopic screening compliance is 75–95%, the overall detection rate of carcinoma is 0.5% and that of adenomas 5%, a rate higher than that reported from FOB screening and only slightly less than full colonoscopy (Cauffman *et al.* 1994; Wherry and Thomas 1994, Nelson 1996; Ackermann 1997).

Faecal occult bloods

Normal blood loss from the gastrointestinal tract is about 1 ml/day, the additional blood loss from colorectal tumours varying from 2.5 to 25 ml/day depending on the site and size of the tumour (Brydon and Ferguson 1992). Guaiac-based tests can detect blood losses of 10 ml/day in two-thirds of cases. Products of blood (haematin) in the faeces catalyses, in the presence of hydrogen peroxide, the oxidation of a naturally occurring gum, guaiac acid. In the presence of blood the test turns blue, the assessment of this change being reproducible (Adamsen *et al.* 1985; Allison *et al.* 1996). False-positives occur with animal haemoglobin (red meat) and certain vegetables (broccoli, cauliflower, parsnips), which contain naturally occurring peroxidases. This accounts for the poor positive predictive value of 45% (Favennec *et al.* 1992; Winawer *et al.* 1995). However,

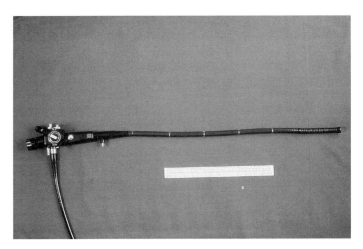

Figure 9.2 The 60-cm flexible sigmoidoscope, which may detect up to half of all colorectal neoplasms.

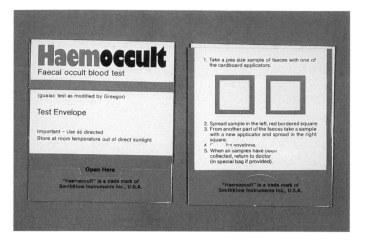

Figure 9.4 The Haemoccult kit which is a faecal occult blood test using guaiac acid.

some claim that dietary restrictions for guaiac occult blood testing are unnecessary in more than 90% of patients (Coughlin and Friend 1987) (Figure 9.4).

FOB tests lose sensitivity during storage due to dehydration. Rehydration immediately before use increases sensitivity at the expense of specificity. Consequently, although more cancers are detected, the costs of screening and of cancer detection are higher with a rehydration than non-hydration regimen (Walker *et al.* 1991*a*). Offering tests over 6 instead of 3 days increases costs without significant improvement in sensitivity and is associated with decreased compliance and a higher rate of colonoscopy (Thomas *et al.* 1990). Cost-effectiveness may be improved by offering FOBs to patients attending out-patients with symptoms suggestive of colorectal disease. In one study the diagnostic yield for neoplasia in those attending out-patients was 60%, associated with a sensitivity of 100% and specificity of 84% (Farrands *et al.* 1985). In this context, there is no firm evidence that a positive FOB found at the time of digital examination should be discounted as a false-positive because of trauma to haemorrhoids or other lesions by the digital examination (Eisner and Lewis 1991). Immunological tests avoid the problems of dietary interference by specifically detecting human haemoglobin (Iida *et al.* 1995; Allison *et al.* 1996). A technician is required to perform the test, so it is unsuitable for population screening. False-positive reactions from upper intestinal bleeding is reduced, although this is partly offset by increased detection of innocent perianal bleeding. Three-day immunochemical testing is not recommended for screening purposes due to its very low specificity. Nevertheless, 1-day immunochemical testing is almost as specific as 3-day guaiac testing (Castiglione *et al.* 1992). Sensitivity is claimed to be 70%, specificity 98%, with both positive and negative predictive values of over 90% (Favennec *et al.* 1992; Shibata et 1993; Iida *et al.* 1995). In one study the detection rate of small relative to large (>1 cm) adenomatous polyps was: Hemoccult II 31% versus 60%, Hemoccult Sensa 73% versus 80% and HemeSelect 34% versus 57% (Petrelli *et al.* 1994; Allison *et al.* 1996). Others suggest that immunological FOBs are not reliable for screening of premalignant adenomas, but valuable for detecting early stage colorectal cancers (Yoshinga *et al.* 1995; Hunt *et al.* 1997).

Although the radial immunodiffusion technique is claimed to be more sensitive, it is less specific than either the rehydrated or non-rehydrated Hemoccult II tests for detecting occult blood in patients with cancer or adenoma (Walter *et al.* 1991, Winawer *et al.* 1995).

The reverse passive haemagglutination test has a slightly lower sensitivity (65% versus 75%) but higher specificity (85% versus 60%) than Haemoccult (Yu 1990; Allison *et al.* 1996). Combining guaiac and immunological tests (Fecatwin/Feca EIA) improves specificity for colorectal cancer from 80% to 90% and increases the positive predictive value of the test for colorectal cancer from 14% to 24% (Pye *et al.* 1989). However, there is a fall in sensitivity from 75% to 67%. Therefore there appears to be no substantial advantage in the addition of the immunological part of the test to justify the extra laboratory work-load incurred (Pye *et al.* 1989).

A haem-porphyrin assay (Hemoquant) is a quantitative measure of total blood loss into the gastrointestinal tract based on the fluorescence of haem-derived porphyrins. It is useful in determining iron-deficiency anaemia but requires a meat-free diet and upper intestinal bleeding reduces the sensitivity for colorectal cancer. Hemoquant provides a precise measurement of faecal haem and its porphyrin degradation products. Although it has a similar sensitivity to Haemoccult for polyps and cancers proximal to the splenic flexure, its sensitivity is substantially lower for more distal cancers (St John *et al.* 1992).

Screening the average-risk population

The detection of occult blood in the stools is the only simple mass screening method for colorectal cancer (Niv 1992; Ferrante 1996; Bond 1997). Although its sensitivity is not ideal, particularly for rectal and caecal tumours, more sensitive tests are likely to result in a loss of specificity with higher costs and overwhelming diagnostic facilities (Hardcastle *et al.* 1989; Trowers *et al.* 1997). Other problems of mass screening with FOBs include compliance, cancer yield, performance, effect on mortality, and cost (Macrae 1996; Mulcahy *et al.* 1997).

Compliance

Poor compliance is a problem in population screening using FOBs. Compliance ranges from 50 to 80% (Table 9.2). Among those who do take the test, 95% are prepared to take it again; while one-third of those who do not take it would accept it if offered a second screening (Arveux *et al.* 1992). The additional investigations associated with a false-positive result does not generally put patients off the screening procedure, colorectal screening being equally acceptable (98%) to patients who experience false-positive results as to those with negative results (Mant *et al.* 1990, Robinson *et al.* 1996). However, increasing the period of Haemoccult testing from 3 to 6 days only reduces compliance while increasing the colonoscopy rate without an increase in neoplastic yield (Thomas *et al.* 1990; Rosinson *et al.* 1996). Those who comply with the test have more positive attitudes to the implications of a positive test, to treatment, and to the value of screening in general (Hunter *et al.* 1991; Thomas *et al.* 1995). The principal reasons for poor compliance are the perceived inconvenience or 'dirtiness' of the FOB testing procedure and unwillingness to know more about their health status (Hunter *et al.* 1991; Myers *et al.* 1991; Arveux *et al.* 1992). Of the factors credited with encouraging persons to perform the test, the most important ones are the practitioner's explanations and sending a leaflet by mail (Thomas *et al.* 1990; Arveux *et al.* 1992; King *et al.* 1992). However, attempts at improving compliance, including television campaigns, among those who refuse the test have generally been

Table 9.2 Features of faecal occult blood tests

Feature	Frequency	Authors
Compliance	50–80%	Hardcastle *et al.* 1989 Kewenter 1990 Hunter *et al.* 1991 Caffarey 1993 Robinson *et al.* 1996 Schnell *et al.* 1994
Positive rate *Unrehydrated*	2%	Hardcastle *et al.* 1989 Thomas *et al.* 1990
Rehydrated	2–6%	Kewenter *et al.* 1990 McGarrity *et al.* 1990 Gregorio *et al.* 1992 Caffarey *et al.* 1993
Positive pre- dictive value	10% (polyps 9% cancer 1%)	Fujita *et al.* 1990 Thomas *et al.* 1989 Kewenter 1990 McGarrity *et al.* 1990 Gregorio *et al.* 1992 Caffarey *et al.* 1993
Sensitivity	67% range 30–95%	Pye *et al.* 1989 Kewenter 1990 Favennec *et al.* 1992 Thomas *et al.* 1992 Caffarey 1993
False negative	1%	Kewenter *et al.* 1990 Jensen *et al.* 1992 Thomas *et al.* 1992
Mortality	reduced by 30%	Kronborg *et al.* 1992 Fujita *et al.* 1990 Mandel *et al.* 1993

poor (Klaaborg 1986; McGarrity *et al.* 1990, Slusser *et al.* 1996). Telephone reminders result in only a 5% increase in compliance rate, while a self-held screening booklet and repeated phone calls result in a 15% increase in compliance (Lee *et al.* 1991; Myers *et al.* 1991). Compliance is also not significantly increased by associating it with a health check, although enclosing the FOB kit with the health check invitation may improve response (Mant *et al.* 1992).

Positivity rate, cancer, and polyp yield

The rate of positive tests has important cost implications as secondary investigation accounts for 30% of the expenditure of a screening programme (Walker *et al.* 1991*b*). About 2% of un-rehydrated tests will have a positive FOB and this is strongly age-related (Table 9.2). Rehydrating the slide increases the positivity rate from 2 to 6% at the cost of reduced specificity and predictive value. The number of secondary examinations can be reduced by a half if further investigations are restricted to only those with a positive repeat FOB test (Thomas *et al.* 1989; Kewenter 1990). Rescreening results in a fall in the positivity rate for rehydration tests from 5 to 2%. A colorectal neoplasm is found in one in three

of those with a positive repeat test, compared with one in seven of those with a negative repeat test (Kewenter 1990). Such a procedure will reduce the work-load by 60% without reducing sensitivity (Kewenter *et al.* 1990). Rescreening of subjects with negative results every 2 years results in a significant fall in the rate of positive results from 2 to 0.3% (Hardcastle *et al.* 1989).

Of those with positive FOBs only 10% will have colorectal cancer or polyps (i.e. positive predictive value is about 10%; 9% polyps larger than 1 cm and 1% carcinoma). The detection rate for cancer is about 3/1000 persons screened compared with 0.9/1000 population in the control group (Kronborg *et al.* 1989; Thomas *et al.* 1990; Ferrante 1996). Large adenomas over 1 cm are detected in 2.6 per 1000 completing FOB tests (Thomas *et al.* 1990). The predictive value of a positive test varies according to the screened person's age and the number of positive tests obtained from that person. In one study a significant trend was observed with positive predictive values ranging from 3% for individuals with only one positive test to 40% for individuals with seven or more positive tests (Petrelli *et al.* 1994). The size of the lesion is also important. While there is no increase in the positive predicted value for adenomatous polyps under 1 cm, there is a direct linear increase for adenomatous polyps over 1 cm (Petrelli *et al.* 1994). Among those 60 years or older, positive predictive value is 10%, compared with 3% for persons younger than 60 years. Having more than one positive test is associated with a positive predictive value of 12%, compared with 5% for one positive test (Gregorio *et al.* 1992). Retesting with dietary restriction reduces the false-positive rate for colorectal cancer but if the retest is negative a further test should be performed after 3 months to maximize compliance (Thomas *et al.* 1989).

Test performance

The overall sensitivity of guaiac tests for colorectal neoplasia (polyps and cancer) varies widely from 30% to 95% depending on the individual test used and the population screened (Table 9.2). There is no correlation between sensitivity and tumour stage or site, or patient age or sex (Castiglione *et al.* 1991). In large unselected population based studies sensitivity is 35% for polyps and 67% for cancer (Thomas *et al.* 1992; Caffarey 1993; Schnell *et al.* 1994). Guaiac occult blood tests therefore fail to detect 65% of polyps and 33% of colorectal cancers (Reilly *et al.* 1990). Haemoccult is more sensitive for carcinoma of the sigmoid and descending colon than for rectal or right-sided cancers (81% versus 45% and 47%, respectively) (Thomas *et al.* 1992) (Figure 9.5). Sensitivity for neoplasia can be increased, but not significantly, by extending the test period to 6 days (Thomas *et al.* 1992). Specificity varies from 67% to 95%, false-negative rate is 10% and negative predictive value 95% (Favennec *et al.* 1992; Caffarey *et al.* 1993).

Effect on mortality

Owing to the size of the population required to produce statistically significant findings there is no firm evidence that FOB testing results in a reduction in colorectal cancer mortality (Ferrante 1996). Assuming a compliance rate of 60%, a study population of 600 000 is required to prove a 25% reduction in mortality with 90% power (Carlsson *et al.* 1986). Current evidence suggests that FOB screening results in detection of tumours at an earlier stage and that this is associated with some, although not necessarily significant, reduction in mortality (Hardcastle *et al.* 1989). Most are potentially curable and over two-thirds are limited to the bowel wall (carcinoma

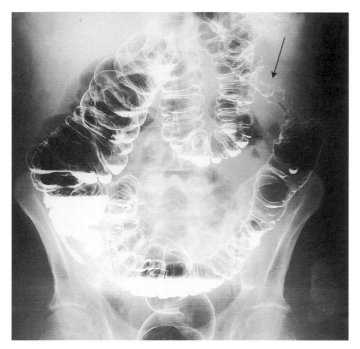

Figure 9.5 Routine screening barium enema in an asymptomatic patient with positive fobs showing a large tumour in the left colon (arrow).

in situ 30%, Dukes' A 35%, Dukes' B 12%, and Dukes' C 8%) (Kronborg 1989; Morris *et al.* 1991; Gregorio *et al.* 1992). Screen-detected tumours are also smaller, often more mobile at surgery, rarely present as emergencies, and are more often resected endoscopically (Hardcastle *et al.* 1989). That a significantly higher proportion of control cancers are poorly differentiated suggests the importance of lead time bias (the possibility that screening moves forward the time of diagnosis without necessarily delaying time of death). However, the high proportion of Dukes' A tumours is maintained in later screening rounds when the majority of prevalent cancers will already have been diagnosed (Hardcastle *et al.* 1989).

Although cancers detected by screening are at a less advanced pathological stage, it is too early to show any effect of screening on mortality from colorectal cancer. The early results from the Danish group suggest a 27% (not significant) reduction in colorectal cancer deaths (Kronborg *et al.* 1989). Death rates were higher among non-responders to screening than among controls or those in whom Hemoccult-II had been performed at least once while persons with negative Hemoccult-II had a lower death rate than controls (Kronborg *et al.* 1992). In the Minnesota study, the 13-year cumulative mortality per 1000 from colorectal cancer was 5.8 in the annually screened group, 8.3 in the biennially screened group, and 8.8 in the control group (Mandel *et al.* 1993). Reduced mortality in the annually screened group was accompanied by improved survival in those with colorectal cancer and a shift to detection at an earlier stage of cancer. Annual faecal occult-blood testing with rehydration of the samples decreased the 13-year cumulative mortality from colorectal cancer by 33% (Mandel *et al.* 1993). Another study compared FOB screening of an asymptomatic population with those attending out-patients (Fujita *et al.* 1990). In the asymptomatic group, more than 60% of the patients had Dukes' A or B1 cancers compared with only 20% in the symptomatic population attending out-patients. The 5-year survival rate of the screened group of 92% was significantly higher than the 60% survival rate for the out-patient group (Fujita *et al.* 1990).

There is concern that a false-negative result and interval cancers (tumours diagnosed in spite of one or more negative screening tests) may adversely affect patient survival. Under 1% of screened patients have a false-negative result (Kewenter 1990). The Nottingham group suggest there is no evidence for a detrimental effect on tumour stage of a false-negative Haemoccult test; indeed, they found a higher proportion of the interval cancers were Dukes' A tumours than cancers in the control group (Thomas *et al.* 1992). In contrast, others have found that interval cancers comprise half of all the cancers detected after doing at least one FOB test (Jensen *et al.* 1992). In this study interval cancers were more advanced than tumours diagnosed after a positive Haemoccult-II test, of larger size, less frequently Dukes' stage A, more often invading neighbouring organs, and less often resectable for cure (Jensen *et al.* 1992). However, these authors suggested that no delay in diagnosis resulted from one or more negative Haemoccult-II tests, compared with controls.

Cost

It is claimed that the guidelines of the American Cancer Society and the National Cancer Institute (annual testing for occult faecal blood and flexible sigmoidoscopy every 5 years) could result in a 40% decrease in colon cancer mortality for those aged between 50 and 75 years provided they comply with screening (Byers *et al.* 1992). The average cost of this policy is estimated as $50 per person per year for screening including follow-up testing of all positive results (Bryers *et al.* 1992). FOB testing alone, although less effective, costs only $20 per person per year, including follow-up testing of all positive findings (Byers *et al.* 1992). The estimated cost per colon cancer diagnosed is $15 200 and $7600 per polyp discovered (Trehu and Cooper 1992). The projected extra life per person screened is an average of 44 days at a net cost of $57 per day of life gained (Byers *et al.* 1992). Subsequent colonoscopic surveillance for those found to have polyps doubles these cost estimates. Applying annual FOB testing to those 65–85 years would detect one-fifth of the expected cases of cancer and could cost $35 000 per year of life saved (Wagner *et al.* 1991). In this age group, screening schedules that include periodic sigmoidoscopy would prevent more cases of cancer but could cost between $43 000 and $47 000 per year of life gained (Wagner *et al.* 1991). In the UK it is estimated that, for an average family practice area with a target population of 75 000 subjects aged 50–74 years, an initial screening round of FOB might be expected to detect 85 cancers at a total cost of approximately £250 000 (Walker *et al.* 1991b). This represents a cost per cancer detected of £2700 and a cost per person screened of approximately £5 (Walker *et al.* 1991b).

Screening policies for average-risk groups (Table 9.3)

In 1980 the American Cancer Society recommended a screening programme for colorectal cancer consisting of digital rectal examination yearly beginning at age 40 years, yearly FOBs, and 3–5 yearly flexible sigmoidoscopy, both beginning at age 50 years (Ferrante 1996, Ozynyk *et al.* 1996; Winawer *et al.* 1997). In addition to having annual FOB tests, persons with first-degree relatives with colorectal cancer can be offered barium enemas instead of sigmoidoscopies every 3–5 years (Winawer *et al.* 1990; Dodd 1992, Macrae 1996) (Figure 9.5). Barium examination is almost as cheap as flexible sigmoidoscopy while giving similar results to colonoscopy, as 90% of polyps under 5 mm missed by radiology will have a neg-

Table 9.3 Proposed screening policies for average-risk populations

Author	Screening policy
American Cancer Society (ACS)	(1) Yearly rectal examination > 40 years (2) Yearly FOB > 50 years (3) 3–5 yearly flexible sigmoidoscopy > 50 years
Winawer et al. 1990, 1997	Same as ACS except 3–5 yearly barium enema if 1st degree relative with colorectal cancer
Dodd 1992	Same as ACS except 2 yearly FOBs > 50 years
Castiglione et al. 1992	
Ransohoff 1994	Same as ACS except 5–10 yearly flexible sigmoidoscopy > 50 years
Sakamoto et al. 1994	
Rex 1994	Single screening colonoscopy for those > 60 years

ligible incidence of malignant transformation (Dodd 1992). However, some feel that screening by FOB every year achieves too limited an increase in sensitivity (70% at 1 year, 60% at both 2 and 3 years) compared with biennial screening, to be worth the difficulties of doubling organizational efforts and costs (Castiglione et al. 1991).

There is also considerable debate about the value of FOBs in population screening (Young and Levin 1995; Trowers et al. 1997). Some feel that these tests merely cause lead time bias. Others feel that subjects who accept the offer of screening are more health conscious than those who do not come forward so that tumours may behave differently between these groups (Farrands et al. 1985). It is also possible that screening may preferentially detect more slow-growing well differentiated tumours because they remain in the population longer. Up to half of all colorectal cancers detected at post mortem are incidental so that a proportion of asymptomatic screen-detected cancers will not present clinically because of death from other causes. Some claim that the detection of small adenomas in FOB screening is often by chance when a falsely positive result due to diet leads to colonoscopic discovery of a non-bleeding small adenoma (Ransohoff and Lang 1990). In the Nottingham study more than 90% of prevalent adenomas were smaller than 1 cm, compared with 63% of those detected by screening (Hardcastle et al. 1989). Nevertheless, small adenomas remain undetected in most persons who have them, even if yearly FOB screening is done. The identification of persons with small adenomas should not be assumed to be an important beneficial outcome of FOB screening, because the clinical significance of small adenomas is not clear, the mechanism of detection is serendipity, and only a minority of persons with small adenomas are identified (Ransohoff and Lang 1990).

Despite the guidelines of the American Cancer Society being widely publicized only 40% of family practitioners in America carry out regular rectal examination, half perform FOBs and 20% arrange for sigmoidoscopy (MMWR 1996). There is also no strong evidence that screening by digital examination or FOB reduces mortality from colorectal cancer (Woodward and Weller 1990; Newcomb et al. 1992). In addition, in those who have previously been screened, further screening with flexible sigmoidoscopy has a low yield (1% polyps) (Sakamoto et al. 1994). Some feel that multiple screenings for asymptomatic, low-risk patients at 3–5-year intervals as recom-

mended by the American Cancer Society may therefore be unnecessary (Sakamoto et al. 1994; Uchman et al. 1997). Consequently, others recommend flexible sigmoidoscopy need be performed only once every 5–10 years in patients aged 50–75 years (Ransohoff 1994). Yet others claim that because adenomas over 1 cm take up to 10 years to progress to invasive cancer, a polyp-free colon at this age might mean that no further follow-up is necessary. These authors therefore advocate that a single screening colonoscopy performed in average-risk persons in their early sixties may reduce colorectal cancer mortality as effectively as repeated endoscopy (Rex 1994). As a result Canada and European countries are awaiting the imminent results of six ongoing controlled trials of Haemoccult screening before establishing screening policies (Mulcahy et al. 1997).

Conclusions

Digital rectal examination is relatively cheap and easy but can detect only a small fraction of large-bowel cancers. Sigmoidoscopy is more sensitive, but its low acceptability to patients has been only partially mitigated by the introduction of the 35-cm flexible instrument. Faecal occult blood testing has limited sensitivity because blood from cancers and polyps is neither continuously shed nor uniformly distributed in faeces; specificity and positive predictive value are also low because of other sources of blood in the stool. Prudent judgement suggests that all of these screening tests may prevent death from colorectal cancer in some patients. As most interval cancers are left sided, adding flexible sigmoidoscopy to Haemoccult screening may increase sensitivity and specificity. However, although the yield of adenomas would increase, the majority would be less than 1 cm, leaving a problem of whether and how to survey them. However, none has been proven effective in general use by well-controlled studies (Friedman and Selby 1990). The current lack of strong evidence in support of these screening tests should not be interpreted as evidence against their use and the imminent results of case–control studies are awaited (Ferrante 1996).

Screening of high-risk groups

Polyposis syndromes (Table 9.4)

Familial adenomatous polyposis (FAP), Gardner's syndrome, Peutz–Jeghers' syndrome, familial juvenile polyposis, and Turcot's syndrome account for less than 1% of colorectal cancers, but children of patients with these conditions have a 50% chance of developing the disease (Figure 9.6). A presymptomatic diagnosis reduces

Table 9.4 Screening procedures for polyposis syndromes

Screening procedure	Author
Hypertrophy of retinal pigment	Parker et al. 1990 Schmidt et al. 1994
Gene mutation	Cunningham and Dunlop 1996 Giardello et al. 1997
Sigmoidoscopy (12–40 years of age)	Burt et al. 1992
Orthopantomography	Bulow et al. 1986
Duodenal screening	Unger 1990 Lynch et al. 1993

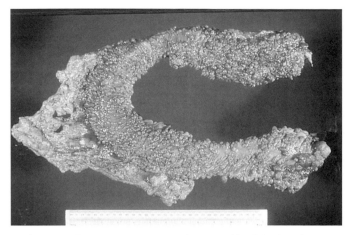

Figure 9.6 Total colectomy specimen in a case of familial polyposis coli.

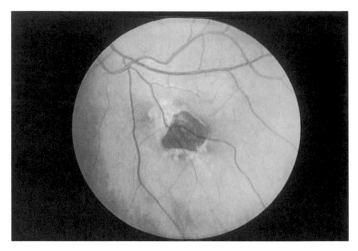

Figure 9.8 Large hyperpigmented CHRPE lesion in polyposis coli (see colour plates).

the need for regular examinations in those who have inherited the disease gene. Formerly, surveillance played an important part in these conditions, but they may now be accurately diagnosed by molecular genetics. Orthopantomography can be useful in identifying affected individuals as mandibular osteomas are more common than normal only in those affected with polyposis coli, unaffected sibs having a similar incidence of osteomas to the normal population (Bulow *et al.* 1986). Unaffected members of FAP families should undergo annual or biennial sigmoidoscopic surveillance beginning at 10–12 years of age and continued to 40 years (Burt *et al.* 1992, Mills *et al.* 1997). Flexible sigmoidoscopy is preferable to the rigid instrument as it detects the few cases with rectal sparing. Duodenal screening is also necessary because of the increased risk of ampullary tumours in those with FAP, multiple colonic polyps, or hereditary flat adenoma syndrome (Unger1990; Lynch *et al.* 1993).

Recently, genotype analysis and fundoscopic examination of retinal pigment anomalies (congenital hypertrophy of retinal pigment epithelium, CHRPE) have been used to detect affected, but still asymptomatic, individuals (Petersen 1994; Parisi 1995) (Figures 9.7–9.9). For screening purposes, fundal anomalies are preferable to gene mutation techniques as they occur in up to 90% of affected individuals and are much less time consuming and expensive (Petersen 1994). Although gene probes have a reliability approaching 100%, in one study a presymptomatic conclusion was achieved in 80% of

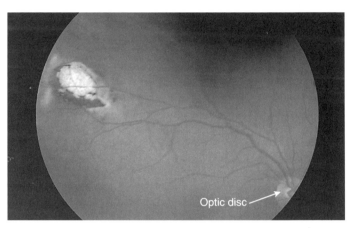

Figure 9.9 Large hypopigmented lesion in polyposis coli (the optic disc is arrowed).

those at risk using ophthalmological examination compared with 32% by direct mutation analysis (Caspai *et al.* 1993). In future these techniques will allow targeting of surveillance in those patients who have fundal anomalies or are gene carriers; reduction of uncertainty for at-risk FAP family members being an important benefit of their introduction. When these tests indicate that an individual does not have the FAP mutation, screening can be decreased. In contrast, for those who are found to be affected no change in the conventional FAP colon screening regimen is recommended (Petersen 1994).

Ulcerative colitis (Table 9.5)

Overall, patients with ulcerative colitis have an eightfold risk of developing colorectal cancer relative to that of the general population (Löfberg *et al.* 1990). The risk is dependent on the extent of the colitis and the duration of disease, there being no increased risk in those with distal disease, a fivefold increase for left-sided disease and a 19-fold risk in those with extensive colitis (Lennard-Jones *et al.* 1990; Löfberg *et al.* 1990) (Figure 9.10). The overall cumulative risk of developing carcinoma in patients with ulcerative colitis is 5% at 20 years and 10% at 25 years, the risk for patients with extensive colitis for over 8 years being 0.5–1% per year (Lashner *et al.* 1989; Löfberg *et al.* 1990). The rectum and sigmoid is the primary site of cancer in over 50% of colitics who develop colorectal malignancy

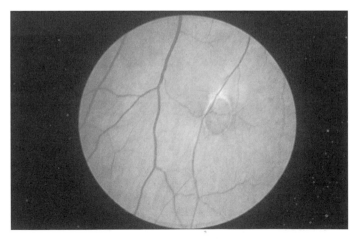

Figure 9.7 Fundoscopic view showing oval CHRPE hyperpigmentation pathognomonic of familial polyposis coli.

Table 9.5 Recommended surveillance programmes for ulcerative colitis

Category	Surveillance schedule
Extent of colitis	
Rectosigmoid only	No surveillance required
Rectosigmoid and left-sided colitis	Surveillance after 20 years of disease
Extensive disease	Surveillance after 10 years of disease Annual sigmoidoscopy Biennial colonoscopy
Age at onset of colitis	
< 40 years	(1) Life-long annual sigmoidoscopy and biennial colonoscopy (2) If disease present > 20 years- restorative proctocolectomy
40–60 years	Annual sigmoidoscopy and biennial colonoscopy up to age 60 years
Over 60 years	No surveillance required
Dysplasia	
Indefinite or low grade	6 monthly colonoscopy and biopsy
High grade	Surgery

with over 80% of tumours arising distal to the splenic flexure (Schneider and Stolte 1993).

Screening of patients with long-standing ulcerative colitis is intended to detect dysplasia before malignancy develops, as in 85% of colitics with colon tumours, dysplasia can be identified at some point in the colon (Schneider and Stolte 1993; Rozen *et al.* 1995). In those with pancolitis for 15 years, low-grade dysplasia is detected in 10%, high-grade dysplasia in 5%, and carcinoma (Dukes' stage A) in 2% (Löfberg *et al.* 1990; Rozen *et al.* 1995). The cumulative risk of developing at least low-grade dysplasia is 15% after 25 years of the disease (Lennard-Jones *et al.* 1990; Löfberg *et al.* 1990).

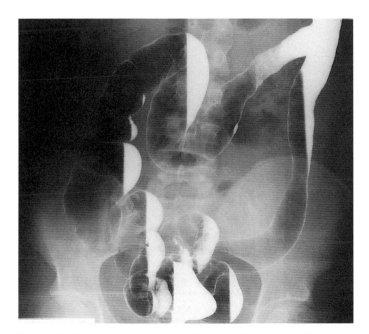

Figure 9.10 Barium enema of a patient with total colitis for 8 years. The patient subsequently entered a colonoscopic surveillance programme.

Sigmoidoscopic biopsies do not substitute for colonoscopic biopsies in a surveillance programme as dysplasia is patchy in one-third of cases. Nevertheless, the ease of obtaining rectal biopsies, the acceptable yield of dysplasia, and the need for frequent sigmoidoscopy in the clinical management of ulcerative colitis suggest a useful supplementary role for rectal biopsies (Fochias *et al.* 1986).

In one colonoscopic study, 8% of patients had dysplasia detected in the initial biopsy specimens and half of these (seven patients) had unsuspected carcinoma (Nugent *et al.* 1991). During a 13-year follow-up 5% of patients developed dysplasia, which was unrelated to the extent of the disease and there was only one Dukes' B carcinoma. No tumour developed in patients without dysplasia on either the initial or subsequent biopsy samples and all cancer-related deaths occurred in patients with high-grade dysplasia in their initial biopsy samples (Nugent *et al.* 1991). However, some authors claim that colonoscopic surveillance in ulcerative colitis is expensive (up to $200 000 per cancer found), compliance is suboptimal, colorectal cancers may be missed and there is little evidence that screening actually improves patient survival (Lashner *et al.* 1990; Vilien *et al.* 1991; Corman 1994). In one study there was no significant improvement in cancer-related survival in those undergoing surveillance despite colectomy being less common and being performed 4 years later than in controls (Lashner *et al.* 1990). In a study from St Mark's Hospital, London, although colonoscopic screening identified patients with dysplasia or early cancers, two of the 400 patients died of colorectal cancer while still under surveillance (Lennard-Jones *et al.* 1990). Others have also reported the development of carcinoma in patients undergoing regular colonoscopy and biopsy (Reiser *et al.* 1994).

Bernstein *et al.* (1994) reviewed 10 prospective studies containing 1225 patients undergoing surveillance colonoscopy. Of 40 patients with dysplasia-associated mass lesion (DALM), almost half already had cancer at immediate colectomy. Of patients found to have high-grade dysplasia after the initial colonoscopy, one-third had cancer. Up to 30% of patients with untreated low-grade dysplasia progressed to DALM, high-grade dysplasia, or cancer. Of patients with indefinite results, almost one-third progressed to high-grade dysplasia and 10% to cancer, so continued surveillance is required in this group of patients. The risk of progression to dysplasia was only 2% for patients whose initial biopsy was negative, so surveillance could perhaps be less frequent for these patients. They concluded that colectomy is required for those with high-grade dysplasia and that a diagnosis of dysplasia does not preclude the presence of invasive cancer (Bernstein *et al.* 1994).

In summary, patients with disease confined to the rectum or sigmoid are unlikely to develop cancer and do not require screening unless, during a relapse, the disease becomes more extensive. Even in those with extensive disease the risk of missing a cancer before it becomes incurable seems to be low (Brostrom *et al.* 1986). Those with extensive colitis therefore require only annual sigmoidoscopy to assess the severity of disease. If extensive disease has been present for over 10 years, patients should enter a screening programme consisting of annual sigmoidoscopy and biennial colonoscopy (Lashner *et al.* 1988; Lennard-Jones *et al.* 1990). However, surveillance may need to begin earlier in young patients with ulcerative colitis as, in one study of young patients with dysplasia, in three-quarters of cases the dysplasia was found before they had the disease for 9 years (Fochias *et al.* 1986). Patients with left-sided colitis should begin surveillance after 20 years. Any abnormal areas should also be biopsied and reported by experienced pathologists (Lashner *et al.* 1989). If this reveals indefinite or low-grade dysplasia short-interval colonoscopy (6 monthly) should be performed. If high-grade dysplasia is identified, surgery should be advised. Patients developing colitis before the age of 40 years should undergo life-long surveillance by annual review and biennial colonoscopy. If the disease has been present for more than 20 years prophylactic restorative proctocolectomy should be considered. Patients aged 40–60 years should undergo annual sigmoidoscopy and biennial colonoscopy as their life-expectancy is less and many asymptomatic patients may wish the surgical alternative of proctocolectomy and ileostomy. Patients developing the disease after the age of 60 years do not require surveillance as they will not become at increased risk of colon cancer for another 10 years, by which time they will be at greater risk of dying from other causes. However, the cost of such screening programmes is considerable and compliance can be poor, two-thirds of patients expressing a reluctance to continue surveillance and 15% actually defaulting (Lennard-Jones *et al.* 1990). Patients should be informed about the limitations of colonoscopic surveillance so that they can take part rationally in decision-making about their management.

Patients with Crohn's disease of the large and small bowel have a fivefold increased risk of colorectal cancer. Cancer can occur in both the small bowel and unaffected segment of large bowel. Routine surveillance may be warranted especially in the presence of symptoms (Korelitz 1990).

Patients with a family history of colorectal cancer

Polyps occur in one-third and cancer in 5% of those with a positive family history of colorectal cancer, 40% of these lesions being multiple (Brzezinski 1990; Orrom *et al.* 1990) (Figure 9.11). The short-term risk of colorectal cancer in Lynch syndrome relatives without adenomas is low, as is the risk in those who have had all adenomas removed (Lanspa *et al.* 1992). Screening of those with a strong family history is associated with a much lower risk of both colorectal cancer and cancer-related death than unscreened populations (Goh and Wong 1992, Nelson 1996; Burke *et al.* 1997). Initial screening should include full colonoscopy as between one-fifth to one-half of subjects have proximal polyps which would be missed by either rigid or flexible sigmoidoscopy (McConnell *et al.* 1990; Guillem

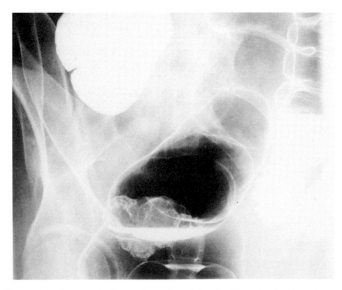

Figure 9.11 Large polyp in a patient whose father had been treated for colon cancer.

1992). Barium enema also misses one-quarter of polyps in these patients, principally because they are less than 0.5 cm diameter, while FOBs detect polyps in only 2% of subjects, compared with the 16% detected by colonoscopy (Baker *et al.* 1990; Houlston 1990).

One-quarter of those under the age of 40 years with a strong family history of colorectal cancer will have colorectal polyps (Orrom *et al.* 1990; Dunlop 1992). In this population acceptance of screening is high (60–90%) (Houlston *et al.* 1990). In those with two or more first-degree relatives with colorectal cancer screening asymptomatic adults by colonoscopy is four times more cost-effective than those with only one relative with colon cancer (Rozen and Ron 1989). It is therefore suggested that all patients over 30 years of age with two or more first-degree relative with colorectal cancer should undergo colonoscopy and, if clear, every 4 years thereafter until at least 65 years (Burt *et al.* 1992; Meagher and Stuart 1992; Vasen 1994). The right colon in particular should be investigated.

Ureterosigmoidostomy

Patients with congenital urinary tract anomalies and those with previous ureterosigmoidostomy are at increased risk of colorectal cancer (Atwell *et al.* 1993). The risk of colon carcinoma in those who have had an ureterosigmoidostomy is 10 times higher than that of the general population (Kalble *et al.* 1992). There is no risk from isolated colon loops used for urinary diversion (Gittes 1986). Regular flexible sigmoidoscopy gives easy access to the area at risk of colorectal cancer (Berg *et al.* 1987).

References

Ackermann RJ. **Performance of gastrointestinal tract endoscopy by primary care physicians. Lessons from the US Medicare database.** Arch. *Fmaily Med.* 1997; 6: 52–8.

Adamsen S, Kronborg O, Hage E, Fenger C. Reproducibility and diagnostic value of Hemoccult II test. A colonoscopic evaluation in asymptomatic patients. *Scand. J. Gastroenterol.* 1985; 20: 1073–7.

Allison JE, Tekawa IS, Ransom LJ, Adrain AL. **A comparison of fecal occult blood tests for colorectal cancer screening. N. Engl. J. Med. 1996; 334: 155–9.**

Andrews HF, Kerner JF, Zauber AG, Mandelblatt J, Pittman J, Struening E. Using census and mortality data to target small areas for breast, colorectal, and cervical cancer screening. *Am. J. Public Health* 1994; 84: 56–61.

Arveux P, Durand G, Milan C, Bedenne L, Levy D, Doan BD, Faivre J. Views of a general population on mass screening for colorectal cancer: the Burgundy Study. *Prev. Med.* 1992; 21: 574–81.

Atwell JD, Taylor I, Cruddas M. Increased risk of colorectal cancer associated with congenital anomalies of the urinary tract. *Br. J. Surg.* 1993; 80: 785–7.

Baker JW, Gathright JB Jr, Timmcke AE, Hicks TC, Ferrari BT, Ray JE. Colonoscopic screening of asymptomatic patients with a family history of colon cancer. *Dis. Colon Rectum* 1990; 33: 926–30.

Bennett JR, Carr Locke DL, Axon ATR, *et al.* Future requirements for colonoscopy in Britain. *Gut* 1987; 28: 772–5.

Berg NO, Fredlund P, Mansson W, Olsson SA. Surveillance colonoscopy and biopsy in patients with ureterosigmoidostomy. *Endoscopy* 1987; 19: 60–3.

Bernstein CN, Shanahan F, Weinstein WM. **Are we telling patients the truth about surveillance colonoscopy in ulcerative colitis?** *Lancet* 1994; 343: 71–4.

Bond JH. Screening for colorectal cancer. *Hospital Practice* (Office Edition). 1997; 32: 59–62.

Brostrom O, Löfberg R, Ost A, Reichard H. Cancer surveillance of patients with longstanding ulcerative colitis: a clinical, endoscopical, and histological study. *Gut* 1986; 27: 1408–13.

Brydon WG, Ferguson A. Haemoglobin in gut lavage fluid as a measure of gastrointestinal blood loss. *Lancet* 1992; 340: 1381–2.

Brzezinski W, Orrom WJ, Wiens E. Prospective and retrospective analysis of colonoscopy findings in patients with a history of colorectal carcinoma in first degree relatives. *Can. J. Surg.* 1990; 33: 314–6.

Bulow S, Holm NV, Sondergaard JO, *et al.* Mandibular osteomas in unaffected sibs and children of patients with familial polyposis coli. *Scand. J. Gastroenterol.* 1986; 21: 744–8.

Burke W, Petersen G, Lynch P *et al.* Recommendations for follow-up care of individuals with an inherited predisposition to cancer. I. Hereditary nonpolyposis colon cancer. Cancer genetics series consortium. *JAMA* 1997; 277: 915–9.

Burt RW, Bishop DT, Cannon Albright L, Samowitz WS, Lee RL, DiSario JA, Skolnick MH. Hereditary aspects of colorectal adenomas. *Cancer* 1992; 70 (Suppl.): 1296–9.

Byers T, Gorsky R. Estimates of costs and effects of screening for colorectal cancer in the United States. *Cancer* 1992; 70: 1288–95.

Caffarey SM, Broughton CI, Marks CG. Faecal occult blood screening for colorectal neoplasia in a targeted high risk population. *Br. J. Surg.* 1993; 80: 1399–400.

Carlsson U, Ekelund G, Eriksson R, *et al.* Evaluation of possibilities for mass screening for colorectal cancer with Hemoccult registered fecal blood test. *Dis. Colon Rectum* 1986; 29: 553–7.

Castiglione G, Grazzini G, Ciatto S. Guaiac and immunochemical tests for faecal occult blood in colorectal cancer screening. *Br. J. Cancer* 1992; 65: 942–4.

Cauffman JG, Rasgon IM, Clark VA, Hara JH. Screening asymptomatic patients for colorectal lesions. *Fam. Pract. Res. J.* 1994; 14: 77–86.

Centers for Disease Control and Prevention. Screening for colorectal cancer—United States, 1992–1993, and new guidelines. *JAMA* 1996; 275: 830–1.

Classen M, Phillip J, Knyrim K, Hertel H. Rectoscope rigid or flexible? A comparison. *Dtsch. Med. Wochenschr.* 1985; 110: 445–8.

Corman ML. Understanding surveillance colonoscopy. *Lancet* 1994; 343: 556–7.

Coughlin RJ, Friend WG. Dietary restrictions and fecal occult blood testing. *Am. Fam. Phys.* 1987; 35: 118–20.

Cunningham C, Dunlop MG. Molecular genetic basis of colorectal cancer susceptibility. *Br J Surg* 1996; 83: 321–9.

Dinning JP, Hixson LJ, Clark LC. Prevalence of distal colonic neoplasia associated with proximal colon cancers. *Arch. Intern. Med.* 1994; 154: 853–6.

Dodd GD. The role of the barium enema in the detection of colonic neoplasms. *Cancer* 1992; 70 (Suppl.): 1272–5.

Dubow RA, Katon RM, Benner KG, *et al.* Short (35 cm) versus long (60 cm) flexible sigmoidoscopy: a comparison of findings and tolerance in asymptomatic patients screened for colorectal neoplasia. *Gastrointest. Endosc.* 1985; 31: 305–8.

Dunlop MG. Screening for large bowel neoplasms in individuals with a family history of colorectal cancer. *Br. J. Surg.* 1992; 79: 488–94.

Eddy DM. Screening for colorectal cancer. *Ann. Intern. Med.* 1990; 113: 373–84.

Eisner MS, Lewis JH. Diagnostic yield of a positive fecal occult blood test found on digital rectal examination. Does the finger count? *Arch. Intern. Med.* 1991; 151: 2180–4.

Farrands PA, O'Regan D, Taylor I. An assessment of occult blood testing to determine which patients with large bowel symptoms require urgent investigation. *Br. J. Surg.* 1985; 72: 835–7.

Favennec L, Kapel N, Meillet D, Chochillon C, Gobert G. Detection of occult blood in stools: comparison of three guaiac tests and a latex agglutination test. *Ann. Biol. Clin.* 1992; 50: 311–3.

Ferrante JM. Colorectal cancer screening. *Med. Clin. North Am.* 1996; 80: 41–3.

Ferrucci JT. Screening for colon cancer: controversies and recommendations. *Radiol. Clin. North Am.* 1993; 31: 1189–95.

Fochios SE, Sommers SC, Korelitz BI. Sigmoidoscopy and biopsy in surveillance for cancer in ulcerative colitis. *J. Clin. Gastroenterol.* 1986; 8: 249–54.

Friedman GD, Selby JV. Colorectal cancer: have we identified an effective screening strategy? *J. Gen. Intern. Med.* 1990; 5 (Suppl.): S23–7.

Fujita M, Sugiyama R, Kumanishi Y, Ota J, Horino T, Nakano Y, Taguchi T. Evaluation of effectiveness of mass screening for colorectal cancer. *World J. Surg.* 1990; 14: 648–52.

Giardiello FM, Brensinger JD, Luce MC et al. Phenotypic expression of disease in families that have mutations in the 5′ region of the adenomatous polyposis coli gene. *Ann. Int. Med.* 1997; 126:514–9.

Gittes RF. Carcinogenesis in ureterosigmoidostomy. *Urol. Clin. North Am.* 1986; 13: 201–5.

Goh HS, Wong J. The Singapore Polyposis Registry. *Ann. Acad. Med. Singapore* 1992; 21: 290–3.

Gregorio DI, Lolachi P, Hansen H. Detecting colorectal cancer with a large scale fecal occult blood testing program. *Public Health Rep.* 1992; 107: 331–5.

Guillem JG, Forde KA, Treat MR, Neugut AI, O'Toole KM, Diamond BE. Colonoscopic screening for neoplasms in asymptomatic first degree relatives of colon cancer patients. A controlled, prospective study. *Dis. Colon Rectum* 1992; 35: 523–9.

Hahn DL. Sex and race are risk factors for colorectal cancer within reach of the sigmoidoscope. *J. Fam. Pract.* 1990; 30: 409–16.

Hardcastle JD, Thomas WM, Chamberlain J, Pye G, Sheffield J, James PD, *et al.* Randomised, controlled trial of faecal occult blood screening for colorectal cancer. Results for first 107349 subjects. *Lancet* 1989; i: 1160–4.

Houlston RS, Murday V, Harocopos C, Williams CB, Slack J. Screening and genetic counselling for relatives of patients with colorectal cancer in a family cancer clinic. *Br. Med. J.* 1990; 301: 366–8.

Hunt LM, Rooney P, Bostock K, Robinson M, Hardcastle J, Armitage N. Chemical and immunological testing for faecal occult blood in screening subjects at risk of familial colorectal cancer. *Gut.* 1997; 40: 110–12.

Hunter W, Farmer A, Mant D, Verne J, Northover J, Fitzpatrick R. The effect of self administered faecal occult blood tests on compliance with screening for colorectal cancer: results of a survey of those invited. *Fam. Pract.* 1991; 8: 367–72.

Iida Y, Munemoto Y, Miura S, Kasahara Y, Saito H, Mitsui T, *et al.* Clinicopathologic studies of immunologic fecal occult blood test for colorectal cancer. *J. Gastroenterol.* 1995; 30: 192–200.

Jensen J, Kewenter J, Asztely M, Lycke G, Wojciechowski J. Double contrast barium enema and flexible rectosigmoidoscopy: a reliable diagnostic combination for detection of colorectal neoplasm. *Br. J. Surg.* 1990; 77: 270–2.

Jensen BM, Kronborg O, Fenger C. Interval cancers in screening with fecal occult blood test for colorectal cancer. *Scand. J. Gastroenterol.* 1992; 27: 779–82.

Kalble T, Mohring K, Waldherr R, Staehler G. Screening study for early detection of intestinal tumours after urinary diversion. *Helv. Chir. Acta* 1992; 59: 507–11.

Kelly RB, Shank JC. Adherence to screening flexible sigmoidoscopy in asymptomatic patients. *Med Care* 1992; 30: 1029–42.

Kewenter J, Engaras B, Haglind E, Jensen J. Value of retesting subjects with a positive Hemoccult in screening for colorectal cancer. *Br. J. Surg.* 1990; 77: 1349–51.

Kewenter J, Brevinge H, Engaras B, Haglind E. The yield of flexible sigmoidoscopy and double contrast barium enema in the diagnosis of neoplasms in the large bowel in patients with a positive Hemoccult test. *Endoscopy* 1995; 27: 159–63.

Kewenter J, Brevinge H. Endoscopic and surgical complications of work-up in screenig for colorectal cancer. *Dis. Colon Rectum* 1996; 39: 676–80.

King J, Fairbrother G, Thompson C, Morris DL. Colorectal cancer screening: optimal compliance with postal faecal occult blood test. *Aust. N.Z. J. Surg.* 1992; 62: 714–9.

Klaaborg K, Stahl Madsen M, Sondergaard O, Kronborg O. Participation in mass screening for colorectal cancer with fecal occult blood test. *Scand. J. Gastroenterol.* 1986; 21: 1180–4.

Korelitz BI. Considerations of surveillance, dysplasia, and carcinoma of the colon in the management of ulcerative colitis and Crohn's disease. Med. Clin. North Am. 1990; 74: 189–99.

Kronborg O, Fenger C, Olsen J, Bech K, Sondergaard O. Repeated screening for colorectal cancer with fecal occult blood test. A prospective randomized study at Funen, Denmark. *Scand. J. Gastroenterol.* 1989; 24: 599–606.

Kronborg O, Fenger C, Worm J, Pedersen SA, Hem J, Bertelsen K, Olsen J. Causes of death during the first 5 years of a randomized trial of mass screening for colorectal cancer with fecal occult blood test. Scand. J. Gastroenterol. 1992; 27: 47–52.

Lanspa SJ, Jenkins JX, Watson P, Smyrk TC, Cavalieri RJ, Lynch JF, Lynch HT. Natural history of at risk Lynch syndrome family members with respect to adenomas. *Nebr. Med. J.* 1992; 77: 310–3.

Lashner BA, Silverstein MD, Hanauer SB. Hazard rates for dysplasia and cancer in ulcerative colitis. Results from a surveillance program. *Dig. Dis. Sci.* 1989; 34: 1536–41.

Lashner BA, Silverstein MD. Evaluation and therapy of the patient with fecal occult blood loss: a decision analysis. *Am. J. Gastroenterol.* 1990; 85: 1088–95.

Lee CY. A randomized controlled trial to motivate worksite fecal occult blood testing. *Yonsei Med J.* 1991; 32: 131–8.

Lennard-Jones JE, Melville DM, Morson BC, Ritchie JK, Williams CB. Precancer and cancer in extensive ulcerative colitis: findings among 401 patients over 22 years. *Gut* 1990; 31: 800–6.

Lieberman DA. Colon cancer screening. The dilemma of positive screening tests. *Arch. Intern. Med.* 1990; 150: 740–4.

Lieberman DA. Targeted colon cancer screening: a concept whose time has almost come. *Am. J. Gastroenterol.* 1992; 87: 1085–93.

Lieberman DA. Screening/early detection model for colorectal cancer. Why screen? Cancer 1994; 74 (Suppl.): 2023–7.

Löfberg R, Brostrom O, Karlen P, Tribukait B, Ost A. Colonoscopic surveillance in long standing total ulcerative colitis a 15 year follow up study. Gastroenterology 1990; 99: 1021–31.

Lush DT. Screening for colorectal cancer. Use of a new protocol may reduce death rates. *Postgrad. Med.* 1994; 96: 99–106.

Lynch HT, Smyrk TC, Lanspa SJ, Jenkins JX, Lynch PM, Cavalieri J, Lynch JF. Upper gastrointestinal manifestations in families with hereditary flat adenoma syndrome. *Cancer* 1993; 71: 2709–14.

Macrae FA. Screening for colorectal cancer, 1996. Med. J. Aust. 1996; 165: 102–5.

Mandel JS, Bond JH, Church TR, Snover DC, Bradley GM, Schuman LM, Ederer F. Reducing mortality from colorectal cancer by screening for fecal occult blood. Minnesota Colon Cancer Control Study. N. Engl. J. Med. 1993; 328: 1365–71.

Mant D, Fitzpatrick R, Hogg A, Fuller A, Farmer A, Verne J, Northover J. Experiences of patients with false positive results from colorectal cancer screening. *Br. J. Gen. Pract.* 1990; 40: 423–5.

Mant D, Fuller A, Northover J, Astrop P, Chivers A, Crockett A, *et al.* Patient compliance with colorectal cancer screening in general practice. *Br. J. Gen. Pract.* 1992; 42: 18–20.

Marshall JB. Colorectal cancer screening: present strategies and future prospects. *Postgrad. Med.* 1996; 99: 253–64.

McCarthy BD, Moskowitz MA. Screening flexible sigmoidoscopy: patient attitudes and compliance. *J. Gen. Intern. Med.* 1993; 8: 120–5.

McConnell JC, Nizin JS, Slade MS. Colonoscopy in patients with a primary family history of colon cancer. *Dis. Colon Rectum* 1990; 33: 105–7.

McGarrity TJ, Long PA, Peiffer LP. Results of a repeat television advertised mass screening program for colorectal cancer using fecal occult blood tests. *Am. J. Gastroenterol.* 1990; 85: 266–70.

Meagher AP, Stuart M. Colonoscopy in patients with a family history of colorectal cancer. *Dis. Colon Rectum* 1992; 35: 315–21.

Mendelson RM, Kelsey PJ, Chakera T. A combined flexible sigmoidoscopy and double contrast barium enema service: initial experience. *Abdom. Imaging.* 1995; 20: 238–41.

Mills SJ, Chapman PD, Burn J, Gunn A. Endoscopic screening and surgery for familial polyposis: dangerous delays. *Br. J. Surg.* 1997; 84: 74–77.

MMWR. Screening for colorectal cancer—United States, 1992–1993, and new guidelines. *MMWR Morb. Mortal. Wkly Rep.* 1996; 45: 107–10.

Morris JB, Stellato TA, Guy BB, Gordon NH, Berger NA. A critical analysis of the largest reported mass fecal occult blood screening program in the United States. *Am. J. Surg.* 1991; 161: 101–5.

Mulcahy HE, Farthing MJ, O'Donoghue DP. Screening for asymptomatic colorectal cancer. Brit. Med. J. 1997; 314: 285–91.

Myers RE, Ross EA, Wolf TA, Balshem A, Jepson C, Millner L. Behavioral interventions to increase adherence in colorectal cancer screening. *Med Care* 1991; 29: 1039–50.

Nelson RL. Screening of average-risk individuals for colorectal cancer and postoperative evaluation of patients with colorectal cancer. Surg. Clin. North Am. 1996; 76: 35–45.

Newcomb PA, Norfleet RG, Storer BE, Surawicz TS, Marcus PM. Screening sigmoidoscopy and colorectal cancer mortality. *J. Natl Cancer Inst.* 1992; 84: 1572–5.

Niv Y. Does a risk questionnaire add anything to a colorectal screening project? Report of a 3 year screening experience. *J. Clin. Gastroenterol.* 1992; 15: 33–6.

Nugent FW, Haggitt RC, Gilpin PA. Cancer surveillance in ulcerative colitis. *Gastroenterology* 1991; 100: 1241–8.

Olynyk JK, Aquila S, Fletcher DR, Dickinson JA. Flexible sigmoidoscopy screening for colorectal cancer in a average-risk subjects in community-based pilot project. *Med. J. Aust.* 1996; 165: 74–6.

Orrom WJ, Brzezinski WS, Wiens EW. Heredity and colorectal cancer. A prospective, community based, endoscopic study. *Dis. Colon Rectum* 1990; 33: 490–3.

Parisi ML. Congenital hypertrophy of the retinal pigment epithelium serves as a clinical marker in a family with familial adenomatous polyposis. *J. Am. Optom. Assoc.* 1995; 66: 106–12.

Parker JA, Kalnins VI, Deck JH, Cohen Z, Berk T, Cullen JB, Kiskis AA. Ke WJ. Histopathological features of congenital fundus lesions in familial adenomatous polyposis. *Can. J. Ophthalmol.* 1990; 25: 159–63.

Petersen GM. Knowledge of the adenomatous polyposis coli gene and its clinical application. *Ann. Med.* 1994; 26: 205–8.

Petrelli N, Michalek AM, Freedman A, Baroni M, Mink I, Rodriguez Bigas M. Immunochemical versus guaiac occult blood stool tests: results of a community based screening program. *Surg. Oncol.* 1994; 3: 27–36.

Pye G, Marks CG, Martin S, Marks V, Jackson J, Hardcastle JD. An evaluation of Fecatwin/Feca EIA, a faecal occult blood test for detecting colonic neoplasia. *Eur. J. Surg. Oncol.* 1989; 15: 446–8.

Ransohoff DF. The case for colorectal cancer screening. *Hosp. Pract. Off. Edn* 1994; 29: 25–32.

Ransohoff DF, Lang CA. Small adenomas detected during fecal occult blood test screening for colorectal cancer. The impact of serendipity. *JAMA* 1990; 264: 76–8.

Reilly JM, Ballantyne GH, Fleming FX, Zucker KA, Modlin IM. Evaluation of the occult blood test in screening for colorectal neoplasms. A prospective study using flexible endoscopy. *Am. Surg.* 1990; 56: 119–23.

Reiser JR, Waye JD, Janowitz HD, Harpaz N. Adenocarcinoma in strictures of ulcerative colitis without antecedent dysplasia by colonoscopy. *Am. J. Gastroenterol.* 1994; 89: 119–22.

Rex DK. Endoscopic screening for colorectal cancer: recent studies from Indiana University. *Indiana Med.* 1994; 87: 68–73.

Rex DK, Lehman GA, Hawes RH, O'Connor KW, Smith JJ. Performing screening flexible sigmoidoscopy using colonoscopes: experience in 500 subjects. *Gastrointest. Endosc.* 1990; 36: 486–8.

Robinson MH, Marks CG, Ferrands PA, Bostock K, Hardcastle JD. Screening for colorectal cancer with an immunological faecal occult blood-test: 2-year follow-up. *Brit. J. Surg.* 1996; 83: 500–1.

Robinson RJ, Stone M, Mayberry JF. Sigmoidoscopy and rectal biopsy: a survey of current UK practice. *Eur. J. Gastroenterol. Hepatol.* 1996; 8: 149–51.

Rodriguez-Bigas MA, Palmer M, Petrelli NJ. Problems encountered in teaching the use of the 65 cm flexible sigmoidoscope in a surgical oncology training program. *J. Cancer Educ.* 1993; 8: 213–6.

Rogge JD, Elmore MF, Mahoney SJ, Brown ED, Troiano FP, Wagner DR, et al. Low cost, office based, screening colonoscopy. *Am. J. Gastroenterol.* 1994; 89: 1775–80.

Rozen P, Ron E. A cost analysis of screening methodology for family members of colorectal cancer patients. *Am. J. Gastroenterol.* 1989; 84: 1548–51.

Rozen P, Baratz M, Fefer F, Gilat T. Low incidence of significant dysplasia in a successful endoscopic surveillance program of patients with ulcerative colitis. *Gastroenterology* 1995; 108: 1361–70.

Sakamoto MS, Hara JH, Schlumpberger JM. Screening flexible sigmoidoscopy in a low risk, highly screened population. *J. Fam. Pract.* 1994; 38: 245–8.

Schmidt D, Jung CE, Wolff G. Changes in the retinal pigment epithelium close to retinal vessels in familial adenomatous polyposis. *Graefes. Arch. Clin. Experimental Ophthalmol.* 1994; 232: 96–102.

Schneider A, Stolte M. Clinical and pathomorphological findings in patients with colorectal carcinoma complicating ulcerative colitis. *Z. Gastroenterol.* 1993; 31: 192–7.

Schnell T, Aranha GV, Sontag SJ, Tode R, Reid S, Chejfec G, et al. Fecal occult blood testing: a false sense of security? *Surgery* 1994; 116: 798–802.

Shibata S, Shiroma T, Tsukiji M, Moroto K, Horimukai F, Miyaoka M, Saito T. Report of colon cancer detection in mass surveys using immunological occult blood test (Latex method). *J. Med. Syst.* 1993; 17: 153–6.

Slusser SO, Liberski SM, McGarrity TJ. Survival of patients diagnosed with colorectal cancer through a television-advertised screening program. *Am. J. Gastroenterol.* 1996; 91: 1563–6.

St John DJ, Young GP, McHutchison JG, Deacon MC, Alexeyeff MA. Comparison of the specificity and sensitivity of Hemoccult and HemoQuant in screening for colorectal neoplasia. *Ann. Intern. Med.* 1992; 117: 376–82.

Thomas WM, White CM, Mah J, Geisser MS, Church TR, Mandel JS. Longitudinal compliance with annual screening for fecal occult blood. Minnesota Colon Cancer Control Study. *Am. J. Epidemiol.* 1995; 142: 176–82.

Thomas WM, Pye G, Hardcastle JD, Chamberlain J, Charnley RM. Role of dietary restriction in Haemoccult screening for colorectal cancer. *Br. J. Surg.* 1989; 76: 976–8.

Thomas WM, Pye G, Hardcastle JD, Mangham CM. Faecal occult blood screening for colorectal neoplasia: a randomized trial of three days or six days of tests. *Br. J. Surg.* 1990; 77: 277–9.

Thomas WM, Pye G, Hardcastle JD, Walker AR. Screening for colorectal carcinoma: an analysis of the sensitivity of haemoccult. *Br. J. Surg.* 1992; 79: 833–5.

Trehu EG, Cooper JN. Cost of screening for colorectal cancer: results of a community mass screening program and review of the literature. *South Med. J.* 1992; 85: 248–54.

Trowers E Jr, Nguyen W, Cobos E. Decision making in colorectal cancer screening. *J. Nat. Med. Assoc.* 1997; 89: 9–12.

Uchman S, Cashel L, Lindenmayer JM. Proposed colorectal cancer screening recommendations. *Medicine & Health.* 1997; 80: 65–7.

Unger SW, Saranto JR, Furlong RJ, Scott JS. Single session panendoscopy. Indications and expectations for yield. *Am. Surg.* 1990; 56: 144–7.

Vasen HF. Periodic examination of families with hereditary nonpolyposis colorectal carcinoma in the Netherlands: a study of 41 families. *Ned. Tijdschr. Geneeskd.* 1994; 138: 77–81.

Vilien M, Jorgensen MJ, Ouyang Q, Schlichting P, Linde J, Riis P, Binder V. Colonic epithelial dysplasia or carcinoma in a regional group of patients with ulcerative colitis of more than 15 years duration. *J. Int. Med.* 1991; 230: 259–63.

Vipond MN, Moshakis V. Four-year evaluation of a direct-access fibreoptic sigmoidoscopy service. *Ann. Roy. Coll. Surg. Eng.* 1996; 78: 23–6.

Wagner JL, Herdman RC, Wadhwa S. Cost effectiveness of colorectal cancer screening in the elderly. *Ann. Intern. Med.* 1991; 115: 807–17.

Walker AR, Whynes DK, Hardcastle JD. Rehydration of guaiac based faecal occult blood tests in mass screening for colorectal cancer. An economic perspective. *Scand. J. Gastroenterol.* 1991*a*; 26: 215–8.

Walker A, Whynes DK, Chamberlain JO, Hardcastle JD. The cost of screening for colorectal cancer. *J. Epidemiol. Community Health* 1991*b*; 45: 220–4.

Walter SD, Frommer DJ, Cook RJ. The estimation of sensitivity and specificity in colorectal cancer screening methods. *Cancer Detect. Prev.* 1991; 15: 465–9.

Wherry DC, Thomas WM. The yield of flexible fiberoptic sigmoidoscopy in the detection of asymptomatic colorectal neoplasia. *Surg. Endosc.* 1994; 8: 393–5.

Wilking N, Petrelli NJ, Herrera Ornelas L, et al. A comparison of the 25 cm rigid proctosigmoidoscope with the 65 cm flexible endoscope in the screening of patients for colorectal carcinoma. *Cancer* 1986; 57: 669–71.

Winawer SJ, O'Brien MJ, Waye JD, Kronborg O, Bond J, Fruhmorgen P, et al. Risk and surveillance of individuals with colorectal polyps. WHO Collaborating Centre for the Prevention of Colorectal Cancer. *Bull. WHO* 1990; 68: 789–95.

Winawer SJ, St John DJ, Bond JH, Rozen P, Burt RW, Waye JD, et al. Prevention of colorectal cancer: guidelines based on new data. WHO Collaborating Center for the Prevention of Colorectal Cancer. *Bull. WHO* 1995; 73: 7–10.

Winawer SJ, Fletcher RH, Miller L, Godlee F, Stolar MH, Mulrow CD, Woolf SH, Glick SN, Ganiats TG, Bond JH, Rosen L, Zapka JG, Olsen SJ, Giardiello FM, Sisk JE, Van Antwerp R, Brown-Davis C, Marciniak DA, Mayer RJ. Colorectal cancer screening: clinical guidelines and rationale. *Gastroenterol.* 1997; 112: 594–642.

Woodward A, Weller D. Colorectal cancer: implications of mass screening for public health. *Med. J. Aust.* 1990; 153: 81–2, 85–8.

Yoshinaga M, Motomura S, Takeda H, Yanagisawa Z, Ikeda K. Evaluation of the sensitivity of an immunochemical fecal occult blood test for colorectal neoplasia. *Am. J. Gastroenterol.* 1995; 90: 1076–9.

Young G, Levin B. Report of UICC colorectal cancer screening workshop. Meeting held in Genoa, Italy, September 29 October 1, 1995. *Int. J. Cancer* 1996; 65: 567–8.

Yu H. Evaluation of RPHA fecal occult blood test in screening for colorectal cancer. *Chung. Hua. Chung. Liu. Tsa. Chih.* 1990; 12: 108–10.

10 Aetiology of colorectal cancer

Incidence

World-wide, colorectal carcinoma accounts for at least 200 000 deaths each year, making it one of the commonest global causes of death from cancer. After carcinoma of the bronchus, cancer of the colon and rectum combined kills more people than any other malignancy in the Western world, accounting for 60 000 deaths each year in the USA (Cresanta 1992; Lieberman 1994). In Western countries colorectal cancer occurs in 5% of the population and accounts for 15% of all deaths from cancer in both men and women (Arbman *et al.* 1995). In America colorectal cancer accounts for one in six of all cancers and affects 150 000 people annually (Lytle 1989). Each year 25 000 new cases and 17 000 deaths are reported in England and Wales. Between 2% and 11% of patients with colorectal cancer will have a synchronous colorectal tumour and 2% will develop a metachronous tumour (Cali *et al.* 1993; Kimura *et al.* 1994) (Figure 10.1).

Age and sex distribution

The incidence of colorectal cancer increases exponentially with age, those over 50 years comprising only 37% of the population yet accounting for over 95% of both colorectal cancer cases and deaths (Figure 10.2). One-quarter of all major laparotomies in those over 70 years are for colorectal cancer. Patients under 40 years account for between 2% and 15% of all cases of large bowel cancer (Yong *et al.* 1990). A 50-year-old American has a 5% risk of developing colorectal cancer by the age of 80 years and a 2.5% chance of dying from it. In those aged under 40 years, the condition is uncommon (3/100 000 population). The incidence rapidly increases over the age of 40, doubling every 5 years until the age of 60 to reach a peak incidence of 500/100 000 in those over 80 years (Neilan 1987; Schatzkin *et al.* 1988; Cooper *et al.* 1995). The average age at presentation, for both sexes, is 65 years (Weaver *et al.* 1991). The mean age at presentation of patients with right colon lesions (71 years) is higher than for either patients with left colon lesions (68 years) or rectal lesions (65 years), largely due to the later presentation of females with caecal or ascending colon cancers (Fleshner *et al.* 1989). Patients with synchronous tumours also tend to be slightly

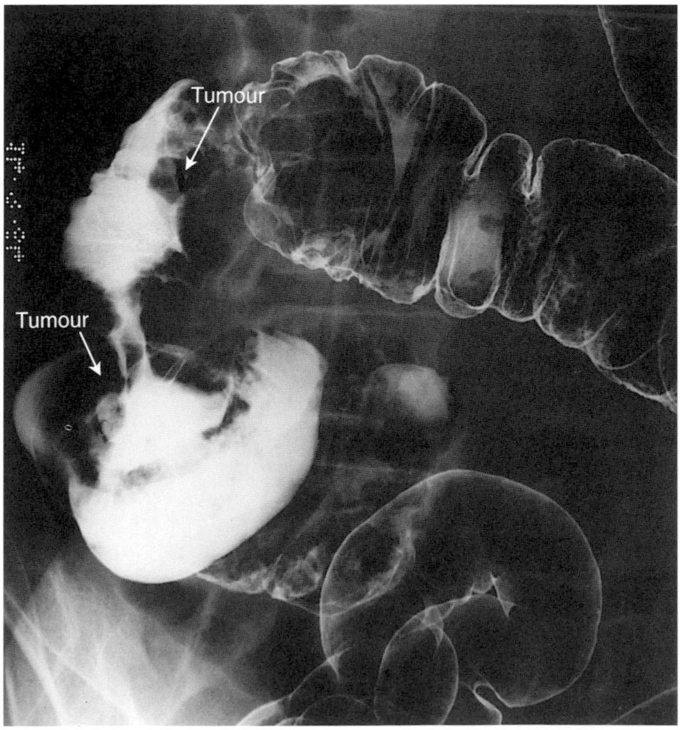

Figure 10.1 Barium enema showing synchronous tumours of the caecum and hepatic flexure.

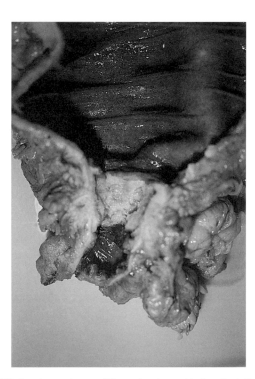

Figure 10.2 Annular carcinoma of the rectum in an elderly patient. Note the dark proximal mucosa of melanosis coli.

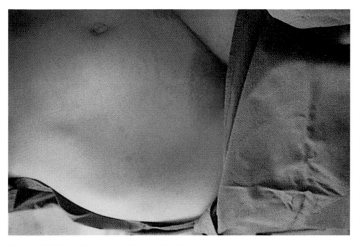

Figure 1.9 Transillumination in the right iliac fossa during colonoscopy signifying the caecum has been reached.

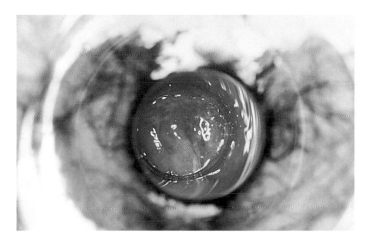

Figure 4.11 Inflamed rectal mucosa due to *C.trachoma*.

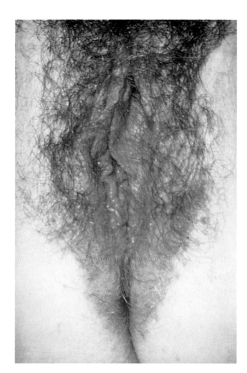

Figure 4.23 Vulval and perianal acute candidiasis. Note the satellite lesions at the margin.

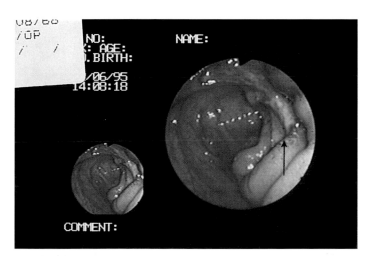

Figure 4.42 Cytomegalovirus ulceration of colon on sigmoidoscopy.

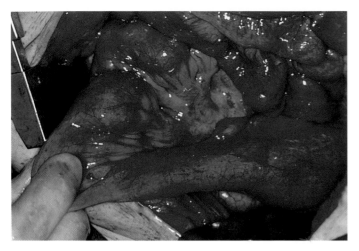

Figure 5.21 'J' pouch following completion.

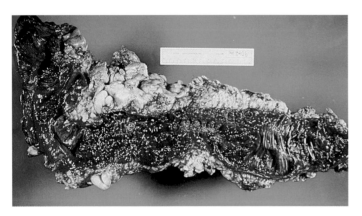

Figure 6.2 Resected Crohn's specimen showing mucosal ulceration, thickening, and mesenteric encroachment.

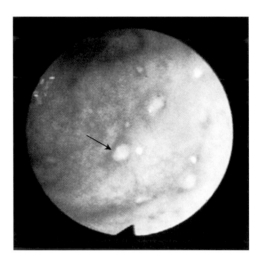

Figure 6.8 Aphthous ulceration in Crohn's disease seen on colonoscopy.

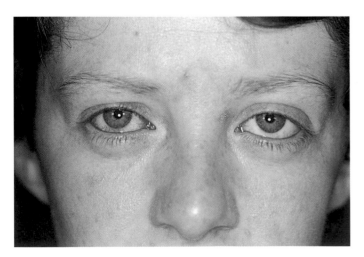

Figure 6.20 Conjunctivitis associated with Crohn's disease.

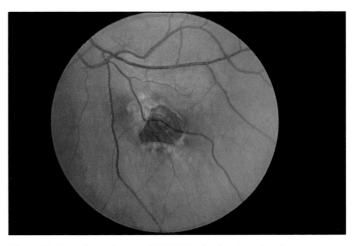

Figure 9.8 Large hyperpigmented CHRPE lesion in polyposis coli.

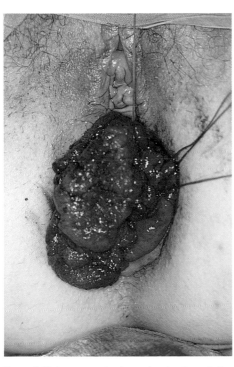

Figure 8.10 Large rectal polyp prolapsing through the anus.

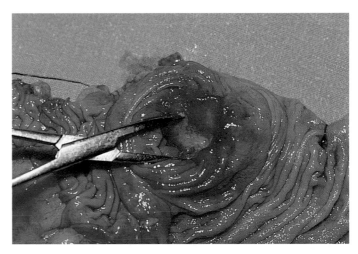

Figure 11.10 Colonic adenocarcinoma involving a lymph node.

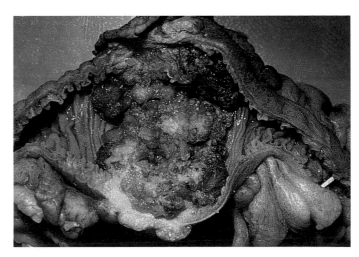

Figure 11.7 Mucinous secreting adenocarcinoma of colon showing the typical colloid appearance.

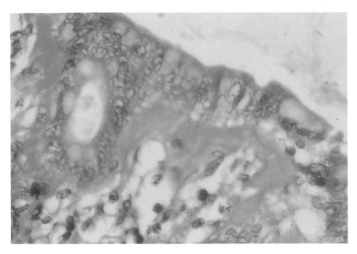

Figure 16.5 Collagenous colitis. Note the marked thickening of the subepithelial collagen band (arrowed).

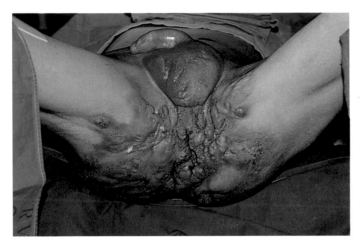

Figure 18.19 Case of extensive hidradenitis suppurativa.

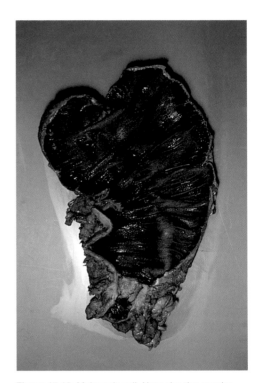

Figure 17.13 Melanosis coli. Note also the annular carcinoma of the rectum (arrowed).

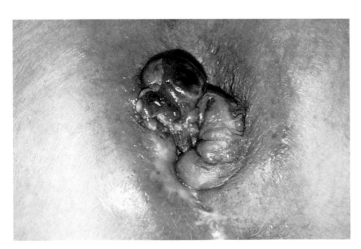

Figure 19.10 Malignant melanoma of the anus referred as a possible thrombosed haemorrhoid. H&E×100.

older (mean age 72 years) and have a higher incidence of associated benign polyps (70%) than those without synchronous carcinomas (Slater *et al.* 1990).

There is a tendency for rectal cancer and left-sided colon cancer to be more common in men, while right-sided colon cancer is more frequently found in older women (DeCosse *et al.* 1993; Howe *et al.* 1993; Stein *et al.* 1993) (Figure 10.2). In America, the age-adjusted incidence of rectal cancer is about 23/100 000 per year for men and 14 cases/100 000 per year for women (Vukasin *et al.* 1990). As the majority of all colorectal tumours are distal, there is a small overall preponderance of men (Stein *et al.* 1993; Deans *et al.* 1994). The distal colon cancer excess among men increases with increasing age, being less apparent, or even reversed, in younger patients. However, with the 'left-to-right' shift that has been noted in colorectal cancer, the incidence of caecal cancer is rising, such that it is now about 15/100 000 per year for both sexes (Vukasin *et al.* 1990; Loffeld *et al.* 1996).

Geographical, social, and racial distribution

Incidence rates, irrespective of sex, tend to be higher in developed countries (age-standardized annual incidence rates of 10–52 per 100 000), than in non-developed countries (less than 10 per 100 000). There is a 50-fold variation in the annual incidence between areas of high incidence (the USA) and those of low incidence (West Africa). Variations in the incidence of colorectal cancer also exist within continents. In Europe the risk is consistently higher in Western than in Eastern and in Northern than in Southern Europe (Ziegler *et al.* 1986). In Asia incidence rates vary, the most Westernized of Asian populations now having risks similar to those of Western Europe (Kuramoto *et al.* 1993). China experiences an intermediate risk (about 25/100 000), similar to those of Eastern Europe, whereas the lowest risk in Asia occurs in Indians. Not only do the incidence rates of colorectal cancer vary within continents, but also within a single country. These differences may be due to racial and environmental (principally dietary) differences within the country (Guo *et al.* 1993). A high incidence of colonic cancer is generally associated with a high incidence of rectal cancer within a particular country. Internationally, however, the incidence of colonic cancer varies to a greater extent than does that of rectal cancer, such that in many countries with low rates of colorectal cancer, the incidence of colonic cancer is less than that of rectal cancer. As the risk of colorectal cancer rises, colonic cancer becomes more frequent than rectal cancer, so that in one of the areas of highest risk (Connecticut), colonic cancer is 1.8 times as common as rectal cancer among men and 2.4 times as common among women (Ziegler *et al.* 1986). It therefore appears that rectal cancer is not as influenced by geographic and epidemiological factors as colonic cancer.

Studies from several countries suggest that poor living conditions in socio-economically less privileged communities contributes to the development of colorectal cancer (Hayes *et al.* 1993; Lindsay *et al.* 1993; van Loon *et al.* 1995). After adjustment for potential biological and other sociogeographical risk factors, relative hazard of death associated with low compared with high socio-economic class is 1.2 for colon cancer and 1.3 for rectal cancer (Brenner *et al.* 1991). Formerly, colorectal cancer rates were consistently reported

higher among urban than rural residents. This has changed over the last 30 years in Western and in African countries that are becoming more westernized due to socio-economic changes (Mayor-Davies *et al.* 1992; Howe *et al.* 1993).

Improved socio-economic factors may explain the rising incidence of colorectal cancer among American black people. This group, who had a low incidence of colorectal cancer in the 1930s, now have an equal incidence of colorectal cancer to their white counterparts. However, despite the similar overall incidence, the prognosis of colorectal cancer has not improved to the same extent in black as in white people (Cordice and Johnson 1991; Weaver *et al.* 1991; Thomas *et al.* 1992). The incidence of right-sided tumours display little difference between blacks and whites. However, tumours of the transverse and descending colon are more frequent in black people while cancer of the sigmoid, rectosigmoid, and rectum is 1.7 times more common in white people (Thomas *et al.* 1992). There is no evidence that colorectal cancer is a more aggressive disease in black than in white people, as outcomes are similar among black and white patients who receive equal access to comparable medical care in spite of socio-economic differences (Thomas *et al.* 1992; Akerley *et al.* 1993; Coates *et al.* 1995; van't Hof *et al.* 1995).

Time trends

World-wide, colonic cancer incidence rates are increasing 1.5–3% annually, with the incidence of rectal cancer increasing more rapidly in low, rather than in high, incidence areas (De Stefani *et al.* 1994). In America over the last 50 years, the age-adjusted incidence for all colorectal cancers has increased from 35 to 70 cases/100 000 per year for men and from 32 to 49 cases/100 000 per year for women (Vukasin *et al.* 1990; Beard *et al.* 1995). From 1973 to 1986 the incidence of colorectal cancer in the USA rose by 9.4%, with an estimated annual percentage change of 0.7% (Schatzkin *et al.* 1988). Similar changes have been noted in Australia, New Zealand, and Denmark and are thought to be related to dietary changes and improvements in reporting (Cox and Little 1992; Johansen *et al.* 1993). The incidence in Japan has also been rising over the last 30 years (Nomiyama *et al.* 1996).

Formerly, about one-half of all large bowel cancers occurred in the rectum or rectosigmoid, 25% in the sigmoid with the remainder spread evenly throughout the more proximal colon. There is considerable evidence suggesting a 'left-to-right' shift in colorectal cancer over the last few decades, so that about one-third of tumours now arise in the right colon (Beart *et al.* 1995; Loffeld *et al.* 1996). Currently, the right colon and rectosigmoid regions each harbour approximately 25% of colon tumours. Therefore, the classic medical teaching that over 50% of colorectal cancers would be detectable by digital examination and/or proctosigmoidoscopy is no longer accurate (Vukasin *et al.* 1990).

A Swiss study revealed the percentage of tumours in the ascending colon increased significantly from 27% in 1978–83 to 33% 1984–88, while rectal cancer declined by 10% over the same period (Levi *et al.* 1993). Other European studies have also identified a recent increase in the proportion of proximal, and decrease in the number of rectal tumours (Sariego *et al.* 1992). This shift to the right may be partially due to the general ageing of the population, as the elderly tend to be more prone to develop right colon tumours (Fleshner *et al.* 1989) (Figure 10.3). Time trend studies indicate

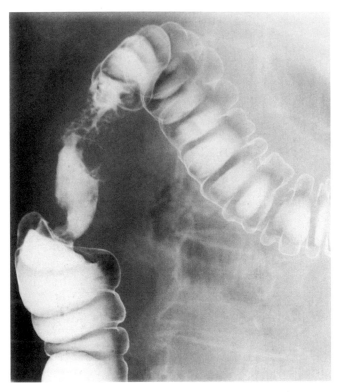

Figure 10.3 Barium enema showing typical 'apple-core' deformity of carcinoma of the ascending colon.

Table 10.1 Enviromental factors known to increase the risk of developing colorectal adenomas or carcinoma

Factor	Author
Low-fibre, high-saturated fat diet	Giovannucci *et al.* 1992 Hoff *et al.* 1992 Kono *et al.* 1993
Obesity	Neugut *et al.* 1991
Bile acids	Ponz *et al.* 1987
Cholecystectomy	Neugut *et al.* 1991 Giovannucci *et al.* 1993 Reid *et al.* 1996
Alcohol and smoking	Zahm *et al.* 1991 Honjo *et al.* 1992 Sandler *et al.* 1993
Non-steroidal anti-inflammatory drugs	Hixson *et al.* 1993 Waddell 1994
Calcium	Barsoum *et al.* 1992 Kleibeuker *et al.* 1993 Kampman *et al.* 1994 Neugut *et al.* 1996
Physical activity	Kono *et al.* 1991

that the skewed subsite distribution of large bowel cancer in different age groups may increase with time. In one study, subsite distribution (right colon, left colon, rectum) for different age groups (25–49, 50–69, over 70 years) was significantly skewed, with an excess of right colonic cancer in individuals aged 25–49 years and over 70 years (Jass 1991). This right colonic excess was accompanied by a relative reduction in left colonic cancer. There was a marked reduction in the incidence of left colonic cancer and rectal cancer in individuals under 50 years. In contrast, the incidence of right colonic cancer remained relatively stable in young individuals (Jass 1991). A characteristic of the cancer family syndrome (three or more first-degree relatives affected by cancer) is a significantly larger proportion of patients with neoplasms located in proximal colonic segments. Similarly, colorectal tumours among relatives are more frequent in patients with right-side cancer. Some suggest that the differences in sex ratio at different colonic subsites, the higher fraction of adenocarcinomas with adenomas in cancer of the more distal tracts of the large bowel, and the more marked familial occurrence of colorectal cancer in patients with right-side neoplasms tend to support the view that cancer of the proximal colon, cancer of the distal colon, and cancer of the rectum may actually be three different types of tumours (Ponz de Leon 1990).

Aetiology

The exact cause of colorectal cancer is unknown but it most likely results from a multifactorial interaction between environmental and genetic factors (Table 10.1). Environmental and dietary factors are considered responsible for 90% of all cases and genetic causes for about 10% (Vargas and Alberts 1992).

Environmental factors

Diet

Diet is thought to be a major environmental factor in the aetiology of colorectal cancer, the risk of colon cancer increasing with the amount of food consumed (Kune *et al.* 1992; Suadicani *et al.* 1993). Meal frequency may act by influencing the enterohepatic circulation of bile and, consequently, the exposure time of intestinal mucosa to bile acids (Franceschi *et al.* 1992). Although several dietary factors have been implicated in colorectal cancer, two principal theories have arisen, the fat theory and the fibre theory.

The fat theory
This is derived from the knowledge that the incidence of bowel cancer closely correlates with the amount of dietary fat (Reddy 1995). The diet also controls the composition of colonic bacterial flora which is known to produce carcinogens from biliary steroids.

There is a correlation between the incidence of large bowel cancer and fat consumption, suggesting that dietary fat, including cholesterol, may play a part in large bowel carcinogenesis (Reddy 1993). A high proportion of fat is normally derived from meat and there is a strong association between large bowel cancer and overall meat consumption (Macrae 1993). This has been linked to mutagenic compounds including polycyclic aromatic hydrocarbons and heterocyclic amines produced by cooking (Nagao and Sugimura 1993). Their precursors are amino acids in meat and fish as well as sugars. Intake of red meat is associated with an increased risk of developing colorectal cancer of between 1.5 and 2.5 times that of non-meat-eaters, (sugars also having been linked to an increased risk of colorectal cancer) (Bruce *et al.* 1993; Steinmetz and Potter 1993). In addition to frequent meat intake, the method of cooking is important (frying being associated with a greater risk than boiling) (Gerhardsson *et al.* 1991). Saturated fat, the ratio of red meat to chicken and fish and carbohydrate intake have also been associated with colorectal polyp formation, particularly in women. However, some large studies have failed to show a relationship between either meat or fat consumption and the incidence of colorectal cancer. While most epidemiological and experimental data indicate a direct relationship between dietary fat, caloric intake and the development of colon cancer, the effect of dietary cholesterol is still unclear (Schatzkin *et al.* 1988). There is a developing literature concerning a relationship between serum cholesterol levels and the risk for colon cancer (Broitman *et al.* 1993). One such study suggested an aetiological role for cholesterol by finding a link between egg consumption and colorectal cancer, particularly proximal colon cancer in females (Steinmetz and Potter 1993). While the relationship between serum cholesterol and colonic or intestinal cholesterol metabolism is presently not understood, genetic studies provide a promising, although as yet unexplored, potential association. Alterations which occur during the developmental progression of colonic cancer include changes in chromosome 5, which also carries two genes vital to the biosynthesis and regulation of systemic and cellular cholesterol metabolism. Colonic cancer cells possess a diminished ability to use low-density lipoproteins to support cellular growth and such a loss would provide a growth advantage to tumour cells (Broitman *et al.* 1993).

Bile acids

Faecal bile acid concentration is increased by dietary fat and meat and is decreased by cereal fibre. In populations who are at risk for colonic cancer, faecal bile acid concentration and excretion of neutral sterols in stools correlates with colorectal cancer incidence and mucosal proliferative index, both being higher in colonic cancer cases than in controls (Gregoire *et al.* 1992; Imray *et al.* 1992). Bile acids have therefore been proposed as potential carcinogens capable of modifying DNA (Alberts *et al.* 1996).

As a consequence of the increased levels of secondary bile acids in the enterohepatic circulation there has been speculation concerning a link between colorectal cancer and both previous peptic ulcer surgery and cholecystectomy. Peptic ulcer surgery favours the formation of carcinogenic N-nitroso compounds in the gastric remnant which may explain the increased risk of cancer at sites in the gastrointestinal tract distant from the stomach (Offerhaus *et al.* 1988). In one study, the incidence of neoplasms greater than 1 cm in patients who had undergone vagotomy was 14% compared with 3% in those who had had no gastric surgery (Mullan *et al.* 1990). This increased risk of colorectal neoplasia 10 years after truncal vagotomy was attributed to altered bile acid metabolism. Some studies have shown that patients who have previously undergone gastrectomy are at a significantly increased risk of developing colorectal carcinoma (Mizusawa *et al.* 1990). Others have failed to support this and suggest that, both conditions being common some years ago, any association between vagotomy and colorectal cancer is purely coincidental (Tersmette *et al.* 1990).

Over 60 studies have investigated the hypothesis that the risk of colorectal cancer is increased following cholecystectomy and have yielded inconsistent findings (Dubrow *et al.* 1992; Jorgensen and Rafaelsen 1992; Ekbom *et al.* 1993; Zuccato *et al.* 1993) (Figure 10.4). In a review by Giovannucci *et al* (1993), the combined results from 33 case–control studies showed an association between cholecystectomy and risk of colorectal cancer (pooled relative risk 1.3),

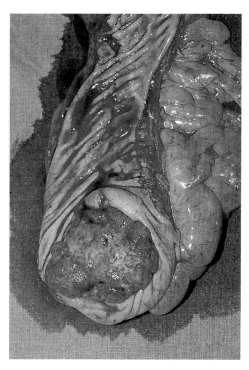

Figure 10.4 Carcinoma of the caecum in a patient who had a cholecystectomy 10 years previously.

particularly when limited to the proximal colon (relative risk 1.9). In most studies, the risk was stronger when the first 5–15 years following the surgery were excluded. The results from six cohort studies, with follow-up to approximately 15 years post-cholecystectomy, were generally null (relative risk 0.97). The authors concluded that because the risks varied substantially by study design and because time since cholecystectomy or potentially confounding factors were often not considered, they could not firmly quantitate the risk of colorectal cancer in cholecystectomized patients. However, the findings were consistent with other evidence suggesting some aspect of bile acid metabolism increases the risk of cancer of the proximal colon (Giovannucci *et al.* 1993).

The fibre theory

In 1971 Denis Burkitt put forward an hypothesis of a fibre-depleted aetiology for colorectal cancer based on the difference in patterns of diseases between Western and traditional African societies. In a meta-analysis of 13 case–control studies, 12 suggested that intake of dietary fibre and the risk of colon cancer were inversely associated (Howe *et al.* 1992; Dwyer 1993). Soluble fibres are metabolized by gut bacteria to yield detoxified products, thus reducing colon carcinogenesis (Weisburger *et al.* 1993). Insoluble fibres increase stool size, the larger bulk diluting carcinogens, especially tumour promoters such as secondary bile acids and lowering the risk of colon cancer (Weisburger *et al.* 1993).

Therefore experimental and clinical evidence suggests that an increase in dietary fibre does have a protective role in colorectal cancer (Lewin 1991; Alberts *et al.* 1996). A high-fibre diet appears to reduce the risk of colorectal cancer in several ways.

1. High dietary fibre content reduces intestinal transit time and dilutes carcinogens therefore decreasing the contact between intestinal mucosa and colonic cancer initiators.

2. Dietary fibre raises the colonic pH with consequent reduction in the bacterial degradation of bile salts (Gregoire *et al.* 1992).
3. Bacterial proliferation resultant on fibre intake, uses up available ammonia so reduces the amount which may predispose to malignant transformation in colonic mucosal cells.
4. Substantial amounts of starch are available for fermentation which may be protective against colorectal cancer.
5. Poorly fermentable fibres such as cellulose appear to inhibit tumour production, although viscous fibres are extensively fermented, producing short chain fatty acids which can stimulate mucosal proliferation leading to colonic cancer.

The fibre content of vegetables may also protect against colorectal cancer (Howe *et al.* 1992). Studies of religious groups support the protective effect of vegetables. In western India an extremely low incidence is seen in strict vegetarian Hindu compared with other religious sects, while in America, Seventh Day Adventists, also strict vegetarians, have incidence rates 60–70% those of the typical white American population (Vogel and McPherson 1989).

While the fat and fibre theories at first appear to be in direct opposition, evidence now suggests that high-fat intake, in conjunction with low-fibre intake may increase the risk of bowel cancer (Macrae 1991), due to their effect on cell replication.

Other dietary factors that have been implicated in the aetiology of colorectal cancer include vitamins, minerals, trace elements, and beverages, particularly alcohol.

Vitamins, minerals, and trace elements

Vitamins 'A', 'E', and 'C' are antioxidant micronutrients which defend the body against free radicals and reactive oxygen molecules. They have been suggested as possible protective factors for colorectal cancer (Bostick *et al.* 1993). However, the influence of these vitamins in the aetiology of colorectal cancer is considerably weakened once the amount of dietary fibre has been taken into account (Dwyer 1993). Vitamin D and calcium have also been linked to colorectal cancer in a protective manner (Kampman *et al.* 1994; Braun *et al.* 1995; Alberts *et al.* 1996). Mechanisms of calcium inhibition are still speculative, but a 'calcium soaps' hypothesis, fatty acid destabilization of cellular membranes and modulation of protein kinase C and K-*ras* mutations have been suggested (Pence 1993). The calcium soap theory suggests that bile acids are bound to calcium, making them insoluble and harmless. The other theories purport that vitamin D and calcium reduce epithelial cell proliferation while inducing differentiation (Govers *et al.* 1994; Bostick *et al.* 1995; Alberts *et al.* 1996). Calcium supplementation affects intestinal bile acids and mucosal cell proliferation without altering the incidence of colorectal cancer (Welberg *et al.* 1993; Cats *et al.* 1995).

Trace elements, notably selenium, have been linked with a reduced risk of colorectal cancer rates (Nelson *et al.* 1996). In one study, patients with low plasma selenium concentrations were significantly more likely to have one or more adenomatous polyps (prevalence odds ratio 4.2) and more adenomatous polyps (3.5 times) per patient than those with normal concentrations (Clark *et al.* 1993). However, other studies have found that, although there is a small inverse association between selenium and colonic cancer, this did not reach statistical significance (van den Brandt *et al.* 1993). The importance of selenium in colorectal cancer may be linked to polyamine biosynthesis by their common requirement for S-adenosylmethionine (McGarrity *et al.* 1993).

Beverages

Coffee and tea, through their effect on serum cholesterol and bile acid metabolism have been implicated with an increased risk of colorectal cancer in some, but not all, studies (Moran 1992; Kohlmeier *et al.* 1997). This may be partly related to the addition of sugar (La Vecchia *et al.* 1993).

A review of the relationship between alcohol consumption and colorectal cancer in 52 major studies has been performed by Kune and Vitetta (1992). These generally support a correlation between alcohol and colorectal cancer. An association was found in five of the seven correlational studies, half of the 31 case–control studies and 10 of the 14 cohort studies. When the type of alcohol consumed was examined separately, beer was the principal type of at-risk alcoholic beverage, with much less risk for spirits and least risk for wine and the association was dose-responsive (Meyer and White 1993; Newcomb *et al.* 1993; Giovannucci *et al.* 1995a). The hypotheses of alcohol as a direct and specific colorectal carcinogen include increased mucosal cell proliferation, the activation of intestinal procarcinogens, and the role of unabsorbed carcinogens, particularly in beer. General or indirect carcinogenic effects of alcohol include immunodepression, activation of liver pro-carcinogens, and changes in bile composition, as well as the nitrosamine content of alcoholic beverages and increased tissue nitrosamine levels (Kune and Vitetta 1992).

Several clinical trials are currently underway to determine if dietary intervention can reduce the risk of colorectal cancer. An intake of calcium of 1.5–2.0 g/day significantly decreases DNA synthesizing cells of high-risk patients while chronic wheat bran supplementation appears to decrease both rectal mucosal DNA synthesis and polyp recurrence (Alberts *et al.* 1990; Vargas and Alberts 1992). Accumulation of DNA methylation abnormalities, observed during progression of human colorectal neoplasia, may be influenced by certain dietary factors. The apparent protective effect of fresh fruits and vegetables, the major folate sources, on colorectal cancer incidence suggests that a methyl-deficient diet contributes to occurrence of this malignancy. Low dietary folate and methionine and high intake of alcohol may reduce levels of S-adenosylmethionine, which is required for DNA methylation (Giovannucci *et al.* 1993). It is estimated that the risk of colorectal cancer in the American population could be reduced by 30% by an average increase in fibre intake of 13 g/day (Howe *et al.* 1992). A diet in which chicken and fish are substituted for red meat with increased intake of vegetables, fruits, and grains has been advocated significantly to reduce the incidence of colorectal cancer (Giovannucci *et al.* 1992; Wynder *et al.* 1992).

Several other factors, known to be implicated in other tumours, have been investigated for their role in colorectal cancer (Table 10.1).

Drugs

Eicosanoids have been implicated in colon carcinogenesis (Turner and Berkel 1993; Paginini-Hill *et al.* 1994). Aspirin and other non-steroidal anti-inflammatory drugs (NSAIDs) which inhibit prostaglandin synthesis are therefore thought to be protective against colorectal cancer (Paginnini-Hill 1994). In one study among patients reporting use of aspirin two or more times a day, the odds ratios for colorectal cancer and polyps were 0.3 and 0.4 compared with those of screening clinic visitors and hospital control subjects, respectively (Su *et al.* 1993; Smigel 1994). In another study, regular users of aspirin had a lower risk for total colorectal cancer (relative risk 0.7) and metastatic or fatal colorectal cancer (Giovannucci *et al.* 1994). Others have reported death rates to be approximately 40% lower among persons who used aspirin regularly compared with those who used no aspirin. (Thun *et al.* 1993). This suggests that the protective effect of aspirin and other NSAIDs in the development of human colon cancer may be mediated, at least in part, through their inhibition of arachidonic acid metabolism by cyclo-oxygenase (Rigas *et al.* 1993). The hypothesis is supported by studies showing that dietary fish oil reduces the rate of proliferation in colorectal epithelium and may protect against colon cancer (Bartram *et al.* 1993).

In one Danish study, use of antihypertensive medicine and minor tranquillizers were highly significantly associated with risk of colon cancer (relative risk 3.5) but not rectal cancer (Suadicani *et al.* 1993). Some studies suggest a statistically significant risk exists for oral contraceptive use and rectal cancer but not for colon cancer (La Vecchia and Franceschi 1991), others that there is no such association (Chute *et al.* 1991; Fernandez *et al.* 1996). There is evidence suggesting that smokers may have a higher risk of developing colorectal adenomas and cancer than non-smokers (Jacobsen *et al.* 1995). In one study, compared with men who had never smoked, the estimated relative risk of adenoma increased with the pack-year smoking number, the average number of cigarettes per day, and the total years smoked (overall relative risk 2.2) (Kikendall *et al.* 1989). In other studies, men and women who smoked were found to have more advanced disease and lower mean age at diagnosis of both colon and rectum cancer than non-smokers (Anton 1991; Kune *et al.* 1992). A review of 18 case–control studies showed an elevated risk for cigar-smoking black males in one study, a statistically non-significant increased risk for current smokers in one of three cohort studies and a statistically significant elevation of risk for smokers in two of three studies of adenomatous large bowel polyps (Kune *et al.* 1992). The authors concluded that although at present there is insufficient evidence to link smoking with large bowel cancer, the possibility that ingested tobacco is in some way carcinogenic for the colorectal mucosa warrants further study.

Physical activity

Increasing physical exercise has been related to decreased risk of developing colorectal cancer (Giovannucci *et al.* 1995*b*). A significantly decreased risk of left-sided colon cancer was observed in persons involved in more than 20 years of physically active work and a significantly decreased risk of rectal cancer in persons involved in more than 20 years of sedentary work (Arbman *et al.* 1993; Chow *et al.* 1993). In one study, relative to males in high physical activity occupations, males in sedentary occupations had an increased incidence of both cancer of the colon (relative risk 1.2) and rectum (relative risk 1.3) (Fraser and Pearce 1993). It is suggested that middle-aged men may reduce their risk of colorectal cancer if they exercise when they are not working (Markowitz *et al.* 1992). However, no relationship with exercise was noted in the Melbourne Colorectal Cancer Study (Kune *et al.* 1990).

Hormones

Sex hormones have been related to colonic cancer, an increased risk of proximal colonic cancer being associated with low parity. More recent studies have also suggested that women who have children are at significantly decreased risk of colon cancer relative to nulliparous females (Cantor *et al.* 1993). A comparison between parity and colorectal cancer risk in America and China revealed no association in China. In America, risks for cancers of both the colon and rectum were lower among parous compared with nulliparous women (odds ratio 0.6), but the trend in risk was not smooth with increas-

ing number of live births (Wu Williams *et al.* 1991). Other reproductive factors, including age at menarche, age at first live birth, and menopausal status, are not significantly associated with an increased risk of colorectal cancer (Chute *et al.* 1991; Wu Williams *et al.* 1991; Jacobsen *et al.* 1995). Among known associations with reduced colorectal cancer risk, women appear to ingest more dietary fibre, seem to benefit more from physical activity, and consume less alcohol. Although these differences may contribute to the risk differential, hormonal events during reproductive years also appear to be important (DeCosse *et al.* 1993). There is no consistent association between oestrogen replacement therapy and the incidence of colorectal cancer (Calle *et al.* 1995; MacLennan *et al.* 1995; Newcomb and Storer 1995).

Gut hormones, particularly gastrin and somatostatin, act as trophic factors in the gastrointestinal tract affecting colon cell proliferation and differentiation (Xu *et al.* 1994). It is suggested that aberrant expression of gastrin may contribute to deregulated proliferation of colorectal carcinomas (Finley *et al.* 1993). Although some believe that fasting serum gastrin concentrations are elevated in colorectal cancer patients and fall following tumour resection, others disagree (Charnley *et al.* 1992; Yapp *et al.* 1992).

Pelvic radiotherapy

There is considerable circumstantial evidence that pelvic irradiation may induce human colorectal cancer, the average interval between radiation and diagnosis of colorectal cancer being 10 years (Tomoda *et al.* 1989; Levitt *et al.* 1990; Kimura *et al.* 1995) (Figure 10.5). In atomic bomb survivors, the risk of colon cancer increased significantly with intestinal dose, but no definite increase of risk was observed for rectal cancer (Natatsuka *et al.* 1992; Ron *et al.* 1995). Radiation probably induces carcinogenesis by a combination of inducing oncogene point mutation and chromosome translocation (Hall and Freyer 1991).

Pathological conditions

Studies on several pathological conditions have given insight into the aetiology of colorectal cancer. These include colorectal adenomas and the adenoma–carcinoma sequence, inflammatory bowel disease,

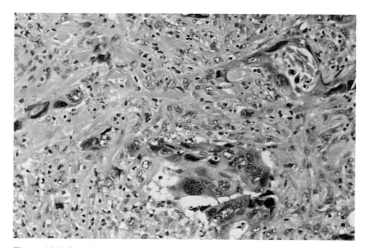

Figure 10.5 Rectal carcinoma in a patient who had received pelvic radiotherapy for cervical carcinoma 11 years previously. H&E×250.

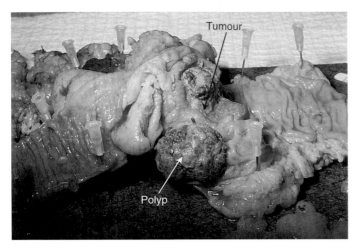

Figure 10.6 Specimen showing colonic carcinoma (arrowed) with adjacent polyp.

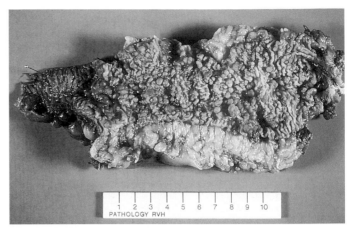

Figure 10.7 Rectal stump in a patient with familial polyposis coli. Several of the polyps showed histological evidence of severe dysplasia.

and recent genetic discoveries in familial polyposis coli and family cancer syndromes.

Carcinomas arising from adenomas (adenoma–carcinoma sequence)

For many years it has been considered that the majority of colonic carcinomas arise in adenomas that have undergone malignant transition (Fearon 1994) (Figure 10.6). Although this hypothesis remains unproven, there is a wealth of circumstantial evidence to support it (Hermanek 1992; Jacoby *et al.* 1995). Many of the factors associated with the aetiology of colorectal cancer are also implicated in the causation of colorectal adenomas.

Studies on site distribution reveal that small polyps tend to be evenly distributed throughout the colon and rectum, while polyps of 1 cm or larger, predominantly occur in the proximal and distal colon. Adenomas located in the left colon have a 1.5 increased frequency of high-grade dysplasia than more proximal polyps (O'Brien *et al.* 1990). There is also a significant increase of cell replication and a marked upward expansion of the proliferative zone in patients with adenomatous polyps, which is most marked in the left colon and rectum (Roncucci *et al.* 1993). This distribution is similar to that of carcinoma, suggesting polyps may be causally related to colorectal cancer.

The risk of colorectal carcinoma in patients or their relatives with polyps is between three and six times that of the general population and patients who develop colorectal cancers often have polyps that pre-date the cancer by many years (Hermanek 1992; Meagher and Stuart 1994; Winawer *et al.* 1996). Between one-third and one half of all bowel cancer specimens contain one or more adenomas and polypectomy does reduce the incidence of colorectal cancer (Winawer *et al.* 1993). The mortality from colorectal cancer in patients with colorectal polyps is almost twice that of the general population, the increase being almost entirely confined to subjects who have adenomatous polyps (Simons *et al.* 1992). In one study severe dysplasia was found in half and malignant transformation in one-fifth of those with adenomatous polyps and coincidental colorectal carcinoma, compared with 20% and 7%, respectively, of those patients with only adenomatous polyps (Zisiadis *et al.* 1993). This association is unlikely to be coincidental as metachronous cancers develop in over 5% of those with a history of polyps, a figure twice

that of those without polyps. In addition, adenomas are found in three-quarters of patients with synchronous colorectal cancers.

Detailed histopathological investigations have documented the transition from adenoma to carcinoma. The risk of malignancy increases with the size, villous architecture, and degree of epithelial dysplasia in a polyp (Muto *et al.* 1975; Bedenne *et al.* 1992; Simons *et al.* 1992). Relative to small adenomas, medium-sized adenomas are three times and large adenomas, eight times, more likely to display high-grade dysplasia, while the risk for villous adenomas is between three and 11 times that of tubular adenomas (O'Brien *et al.* 1990). The number of adenomas affects the risk for high-grade dysplasia patients, with five or more adenomas showing a high risk (15%) of having colon cancer that is particularly prone to arise from the right side (O'Brien *et al.* 1990; Schuman *et al.* 1990). The inevitable development of colorectal cancer in the adenomatous polyps of patients with familial polyposis also supports the concept of the adenoma–carcinoma sequence (Tierney *et al.* 1990) (Figure 10.7).

Recent molecular biology findings also support the concept of the adenoma as a step in the evolution of large bowel cancer (Hamilton 1992; Gerdes *et al.* 1993; Fearon 1994). Chromosomal abnormalities are found in 60% of polyps in patients with a positive family history of colorectal cancer (Dave *et al.* 1993). As in colorectal cancer formation, the adenomatous polyposis (APC) gene mutation plays a part in adenoma progression, its frequency being significantly higher (relative risk 6.7) in lesions with a more villous morphology (Varesco *et al.* 1993; Thomas and Olschwang 1995). A variety of oncogenes and tumour suppressor genes are altered during progression of adenomas. The mutation frequency of K-*ras* increases steadily from flat adenomas (25%) through polypoid adenomas (67%) to cancers (75%) (Yamashita *et al.* 1995). K-*ras* mutations at codon 12 occur in 35% of both sporadic adenomas and carcinomas, the frequency of mutations increasing with the size and severity of dysplastic change in the adenoma (Boughdady *et al.* 1992; Pretlow *et al.* 1993; Yamashita *et al.* 1995). Overexpression of c-*myc* oncogenes also occurs in both colorectal adenomas and cancers (Salem *et al.* 1993). These findings suggest that *ras* and *myc* gene mutations give a selective growth advantage to those polyps with mutations. This allows them to increase in size and prepares the way for malignant transformation (Boughdady *et al.* 1992; Pretlow *et al.* 1993).

Siblings and parents of patients with adenomatous polyps are at increased risk for colorectal cancer. In a recent study, the relative risk of colorectal cancer, adjusted for the year of birth and sex, was

1.8 for the parents and siblings of the patients with adenomas as compared with the spouse controls (Winawer *et al.* 1996). The relative risk for siblings of patients in whom adenomas were diagnosed before 60 years of age was 2.6 as compared with the siblings of patients who were 60 or older at the time of diagnosis and after adjustment for the sibling's year of birth and sex and a parental history of colorectal cancer. The risk increased with decreasing age at the time of the diagnosis of adenoma. The relative risk for the siblings of patients who had a parent with colorectal cancer, as compared with those who had no parent with cancer, was 3.25, after adjustment for the sibling's year of birth and sex and the patient's age at diagnosis (Winawer *et al.* 1996).

Histochemical investigations have demonstrated that abnormalities of DNA content, enzyme activities, carcino-embryonic antigen (CEA) expression, and mucin composition are shared by both adenoma and carcinoma. DNA abnormalities detected by flow cytometry progressively increase from normal mucosa through benign adenomas and early invasive carcinoma to frankly invasive tumours. The proportion and number of antigens expressed (including CEA, CA 19-9, and CA-50) also increase progressively from normal mucosa to carcinoma. Both adenomatous polyps and colorectal carcinoma have significantly increased levels of plasminogen activator activity relative to that of normal colon. Plasminogen activator activity plays an important part in the degradation of epithelial basement membrane, allowing transition of adenomatous polyps to invasive carcinoma.

Not all studies, however, support the existence of the adenoma–carcinoma sequence. In an autopsy study, the lowest proportion of adenomas was found in the rectum, the segment in which cancer is most frequent. In a chromosomal study, the respective frequencies of cytogenetic alterations varied inversely between adenomas and adenocarcinomas, suggesting that they may evolve differently (Longy *et al.* 1993). Another study suggested that it cannot always be assumed that the histological finding of cancer in a polyp that has been observed for many years represents 'malignant degeneration' of a previously benign neoplasm (Koretz 1993). Other pathological studies found that infiltrating and ulcero-infiltrating tumours, which represented 40% of all resected colorectal cancers, very rarely displayed adenomatous tissue (0.5%) (Bedenne *et al.* 1992). It is also suggested that the flat or superficial-type adenocarcinomas also may not progress by the classical adenoma–carcinoma pathway (Jass 1989; Lanspa *et al.* 1992a).

Therefore, although a large number of colorectal cancers do appear to arise from polyps, the numbers may not be as large as was previously thought. Rather the presence of polyps indicates a diffusely abnormal state ('field change') that renders the colorectal mucosa more prone to develop further benign or malignant polyps. The malignant potential of most colorectal adenomas is reflected not only in the overt histological transition to carcinoma, but also in the disruption of the genetic and biochemical control mechanisms of cellular function (Tierney *et al.* 1990).

Inflammatory bowel disease

Ulcerative colitis

Ulcerative colitis accounts for less than 1% of all colorectal cancers, with an estimated incidence of 700 per 100 000 in those with ulcerative colitis affecting the entire colon (Figures 10.8 and 10.9). In most large series, about 3% of patients with ulcerative colitis will develop colorectal carcinoma and over 80% of patients with cancer and colitis exhibit total colonic inflammatory involvement (Sugita

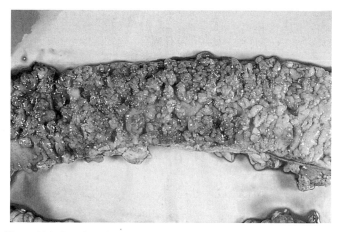

Figure 10.8 Pseudo-polyposis in a patient with long-standing ulcerative colitis.

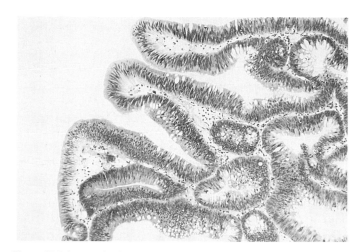

Figure 10.9 Low-grade dysplasia in ulcerative colitis. Note the extensive stratification of nuclei lining the mucosal glands. H&E×100.

et al. 1991; Schneider *et al.* 1993). However, some have found that, although the incidence of colorectal cancer in patients with haemorrhagic proctitis was zero, that for pancolitis and left-sided colitis was equal (Kvist *et al.* 1989). Patients with left-sided colitis develop both their colitis and their cancers about a decade later than those with extensive disease (Sugita *et al.* 1991; Mellemkjaer *et al.* 1995).

A correlation with the duration of colitis has been suggested (Lashner *et al.* 1995; Rhodes 1996). In the first decade of symptoms the risks are negligible, while in the second decade 1–7% of patients will develop carcinoma, representing a 20-fold increased risk relative to age–sex matched controls (Levin and Dozios 1991; Ekbom *et al.* 1992). In most studies colorectal cancer normally develops 12–20 years after the onset of colitis and patients who have had symptoms for more than 30 years have a 10% reported risk of colorectal cancer (Lennard-Jones *et al.* 1990; Sugita *et al.* 1991; Schneider *et al.* 1993). In patients with extensive colitis (at least as far as the hepatic flexure) undergoing colonoscopic surveillance, the cumulative incidence of cancer at 15, 20, and 25 years was 3, 5, and 9% (Lennard-Jones *et al.* 1990). No patient developed cancer if the disease had been present for less than 10 years. With an active approach to medical and surgical treatment, based upon colonoscopic screening, patients whose colons are left intact appear to have no significantly increased risk of colorectal malignancy. With such an approach, the calculated cumulative cancer incidence in a Danish study was 3% after 25 years, the same for colitics as for the normal population (3.5%) (Langholz *et al.* 1992).

The younger the age of onset the greater the likelihood of developing cancer, although the relationship between the activity of the disease and carcinoma at the time of diagnosis appears to be variable (Levin and Dozios 1991; von Herbay *et al.* 1994; Mellemkjaer *et al.* 1995). One population-based study identified age at onset of ulcerative colitis as an independent factor, risk at 35 years after onset being 40% for patients whose colitis began at an early age (Macrae 1991). In another study of 100 cases of carcinoma in ulcerative colitis, there was a strong direct correlation between the age at onset of ulcerative colitis and age at diagnosis of cancer for patients with both extensive and left-sided colitis (Sugita *et al.* 1991). In a recent study of inflammatory bowel disease (IBD) patients who developed colorectal cancer, the cancer developed at a younger age (average 7 years earlier) and was characterized by a more proximal localization when compared with colorectal cancers of non-IBD patients (Bansal and Sonnenberg 1996). Sclerosing cholangitis was a strong risk factor for developing colon cancer while NSAIDs were protective against colon cancer.

The predominant site of adenocarcinoma in ulcerative colitis is the distal colon and rectum, evidence for the 'left to right' shift being less apparent than in other causes of colorectal cancer (Connell *et al.* 1994). Over 80% of carcinomas in colitics are located distal to the splenic flexure, with over half of all tumours occurring in the rectosigmoid region. However, diffuse abnormalities of the epithelium can be detected so that in one in six patients, multiple synchronous tumours are present (Schneider *et al.* 1993; Gibson *et al.* 1995; Fante *et al.* 1996). Almost half the carcinomas are diffusely stenosing lesions with 20% being mucus-producing adenocarcinomas (Schneider *et al.* 1993; von Herbay *et al.* 1994). Formerly, cancers secondary to ulcerative colitis tended to be poorly differentiated. However, with the advent of screening programmes this may be changing. In some studies, 90% of lesions are now well or moderately well differentiated and less than 35% of patients have Dukes' C or D tumours (Lennard-Jones *et al.* 1990; Schneider *et al.* 1993).

Very occasionally squamous cell carcinoma may complicate idiopathic IBD (Kulaylat *et al.* 1995). This carcinoma develops more commonly in females and in patients with pancolonic disease of more than 8 years duration. The rectum is affected in two-thirds of the cases. Squamous cell changes, in the vicinity of the primary adenocarcinoma, are present in 27% of cases (Kulaylat *et al.* 1995). The carcinoma is in a pathologically advanced stage in one-third of the cases. Colectomy is the main therapeutic modality, survival following surgical resection ranging from 7 months to 21 years (Kulaylat *et al.* 1995).

Crohn's disease

Evidence implicating Crohn's disease as a risk factor for colorectal cancer is variable (Nikias *et al.* 1995; Bernstein and Rogers 1996) (see Chapter 6). Some report no association (Fireman *et al.* 1989), others a definite link with an estimated incidence of 270 per 100 000 patients with Crohn's disease. In a Swedish population-based study, patients with Crohn's disease had a 2.5 increased risk for both males and females of developing colorectal cancer relative to the general population (Ekbom *et al.* 1990).

In reports suggesting an association, the risk factors are similar to those in ulcerative colitis (Bernstein and Rogers 1996). The risk increases with the duration of the disease, cancer occurring at an average of 10 years earlier than in the general population and featuring a high percentage of colloid and multifocal carcinomas (Greenstein *et al.* 1989). Tumours tend to arise in those with long-standing perianal disease (Nikias *et al.* 1995; Lumley and Hoffmann 1997). In the Swedish study the relative risk of colorectal cancer for those with Crohn's disease confined to the terminal ileum was 1.0; for terminal ileum and parts of colon 3.2; and for colon alone 5.6 (Ekbom *et al.* 1992). Patients in whom Crohn's disease was diagnosed before age 30 years with any colonic involvement at diagnosis had a higher relative risk than those diagnosed at older ages (Ekbom *et al.* 1990). The prognosis of Crohn's carcinoma is poor, with 5-year survival ranging from 18% to 39% (Greenstein *et al.* 1989). The generally late diagnosis of colorectal cancer is blamed on symptoms being attributed to the underlying IBD, so that all new symptoms should be carefully evaluated in patients with Crohn's disease (Greenstein *et al.* 1989).

Ureteric-colic anastomosis

Ureterosigmoidoscopy increases the risk of colonic adenocarcinoma at or near the site of the anastomosis by 80–550-fold relative to the general population and by 7000-fold in those in whom the operation was performed before the age of 25 years (Beshai and Zimmern 1990; Kalble *et al.* 1990). Cancer develops after an average of 25 years after diversion for benign conditions and 5 years after diversion for urological malignancy.

Genetics

Hereditary syndromes

Advances in molecular genetics have led to patients with colorectal cancer being classified as having sporadic, familial, or hereditary forms of the disease (Lynch *et al.* 1992; Cole *et al.* 1996). Cancer that occurs in the absence of a family history is classified as sporadic. Familial forms include familial adenomatous polyposis (FAP), Gardner's syndrome, Peutz–Jeghers' syndrome, and familial juvenile polyposis (see Chapter 8). Together these account for less than 1% of all colorectal cancers (Burt *et al.* 1992; Cunningham and Dunlop 1996).

The hereditary type is defined as a family history of colorectal cancer occurring in a pattern that indicates autosomal-dominant inheritance, which also may involve certain phenotypic signs (depending on the specific disorder, i.e. florid adenomatous polyps, benign and malignant extracolonic lesions, cancer of unusually early onset, and multiple primary cancer, particularly synchronous and metachronous colorectal cancer) (Fante *et al.* 1996; Beck *et al.* 1997). This hereditary non-polyposis colorectal cancer (HNPCC) accounts for 5–10% of all colorectal cancers (Brewer *et al.* 1993; Mecklin *et al.* 1995; Belacosa *et al.* 1996). There are two clinical subsets, Lynch syndromes I and II (Lynch *et al.* 1992; Vasen *et al.* 1994; Sterm 1996). Lynch syndrome I is characterized by an autosomal dominantly inherited tendency to early-onset colonic cancer with proximal predominance and an excess of multiple primary colonic cancer (Lynch and Lynch 1994). Over half of tumours are located in the proximal colon and one-quarter of patients have multiple primary colorectal cancers (Kee and Collins 1991; Vasen 1994). The mean age at diagnosis of such patients is 40 years (Jass and Stewart 1992). The HNPCC trait has been linked to the D2S123 locus on 2p15–16 (Lynch *et al.* 1997). This HNPCC locus is now designated 'COCA1' and has been localized to an 8-cM region that is consistent with the location of the hMSH2 gene (Froggatt *et al.* 1995; Fishel and Wilson 1997). The HNPCC gene causes DNA replication errors to develop and accumulate within neoplastic but not normal tissues (Vasen *et al.* 1996; Dunlop *et al.* 1997). The effect of the HNPCC gene is to accelerate the progression of adenoma to carcinoma, but not to initiate adenoma development (Sterm 1996).

Patients with a first-degree relative with colorectal cancer have a two- to fourfold increased risk of developing colorectal cancer compared with the rest of the population (Kee and Collins 1992; Hall *et al.* 1996). Relative to subjects with no family history, asymptomatic patients with one first-degree relative with colorectal cancer have nearly double the risk of developing adenomatous polyps, greater frequency of severely dysplastic lesions, and significantly higher frequency of proximal polyp location (Bazzoli *et al.* 1995; Hall *et al.* 1996). Familial aggregation of colorectal cancer decreases as the probands' age increases, the odds ratio increasing from 2 for relatives of those who developed colorectal cancer over 50 years to 8 in those 40–50 years, and 13 if cancer developed in a first-degree relative under 40 years of age (Zhao and Le Marchand 1992*b*). In contrast, spouses of patients with colorectal cancer do not have an increased risk of the disease. One-fifth of patients with a family history of colorectal cancer will have colorectal polyps and 2% colorectal cancers (Orrom *et al.* 1990; Jass and Stewart 1992; Lanspa *et al.* 1992*b*). The risk of rectal cancer in patients who have had a colectomy for HNPCC is 12% at 12 years (Rodrienez-Breias *et al.* 1997). The risk of polyps is increased to 35% if several first-degree relatives have colorectal cancer (Orrom *et al.* 1990). Adenomas do not occur in large numbers in HNPCC, but develop at a young age (mean age 40 years), attain a large size (85% over 1 cm), often show a villous configuration, and are more prone to malignant conversion (55%) than sporadic adenomas (Jass and Stewart 1992; Lynch *et al.* 1997).

The incidence of colorectal polyps or cancer is similar (45%) in those with only one first-degree relative or one or more second-degree relatives affected with the condition (Meagher and Stuart 1992). In those with one first-degree relative afflicted with colon cancer the greatest risk of developing a colonic adenoma is in males over the age of 50 years (Guillem *et al.* 1992). In patients with HNPPC, over half will have polyps detected by colonoscopy, 40% of these having multiple lesions and 4% carcinomas (Orram *et al.* 1990; Meagher and Stuart 1992). A high rate (80%) of synchronous and metachronous lesions is also found. The adenomas are more proximally located (20–40% proximal to splenic flexure), corresponding to the site of cancer distribution in the Lynch syndromes. Adenomas will be found in one-quarter of such subjects under the age of 40 years (Meagher and Stuart 1992). In one-third to one-half of cases synchronous tumours are located in non-adjacent segments of the colon, with rectal lesions accounting for up to 20% of synchronous tumours (Slater *et al.* 1990). Patients with HNPCC also have a 25% cumulative risk of developing metachronous colorectal cancer within 10 years (Svendsen *et al.* 1991; Vasen 1994). These metachronous colorectal cancers are predominantly located in the right colon with a decreasing frequency toward the rectum. Despite this, a positive family history does not independently influence prognosis in patients with bowel cancer, the 5- and 10-year actuarial survival being 85% and 70% (Kee and Collins 1991).

In some families with HNPCC all of these features are present plus a high risk of certain cancers other than colon cancer (Lynch II or cancer family syndrome) (Lynch *et al.* 1992). Up to two-thirds of these families have three or more relatives affected by colorectal cancer in a first-degree kinship (Mecklin and Jarvinen 1991; Kee and Collins 1992). In families with this syndrome, extra-colonic tumours appear in half of the colon cancer patients and in one-fifth of family members (Boyd and Rubin 1997). The common sites of extra-colonic tumours are the endometrium (10%), stomach (5%), biliary–pancreatic tract (5%), and uroepithelium (2%) (Mecklin and Jarvinen 1991; Vasen 1994). This corresponds to a relative risk in these patients for ovarian cancer of 6, stomach cancer of 3, uterine cancer of 3, and cervical cancer of 2 (Houlston *et al.* 1992; Kee and Collins 1992). In female relatives the risk of breast cancer is increased up to fivefold and the lifetime risk of breast cancer is 1 in 4 (Slattery and Kerber 1993).

Patients with extra-colonic cancer family syndrome have a threefold risk of developing colorectal cancer (Houlston *et al.* 1992; Kee and Collins 1992). In women there is a reciprocal association between breast, ovarian, and endometrial cancer and colorectal polyps or cancer (Toma *et al.* 1987). Families with a history of endometrial cancer have more members who develop colon cancer than families without any endometrial cancer (Mecklin and Jarvinen 1991). In one study the incidence of adenomas was 15% in those with breast cancer compared with 5% in controls (Jouin *et al.* 1989). Patients with Barrett's oesophagus are also at an increased risk of colorectal cancer (Robertson *et al.* 1989). These associations are possibly due to shared risk factors between these conditions and colorectal cancer which act at the level of promoting conversion of adenomatous polyps into colorectal cancer (Murray *et al.* 1992).

Chromosomal abnormalities

Allele loss of various segments of chromosome 5q occurs in FAP, Gardner's syndrome, 30% of polyps occurring in non-polyposis patients, and in 20–40% of carcinomas (Neuman *et al.* 1991; Cunningham and Dunlop 1996). It is believed that the changes in the 5q21 region represent the MCC (mutated in colorectal cancer) gene, which encodes an 829 amino acid protein (Kinzler *et al.* 1991; Minchin *et al.* 1993). This MCC gene has been implicated in almost half of sporadic colorectal cancers and 80% of colorectal cancer in patients under 35 years of age (Hamilton 1992; Houlston *et al.* 1992; Goyette *et al.* 1992).

Allele losses commonly occur at other genetic loci. Loss of the short arm of chromosome 17 occurs in up to 75% of colorectal cancers, loss of all of chromosome 18, and part of chromosome 22 have also been implicated in sporadic colorectal cancer and familial polyposis coli (Okamoto *et al.* 1988). Genetic probes have also identified changes to chromosomes 2, 3, 6, 7, 8, 13, 15, and 19 in patients with hereditary non-polyposis syndromes and sporadic cancer (Barletta *et al.* 1993; Lyn *et al.* 1993; Schweinfest *et al.* 1993; van der Bosch *et al.* 1993). It is not yet clear whether these losses in chromosome structure are primary or secondary events in carcinogenesis. It is suggested that oncogenes may be responsible for transmitting these alterations in chromosomal structure into functional changes of the cell which can lead to cancer. Proto-oncogenes act to regulate and oncogenes to deregulate cell proliferation by signal reception, transduction, mediation, and response. Signal transducing proto-oncogenes include *src* and the *ras* gene family. Transcription regulators like the *fos* and *jun* proto-oncogenes would be considered mediators of the transduced signals which induce expression of target genes, such as members of the *myc* proto-oncogene family (Miller *et al.* 1992). Two oncogenes, the c-*myc* and the *ras* have been directly implicated in colonic tumour initiation and/or progression (Rigas 1990).

The c-*myc* gene is located on human chromosome 8q. The gene is expressed at levels five to 40 times those in normal colonic mucosa in up to 80% of colorectal adenocarcinomas (Rew *et al.* 1991). A gene product essential for *myc* regulation is missing in such cases and presumably the deregulation is due to a defect in a gene whose product acts to regulate c-*myc* gene transcription. A colon carcinoma cell expressing such elevated levels of *myc* would be in a constant state of proliferation. *Ras* mutations may also be involved in tumour progression by conferring a strong growth advantage to the cells harbouring them. *Ras* alleles which have been activated through point mutation are found in half of colorectal cancers and 60% of adenomas larger than 1 cm (Pretlow *et al.* 1993). *Ras* gene mutation seems to be an early event, with the recessive changes on chromosomes 5 and 18 possibly occurring later, at the transition from adenoma to carcinoma. The recessive changes on chromosome 17, acting through a 'dominant negative' action of the p53 nuclear oncoprotein, appear to be restricted to cancers (Kanamaru and Ishioka 1992; Losi *et al.* 1992; Yamaguchi *et al.* 1992).

It is probable that for tumour transformation to begin, two processes are necessary (Wildrick 1989). First, the cell cycle regulating pathway is disrupted by, say, deregulation of c-*myc* expression, while the signal transduction pathway is activated by an event such as *ras* point mutation. In addition, the *ras* point mutations and allele loss on 17p and 18q, may be events of progression in some cases and events of initiation in others. The situation is more complicated than this, as *myc* and *ras* are uninvolved in a significant number of tumours. Secondly, progression to a fully invasive carcinoma probably requires disruption of normal cell to cell interactions and local disruption of the architecture of the colonic epithelium to allow transformed cells to reach and penetrate the basement membrane.

Tumour formation therefore requires multiple genetic events. In FAP, the first event is inherited loss of one FAP allele, leading to formation of a pre-neoplastic polyp. Formation of a carcinoma *in situ* requires additional events, such as loss of function of the second FAP allele and mutational activation of *ras*. Disruption of the surrounding normal tissue (pericryptal sheath and lamina propria), dissolution of the basement membrane, and rupture of the muscularis mucosae may then be effected by genetic events that disrupt attachment of the tumour cell to the extracellular matrix. In cases of FAP, these genetic events take an average of 30–40 years to accumulate; for sporadic colonic cancer, an average of six to seven decades is required. During progression from adenoma to carcinoma, *ras* gene mutations and 5q allele deletions are likely to be earlier events, whereas allele losses from chromosomes 18q and 17p seem to occur more often in advanced tumours. Involvement of the genes on 5q (FAP) and 18q (Lynch syndrome II) in hereditary colonic cancer syndromes is supported by linkage studies, but their respective roles (as well as that of the gene on 17p) in familial and sporadic colorectal cancer remain to be precisely defined.

References

Akerley WL 3d, Moritz TE, Ryan LS, Henderson WG, Zacharski LR. Racial comparison of outcomes of male Department of Veterans Affairs patients with lung and colon cancer. *Arch. Intern. Med.* 1993; 153: 1681–8.

Alberts DS, Einspahr J, Rees McGee S, Ramanujam P, Buller MK, Clark L, *et al.* Effects of dietary wheat bran fiber on rectal epithelial cell proliferation in patients with resection for colorectal cancers. *J. Natl Cancer Inst.* 1990; 82: 1280–5.

Alberts DS, Ritenbaugh C, Story JA, Aickin M, Rees McGee S, Buller MK, *et al.* Randomized, double blinded, placebo controlled study of effect of wheat bran fiber and calcium on fecal bile acids in patients with resected adenomatous colon polyps. *J. Natl Cancer Inst.* 1996; 88: 81–92.

Anton CH. Smoking and other risk factors associated with the stage and age of diagnosis of colon and rectum cancers. *Cancer Detect. Prev.* 1991; 15: 345–50.

Arbman G, Axelson O, Fredriksson M, Nilsson E, Sjodahl R. Do occupational factors influence the risk of colon and rectal cancer in different ways? *Cancer* 1993; 72: 2543–9.

Arbman G, Nilsson E, Storgren Fordell V, Sjodahl R. Outcome of surgery for colorectal cancer in a defined population in Sweden from 1984 to 1986. *Dis. Colon Rectum* 1995; 38: 645–50.

Bansal P, Sonnenberg A. Risk factors of colorectal cancer in inflammatory bowel disease. *Am. J. Gastroenterol.* 1996; 91: 44–8.

Barletta C, Scillato F, Sega FM, Mannella E. Genetic alteration in gastrointestinal cancer. A molecular and cytogenetic study. *Anticancer Res.* 1993; 13: 2325–9.

Barsoum GH, Hendrickse C, Winslet MC, Youngs D, Donovan IA, Neoptolemos JP, Keighley MR. Reduction of mucosal crypt cell proliferation in patients with colorectal adenomatous polyps by dietary calcium supplementation. *Br. J. Surg.* 1992; 79: 581–3.

Bartram HP, Gostner A, Scheppach W, Reddy BS, Rao CV, Dusel G, Richter F, *et al.* Effects of fish oil on rectal cell proliferation, mucosal fatty acids, and prostaglandin E2 release in healthy subjects. *Gastroenterology* 1993; 105: 1317–22.

Bazzoli F, Fossi S, Sottili S, Pozzato P, Zagari RM, Morelli MC, *et al.* The risk of adenomatous polyps in asymptomatic first degree relatives of persons with colon cancer. *Gastroenterology* 1995; 109: 783–8.

Beard CM, Spencer RJ, Weiland LH, O'Fallon WM, Melton LJ 3rd. Trends in colorectal cancer over a half century in Rochester, Minnesota, 1940 to 1989. *Ann. Epidemiol.* 1995; 5: 210–4.

Beart RW, Steele GD Jr, Menck HR, Chmiel JS, Ocwieja KE, Winchester DP. Management and survival of patients with adenocarcinoma of the colon and rectum: a national survey of the Commission on Cancer. *J. Am. Coll. Surg.* 1995; 181: 225–36.

Beck NE, Tomlinson IP, Homfray T, Hodgson SV, Harocopos CJ, Bodmer WF. Genetic testing is important in families with a history suggestive of hereditary non-polyposis colorectal cancer even if the Amsterdam criteria are not fulfilled. *Br. J. Surg.* 1997; 84: 233–7.

Bedenne L, Faivre J, Boutron MC, Piard F, Cauvin JM, Hillon P. Adenoma—carcinoma sequence or 'de novo' carcinogenesis? A study of adenomatous remnants in a population based series of large bowel cancers. *Cancer* 1992; 69: 883–8.

Bellacosa A, Genuardi M, Anti M, Viel A, Ponz de Leon M. Hereditary nonpolyposis colorectal cancer: review of clinical, molecular genetics, and counseling aspects. *Am. J. Med. Genet.* 1996; 62: 6353–424.

Bernstein D, Rogers A. Malignancy in Crohn's disease. *Am. J. Gastroenterol.* 1996; 91: 434–40.

Beshai AZ, Zimmern PE. Is evaluation of the right colon necessary prior to cecocystoplasty? *J. Urol.* 1990; 144: 359–61.

Bostick RM, Potter JD, Sellers TA, McKenzie DR, Kushi LH, Folsom AR. Relation of calcium, vitamin D, and dairy food intake to incidence of colon cancer among older women. The Iowa Women's Health Study. *Am. J. Epidemiol.* 1993; 137: 1302–17.

Bostick RM, Fosdick L, Wood JR, Grambsch P, Grandits GA, Lillemoe TJ, *et al.* Calcium and colorectal epithelial cell proliferation in sporadic adenoma patients: a randomized, double blinded, placebo controlled clinical trial. *J. Natl Cancer Inst.* 1995; 87: 1307–15.

Boughdady IS, Kinsella AR, Haboubi NY, Schofield PF. K ras gene mutations in adenomas and carcinomas of the colon. *Surg. Oncol.* 1992; 1: 275–82.

Boyd J, Rubin SC. Hereditary ovarian cancer: molecular genetics and clinical implications. *Gynecol. Oncol.* 1997; 64: 196–206.

Braun MM, Helzlsouer KJ, Hollis BW, Comstock GW. Colon cancer and serum vitamin D metabolite levels 10–17 years prior to diagnosis. *Am. J. Epidemiol.* 1995; 142: 608–11.

Brenner H, Mielck A, Klein R, Ziegler H. The role of socioeconomic factors in the survival of patients with colorectal cancer in Saarland/Germany. *J. Clin. Epidemiol.* 1991; 44: 807–15.

Brewer DA, Bokey EL, Fung C, Chapuis PH. Heredity, molecular genetics and colorectal cancer: a review. *Aust. N.Z. J. Surg.* 1993; 63: 87–94.

Broitman SA, Cerda S, Wilkinson J. Cholesterol metabolism and colon cancer. *Prog. Food Nutr. Sci.* 1993; 17: 1–40.

Bruce WR, Archer MC, Corpet DE, Medline A, Minkin S, Stamp D, *et al.* Diet, aberrant crypt foci and colorectal cancer. *Mutat. Res.* 1993; 290: 111–8.

Burt RW, Bishop DT, Cannon Albright L, Samowitz WS, Lee RL, DiSario JA, Skolnick MH. Population genetics of colonic cancer. *Cancer* 1992; 70 (Suppl.): 1719–22.

Cali RL, Pitsch RM, Thorson AG, Watson P, Tapia P, Blatchford GJ, Christensen MA. Cumulative incidence of metachronous colorectal cancer. *Dis. Colon Rectum* 1993, 36: 388–93.

Calle EE, Miracle McMahill HL, Thun MJ, Heath CW Jr. Estrogen replacement therapy and risk of fatal colon cancer in a prospective cohort of postmenopausal women. *J. Natl Cancer Inst.* 1995; 87: 517–23.

Cantor KP, Lynch CF, Johnson D. Reproductive factors and risk of brain, colon, and other malignancics in Iowa (United States). *Cancer Causes Control* 1993; 4: 505–11.

Cats A, Kleibeuker JH, van der Meer R, Kuipers F, Sluiter WJ, Hardonk MJ, *et al.*. Randomized, double blinded, placebo controlled intervention study with supplemental calcium in families with hereditary nonpolyposis colorectal cancer. *J. Natl Cancer Inst.* 1995; 87: 598–603.

Charnley RM, Thomas WM, Stanley J, Morris DL. Serum gastrin concentrations in colorectal cancer patients. *Ann. R. Coll. Surg. Engl.* 1992; 74: 138–40.

Chow WH, Dosemeci M, Zheng W, Vetter R, McLaughlin JK, Gao YT, Blot WJ. Physical activity and occupational risk of colon cancer in Shanghai, China. *Int. J. Epidemiol.* 1993; 22: 23–9.

Chute CG, Willett WC, Colditz GA, Stampfer MJ, Baron JA, Rosner B, Speizer FE. A prospective study of body mass, height, and smoking on the risk of colorectal cancer in women. *Cancer Causes Control* 1991; 2: 117–24

Clark LC, Hixson LJ, Combs GF Jr, Reid ME, Turnbull BW, Sampliner RE. Plasma selenium concentration predicts the prevalence of colorectal adenomatous polyps. *Cancer Epidemiol. Biomarkers Prev.* 1993; 2: 41–6.

Coates RJ, Greenberg RS, Liu MT, Correa P, Harlan LC, Reynolds P, *et al.* Anatomic site distribution of colon cancer by race and other colon cancer risk factors. *Dis. Colon Rectum* 1995; 38: 42–50.

Cole DE, Gallinger S, McCready DR, Rosen B, Engel J, Malkin D. Genetic counselling and testing for susceptibility to breast, ovarian and colon cancer: where are we today? *Can. Med. Assoc. J.* 1996; 154: 149–55.

Connell WR, Talbot IC, Harpaz N, Britto N, Wilkinson KH, Kamm MA, Lennard Jones JE. Clinicopathological characteristics of colorectal carcinoma complicating ulcerative colitis. *Gut* 1994; 35: 1419–23.

Cooper GS, Yuan Z, Landefeld CS, Johanson JF, Rimm AA. A national population based study of incidence of colorectal cancer and age. Implications for screening in older Americans. *Cancer* 1995; 75: 775–81.

Cordice JW Jr, Johnson H Jr. Anatomic distribution of colonic cancers in middle class black Americans. *J. Natl. Med. Assoc.* 1991; 83: 730–2.

Cox B, Little J. Reduced risk of colorectal cancer among recent generations in New Zealand. *Br. J. Cancer* 1992; 66: 386–90.

Cresanta JL. Epidemiology of cancer in the United States. *Primary Care* 1992; 19: 419–41.

Cunningham C, Dunlop MG. Molecular genetic basis of colorectal cancer susceptibility. *Brit. J. Surg.* 1996; 83: 321–9.

Dave BJ, Hopwood VL, Hughes JI, Mellilo D, Jackson GL, Pathak S. Nonrandom chromosomal abnormalities in lymphocyte cultures of individ-

uals with colorectal polyps and of asymptomatic relatives of patients with colorectal cancer or polyps. *Cancer Epidemiol. Biomarkers Prev.* 1993; 2: 587–91.

De Stefani E, Fierro L, Barrios E, Ronco A. Cancer mortality trends in Uruguay 1953–1991. *Int. J. Cancer* 1994; 56: 634–9.

Deans GT, Heatley M, Moorehead RJ, Rowlands BJ, Parks TG, Spence RAJ. Colorectal carcinoma: the importance of clinical and pathological factors in survival. *Ann. R. Coll. Surg. Engl.* 1994; 76: 59–64.

DeCosse JJ, Ngoi SS, Jacobson JS, Cennerazzo WJ. Gender and colorectal cancer. *Eur. J. Cancer Prev.* 1993; 2: 105–15.

Dubrow R, Kim CS, Eldred AK. Fecal lysozyme: an unreliable marker for colorectal cancer. *Am. J. Gastroenterol.* 1992; 87: 617–21.

Dunlop MG, Farrington SM, Carothers AD, Wyllie AH, Sharp L, Burn J, Liu B, Kinzler KW, Vogelstein B. Cancer risk associated with germline DNA mismatch repair gene mutations. *Hum. Molec. Genet.* 1997; 6: 105–13.

Dwyer J. Dietary fiber and colorectal cancer risk. *Nutr. Rev.* 1993; 51: 147–8.

Ekbom A, Helmick C, Zack M, Adami HO. Increased risk of large bowel cancer in Crohn's disease with colonic involvement. *Lancet* 1990; 336: 357–9.

Ekbom A, Helmick CG, Zack M, Holmberg L, Adami HO. Survival and causes of death in patients with inflammatory bowel disease: a population based study. *Gastroenterology* 1992; 103: 954–60.

Ekbom A, Yuen J, Adami HO, McLaughlin JK, Chow WH, Persson I, Fraumeni JF Jr. Cholccystectomy and colorectal cancer. *Gastroenterology* 1993, 105: 142–7.

Fante R, Roncucci L, Di Gregorio C, Tamassia MG, Losi L, Benatti P, Pedroni M, Percesepe A, De Pietri S, Ponz de Leon M. Frequency and clinical features of multiple tumors of the large bowel in the general population and in patients with hereditary colorectal carcinoma. *Cancer* 1996; 77: 2013–21.

Fearon ER. Molccular genetic studies of the adenoma carcinoma sequence. *Adv. Intern. Med.* 1994; 39: 123–47.

Fernandez E, La Vecchia C, D'Avanzo B, Franceschi S, Negri E, Parazzini F. Oral contraceptives, hormone replacement therapy and the risk of colorectal cancer. *Brit. J. Cancer* 1996; 73: 1431–5.

Finley GG, Koski RA, Melhem MF, Pipas JM, Meisler AI. Expression of the gastrin gene in the normal human colon and colorectal adeno-carcinoma. *Cancer Res.* 1993; 53: 2919–26.

Fireman Z, Grossman A, Lilos P, Hacohen D, Bar Meir S, Rozen P, Gilat T. Intestinal cancer in patients with Crohn's disease. A population study in central Israel. *Scand. J. Gastroenterol.* 1989; 24: 346–50.

Fishel R, Wilson T. MutS homologs in mammalian cells. *Curr. Opinion Genet. Develop.* 1997; 6: 105–13.

Fleshner P, Slater G, Aufses AH Jr. Age and sex distribution of patients with colorectal cancer. *Dis. Colon Rectum* 1989; 32: 107–11.

Franceschi S, La Vecchia C, Bidoli E, Negri E, Talamini R. Meal frequency and risk of colorectal cancer. *Cancer Res.* 1992; 52: 3589–92.

Fraser G, Pearce N. Occupational physical activity and risk of cancer of the colon and rectum in New Zealand males. *Cancer Causes Control* 1993; 4: 45–50.

Froggatt NJ, Koch J, Davies R, Evans DG, Clamp A, Quarrell OW, *et al.* Genetic linkage analysis in hereditary non polyposis colon cancer syndrome. *J. Med. Genet.* 1995; 32: 352–7.

Gerdes H, Gillin JS, Zimbalist E, Urmacher C, Lipkin M, Winawer SJ. Expansion of the epithelial cell proliferative compartment and frequency of adenomatous polyps in the colon correlate with the strength of family history of colorectal cancer. *Cancer Res.* 1993; 53: 279–82.

Gerhardsson de Verdier M, Hagman U, Peters RK, Steineck G, Overvik E. Meat, cooking methods and colorectal cancer: a case referent study in Stockholm. *Int. J. Cancer* 1991; 49: 520–5.

Gibson P, Rosella O, Nov R, Young G. Colonic epithelium is diffusely abnormal in ulcerative colitis and colorectal cancer. *Gut* 1995; 36: 857–63.

Giovannucci E, Stampfer MJ, Colditz G, Rimm EB, Willett WC. Relationship of diet to risk of colorectal adenoma in men. *J. Natl Cancer Inst.* 1992; 84: 91–8.

Giovannucci E, Stampfer MJ, Colditz GA, Rimm EB, Trichopoulos D, Rosner BA, et al. Folate, methionine, and alcohol intake and risk of colorectal adenoma. *J. Natl Cancer Inst.* 1993; 85: 875–84.

Giovannucci E, Rimm EB, Stampfer MJ, Colditz GA, Ascherio A, Willett WC. Aspirin use and the risk for colorectal cancer and adenoma in male health professionals. *Ann. Intern. Med.* 1994; 121: 241–62.

Giovannucci E, Rimm EB, Ascherio A, Stampfer MJ, Colditz GA, Willett WC. Alcohol, low methionine—low folate diets, and risk of colon cancer in men. *J. Natl Cancer Inst.* 1995a; 87: 265–73.

Giovannucci E, Ascherio A, Rimm EB, Colditz GA, Stampfer MJ, Willett WC. Physical activity, obesity, and risk for colon cancer and adenoma in men. *Ann. Intern. Med.* 1995b; 122: 327–34.

Govers MJ, Termont DS, Van der Meer R. Mechanism of the anti-proliferative effect of milk mineral and other calcium supplements on colonic epithelium. *Cancer Res.* 1994; 54: 95–100.

Goyette MC, Cho K, Fasching CL, Levy DB, Kinzler KW, Paraskeva C, et al. Progression of colorectal cancer is associated with multiple tumor suppressor gene defects but inhibition of tumorigenicity is accomplished by correction of any single defect via chromosome transfer. *Mol. Cell. Biol.* 1992; 12: 1387–95.

Greenstein AJ, Meyers S, Szporn A, et al. Colorectal cancer in regional ileitis. *Q. J. Med.* 1989; 62: 33–40.

Gregoire RC, Kashtan H, Stern HS, Yeung KS, Stadler J, Neil GA, et al. The effect of lowering faecal pH on the rate of proliferation of the normal colonic mucosa. *Surg. Oncol.* 1992; 1: 43–7.

Guillem JG, Forde KA, Treat MR, Neugut AI, O'Toole KM, Diamond BE. Colonoscopic screening for neoplasms in asymptomatic first degree relatives of colon cancer patients. A controlled, prospective study. *Dis. Colon Rectum* 1992; 35: 523–9.

Guo W, Zheng W, Li JY, Chen JS, Blot WJ. Correlations of colon cancer mortality with dietary factors, serum markers, and schistosomiasis in China. *Nutr. Cancer* 1993; 20: 13–20.

Hadfield M, Nicholson A, MacDonald A, Farouk R, Lee P, Duthie G, Monson J. Preoperative staging of rectal carcinoma by magnetic resonance imaging with a pelvic phased-array coil. *Br. J. Surg.* 1997; 84: 529–31.

Hall EJ, Freyer GA. The molecular biology of radiation carcinogenesis. *Basic Life Sci.* 1991; 58: 3–19.

Hall NR, Bishop DT, Stephenson BM, Finan PJ, Hereditary susceptibility to colorectal cancer. Relatives of early onset cases are particularly at risk. *Dis. Colon Rectum* 1996; 39: 739–43.

Hamilton SR. The adenoma adenocarcinoma sequence in the large bowel: variations on a theme. *J. Cell Biochem.* 1992; 16G (Suppl.): 41–6.

Hayes RB, Dosemeci M, Riscigno M, Blair A. Cancer mortality among jewelry workers. *Am. J. Indust. Med.* 1993; 24: 743–51.

Hermanek P. The dysplasia carcinoma sequence in the colorectum. *Zentralbl. Chir.* 1992; 117: 476–82.

Hixson LJ, Garewal HS, McGee DL, Sloan D, Fennerty MB, Sampliner RE, Gerner EW. Ornithine decarboxylase and polyamines in colorectal neoplasia and mucosa. Cancer Epidemiol. Biomarkers Prev. 1993; 2: 369–74.

Hoff G, Moen IE, Mowinckel P, Rosef O, Nordbo E, Sauar J, et al. Drinking water and the prevalence of colorectal adenomas: an epidemiologic study in Telemark, Norway. *Eur. J. Cancer Prev.* 1992; 1: 423–8.

Honjo S, Kono S, Shinchi K, Imanishi K, Hirohata T. Cigarette smoking, alcohol use and adenomatous polyps of the sigmoid colon. *Jpn. J. Cancer Res.* 1992; 83: 806–11.

Houlston RS, Collins A, Slack J, Morton NE. Dominant genes for colorectal cancer are not rare. *Ann. Hum. Genet.* 1992; 56: 99–103.

Howe GR, Benito E, Castelleto R, Cornee J, Esteve J, Gallagher RP, et al. Dietary intake of fiber and decreased risk of cancers of the colon and rectum: evidence from the combined analysis of 13 case control studies. *J. Natl Cancer Inst.* 1992; 84: 1887–96.

Howe HL, Keller JE, Lehnherr M. Relation between population density and cancer incidence, Illinois, 1986–1990. *Am. J. Epidemiol.* 1993; 138: 29–36.

Hunerbein M, Schlag P. Three-dimensional endosonography for staging rectal cancer. *Ann. Surg.* 1997; 225: 432–8.

Imray CH, Radley S, Davis A, Barker G, Hendrickse CW, Donovan IA, et al. Faecal unconjugated bile acids in patients with colorectal cancer or polyps. *Gut* 1992; 33: 1239–45.

Jacobsen BK, Vollset SE, Kvale G. Do reproductive factors influence colorectal cancer survival? *J. Clin. Epidemiol.* 1995; 48: 1119–22.

Jacoby RF, Marshall DJ, Kailas S, Schlack S, Harms B, Love R. Genetic instability associated with adenoma to carcinoma progression in hereditary nonpolyposis colon cancer. *Gastroenterology* 1995; 109: 73–82.

Jass JR. Do all colorectal carcinomas arise in preexisting adenomas? *World J. Surg.* 1989, 13: 45–51.

Jass JR. Subsite distribution and incidence of colorectal cancer in New Zealand, 1974–1983. *Dis. Colon Rectum* 1991; 34: 56–9.

Jass JR, Stewart SM. Evolution of hereditary non polyposis colorectal cancer. *Gut* 1992; 33: 783–6.

Johansen C, Mellemgaard A, Skov T, Kjaergaard J, Lynge E. Colorectal cancer in Denmark 1943–1988. *Int. J. Colorectal Dis.* 1993; 8: 42–7.

Jorgensen T, Rafaelsen S. Gallstones and colorectal cancer—there is a relationship, but it is hardly due to cholecystectomy. *Dis. Colon Rectum* 1992; 35: 24–8.

Jouin H, Baumann R, Derlon A, Varra A, Calderoli H, Jaeck D, et al. Is there an increased incidence of adenomatous polyps in breast cancer patients? *Cancer* 1989; 63: 599–603.

Kalble T, Tricker AR, Friedl P, Waldherr R, Hoang J, Staehler G, Mohring K. Ureterosigmoidostomy: long term results, risk of carcinoma and etiological factors for carcinogenesis. *J. Urol.* 1990; 144: 1110–4.

Kampman E, Giovannucci E, van't Veer P, Rimm E, Stampfer MJ, Colditz GA, et al. Calcium, vitamin D, dairy foods, and the occurrence of colorectal adenomas among men and women in two prospective studies. *Am. J. Epidemiol.* 1994; 139: 16–29.

Kanamaru R, Ishioka C. Mutations of the p53 gene and other genes involving in human colorectal carcinogenesis. *Tohoku J Exp Med.* 1992; 168: 159–66.

Kee F, Collins BJ. How prevalent is cancer family syndrome? *Gut* 1991; 32: 509–12.

Kee F, Collins BJ. Families at risk of colorectal cancer: who are they? *Gut* 1992; 33: 787–90.

Kimura T, Iwagaki H, Fuchimoto S, Hizuta A, Orita K. Synchronous colorectal carcinomas. *Hepatogastroenterology* 1994; 41: 409–12.

Kimura T, Iwagaki H, Hizuta A, Nonaka Y, Tanaka N, Orita K. Colorectal cancer after irradiation for cervical cancer case reports. *Anticancer Res.* 1995; 15: 557–8.

Kinzler KW, Nilbert MC, Vogelstein B, Bryan TM, Levy DB, Smith KJ, et al. Identification of a gene located at chromosome 5q21 that is mutated in colorectal cancers. *Science* 1991; 251: 1366–70.

Kleibeuker JH, Welberg JW, Mulder NH, van der Meer R, Cats A, Limburg AJ, et al. Epithelial cell proliferation in the sigmoid colon of patients with adenomatous polyps increases during oral calcium supplementation. *Br. J. Cancer* 1993; 67: 500–3.

Kohlmeier L, Weterings KG, Steck S, Kok FJ. Tea and cancer prevention: an evaluation of the epidemiologic literature. *Nutrit. Cancer.* 1997; 27: 1–13.

Kono S, Shinchi K, Ikeda N, Yanai F, Imanishi K. Physical activity, dietary habits and adenomatous polyps of the sigmoid colon: a study of self defense officials in Japan. *J. Clin. Epidemiol.* 1991; 44: 1255–61.

Kono S, Imanishi K, Shinchi K, Yanai F. Relationship of diet to small and large adenomas of the sigmoid colon. *Jpn. J. Cancer Res.* 1993; 84: 13–9.

Koretz RL. Malignant polyps: are they sheep in wolves' clothing? *Ann. Intern. Med.* 1993; 118: 63–8.

Kulaylat MN, Doerr R, Butler B, Satchidanand SK, Singh A. Squamous cell carcinoma complicating idiopathic inflammatory bowel disease. *J. Surg. Oncol.* 1995, 59: 48–55.

Kune GA, Vitetta L. Alcohol consumption and the etiology of colorectal cancer: a review of the scientific evidence from 1957 to 1991. *Nutr. Cancer* 1992; 18: 97–111.

Kune GA, Bannerman S, Watson LF. Attributable risk for diet, alcohol, and family history in the Melbourne Colorectal Cancer Study. *Nutr. Cancer* 1992; 18: 231–5.

Kune GA, Kune S, Watson LF. Body weight and physical activity as predictors of colorectal cancer risk. *Nutr. Cancer* 1990; 13: 9–17.

Kuramoto K, Matsushita S, Esaki Y, Shimada H. Prevalence, rate of correct clinical diagnosis and mortality of cancer in 4,894 elderly autopsy cases. *Nippon Ronen Igakkai Zasshi* 1993; 30: 35–40.

Kvist N, Jacobsen O, Kvist HK, Norgaard P, Ockelmann HH, Schou G, Jarnum S. Malignancy in ulcerative colitis. *Scand. J. Gastroenterol.* 1989; 24: 497–506.

La Vecchia C, Franceschi S. Reproductive factors and colorectal cancer. *Cancer Causes Control* 1991; 2: 193–200.

La Vecchia C, Negri E, Franceschi S, D'Avanzo B. Moderate beer consumption and the risk of colorectal cancer. *Nutr. Cancer* 1993; 19: 303–6.

Langholz E, Munkholm P, Davidsen M, Binder V. Colorectal cancer risk and mortality in patients with ulcerative colitis. *Gastroenterology* 1992; 103: 1444–51.

Lanspa SJ, Rouse J, Smyrk T, Watson P, Jenkins JX, Lynch HT. Epidemiologic characteristics of the flat adenoma of Muto. A prospective study. *Dis. Colon Rectum* 1992a; 35: 543–6.

Lanspa SJ, Jenkins JX, Watson P, Smyrk TC, Cavalieri RJ, Lynch JF, Lynch HT. Natural history of at risk Lynch syndrome family members with respect to adenomas. *Nebr. Med. J.* 1992b; 77: 310–3.

Lashner BA, Provencher KS, Bozdech JM, Brzezinski A. Worsening risk for the development of dysplasia or cancer in patients with chronic ulcerative colitis. *Am. J. Gastroenterol.* 1995; 90: 377 80.

Lennard-Jones JE, Melville DM, Morson BC, Ritchie JK, Williams CB. Precancer and cancer in extensive ulcerative colitis: findings among 401 patients over 22 years. *Gut* 1990; 31: 800–6.

Levi F, Randimbison L, La Vecchia C. Trends in subsite distribution of colorectal cancers and polyps from the Vaud Cancer Registry. *Cancer* 1993; 72: 46–50.

Levin KE, Dozois RR. Epidemiology of large bowel cancer. *World J. Surg.* 1991; 15: 562–7.

Levitt MD, Millar DM, Stewart JO. Rectal cancer after pelvic irradiation. *J. R. Soc. Med.* 1990; 83: 152–4.

Lewin MR. Is there a fibre depleted aetiology for colorectal cancer? Experimental evidence. *Rev. Environ. Health* 1991; 9: 17–30.

Lieberman D. Screening/early detection model for colorectal cancer. Why screen? *Cancer* 1994; 74 (Suppl.): 2023–7.

Lindsay JP, Stavraky KM, Howe GR. The Canadian Labour Force Ten Percent Sample Study. Cancer mortality among men, 1965–1979. *J. Occup. Med.* 1993; 35: 408–14.

Loffeld R, Putten A, Balk A. Changes in the localization of colorectal cancer: implications for clinical practice. *J. Gastroenterol. Hepatol.* 1996; 11: 47–50.

Longy M, Saura R, Dumas F, Leseve JF, Taine L, Goussot JF, Couzigou P. Chromosome analysis of adenomatous polyps of the colon: possible existence of two differently evolving cytogenetic groups. *Cancer Genet. Cytogenet.* 1993; 67: 7–13.

Losi L, Benhattar J, Costa J. Stability of K ras mutations throughout the natural history of human colorectal cancer. *Eur. J. Cancer* 1992; 28A: 1115–20.

Lumley JW, Hoffmann DC. Adenocarcinoma complicating an anorectal sinus in a patient with Crohn's disease. *Aust. N. Z. J. Surg.* 1997; 67: 66–72.

Lyn D, Cherney BW, Lalande M, Berenson JR, Lichtenstein A, Lupold S, et al. A duplicated region is responsible for the poly(ADP ribose) polymerase polymorphism, on chromosome 13, associated with a predisposition to cancer. *Am. J. Hum. Genet.* 1993; 52: 124–34.

Lynch HT, Lynch JF. 25 years of HNPCC. *Anticancer Res.* 1994; 14: 1617–24.

Lynch HT, Watson P, Smyrk TC, Lanspa SJ, Boman BM, Boland CR, et al. Colon cancer genetics. *Cancer* 1992; 70 (Suppl.): 1300–12.

Lynch HT, Smyrk T, Lynch J. An update of HNPCC (Lynch syndrome). *Cancer Genet. Cytogenet.* 1997; 93: 84–99.

Lytle GH. Screening for colorectal carcinoma. *Semin. Surg. Oncol.* 1989; 5(3): 194–200.

MacLennan SC, MacLennan AH, Ryan P. Colorectal cancer and oestrogen replacement therapy. A meta analysis of epidemiological studies. *Med. J. Aust.* 1995; 162: 491–3.

Macrae FA. Epidemiology and early detection of colorectal cancer. *Curr. Opin. Oncol.* 1991; 3: 711–8.

Macrae FA. Fat and calories in colon and breast cancer: from animal studies to controlled clinical trials. *Prev. Med.* 1993; 22: 750–66.

Mallo GV, Rechreche H, Frigerio JM, Rocha D, Zweibaum A, Lacasa M, Jordan BR, Dusetti NJ, Dagorn JC, Iovanna JL. Molecular cloning, sequencing and expression of the mRNA encoding human Cdx1 and Cdx2 homeobox. Down-regulation of Cdx1 and Cdx2 mRNA expression during colorectal carcinogenesis. *Int. J. Cancer.* 1997; 74: 35–44.

Markowitz S, Morabia A, Garibaldi K, Wynder E. Effect of occupational and recreational activity on the risk of colorectal cancer among males: a case control study. *Int. J. Epidemiol.* 1992; 21: 1057–62.

Mayor-Davies J, Britz RS, Menashe L. A review of carcinoma of the colon and rectum over a 3-year period at Hillbrow Hospital, Johannesburg. *S. Afr. J. Surg.* 1992; 30: 147–50.

McGarrity TJ, Peiffer LP, Hartle RJ. Effect of selenium on growth, S adenosylmethionine and polyamine biosynthesis in human colon cancer cells. *Anticancer Res.* 1993; 13: 811–5.

Meagher AP, Stuart M. Colonoscopy in patients with a family history of colorectal cancer. *Dis. Colon Rectum* 1992; 35: 315–21.

Meagher AP, Stuart M. Does colonoscopic polypectomy reduce the incidence of colorectal carcinoma? *Aust. N.Z. J. Surg.* 1994; 64: 400–4.

Mecklin JP, Jarvinen HJ. Tumor spectrum in cancer family syndrome (hereditary nonpolyposis colorectal cancer). *Cancer* 1991; 68: 1109–12.

Mecklin JP, Jarvinen HJ, Hakkiluoto A, Hallikas H, Hiltunen KM, Harkonen N, et al. Frequency of hereditary nonpolyposis colorectal cancer. A prospective multicenter study in Finland. *Dis. Colon Rectum* 1995; 38: 588–93.

Mellemkjaer L, Olsen JH, Frisch M, Johansen C, Gridley G, McLaughlin JK. Cancer in patients with ulcerative colitis. *Int. J. Cancer* 1995; 60: 330–3.

Meyer F, White E. Alcohol and nutrients in relation to colon cancer in middle aged adults. *Am. J. Epidemiol.* 1993; 138: 225–36.

Miller F, Heimann TM, Quish A, Pyo DJ, Szporn A, Martinelli G, Fasy TM. ras and c myc protein expression in colorectal carcinoma. Study of cancer prone patients. *Dis. Colon Rectum* 1992; 35: 430–5.

Minchin RF, Kadlubar FF, Ilett KF. Role of acetylation in colorectal cancer. *Mutat. Res.* 1993; 290: 35–42.

Mizusawa K, Kaibara N, Yonekawa M, Ohta M, Sumi K, Kimura O, et al. A prospective cohort study on the development of colorectal cancer after gastrectomy. *Dis. Colon Rectum* 1990; 33: 298–301.

Moran EM. Epidemiological factors of cancer in California. *J. Environ. Pathol. Toxicol. Oncol.* 1992; 11: 303–7.

Mullan FJ, Wilson HK, Majury CW, Mills JO, Cromie AJ, Campbell GR, McKelvey ST. Bile acids and the increased risk of colorectal tumours after truncal vagotomy. *Br. J. Surg.* 1990; 77: 1085–90.

Murray TI, Neugut AI, Garbowski GC, Waye JD, Forde KA, Treat MR. Relationship between breast cancer and colorectal adenomatous polyps. A case control study. *Cancer* 1992; 69: 2232–4.

Muto T, Bussey HJR, Morson BC. The evolution of cancer of the colon and rectum. *Cancer* 1975; 36: 2251–70.

Nagao M, Sugimura T. Carcinogenic factors in food with relevance to colon cancer development. *Mutat Res.* 1993; 290: 43–51.

Nakatsuka H, Shimizu Y, Yamamoto T, Sekine I, Ezaki H, Tahara E, et al. Colorectal cancer incidence among atomic bomb survivors, 1950–80. *J. Radiat. Res.* 1992; 33: 342–61.

Neilan BA. Colorectal cancer. *Clinics Geriatr. Med.* 1987; 3(4): 625–35.

Nelson RL, Abcarian H, Nelson TM, Misumi A, Kako H, Rizk S, Sky-Peck H. The effect of dietary selenium deficiency on acute colorectal mucosal nucleotoxicity induced by several carcinogens in the rodent. *Am. J. Surg.* 1996; 172: 85–8.

Neugut AI, Horvath K, Whelan RL, Terry MB, Garbowski GC, Bertram A, Forde KA, Treat MR, Waye J. The effect of calcium and vitamin supplements on the incidence and recurrence of colorectal adenomatous polyps. *Cancer* 1996; 78: 723–8.

Neuman WL, Wasylyshyn ML, Jacoby R, Erroi F, Angriman I, Montag A, *et al.* Evidence for a common molecular pathogenesis in colorectal, gastric, and pancreatic cancer. *Genes Chromosomes Cancer* 1991; 3: 468–73.

Newcomb PA, Storer BE. Postmenopausal hormone use and risk of large bowel cancer. *J. Natl Cancer Inst.* 1995; 87: 1067–71.

Newcomb PA, Storer BE, Marcus PM. Cancer of the large bowel in women in relation to alcohol consumption: a case control study in Wisconsin (United States). *Cancer Causes Control* 1993; 4: 405–11.

Nikias G, Eisner T, Katz S, Levin L, Eskries D, Urmacher C, McKinley M. Crohn's disease and colorectal carcinoma: rectal cancer complicating longstanding active perianal disease. *Am. J. Gastroenterol.* 1995; 90: 216–9.

Nomiyama K, Ueda K, Kiyohara Y, Kato I, Ohmura T, Iwamoto H, *et al.* Malignant neoplasms in the Japanese community of Hisayama: mortality and changing pattern during a 30 year observation period based on a consecutive autopsy series. *J. Clin. Epidemiol.* 1996; 49: 45–50.

Nugent FW, Haggitt RC, Gilpin PA. Cancer surveillance in ulcerative colitis *Gastroenterology* 1991; 100: 1241–8.

O'Brien MJ, Winawer SJ, Zauber AG, Gottlieb LS, Sternberg SS, Diaz B, et al. The National Polyp Study. Patient and polyp characteristics associated with high grade dysplasia in colorectal adenomas. Gastroenterology 1990; 98: 371–9.

Offerhaus GJ, Tersmette AC, Tersmette KW, Tytgat GN, Hoedemaeker PJ, Vandenbroucke JP. Gastric pancreatic and colorectal carcinogenesis following remote peptic ulcer surgery. Review of the literature with the emphasis on risk assessment and underlining mechanism. J. Mod. Pathol. 1988; 1(5): 352–6.

Okamoto M, Sasaki M, Sugio K, Sato C, Iwama T, Ikeuchi T, *et al.* Loss of constitutional heterozygosity in colon carcinoma from patients with familial polyposis coli. *Nature* 1988; 331: 273–7.

Orrom WJ, Brzezinski WS, Wiens EW. Heredity and colorectal cancer. A prospective, community based, endoscopic study. *Dis. Colon Rectum* 1990; 33: 490–3.

Pence BC. Role of calcium in colon cancer prevention: experimental and clinical studies. *Mutat. Res.* 1993; 290: 87–95.

Ponz de Leon M, Sacchetti C, Sassatelli R, Zanghieri G, Roncucci L, Scalmati A. Evidence for the existence of different types of large bowel tumor: suggestions from the clinical data of a population based registry. *J. Surg. Oncol.* 1990; 44: 35–43.

Pretlow TP, Brasitus TA, Fulton NC, Cheyer C, Kaplan EL. K ras mutations in putative preneoplastic lesions in human colon. *J. Natl Cancer Inst.* 1993; 85: 2004–7.

Reddy BS. Dietary fat, calories, and fiber in colon cancer. *Prev. Med.* 1993; 22: 738–49.

Reddy BS. Nutritional factors and colon cancer. Crit. Rev. Food Sci. Nutr. 1995; 35: 175–90.

Reid FD, Mercer PM, Harrison M, Bates T. Cholecystectomy as a risk factor for colorectal cancer: a meta-analysis. *Scand. J. Gastroenterol.* 1996; 31: 160–9.

Rew DA, Taylor I, Cox H, Watson JV, Wilson GD. c myc protein product is a marker of DNA synthesis but not of malignancy in human gastrointestinal tissues and tumours. *Br. J. Surg.* 1991; 78: 1080–3.

Rhodes JM. Unifying hypothesis for inflammatory bowel disease and associated colon cancer: sticking the pieces together with sugar. Lancet 1996; 347: 40–4.

Rigas B. Oncogenes and suppressor genes: their involvement in colon cancer. J. Clin. Gastroenterol. 1990; 12(5): 494–9.

Rigas B, Goldman IS, Levine L. Altered eicosanoid levels in human colon cancer. *J. Lab. Clin. Med.* 1993; 122: 518–23.

Robertson AJ, Anderson JM, Swanson Beck J, Burnett RA, Howatson SR, Lee FD, *et al.* Observer variability in histopathological reporting of cervical biopsy specimens. *J. Clin. Pathol.* 1989; 42: 231–8.

Ron E, Wong FL, Mabuchi K. Incidence of benign gastrointestinal tumors among atomic bomb survivors. *Am. J. Epidemiol.* 1995; 142: 68–75.

Roncucci L, Pedroni M, Fante R, Di Gregorio C, Ponz de Leon M. Cell kinetic evaluation of human colonic aberrant crypts (Colorectal Cancer Study Group of the University of Modena and the Health Care District 16, Modena, Italy). *Cancer Res.* 1993; 53: 3726–9.

Salem RR, Wolf BC, Sears HF, Lavin PT, Ravikumar TS, DeCoste D, *et al.* Expression of colorectal carcinoma associated antigens in colonic polyps. *J. Surg. Res.* 1993; 55: 249–55.

Sandler RS, Lyles CM, McAuliffe C, Woosley JT, Kupper LL. Cigarette smoking, alcohol, and the risk of colorectal adenomas. *Gastroenterology* 1993; 104: 1445–51.

Sariego J, Byrd ME, Kerstein M, Sano C, Matsumoto T. Changing patterns in colorectal carcinoma: a 25-year experience. *Am. Surg.* 1992; 58: 686–91.

Schatzkin A, Baranovsky A, Kessler LG. Diet and cancer: evidence from asociations of multiple primary cancers in the SEER programme. *Cancer* 1988; 62: 1451–7.

Schneider H, Fiander H, Latta RK, Ross NW. Bile acid inhibition of xenobiotic metabolizing enzymes is a factor in the mechanism of colon carcinogenesis: tests of aspects of the concept with glucuronosyltransferase. *Eur. J. Cancer Prev.* 1993; 2: 393–400.

Schuman BM, Simsek H, Lyons RC. The association of multiple colonic adenomatous polyps with cancer of the colon. *Am. J. Gastroenterol.* 1990; 85: 846–9.

Schweinfest CW, Henderson KW, Suster S, Kondoh N, Papas TS. Identification of a colon mucosa gene that is down regulated in colon adenomas and adenocarcinomas. *Proc. Natl Acad. Sci. USA* 1993; 90: 4166–70.

Shepherd N, Baxter KJ, Love SB. The prognostic importance of peritoneal involvement in colonic cancer: a prospective evaluation. *Gastroenterol.* 1997; 112: 1096–1102.

Simons BD, Morrison AS, Lev R, Verhoek Oftedahl W. Relationship of polyps to cancer of the large intestine. *J. Natl Cancer Inst.* 1992; 84: 962–6.

Slater G, Aufses AH Jr, Szporn A. Synchronous carcinoma of the colon and rectum. *Surg. Gynecol. Obstet.* 1990; 171: 283–7.

Slattery ML, Kerber RA. A comprehensive evaluation of family history and breast cancer risk. The Utah Population Database. *JAMA* 1993; 270: 1563–8.

Stein W, Farina A, Gaffney K, Lundeen C, Wagner K, Wachtel T. Characteristics of colon cancer at time of presentation. *Fam Pract Res J.* 1993; 13: 355–63.

Steinmetz KA, Potter JD. Food group consumption and colon cancer in the Adelaide Case Control Study. II. Meat, poultry, seafood, dairy foods and eggs. *Int. J. Cancer* 1993; 53: 720–7.

Sterm HS. Contributions of molecular genetics to the clinical management of colorectal cancer. Am. J. Surg. 1996; 171: 10–5.

Suadicani P, Hein HO, Gyntelberg F. Height, weight, and risk of colorectal cancer. An 18-year follow up in a cohort of 5249 men. *Scand. J. Gastroenterol.* 1993; 28: 285–8.

Sugita A, Sachar DB, Bodian C, Ribeiro MB, Aufses AH Jr, Greenstein AJ. Colorectal cancer in ulcerative colitis. Influence of anatomical extent and age at onset on colitis cancer interval. *Gut* 1991; 32: 167–9.

Svendsen LB, Bulow S, Mellemgaard A. Metachronous colorectal cancer in young patients: expression of the hereditary nonpolyposis colorectal cancer syndrome? *Dis. Colon Rectum* 1991; 34: 790–3.

Tersmette AC, Offerhaus GJ, Giardiello FM, Tersmette KW, Vandenbroucke JP, Tytgat GN. Occurrence of non gastric cancer in the digestive tract after remote partial gastrectomy: analysis of an Amsterdam cohort. *Int. J. Cancer* 1990; 46: 792–5.

Thomas MG, Olschwang S. Genetic predispositions to colorectal cancer. *Pathol. Biol.* 1995; 43: 159–64.

Thomas MG, Tebbutt S, Williamson RC. Vitamin D and its metabolites inhibit cell proliferation in human rectal mucosa and a colon cancer cell line. *Gut* 1992; 33: 1660–3.

Thun MJ, Namboodiri MM, Calle EE, Flanders WD, Heath CW. Aspirin use and risk of fatal cancer. *J. Cancer Res.* 1993; 53: 1322–7.

Tierney RP, Ballantyne GH, Modlin IM. The adenoma to carcinoma sequence. *Surg. Gynecol. Obstet.* 1990; 171: 81–94.

Toma S, Giacchero A, Bonelli L, Graziani, De Lorenzi R, Aste H. Association between breast and colorectal cancer in a sample of surgical patients. *Eur. J. Surg. Oncol.* 1987, 13: 429–32.

Tomoda H, Furusawa M, Hayashi I. Development of a cancer of the large bowel following radiotherapy for cancer of the uterine cervix. *Gan No Rinsho* 1989; 35: 1749–52.

Turner D, Berkel HJ. Nonsteroidal anti inflammatory drugs for the prevention of colon cancer. *Can. Med. Assoc. J.* 1993; 149: 595–602.

van den Brandt PA, Goldbohm RA, van't Veer P, Bode P, Dorant E, Hermus RJ, Sturmans F. A prospective cohort study on toenail selenium levels and risk of gastrointestinal cancer. *J. Natl Cancer Inst.* 1993; 85: 224–9.

van Loon AJ, van den Brandt PA, Golbohm RA. Socioeconomic status and colon cancer incidence: a prospective cohort study. *Br. J. Cancer* 1995; 71: 882–7.

van't Hof A, Gilissen K, Cohen RJ, Taylor L, Haffajee Z, Thornley AL, Segal I. Colonic cell proliferation in two different ethnic groups with contrasting incidence of colon cancer: is there a difference in carcinogenesis? *Gut* 1995; 36: 691–5.

Varesco L, Gismondi V, James R, Robertson M, Grammatico P, Groden J, *et al.* Identification of APC gene mutations in Italian adenomatous polyposis coli patients by PCR SSCP analysis. *Am. J. Hum. Genet.* 1993; 52: 280–5.

Vargas PA, Alberts DS. Primary prevention of colorectal cancer through dietary modification. *Cancer* 1992; 70: 1229–35.

Vasen HF. Periodic examination of families with hereditary nonpolyposis colorectal carcinoma in The Netherlands: a study of 41 families. *Ned. Tijdschr. Geneeskd.* 1994; 138: 77–81.

Vasen HF, Mecklin JP, Khan PM, Lynch HT. The International Collaborative Group on HNPCC. *Anticancer Res.* 1994; 14: 1661–4.

Vasen HF, Wijnen JT, Menko FH, Kleibeuker JH, Taal BG, Griffioen G. Nagengast FM, Meijers-Heijboer EH, Bertario L, Varesco L, Bisgaard ML, Mohr J, Fodde R, Khan PM. Cancer risk in families with hereditary nonpolyposis colorectal cancer diagnosed by mutation analysis. *Gastroenterol.* 1996; 110: 1020–7.

Vogel VG, McPherson RS. Dietary epidemiology of colon cancer. *Hematol. Oncol. Clin. North Am.* 1989; 3:1 35–63.

von Herbay A, Herfarth C, Otto HF. Cancer and dysplasia in ulcerative colitis: a histologic study of 301 surgical specimen. *Z. Gastroenterol.* 1994; 32: 382–8.

Vukasin AP, Ballantyne GH, Flannery JT, Lerner E, Modlin IM. Increasing incidence of cecal and sigmoid carcinoma. Data from the Connecticut Tumor Registry. *Cancer* 1990; 66: 2442–9.

Waddell WR. The effect of sulindac on colon polyps: circumvention of a transformed phenotype—a hypothesis. *J. Surg. Oncol.* 1994; 55: 52–5.

Weaver P, Harrison B, Eskander G, Jahan MS, Tanzo V, Williams W, *et al.* Colon cancer in blacks: a disease with a worsening prognosis. *J. Natl Med. Assoc.* 1991; 83: 133–6.

Weisburger JH, Reddy BS, Rose DP, Cohen LA, Kendall ME, Wynder EL. Protective mechanisms of dietary fibers in nutritional carcinogenesis. *Basic Life Sci.* 1993; 61: 45–63.

Welberg JW, Kleibeuker JH, Van der Meer R, Kuipers F, Cats A, Van Rijsbergen H, *et al.* Effects of oral calcium supplementation on intestinal bile acids and cytolytic activity of fecal water in patients with adenomatous polyps of the colon. *Eur. J. Clin. Invest.* 1993; 23: 63–8.

Wildrick DM. Molecular genetic studies of colon cancer. *Hematol. Oncol. Clin. North Am.* 1989. 3: 11–18.

Winawer SJ, Zauber AG, Ho MN, O'Brien MJ, Gottlieb LS, Sternberg SS, *et al.* Prevention of colorectal cancer by colonoscopic polypectomy. The National Polyp Study Workgroup. *N. Engl. J. Med.* 1993; 329: 1977–81.

Winawer SJ, Zauber AG, Gerdes H, O'Brien MJ, Gottlieb LS, Sternberg SS, *et al.* Risk of colorectal cancer in the families of patients with adenomatous polyps. National Polyp Study Workgroup. *N. Engl. J. Med.* 1996; 334: 82–7.

Wu Williams AH, Lee M, Whittemore AS, Gallagher RP, Jiao DA, Zheng S, *et al.* Reproductive factors and colorectal cancer risk among Chinese females. *Cancer Res.* 1991; 51: 2307–11.

Wynder EL, Reddy BS, Weisburger JH. Environmental dietary factors in colorectal cancer. Some unresolved issues. *Cancer* 1992; 70: 1222–8.

Xu Z, Dai B, Dhruva B, Singh P. Gastrin gene expression in human colon cancer cells measured by a simple competitive PCR method. *Life Sci.* 1994; 54: 671–8.

Yamaguchi A, Kurosaka Y, Fushida S, Kanno M, Yonemura Y, Miwa K, Miyazaki I. Expression of p53 protein in colorectal cancer and its relationship to short term prognosis. *Cancer* 1992; 70: 2778–84.

Yamashita N, Minamoto T, Ochiai A, Onda M, Esumi H. Frequent and characteristic K ras activation in aberrant crypt foci of colon. Is there preference among K ras mutants for malignant progression? *Cancer* 1995; 75: 1527–33.

Yapp R, Modlin IM, Kumar RR, Binder HJ, Dubrow R. Gastrin and colorectal cancer. Evidence against an association. *Dig. Dis. Sci.* 1992; 37: 481–4.

Yong CK, Ng BK. Large bowel cancer in the young adult. *Ann. Acad. Med. Singapore* 1990, 19: 385–8.

Zahm SH, Cocco P, Blair A. Tobacco smoking as a risk factor for colon polyps. *Am. J. Public Health.* 1991; 81: 846–9.

Zhao LP, Le Marchand L. An analytical method for assessing patterns of familial aggregation in case control studies. *Genet. Epidemiol.* 1992; 9: 141–54.

Ziegler RG, Devesa SS, Fraumeni JF. Epidemiologic patterns of colorectal cancer. *Important Adv. Oncol.* 1986; 2: 209–231.

Zisiadis A, Harlaftis N, Zaraboukas T, Basdanis G, Aletras H. The significance of dysplasia in colorectal adenomatous polyps associated with carcinoma. *J. Med. Assoc. Ga.* 1993; 82: 247–9.

Zuccato E, Venturi M, Di Leo G, Colombo L, Bertolo C, Doldi SB, Mussini E. Role of bile acids and metabolic activity of colonic bacteria in increased risk of colon cancer after cholecystectomy. *Dig. Dis. Sci.* 1993; 38: 514–9.

11 Clinicopathological features of colorectal cancer

Pathology

Macroscopic appearance

Colorectal tumours may have an ulcerating, polypoid or annular appearance. Ulcerating tumours are the most common and have raised, everted edges with slough in the base (Figure 11.1). Annular tumours also tend to occur in the left colon. Despite their small

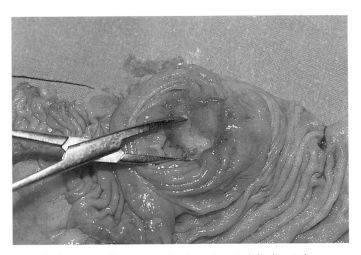

Figure 11.1 Tumour of the caecum showing a characteristic ulcerated appearance (see colour plates).

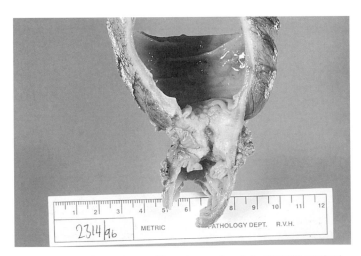

Figure 11.2 Annular carcinoma of the colon causing obstruction with proximal dilatation of the bowel.

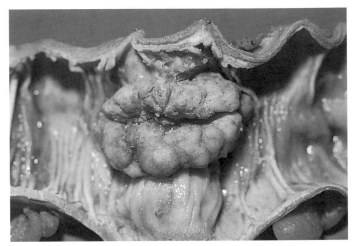

Figure 11.3 Colonic carcinoma displaying a fungating appearance.

size, they often markedly constrict the bowel causing obstruction or perforation (Figure 11.2). Polypoid tumours have a villous or papillary appearance (Figure 11.3).

Other macroscopic appearances have been described. About 10% of colorectal tumours have a colloid appearance due to mucin. A diffusely infiltrative linitis plastica form, extending submucosally for over 5 cm, is recognized, classically superimposed on ulcerative colitis. Recently, a flat form of colorectal cancer has been described (Kasumi *et al.* 1992). This cancer invades deeply into the submucosa, even in its early stages and has characteristics quite different from cancers which follow the adenoma–cancer sequence (Kasumi *et al.* 1992).

Microscopic appearance

Adenocarcinomas comprise 97% of all colorectal tumours (DiSario *et al.* 1994). In well differentiated adenocarcinomas the tubular pattern is preserved and nuclei are uniform in size and shape. The nuclei may display stratification but polarity is maintained so that the apex and base of the cells are easily identified (Figure 11.4). In moderately differentiated adenocarcinomas, glandular structures are still apparent but irregular with pleomorphic nuclei and poorly discerned polarity (Figure 11.5). In poorly differentiated tumours tubular structures are irregular or completely absent with cells in clumps or sheets. About 20% of adenocarcinomas are well differentiated, 60% moderately and 20% poorly. Correlation between histological grading of pre-operative biopsy specimens and the corresponding resected tumour is about 60% (Kato *et al.* 1989). Undifferentiated tumours show no attempt at tubular differentiation or mucin secretion but do contain scanty agryophilic cells (Figure

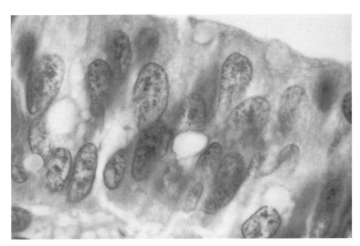

Figure 11.4 Well differentiated colonic adenocarcinoma. The nuclei are stratified, but polarity is maintained resulting in the apex and base of the cells being easily seen (H&E×250).

11.6). Such tumours can be differentiated from anaplastic carcinomas by their lack of pleomorphism and bizarre mitotic figures.

About 10–15% of colorectal tumours contain large amounts of mucin (mucinous or colloid tumours) (Blank *et al.* 1994) (Figure 11.7). Histologically, these appear as mucin-filled glands associated with interstitial mucin or as clumps of cells surrounded by mucin (Figure 11.8). Although the degree of mucin may be so great as to make the assessment of differentiation difficult, entirely signet cell tumours are rare in countries with a high incidence of colorectal cancer. Although patients present with more advanced disease, stage-for-stage survival is similar to other types of colorectal cancer (Green *et al.* 1993). In contrast, mucinous carcinomas of the rectum not only present at a more advanced stage but also have a worse 5-year survival (10% versus 60%) than non-mucinous rectal carcinomas (Green *et al.* 1993). This may be related to their greater tendency to metastasize (Schwartz *et al.* 1992).

It is routine to examine the resection margins of the excised specimen for residual tumours. However, this policy has been challenged if, on macroscopic appearance, the tumour is not within 2 cm of the resection margin as recurrence is then extremely unlikely (Cross *et al.* 1989). It is claimed that assessment of the

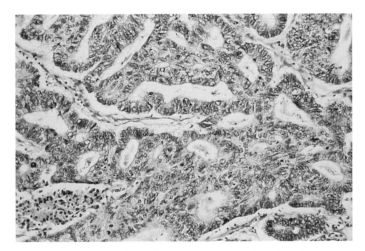

Figure 11.5 Moderately differentiated adenocarcinoma. The glandular structure is present but irregular with loss of nuclear polarity. H&E×100.

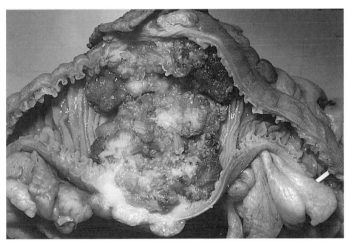

Figure 11.7 Mucinous secreting adenocarcinoma of colon showing the typical colloid appearance (see colour plates).

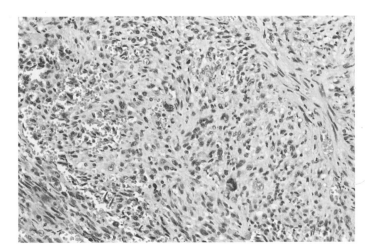

Figure 11.6 Poorly differentiated adenocarcinoma. There is no attempt at glandular formation. H&E×100.

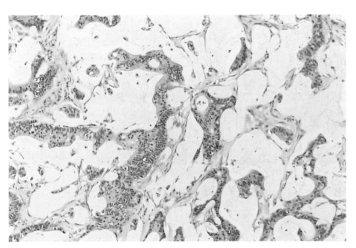

Figure 11.8 Mucinous carcinoma showing large clumps of cells surrounded by mucin. H&E×100.

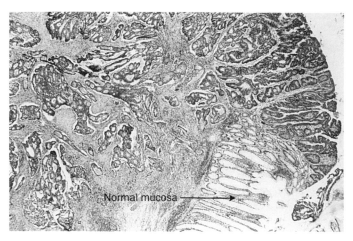

Figure 11.9 Normal colonic mucosa (arrowed) adjacent to an infiltrating adenocarcinoma Note the elongation of the crypts in this transitional mucosa.

Table 11.1 Features of histological grading	
Categories	Well: 20%
	Moderate: 60%
	Poor: 20%
	Uniform nuclei and well formed tubules
	Nuclei in clumps and tubules irregular
Advantages	Widely performed and accepted
	Independent prognostic variable
Disadvantages	Assessment consistent in only 30% of specimens
	Poor inter-observer variation among pathologists
Five-year survival	Well: 80%
	Moderately: 60%
	Poor: 25%

lateral resection margins and distal intramural spread would be a more effective use of histopathological resources as this is strongly related to tumour recurrence (Quirke and Dixon 1988; Sidoni *et al.* 1991).

Transitional mucosa

The transitional mucosa adjacent to colorectal cancer frequently displays abnormalities, reflecting the 'field change' recognized to occur in colorectal mucosa (Xiang *et al.* 1997). Such changes can be detected by mucin histochemical staining, staining with high iron diamine–alcian blue distinguishing sulphomucin from sialomucin. Normal mucosa shows a predominantly sulphated mucin pattern while tumours display marked sialomucin staining. Colorectal carcinomas displaying a loss of an organ-specific mucin (sulphomucin), an increased expression of non-intestinal sialomucins, or an ectopic expression of adhesion ligands (sialyl-dimeric Lex antigens) on mucin staining have increased metastatic potential and poor prognosis (Irimura *et al.* 1991). Alternatives are monoclonal antibodies, diastase PAS, and lectin histochemistry using peanut agglutinin which are specific for O-acetylated sialomucins (Milton *et al.* 1993).

Transitional mucosa shows elongation of crypts, marked sialomucin secretion accompanied by a significant reduction in the normal sulphomucin content (Mori *et al.* 1990) (Figure 11.9). Such changes are found in 95% of carcinomas, one-half of adenomas and one-third of metaplastic polyps (Mori *et al.* 1990). In addition, multiple patch lesions of increased sialomucin production, suggesting a field change in the mucosa, can be identified in up to one-third of colorectal cancers. Sialomucin staining reveals the transitional zone can extend for 20 cm (mean 3 cm) from either resection margin (Mori *et al.* 1990). DNA flow cytometry also provides evidence for a field change, aneuploid changes, and significantly increased proliferative activity being apparent up to 10 cm from a colorectal cancer (Ngoi *et al.* 1990).

Prognostic factors in colorectal cancer

Histological grading (Table 11.1)

In 1928, Rankin and Broders related the degree of tumour differentiation to patient survival in rectal cancer. Mortality in those with grade 1 tumours (in which at least 75% of the cells were differentiated) was considerably less than in those with grade 4

tumours (in which less than 25% of the cells were differentiated). This was subsequently simplified into three grades: well, moderate, and poorly differentiated, according to the degree of invasive tendency, glandular arrangement, nuclear polarity, and frequency of mitosis. These features are still used today.

The degree of differentiation within the same specimen is entirely consistent throughout the tumour in only one-third of cases so that several areas of the specimen need to be examined, with the most anaplastic being taken as the grade for the tumour as a whole (Halvorsen and Seim 1988). This results in a subjective, poorly reproducible assessment of tumour differentiation (Thomas *et al.* 1983). Grading by the same observer is reasonably reproducible, whereas grading of the same specimen by different observers is more variable, with haphazard agreement of up to 40% occurring between some pathologists (Thomas *et al.* 1983; Halvorsen and Seim 1988). In one study of pathologists assessing colorectal cancers, the proportion of tumours classified as well differentiated varied from 3% to 93%, moderately differentiated from 8% to 82%, and poorly differentiated from 5% to 30% (Blenkinsopp *et al.* 1981). Pathologists are better at distinguishing poorly differentiated from the other types of tumours, the distinction between well and moderately differentiated tumours being poorly reproducible (Quirke and Dixon 1988). There is also an unwillingness for pathologists to depart from the middle ground and allocate extreme grades, resulting in most large series reporting about 60% of all colorectal tumours as being moderately differentiated.

Despite this poor reproducibility, histological grading of colorectal tumours is of independent prognostic significance in the presence of other clinicopathological variables (Halvorsen and Seim 1988; Deans *et al.* 1994a). Five-year survival for well, moderately, and poorly differentiated tumours is 80, 60, and 25%, respectively. Stipulating only two grades (poor and 'not poor' differentiation) maintains the prognostic value while improving reproducibility (Quirke and Dixon 1988).

Pathological staging

In 1932 Dukes developed a system for the pathological staging of carcinoma of the rectum which correlated with prognosis. Three stages of extension of tumours were described: 'A—Growth limited to wall of rectum; B—Extension of growth to extrarectal tissues but no metastases in regional lymph nodes; C—Metastases in regional lymph nodes' (Figure 11.10). Dukes also correlated his pathological

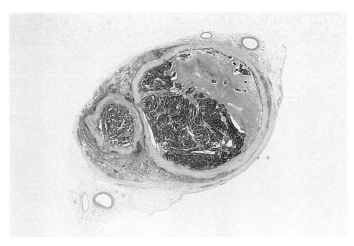

Figure 11.10 Metastastic colonic adenocarcinoma.

classification with Broder's histological grading. Nearly all Broder's grade 1 tumours occurred in Dukes' stage A cases, while most of the grade 3 and 4 tumours occurred in stage C cases. Stage C was subsequently subdivided into: 'C1—Regional lymph glands only are involved; C2—glandular spread has reached to the level of the point of ligature of the blood vessels'. Despite skip metastases (distant node metastases without local node involvement) occurring in one-third of Dukes' C cases, the prognostic value of this subdivision has been repeatedly shown: 5-year disease-free survival for stage C1 is 70% compared with 40% for C2 cases (Shida *et al.* 1992). However, rectal cancers within 6 cm from the anal verge have a high risk of

lateral lymph node metastases. Although Dukes' confined his classification to rectal carcinoma, it soon became applied to colonic cancers, becoming the standard prognostic classification for all colorectal tumours (Table 11.2).

In America, Dukes' system was subclassified into: 'A—Lesion limited to the mucosa; B1—Lesion extends into muscularis propria, but does not penetrate through it; B2—Lesion penetrates through muscularis propria; C—Lesion of either B1 or B2 with involvement of lymph nodes'. The C group of this system was then modified in 1954 by Astler and Coller into: 'C1—Lesion limited to (bowel) wall with positive nodes; C2—Lesion through all layers (of bowel) with positive nodes'. These modifications have created more confusion than clarity, making it difficult to compare reported series. A modified B1 lesion corresponds to Dukes' stage A. Tumours staged as A, as designated by Astler and Coller are rare, accounting for less than 1% of the tumours in their series. In contrast, the reported frequency of Dukes' stage A in tumours of the colon and rectum varies widely from 6% to over 25%, largely due to different interpretations of what constitutes a Dukes' A lesion (Deans *et al.* 1992).

The C1 and C2 categories proposed by Astler and Coller are different from those described by Dukes. The use of the muscularis propria in the Astler and Coller staging system, has subsequently been incorrectly interpreted to mean muscularis mucosa. The result is that both B1 and B2 staging by the modified Dukes' system would correspond to a Dukes' stage A lesion and neither modified system would have a category for tumours that penetrate the wall of the intestine but have no lymph node spread, that is, Dukes' stage B.

There are other deficiencies in the Dukes' system. Analysis based on small numbers of tissue samples may miss breakthrough of the muscularis propria, the thoroughness with which the pathologist searches for lymph nodes is also important. Consequently, some patients who have been misclassified as having good prognosis stage A tumours may die fairly rapidly. In Dukes' own series 5-year survival of stage A lesions was 81%, instead of the 100% expected if the classification were perfect. Blenkinsopp *et al.* (1981) noted inter-observer variation in pathologists' assessment of the extent of tumour penetration between institutions to be 5–30%. Significant differences also existed in the proportion of cases with no nodes identified and the number of nodes harvested per specimen. As the microscopic appearances are rarely difficult to interpret, these differences are most likely due to errors in the macroscopic assessment of the specimen. Caution is therefore necessary in interpreting reports of Dukes' stages between institutions. Further problems are that histological grade and the number of involved nodes are not considered in Dukes' classification, although they are known to be of prognostic significance. Despite these problems, Dukes' classification remains an extremely powerful prognostic tool. In addition, the reproducibility of Dukes' stage is better than for any of the other staging systems (Deans *et al.* 1994*a*). Dukes' classification is also less affected by pre-operative radiotherapy than other pathological variables and remains the most important predictive variable for survival and pelvic recurrence (James *et al.* 1991).

Dukes and Bussey reported crude 5-year survival of 81%, 64%, and 27.5% for patients with Dukes' stage A, B and C tumours, respectively, figures similar to most modern series (Deans *et al.* 1992). Tumour staging has been repeatedly shown to be the major determinant of prognosis in studies employing both univariate and multivariate analysis (Deans *et al.* 1992). Some therefore claim that the only improvement required on Dukes' own classification is the use of Astler–Coller stages C1 and C2. Multivariate analysis has

Table 11.2 Features of Duke's classification	
Categories	
A: 15% (6–25%)	Growth confined to bowel wall
B: 25%	Involvement of extra-intestinal tissues without nodes
C: 45%	Metastases in regional lymph nodes (subdivided as C1 and C2)
D: 15%	Distant or hepatic metastases
Advantages	Widely performed and accepted
	Reasonable inter-observer variation among pathologists
	Reproducibility better than for other staging systems
	Assessment less affected by radiotherapy than other staging systems
	Highly independent prognostic variable
Disadvantages	Several variations in classification:
	Astler Coller B1(and B2) corresponds to original Dukes' A
	Astler Coller C1 and C2 do not correspond to original Dukes' C
	Thoroughness of lymph node assessment by pathologist important
	Number of involved lymph nodes not included
Five-year survival	A: 85%
	B: 65%
	C: 25%
	D: < 10%

shown this to be superior to a single Dukes' C class, and to be independent of the number and site of nodal metastases and the degree of tumour differentiation (Fisher *et al.* 1989). The Japanese Society for Cancer of the Colon and Rectum (JRSCCR) have devised a system very similar to Dukes' stage, which is highly related to prognosis (Onodera *et al.* 1989). Dukes' stage therefore remains the 'gold standard' against which all other prognostic classifications should be compared (Deans *et al.* 1992).

Clinicopathological staging

The Tumour Node Metastasis system (TNM)

As a result of the deficiencies and confusion over modifications of Dukes' classification, a clinicopathological TNM classification was proposed. It has been agreed that the extent of colonic carcinoma cannot be fully assessed clinically at the time of surgery and several modifications of the TNM classification have ensued. The American Joint Committee on Cancer therefore developed a series of prefixes to relate to the extent of disease at various sites and times (Payne 1989). These are: cTNM, clinical diagnostic staging; sTNM, surgical staging; pTNM, postsurgical staging; rTNM, retreatment staging (at second laparotomy); and aTNM, autopsy staging (Table 11.3). Some studies, however, found the clinical and postoperative assessment of TNM stages diverged, indicating a low precision for clinical staging. A recent study found that on multivariate analysis the most independent prognostic factors were lymph node metastases, TNM stage and lymphatic invasion (Tanaka *et al.* 1994).

In Australia it was felt that this American classification was too complex and another clinicopathological version of the TNM classification developed (Chapuis *et al.* 1990; D'eredita *et al.* 1996). This combined clinical information, curative or palliative operation status, and a pathological subdivision of Dukes' stages into a final A, B, C, and D grade. The Australian clinicopathological system is claimed to be better than the American system as the pTNM classification is only partially able to separate patients into different survival groups, is complicated and difficult to memorize, and does not give useful prognostic information beyond that provided by the simpler Australian system. Despite attempts to produce a standardized clinicopathological classification, the TNM system is complex relative to Dukes' classification (Ponz de Leon *et al.* 1992).

Jass' classification (Table 11.4)

The advent of multivariate survival analysis allowed Jass and colleagues (1987) to develop a grading system based on tumour stage and a series of pathological variables related to histological grade. This classification was claimed to be superior to that of Dukes. All of the grade-related variables investigated by Jass *et al.* (1987) were related to survival on univariate analysis, but only three remained important after Cox's regression analysis. After correction for Dukes' stage, the extent of lymphocytic infiltration was the only grade-related variable that remained significantly correlated with survival. Other studies have confirmed these findings, a poorer prognosis being detected in patients with minor or no lymphocytic infiltration (Ponz de Leon *et al.* 1992; Deans *et al.* 1994*a*). Nevertheless, the prognostic power of lymphocytic infiltration, although exceeding that of growth pattern and fibrous proliferation, is less than that of tumour penetration and histological grade (Offerhaus *et al.* 1991; Deans *et al.* 1994*a*) (Figure 11.11).

Table 11.3 TNM classification of colorectal tumours

T—Primary tumour
TX: Primary tumour cannot be assessed
T0: No evidence of primary tumour
T1: Involvement confined to the mucosa or submucosa
T2: Involvement confined to the muscular wall or serosa
T3: Involvement of all layers with extension to immediately adjacent structures
T4: Fistula present with any degree of penetration

N—Regional lymph nodes
NX: Regional nodes not assessed
N0: No regional node metastasis
N1: Nodes involved
M–-Distant metastasis
MX: Distant metastases not assessed
M0: No known distal metastases
M1: Distant metastases present

G—Pathological grade
GX: Grade of differentiation cannot be assessed
G1: Well differentiated tumour
G2: Moderately differentiated tumour
G3: Poorly differentiated tumour
G4: Undifferentiated tumour

Stage

Stage			
Stage 0	Tis	N0	M0
Stage I	T0/T1	N0/NX	M0
Stage II	T2-T4	N0/NX	M0
Stage III	Any T	N1	M0
Stage IV	Any T	Any N	M1

Table 11.4 The variables assessed by Jass *et al.*. (1987)

Variable assessed	Categories
Tumour type	tubular
	mucinous
	papillary
Tumour differentiation	well
	moderate
	poor
Nuclear polarity	easily discerned
	just discerned
	lost
Tubule configuration	complex
	irregular
	simple
	no tubules
Lymphocytic infiltration	little
	moderate
	marked
Growth pattern	expanding
	infiltrating
Fibrosis	extensive
	moderate
	little
Tumour infiltration	mucosa/submucosa
	serosa
	nodes
	distant spread

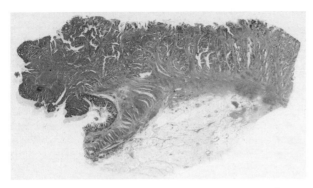

Figure 11.11 Tissue section mount of a tumour showing an expanding, as opposed to an infiltrating, growth pattern.

A problem is that assessment of the component variables among pathologists is subjective. Jass *et al.* (1987) initially assessed intra-observer variation by one pathologist and subsequently reported fair to excellent levels of interobserver agreement for tumour type, differentiation, growth pattern, and lymphocytic infiltration (Shepherd *et al.* 1989). These assessments were performed by specialist pathologists from a centre dealing almost entirely with colorectal cancer. Reports using non-specialist general pathologists, which may be more relevant to the majority of pathology departments nation-wide, have shown poor observer variation for many of the components of Jass' classification (Deans *et al.* 1994a). The reproducibility of lymphocytic infiltration, which is the only variable of Jass' classification

independently associated with survival, can be little better than chance (Deans *et al.* 1994a). This may be related to inter-relationships between the component grade-related variables and casts doubt on the clinical relevance of Jass' classification for non-specialist colorectal units.

Studies employing multivariate analysis suggest that Dukes' classification is to be preferred to Jass' system. Others have found that lymphocytic infiltration is of less importance than Dukes' stage. In studies comparing clinicopathological variables, including the components of Jass' classification and patient age, staging was the strongest variable of independent prognostic significance (Ponz de Leon *et al.* 1992; Deans *et al.* 1994a). Large studies directly comparing Dukes' and Jass' classifications have suggested that the former is significantly more related to survival on multivariate analysis (Fisher *et al.* 1989; Deans *et al.* 1994a). In one study of over 700 patients, Jass' system allowed for only two major prognostic systems, whereas five were noted by Dukes' stage (Fisher *et al.* 1989). These studies conclude that the more objective nature, and greater prognostic power of Dukes' classification warrant its continued use in preference to Jass' system in patients with colorectal cancer (Fisher *et al.* 1989; Deans *et al.* 1994a).

Tumour recurrence can be expected in about one-quarter of patients and is related to Dukes' stage, histological grade, involvement of the lateral margins and tumour perforation (Quirke and Dixon 1988; Jensen *et al.* 1996). Local involvement of the peritoneum is a consistent predictor of subsequent intraperitoneal recurrence (Shepherd *et al.* 1997). It is suggested that the pathological criteria that should be routinely assessed include tumour spread

Table 11.5 Prognostic value of clinicopathological variables

Variable	Comments	Authors
Venous invasion	Classified as: Extra- or intramural Thick- or thin-walled vessel	Talbot *et al.* 1980
	Not a major independent prognostic variable	Minsky *et al.* 1989 Offerhaus *et al.* 1991 Deans *et al.* 1994b
Lymphatic vessel invasion	Related to Dukes' stage and both local and distant nodal involvement Related to survival	Minsky *et al.* 1989
HLA class I antigen expression	HLA expression lost in tumours Relationship to survival variable	Tsioulias *et al.* 1993 Nakagoe *et al.* 1994
Blood transfusion	Retrospective studies: Recurrence twice as common and 5 year disease-free survival reduced by 20% with transfusion	Liewald *et al.* 1990 Modin *et al.* 1992 Tartter 1992 Leite *et al.* 1993
	This might be explained by other factors necessitating transfusion Prospective studies:	Busch *et al.* 1994 Bentzen *et al.* 1990 Jakobsen *et al.* 1990
	Effect on recurrence and survival variable	Garau *et al.* 1994 Donohue *et al.* 1995
	Autologous blood of no benefit	Molland *et al.* 1995 Faenza *et al.* 1992 Sibbering *et al.* 1994 Busch *et al.* 1994 Heiss *et al.* 1994 Houbiers *et al.* 1994
Ornithine decarboxylase	Little prognostic value May help in assessing response to treatment	Moorehead *et al.* 1987 Hixson *et al.* 1993 Phillips *et al.* 1993 Braverman *et al.* 1990

Table 11.6 Prognostic value of other clinicopathological variables

Variable	Comments	Authors
Patient age	Independent prognostic variable Elderly high mortality More associated medical conditions More emergency operations Under 40s high mortality Diagnosed late but stage for stage survival similar to older patients	Hermanek *et al.* 1994 Ponz de Leon *et al.* 1992 Deans *et al.* 1994b Catalano and Levin 1991 Cozart *et al.* 1993 Heys *et al.* 1994
Intestinal obstruction and perforation	Occurs in 15% of patients Associated with worse prognosis but not independent prognostic variables on multivariate survival analysis	Catalano and Levin 1991 Crucitti *et al.* 1991 Garcia-Peche *et al.* 1991 Deans *et al.* 1994b
Sex, symptom duration, tumour size, tumour site, multiple tumours	Not independent prognostic variables on multivariate survival analysis	Adloff *et al.* 1989 Garcia-Peche *et al.* 1991 Cali *et al.* 1993 Deans *et al.* 1994b
Tumour DNA content	Aneuploid tumours associated with poorer prognosis Not consistently an independent prognostic variable on multivariate survival analysis	Rowley *et al.* 1990 Kim *et al.* 1991 Deans *et al.* 1993a,b Ensley *et al.* 1993 Yamazoe *et al.* 1994
Epithelial cell turnover	No independent prognostic benefit	Deans *et al.* 1993a Buchsbaum *et al.* 1994 Pagangili *et al.* 1994
Argyrophil nucleolar organiser regions (AgNORs)	Numbers increased in colon tumours Considerable observer variation Variable relationship to survival	Kawasaki *et al.* 1990 Joyce *et al.* 1992 Rayter *et al.* 1992

(Dukes' stage), involvement of the deep (lateral) excision margin, incomplete removal (histologically confirmed, or bowel perforation should constitute cases being classified as non-curative), the number of positive lymph nodes (0, 1–4, greater than 4, as only 10% of patients with no positive lymph nodes die as a result of cancer), venous invasion, tumour type, tumour differentiation (classified as 'poorly differentiated' and 'other' to minimize the subjective nature of grading), and possibly invasive margin and lymphocytic infiltration (Quirke and Dixon 1988; Garcia-Peche *et al.* 1991).

Other clinicopathological variables (Tables 11.5 and 11.6)

The prognostic value of several other clinicopathological criteria have been assessed in an attempt to improve on the prediction of prognosis and recurrence.

Venous and lymphatic invasion

It has been known for many years that liver metastases occur via the portal vein, the incidence of venous invasion by tumour in early series ranging from 10% to 60%. These series recorded 5-year survival rates less than 50% if venous invasion was present compared to up to 73% when venous invasion was absent. In 1980, Talbot and colleagues finding venous invasion in half of cases, emphasized that venous invasion should be classified into extra- versus intramural and thick-walled as opposed to thin-walled veins; thick-walled extramural vein involvement having the poorest prognosis (Figure 11.12). Venous spread was related to local spread (Dukes' stage) and lymph node metastases and appeared to have an independent influence on

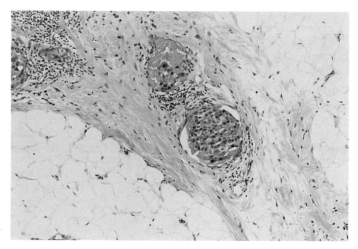

Figure 11.12 Vascular invasion of the vessels in the fat by an adenocarcinoma of the rectum. H&E×250.

prognosis. More recent studies, while supporting the role of venous invasion in survival in colorectal cancer, have shown considerable overlap in survival rates between patients with and without venous invasion (Offerhaus *et al.* 1991; Deans *et al.* 1994b).

Lymphatic vessel invasion is detected in 15% of colorectal cancers. Relative to tumours without lymphatic vessel invasion, its presence is associated with blood vessel invasion, increased incidence of positive nodes (60% versus 25%) and average number of positive nodes (5 versus 2) (Minsky *et al.* 1989). Lymphatic vessel invasion is also associated with significantly greater local (15% versus 5%), abdominal (33% versus 10%), and distant (15% versus 5%) lymph node metastases (Minsky *et al.* 1989). Lymphatic vessel invasion is also claimed to be an independent prognostic factor for survival (5-year survival rate: colon 60%; rectosigmoid/rectum, 40%) (Minsky *et al.* 1989).

Tumour markers

Pre-operative carcino-embryonic antigen (CEA) is claimed to be still the best tumour marker (Wang *et al.* 1994). However, its concentration is dependent on the bulk of tumour present, so that levels are often not elevated until disease is advanced (Einspahr *et al.* 1994). Consequently, CEA is not significantly associated with survival among patients with Dukes' A and B lesions or Dukes' C lesions with one to three nodes involved (Moertel *et al.* 1986; Wang *et al.* 1997). Some claim that the prognostic value of CEA is limited because of a lack of sensitivity in identifying good prognosis patients, others claim that CEA levels >5 ng/ml are significantly related to survival of Dukes' B and C cases (Wang *et al.* 1994; Plebani *et al.* 1996). CEA is discussed in more detail in the section on diagnosis of colorectal cancer.

Immunohistochemistry for collagen IV, epidermal growth factor receptors, and oncogene mutations have all been claimed to be related to survival to varying extents (Hemming *et al.* 1992; Tanaka *et al.* 1994). Increased sialomucin at the surgical resection margins is detected in 15–30% of patients with colorectal cancers and is an independent prognostic variable for the development of local tumour recurrence, metachronous tumour development and of subsequent survival for patients with colorectal carcinoma (Wang *et al.* 1991). There is no correlation with the amount of sialomucin present and tumour site, Dukes' stage, distance of the resection margins from the tumour and clinical variables. The presence of sialomucin is significantly related to both survival and recurrence with Dukes' classification and histological differentiation (Dawson *et al.* 1987).

Blood group antigens

The loss of human leucocyte antigens (HLAs) by neoplastic cells is thought to allow tumours to escape immune surveillance. HLA class I antigen expression is reduced in half of adenomas and is related to the grade of dysplasia (Tsioulias *et al.* 1993). HLA class I antigens have been described in colorectal carcinomas, but their relationship to metastases and hence prognostic significance is variable (Nakagoe *et al.* 1994). It may be that class I HLA-ABC deficient, poorly differentiated tumours evade lethal immune aggression by HLA-restricted cytotoxic T cells and thus progress to overt malignancy. Thus negative expression may provide an explanation for the poorer prognosis observed among patients afflicted by a poorly differentiated adenocarcinoma or mucin-producing adenocarcinoma of the colon (Eyal *et al.* 1990).

Blood transfusion

Several retrospective reports suggest that perioperative blood transfusion results in a higher recurrence and death rate after colorectal cancer surgery, some claiming blood transfusion to be an adverse independent prognostic variable (Liewald *et al.* 1990; Tartter 1992; Leite *et al.* 1993; Busch *et al.* 1994). These reports suggest that recurrence is twice as common and 5-year disease-free survival 20% less patients in patients receiving blood transfusion, even after other factors have been taken into account (Modin *et al.* 1992; Tartter 1992). Against this, others report that the observed association between transfusion status and prognosis is adequately explained by

a multivariate prognostic model including well-established prognostic factors (Bentzen *et al.* 1990; Jakobsen *et al.* 1990; Garau *et al.* 1994; Donohue *et al.* 1995; Molland *et al.* 1995).

Studies that are claimed to be prospective also fail to provide a definitive answer. Some report that transfused patients developed significantly more recurrences and had a higher death rate (Laffer *et al.* 1989; Faenza *et al.* 1992), others that transfusion has no significant effect on prognosis (Sibbering *et al.* 1994).

The possible adverse effect from transfusion has been related to immunosuppression, which may be reduced by autologous blood transfusions (Heiss *et al.* 1994). A study employing autologous blood transfusions did not improve prognosis (Busch *et al.* 1994). The risk of recurrence was significantly increased for patients transfused with allogeneic, or with autologous, or with both types of blood relative to those not requiring transfusion. The authors conclude that it is not blood transfusion but the circumstances that necessitate the transfusion that are the real determinants of prognosis (Busch *et al.* 1994). However, leucocyte-depleted blood is not associated with a significant improvement in overall survival, disease-free survival, cancer recurrence rates, or overall infection rates (Houbiers *et al.* 1994). Patients who received blood of any sort had a lower 3-year survival, but not higher recurrence rates, than non-transfused patients, suggesting that the poorer survival in those receiving transfusion is not due to the promotion of cancer. Although the evidence is still equivocal, it seems prudent to minimize blood transfusions in those undergoing colorectal cancer surgery (Faenza *et al.* 1992).

Ornithine decarboxylase

Polyamines are intimately involved in normal cellular proliferation and are likely to play a part in carcinogenesis (Giardiello *et al.* 1997). In tumours, concentrations of polyamines are increased 120–200% compared with normal mucosa; while those of spermine vary inversely with the histological grade of the tumour (LaMuraglia *et al.* 1986). Ornithine decarboxylase (ODC) is the first and probably rate-limiting enzyme in polyamine synthesis, some studies implying that ODC may be a useful marker in screening for colorectal neoplasia (Moorehead *et al.* 1987). However, although ODC and polyamines are elevated in the majority of colorectal neoplasms, there is considerable overlap such that amounts in normal mucosa do not differentiate between patients with cancer, benign neoplastic polyps, and normal subjects (Love *et al.* 1992; Hixson *et al.* 1993; Giardello *et al.* 1977). ODC activity in normal-appearing mucosa also varies throughout the large intestine, the higher activities in the sigmoid colon and rectum correlating with the higher incidence of tumours in this region (Nishioka *et al.* 1991). Neither ODC activity nor polyamine contents of normal mucosa appear to be discriminatory markers of colorectal carcinogenesis possibly due to poor reproducibility in assessment of tissue levels (Braverman *et al.* 1990; Hixson *et al.* 1994). Although ODC activity is of little prognostic value, it may be helpful in assessing response to treatment (Phillips *et al.* 1993).

Clinical variables

Patient age is the most important clinical variable related to survival, although it is unclear whether older or younger patients are at greater risk. In most large studies the overall 5-year survival rate of colorectal cancer is 50%, age-corrected survival being 60% (Hermanek *et al.* 1994). Many series have reported that increasing age is associated with a poorer prognosis (Ponz de Leon *et al.* 1992; Deans *et al.* 1994*b*). Surgery for colorectal carcinoma in the over 75 year olds has a hospital mortality of 10–15%, which is higher than that of younger patients (5%) (Payne *et al.* 1986). This is not just related to cardiorespiratory causes but a greater number of emergency operations (20%) in elderly patients, suggesting a tendency to delay treatment in older patients (Catalano and Levin 1991). The mortality of elective colorectal cancer surgery in the over 70s is 8%, compared with up to 25% in emergency cases (Mulcahy *et al.* 1994). Other factors resulting in high mortality in the elderly are the presence of liver metastases; age over 80 years, and patients with a markedly reduced vital capacity; the presence of more than one of these factors being associated with mortality rates about 50% (Nudelmann *et al.* 1986). Despite up to 90% of deaths in the elderly being attributable to complications of coexisting medical disorders, age is an independent prognostic factor in colorectal cancer (Di Giorgio *et al.* 1990; Ponz de Leon *et al.* 1992; Deans *et al.* 1994*b*). However, ability to resect a tumour is not dependent on age so that elderly patients should not be denied surgery for large bowel cancer for fear of increased operative mortality (Mulcahy *et al.* 1994).

In contrast, some have noted that patients under 40 years at presentation have a particularly poor prognosis. Recio and Bussey (1965) found that 45% of patients with rectal cancer under the age of 30 years died in the first year, crude 5-year survival being only 20%. They stated, however, that the 'accepted gloomy prognosis for young patients with rectal cancer is confirmed only for those with lymphatic metastases; for those without, the outlook is hopeful'. It is likely that late diagnosis may be the reason for the poor prognosis in younger patients. In support of this, the proportion of those under 40 years presenting as Dukes' stage A being 5%, stage B 35%, stage C 35%, and stage D 25% with a preponderance of poorly differentiated and mucinous tumours (Cozart *et al.* 1993; Heys *et al.* 1994). Others have found the incidence of lymph node and distant metastases to be twice that of the over 40s with colorectal cancer (Heimann *et al.* 1989). Consequently, the 5-year survival rate is 25% and the 5-year disease-free survival 20%. Stage for stage survival is similar in those under and over 40 years of age, overall 5-year survival being 60% (Lee *et al.* 1994; McGahren *et al.* 1995; Cusack *et al.* 1996).

Intestinal obstruction is also thought to have a poor prognosis (Garcia-Peche *et al.* 1991). Individuals with obstructed carcinoma of the colon have a higher operative mortality and a shorter long-term survival which may be explained by the choice of operative procedure (Fitchett and Hoffman 1986). Obstructing right colon tumours have a three times poorer prognosis than non-obstructing carcinomas of the right colon, while obstructing tumours in the rectum have a very poor prognosis (Fitchett and Hoffman 1986). However, studies using multivariate analysis show only a weakly adverse prognostic relationship which is present for colorectal cancer deaths, but not overall survival (Crucitti *et al.* 1991; Deans *et al.* 1994*b*). Perforation and emergency surgery are also related with a poor prognosis, about 15% of patients presenting with colonic obstruction (Catalano and Levin 1991) (Figure 11.13). Despite right-sided tumours being more advanced at presentation, tumour site is not a major prognostic variable (Stebbing and Nash 1995). Sex, duration of symptoms, tumour extension within the circumference of the bowel lumen, tumour size, and the surgical technique employed, all show differences in terms of 5-year survival, but without reaching statistical significance (Garcia-Peche *et al.* 1991; Deans *et al.* 1994*b*). In patients with synchronous tumours, the 5-year survival is no different from that of single lesions, despite a higher incidence of lymph node involvement and a greater frequency of mucinous adenocarcinoma (Adloff *et al.* 1989). The cumulative probability of sur-

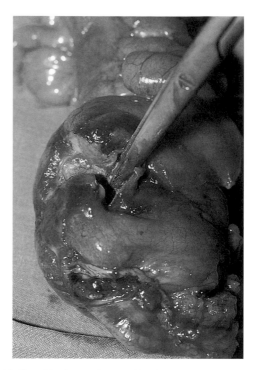

Figure 11.13 Sigmoid colon carcinoma which had perforated (indicated by the scissors).

vival shows a better prognosis for metachronous carcinomas than for synchronous carcinomas as metachronous tumours tend to be detected at an earlier stage (Cali *et al.* 1993).

Quantitative pathology

The knowledge that cancer cells are characterized by enlarged nuclei and abnormal DNA content (ploidy) has led to investigation as to whether techniques, such as flow cytometry, may improve on the deficiencies in the present pathological grading systems (Figure 11.14). Reports on both fresh and paraffin-embedded material consistently suggest that tumours with normal (diploid) DNA content are associated with a survival advantage over DNA aneuploid tumours (Rowley *et al.* 1990; Nori *et al.* 1995). However, the importance of DNA ploidy as an independent prognostic variable in colorectal cancer varies enormously, possibly due to differences in

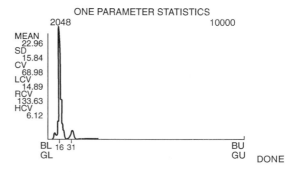

Figure 11.14 DNA flow cytometry analysis of a colon tumour showing the typical two (diploid) peaks representing cells in the G_0/G_1 and G_2/M phases of the cell cycle.

specimen preparation and sampling (Kim *et al.* 1991; Ensley *et al.* 1993).

Many studies reveal DNA content to be a prognostic variable on univariate analysis (Rowley *et al.* 1990). Studies employing multi-variate analysis, however, reveal the prognostic significance of DNA ploidy to be much less than that of Dukes' stage (Deans *et al.* 1993*a*; Yamazoe *et al.* 1994). Some of these studies have found that ploidy is significantly related to survival only in patients with a better survival according to Dukes' classification (Witzig *et al.* 1991). Still others report that, on multivariate analysis, DNA ploidy is not significantly related to survival in any group of patients (Deans *et al.* 1993*a*; Yamazoe *et al.* 1994).

DNA densitometry may be more specific than flow cytometry at assessing DNA content. However, results are similar to those obtained using flow cytometry in that, although diploidy confers a better survival advantage than aneuploidy, DNA ploidy status is not of independent prognostic significance (Bottger *et al.* 1993). Reports on both flow cytometry and densitometry suggest that the relationship between survival and ploidy seen on univariate analysis, disappears on subsequent multivariate analysis (Deans *et al.* 1993*b*). The assessment of nuclear DNA content by flow cytometry or DNA densitometry appears to be too crude a measure to be of prognostic significance relative to Dukes' classification in colorectal cancer (Deans *et al.* 1992). In future *in situ* hybridization using centromere-specific DNA probes to specific chromosomes may provide more specific information on DNA ploidy that may prove of greater prognostic value (Steiner *et al.* 1993).

Epithelial cell turnover is known to be increased in patients with colorectal cancer. Cell turnover may be assessed by flow cytometry quantifying the proportion of cells in the replicating (S phase) of the cell cycle or by determining the thymidine labelling index, either using microautoradiography or dual parameter flow cytometry with the thymidine analogue bromodeoxyuridine (BrdUrd) (Qin and Willems 1993). Although these techniques may be useful in screening or treating patients at high risk of developing colorectal cancer, they are of little benefit in predicting prognosis or tumour recurrence (Buchsbaum *et al.* 1994). The relative proportion of cells in various phases of the cell cycle is increased in patients with colorectal carcinoma but is not related to the degree of dysplasia or survival (Deans *et al.* 1993*a*; Paganelli *et al.* 1994). Combining ploidy with an assessment of the proportion of actively dividing cells (pro-liferative index), c-*myc* oncogene or CEA expression improves the prediction of survival over ploidy alone, but stills falls short of that of Dukes' stage (Witzig *et al.* 1991; Deans *et al.* 1993*a*). Ki-67, a monoclonal antibody marker of cell proliferation can be used to characterize the proliferative characteristics of normal colonic mucosa, adenomas, and carcinomas but does not correlate with any clinicopathological variables and is of limited prognostic value (Hemming *et al.* 1992). Similarly, quantitative assessment of nuclear size and shape using morphometric image analysis, can accurately distinguish normal from malignant colorectal tissue and categorize the degree of dysplasia and tumour ploidy (Levi *et al.* 1991). However, on univariate and multivariate analysis nuclear morpho-metric features bear no correlation with Dukes' stage or patient survival (Deans *et al.* 1993*c*).

Mitotic activity within the tumour has been claimed to be an independent prognostic variable, patients with a mitotic index less than 20% having a significantly better survival than those with mitotic activity above this figure (Kawasaki *et al.* 1990). Argyrophil nucleolar organizer regions (AgNORs) are increased in a variety of malignant cells. AgNORs are loops of ribosomal DNA which reflect the cellular activity or malignant potential of the cell and are identified by a specific staining technique. AgNOR count per cell is significantly increased in colorectal tumours relative to normal mucosa, but is not related to Dukes' stage or degree of dif-ferentiation (Rayter *et al.* 1992). The prognostic value of AgNORs is variable. Some claim that survivors have significantly lower nucle-olar organizer region counts in primary tumours and lymph node metastases than non-survivors, with AgNORs being the most im-portant of any pathological variable for predicting survival (Joyce *et al.* 1992). Others state that AgNORs have no prognostic value in colorectal cancer (Rayter *et al.* 1992). This discrepancy may be due to observer variation and problems in accurately counting the number of AgNORs per cell.

Clinical presentation

Symptoms

Symptoms and signs have a sensitivity and specificity of 44% and 80% for colonic neoplasms (McIntyre and Long 1993). Over 85% of patients with colorectal cancer will have symptoms at diagnosis, the remaining 15% being detected from asymptomatic screening programmes (Speights *et al.* 1991). Some suggest that almost half of colonic malignancies detected by colonoscopy are not predicted on clinical grounds (Brenna *et al.* 1990). Asymptomatic tumours are more common in the right colon and account for 80% of tumours detected at this site by screening programmes (Stein *et al.* 1993). In those not undergoing screening, delay in diagnosis (usually about 6 months) is common, being reported in one-fifth of all colorectal tumours. In almost one-third of cases the delay is due to false-negative X-rays or doctors neglecting to perform rectal examination or rectosigmoidoscopy. Despite this, patients with longer symptoms do not have a more adverse tumour stage, tumour differentiation or survival (Barillari *et al.* 1989).

In one study, significant clinical predictors of colorectal cancer were age over 60 years (odds ratio 15), rectal bleeding (odds ratio 3), loss of weight (odds ratio 2), and male sex (odds ratio 2) (Steine *et al.* 1994). Fatigue and abdominal pain were nearly significant negative predictors for cancer but no association was found between patient delay and the detection of polyps or cancer (Steine *et al.* 1994). Others have also found age to be one of the most important predictors of both polyps and cancer (McIntyre and Long 1993). In patients under 40 years old a positive family history for colorectal cancer will be found in 15% with a further 10% having a first-degree relative with another form of cancer (Heimann *et al.* 1989).

Clinical presentation is similar irrespective of age with rectal bleeding and abdominal pain being the most common symptoms (Figure 11.15). Of patients over the age of 40 years presenting to general practitioners with rectal bleeding, investigation will reveal 10% to have colorectal cancer and a further 10% to have polyps (Goulston *et al.* 1986). In those under 20 years old with colorectal cancer, rectal bleeding is noticed by three-quarters of patients with pain, anaemia, and abdominal distension occurring in two-thirds (Lewis *et al.* 1990). Overall about half of patients with colorectal cancer or polyps notice overt rectal bleeding (Griffioen *et al.* 1989). Although, the passage of blood per rectum is not specific for colorectal cancer, rectal bleeding in all patients, and particularly in those on anticoagulants requires investigation (Helfand *et al.* 1997; Norton and Armstrong 1997). Rectal bleeding is common

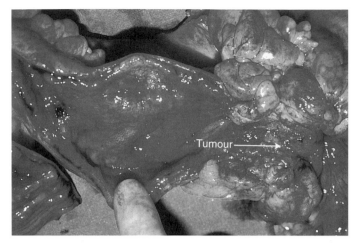

Figure 11.15 A colonic carcinoma (arrowed) which presented with heavy intestinal bleeding.

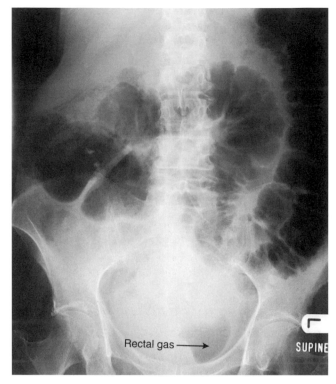

Figure 11.16 Plain abdominal X-ray in patient with a sigmoid colon tumour. Note the presence of gas in the rectum (arrowed) indicating partial obstruction.

among the general population, 70% of all rectal bleeding being accounted for by minor anorectal conditions such as haemorrhoids or fissures (Hixson *et al.* 1989). The predictive value of rectal bleeding for colorectal cancer is not improved by distinguishing between bright and dark red blood and whether or not the blood is mixed with the stool (Farrands and Hardcastle 1984; Helfand *et al.* 1997). In one-half of patients presenting to their general practitioner with rectal bleeding, the bleeding is attributed to haemorrhoids, yet one-sixth of these will ultimately be found to have a colonic or rectal cause for the blood loss. After a rigid sigmoidoscopy, gastro-enterologists predict an anal source in two-thirds of patients with rectal bleeding and 5% of these are ultimately found to be due to colorectal disease (Goulston *et al.* 1986). Up to one-quarter of patients over 40 years presenting with rectal bleeding have an adenoma or carcinoma, so that it is suggested that all patients over 40 years require investigation (Goulston *et al.* 1986). The incidence of symptoms such as rectal bleeding is not increased in those with synchronous tumours so that pre-operative diagnosis of such lesions is obtained in only one-third of cases (Adloff *et al.* 1989).

Up to two-thirds of patients undergoing emergency operation for obstructed colon cancer have had previous symptoms which have often not been investigated (Figure 11.16). These include altered bowel habit, flatulent distension and audible borborygmi. Alteration in bowel habit may take the form of diarrhoea, constipation or a combination of the two and becomes increasingly common the more distally the tumour is situated. Abdominal pain lacks sensitivity for colon cancer, being a prominent symptom of benign conditions and often only occurring in the presence of considerable stenosis. Anorexia and weight loss are normally ominous symptoms signifying advanced disease. Right bowel tumours more often present with advanced disease, intestinal obstruction being rare as the liquid stool can flow around even large tumours. Symptoms or signs of iron deficiency anaemia are common in occult right-sided tumours so that colonic pathology should be excluded before anaemia is attributed to other causes such as menstrual loss or minor upper intestinal lesions (Rockey and Cello 1993). The incidence of neoplasm in patients with iron deficiency anaemia is 15% compared with 2% in non-anaemic patients and is more common (20%) in iron-deficient males than females (9%) (Gordon *et al.* 1994; Guthrie *et al.* 1994). Tenesmus and rectovesical or vaginal fistula may be a feature of rectal cancer, sacral pain usually signifying advanced disease. In

pregnant patients, early diagnosis is difficult because the initial symptoms of colorectal cancer, such as abdominal pain, nausea and vomiting, constipation, and abdominal distension, are often attributed to a normal pregnancy (Heise *et al.* 1992).

Signs

In the vast majority of patients with colon cancer no abnormality is detected on clinical examination. The presence of advanced disease

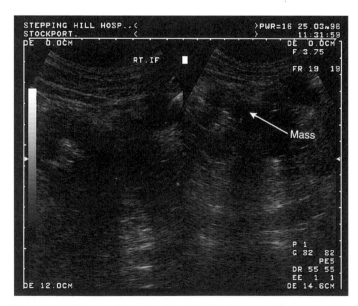

Figure 11.17 Ultrasound scan showing a right iliac fossa mass from a caecal tumour with nodes on the iliac artery.

is associated with cachexia and a deterioration in general health. Right-sided lesions have a tendency to present with anaemia or a palpable mass (Figure 11.17). Left colonic masses due to tumours can be distinguished from faecal loading by their firm, irregular border which cannot be indented (Bryan *et al.* 1997). Intestinal obstruction is also a feature of left colon tumours. Rectal examination identifies about three-quarters of rectal tumours. The accuracy of rectal examination in determining the depth of invasion of rectal carcinoma ranges from 50% to 80%. The accuracy of this examination in assessing tumour stage depends on the experience of the examiner, varying from 67% to 83% for consultants compared with 45–75% when performed by registrars (Nicholls and Dube 1982). Observer variation and poor assessment of lymph node involvement are further problems of rectal examination. The presence of deep venous thrombosis should alert the clinician to a possible visceral malignancy, colorectal cancer being detected in 2% of patients who present with venous thrombosis (Monreal *et al.* 1991). Patients with *Streptococcus bovis* endocarditis should also undergo large bowel investigation, even in the absence of symptoms of bowel disease, as colonic cancers are found in 10% and polyps in 67% of patients with this condition (Grinberg *et al.* 1990; Siegert and Overbosch 1995).

Diagnosis

A careful history and examination may suggest the diagnosis but are usually insufficiently specific to diagnose colorectal cancer

confidently. Symptoms without objective indicators or pertinent risk factors do not correlate well with abnormal findings on subsequent colonic investigation. In one study, logistic regression analysis revealed four variables to be significant predictors of colon cancer: abnormal sigmoidoscopy (odds ratio 3.7), iron deficiency anaemia (odds ratio 2.8), positive faecal occult bloods (odds ratio 2.8), and a relevant history (odds ratio 1.9) (Zarchy and Ershoff 1991). In a patient without any of these indicators, the predicted probability of having colon cancer was only 0.7%, while in a patient with at least two objective indicators, the probability of having colon cancer was greater than 15%. Investigations that may therefore be performed to diagnose colorectal cancer consist of haematological tests, including tumour markers, barium enema, and endoscopy.

Haematological tests

Iron deficiency anaemia may often be the only clue to an occult tumour, particularly in the right colon and requires further investigation. This may take the form of faecal occult blood tests (FOBs) (see section on screening, Chapter 9). FOBs have a positive predictive value of 30–45% for colorectal neoplasia which increases to 60% when combined with one or more colorectal symptoms such as dark red rectal bleeding or altered bowel habit (Silman *et al.* 1983). Sensitivity is about 70%, so that a negative result does not exclude a neoplastic lesion. The test is well accepted by the symptomatic patient in the general practice setting and, if positive, allows early referral for investigation. Low serum ferritin, an indicator of iron deficiency without anaemia, may improve the detection of colonic malignancies and polyps when used in combination with stool occult

Table 11.7 Tumours markers in colorectal cancer

Tumour marker	Comments
Tissue carcino-embryonic antigen (CEA)	Staining dependent on histological grade (85% of well-differentiated tumours stain positive)
	Not related to serum CEA levels
	Transitional zone stains positive in 66%
	No benefit over light microscopy in identifying nodal involvement
Tissue epithelial membrane antigen (EMA)	Does not detect transitional zone
	Discontinuous staining related to advanced Dukes' stage, poor differentiation and lymph node metastases
	No benefit over light microscopy in identifying nodal involvement
Serum CEA	Detectable in 60% of all colon cancers but elevated in only 25%
	Most specific tumour marker for colon cancer
	Also elevated in 20% of benign gastrointestinal tract conditions and 25% of gastric cancers
	Elevated principally in advanced disease
	Lacks sensitivity in detecting good prognosis cases
	For colon cancer:
	overall sensitivity 55%, specificity 95%
	Sensitivity for curative disease 25%
	Sensitivity for incurable disease 75%
	Not related to tissue CEA staining
Serum CA19-9	Detectable in 55% of all colon cancers but elevated in only 15%
	Also elevated in 10% of benign gastrointestinal tract conditions and 50% of gastric cancers
	Elevated principally in advanced disease
	Lacks sensitivity in detecting good prognosis cases
	For colon cancer:
	overall sensitivity 35%, specificity 95%
	Sensitivity for curative disease 10%
	Sensitivity for incurable disease 80%
Serum gastrointestinal cancer antigen	Provides less information than CEA in 42% of cases
	True positive rate 18%
	False negative 38%

blood testing (Griffiths *et al.* 1991). Liver function tests are of little benefit in detecting metastatic disease, less than half of patients with elevated results having proven hepatic involvement at operation

Tumour markers

Antigens secreted by colorectal mucosa have been used to detect primary tumours or their recurrence (Table 11.7). The most common of these are derived from a non-specific cross-reacting antigen and include CEA and CA19-9 (Northover 1995). These antigens may be assessed on either blood or histological samples and show a steady increase in concentration from normal tissue, through pre-cancerous lesions or polyps to tumours (Figure 11.18). CEA levels in portal blood are significantly higher than those of peripheral blood, being correlated with the presence of venous invasion by the tumour and, to a lesser extent, survival (Deguchi *et al.* 1990). Faecal CEA measurements are of little benefit as considerable overlap occurs between the results obtained from colorectal cancer patients and controls (Stubbs *et al.* 1986).

Tissue CEA expression using immunohistochemical examination stains positive in virtually all colorectal tumours and epithelial membrane antigen (EMA) in 90% (Davidson *et al.* 1989). An increase in tissue CEA is not paralleled by a simultaneous increase in serum CEA (Imamura *et al.* 1990). Tissue CEA concentrations are significantly lower in poorly differentiated carcinomas, whereas serum CEA concentrations are not related to histological grade (Davidson *et al.* 1989). CEA, but not EMA, may also be used to detect transitional zones as it is elevated in two-thirds of normal mucosa adjacent to the tumour (Mori *et al.* 1990). An association has been found between lack of EMA immunostaining in the tumour centre and more extensive malignant spread (Hewitt *et al.* 1991). However, immunohistochemical staining for CEA and EMA is of no advantage in detecting lymph node spread as these techniques detect only 2% more lymph node metastases than light microscopy (Davidson *et al.* 1989).

Current serum tumour markers are relatively inadequate for presymptomatic diagnosis because they are not specific for colorectal cancer (Slentz *et al.* 1994). CEA is the most specific antigen for colorectal cancer. However, it is also elevated in one-quarter of gastric carcinomas, while CA19-9 is elevated in one-half and CA72-4 in 60% of stomach tumours (Heptner *et al.* 1989). In addition, CA19-9

has a higher sensitivity for pancreatic than for gastric and colorectal carcinoma. CEA can be detected in 60% of colorectal carcinomas and CA19-9 in 55%, with elevated serum levels observed in 25% and 15%, respectively (Ueda *et al.* 1994). Elevated serum CEA levels also occur in 20% and CA19-9 levels in 10% of benign gastrointestinal conditions (Ueda *et al.* 1994). In the detection of colorectal cancer, serum CEA and CA19-9 both have a sensitivity of about 25% and specificity of 95% if benign conditions are grouped with patients without colorectal disease (Imamura *et al.* 1990). When patients with adenomatous polyps are included in the malignant category, the sensitivity and specificity of CEA and CA19-9 are both about 10% and 95%, respectively (Goldberg *et al.* 1989) (Table 11.7).

Both pre-operative CEA and CA19-9 levels are proportional to the amount of tumour present, so that the tests are more frequently positive in patients with advanced stage disease or with large primary tumours. In the presence of liver metastases, serum CEA levels are elevated in 90% of all patients and CA19-9 in 60% (Lorenz *et al.* 1989). Consequently, serum CEA is insensitive (25%) in diagnosing curable colorectal cancers and only reasonably reliable (sensitivity 75%) in detecting unresectable and metastatic disease (Moertel *et al.* 1986). CA19-5 levels may be elevated in some patients with hepatocellular disease so that its overall sensitivity (35%) is less than that of CEA (50%). CA 72-4 is also inferior to CEA in detecting colorectal cancer (sensitivity in all stages 30% compared with 55%) (Heptner *et al.* 1989). CA-242 alone is not superior to CEA, although their combined use (either abnormal) has a high sensitivity (88%), specificity (78%), and negative predictive value (97%) (Hall *et al.* 1994; Holmström 1996).

Serum gastrointestinal cancer antigen (GICA) offers little advantage in tumour detection over serum CEA. The test gives more information than CEA in only 2% of colorectal cancer patients, with a true-positive rate of 18% and false-negative rate of 38%. Tumour-associated glycoprotein (TAG-72) is expressed in two-thirds of colorectal cancers and may be useful in patients who are CEA or CA19-9 negative (Ochuchi *et al.* 1989). Antitumour immune response to colorectal cancer extracts by leucocyte adherence inhibition (LAI) assay is claimed to be positive in 70% of colorectal cancers, compared with 5% of benign gastrointestinal conditions and other malignancies. However, direct comparison of the LAI and haemoccult tests reveals that the predictive value of a positive haemoccult test is 33% compared with 16% for the LAI test. The total sialic acid to total protein ratio is claimed to detect colorectal cancer patients at an earlier stage than CEA (Verazin *et al.* 1990).

Attempts at improving the detection of colorectal cancer by using a 'panel' of tumour markers has generally been unsatisfactory in either early or advanced disease (Heptner *et al.* 1989; Lorenz *et al.* 1989). If patients are CEA negative, using CA19-9 will detect only a further 6% of patients with colorectal cancer. A cocktail of CA72-4, CA19-9 and CEA increases positivity rates to 85% from 60% with CEA alone, although the positive rate for benign disease is also increased to 30% (Ohuchi *et al.* 1989). One study revealed that of four tumour-associated markers (CEA, CA 19-9, CA 125, and SLEX [sialylated Lewis(x) epitope]), no patient with early disease, and only 13% of those with hepatic metastases, reacted to all four markers (Kawahara *et al.* 1986). In another study of 11 biochemical markers, the five most-sensitive markers were CEA, C-reactive protein, alpha-1-glycoprotein, macrocreatine kinase type 2, and homoarginine-sensitive alkaline phosphatase. A combination of these markers instead of CEA alone increased sensitivity by 17% for late- and 64% for early-stage cancer, although specificity decreased by 30% (Mercer *et al.* 1985).

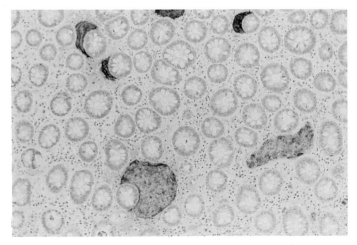

Figure 11.18 Immunohistochemical staining of rectal tissue. This particular stain was Prostatic Specific Antigen and in fact identified the rectal mass as prostatic carcinoma invading the rectum.

Biochemical tests are useful in detecting liver metastases only in combination. It is suggested that if CEA, alkaline phosphatase, gamma-glutamyltranspeptidase, lactic dehydrogenase, and cholinesterase are all normal, liver metastases can confidently be excluded (negative predictive value 97%), so that radiological investigations are unnecessary (Bonfanti *et al.* 1990). Although CEA is the most sensitive at predicting liver metastases, no single tumour marker can confidently detect hepatic involvement.

This only becomes possible when four or five of these markers are abnormal, by which time there is often gross replacement of the liver by the tumour (Bonfanti *et al.* 1990).

Endoscopy

Patients with suspected colorectal tumours normally undergo rigid sigmoidoscopy and proctoscopy. Proctoscopy allows adequate inspection of the anorectal region and assessment of haemorrhoids. The 25 cm rigid sigmoidoscope is rarely passed beyond 17–20 cm, allowing at most, visualization of 40% of all colorectal cancers (Wilking *et al.* 1986). The examination also provides information about the consistency of stool, presence of blood, and mucosal appearance. Rigid sigmoidoscopy is less likely to miss lesions in a capacious rectum than flexible instruments but is more unpleasant and carries a small but definite risk of perforation. A controlled study of multiphasic health checks failed to show a reduction in mortality from repeated sigmoidoscopy, because the sample size was aimed at the benefits of health checks as a whole rather than just sigmoidoscopy (Selby *et al.* 1988).

Flexible sigmoidoscopy may be performed on an out-patient basis after preparation with phosphate enemas. Although more costly, it is better tolerated than rigid sigmoidoscopy and the yield is significantly greater (Wilking *et al.* 1986). Patient compliance with screening programmes using flexible sigmoidoscopy is over 90% (Wherry and Thomas 1994). Screening with the 60 cm flexible sigmoidoscope identifies polyps in five per 100 and carcinomas in three per 1000 subjects screened, which is higher than with faecal occult blood screening (Wherry and Thomas 1994). Flexible sigmoidoscopy is quicker and easier to learn than colonoscopy and can be performed with minimum or no sedation. The 60 cm instrument visualizes the entire sigmoid colon in 80% and the entire left colon in 45% of patients, where about 60% of colorectal neoplasms and 90% of polyps may be expected to occur. Although in future logistical problems of population screening may be overcome by training nurse or GP endoscopists in the use of the shorter and safer 35 cm endoscopes, the trend for a left-to-right shift in colon cancer may necessitate more total colonoscopies (Kee *et al.* 1992; Beart *et al.* 1995). The combination of flexible sigmoidoscopy and selective barium enema is claimed to have a sensitivity of 100%, a specificity of 82%, a negative predictive value of 1.0 and a positive predictive value of 0.62 (Hough *et al.* 1994). It is reported that using this combination only one-third of patients would require colonoscopy (Hough *et al.* 1994).

Colonoscopy is the 'gold-standard' for detecting colorectal neoplasms, the overall accuracy relative to pathology of excised specimens being over 95%. Blind areas in the colon, plus misjudgement that the scope had reached the caecum, are responsible for the majority of colonoscopic errors. It is therefore important to verify that the colonoscope has reached the caecum (Figure 11.19). Interobserver agreement is almost 100% for lesions over 1 cm and 85% for lesions smaller than this (Hixson *et al.* 1991). In comparison, the sensitivity of single contrast barium enema can be as

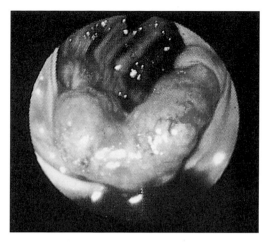

Figure 11.19 Carcinoma of the right colon detected on colonoscopy.

low as 13%, and that of double contrast enema 26% (Norfleet *et al.* 1991). Relative to barium enema, colonoscopy has fewer negative results (40% versus 75%), fewer inconclusive examinations requiring repeat procedures (5% versus 20%), and more positive correct findings to explain the cause of bleeding (55% versus 5%) (Maxfield *et al.* 1986). The greatest benefit of colonoscopy is in the investigation of occult or overt rectal bleeding and abnormal barium enema or sigmoidoscopy findings (Metcalf *et al.* 1996). In patients with intestinal bleeding and a normal barium enema, colonoscopy may identify a carcinoma in 15%, polyps larger than 1 cm in 20%, and other causes in 20% (Maxfield *et al.* 1986). However, colonoscopy is less sensitive than double contrast barium enema at detecting diverticular disease and is claimed to be slower, three times more expensive, and 10 times more dangerous. If colonoscopy fails to detect a colonic tumour suspected on an initial barium enema, a repeat barium enema is indicated. Glick *et al.* (1989) presented a series of 18 colonic neoplasms 2–8 cm in diameter that were detected by barium enema but overlooked on initial endoscopy. All of the lesions were relatively flat with little intraluminal protuberance.

Routine pre-operative colonoscopy has been recommended to identify synchronous polyps and/or cancers which might otherwise be undetected on barium enema or at the time of operation. Preoperative colonoscopy demonstrates synchronous carcinomas in 4–7% and synchronous polyps in 15–55% of those with colorectal cancer (Barillari *et al.* 1990). It is claimed that 10–40% of synchronous cancers and up to 70% of synchronous polyps would not have been included in the standard surgical resection for the index cancer if the additional information provided by colonoscopy had not been available (Slater *et al.* 1990). The majority of synchronous tumours detected by colonoscopy are also early (Dukes' stage A or B). In contrast, barium enema may fail to identify synchronous cancers in up to one-half of patients, many of the lesions subsequently detected showing metastatic disease (Barillari *et al.* 1990). Synchronous polyps are missed by single contrast enemas in 60% of patients and by double-contrast enemas in 25% (Barillari *et al.* 1990). Patients who undergo pre-operative colonoscopy also have a reduced incidence (under 1%) of metachronous cancer within 3 years from surgery (Barillari *et al.* 1990). Pre-operative colonoscopy may not be possible in those with a stenosing lesion (Tate *et al.* 1988). Such patients should be investigated postoperatively within 3–6 months as synchronous cancers, if treated early, have little effect on overall prognosis.

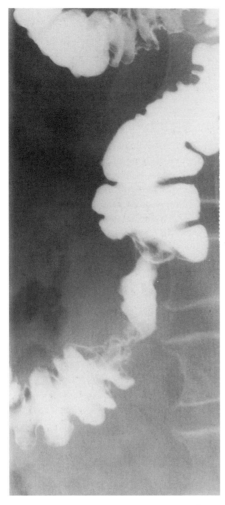

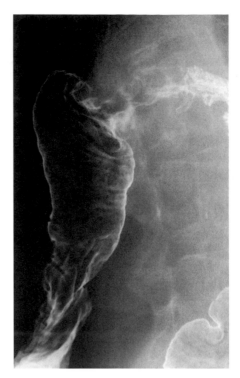

Figure 11.21 Double contrast barium enema showing mucosal detail of the 'shoulder' of the tumour.

Figure 11.20 Barium enema showing the typical 'apple core' appearance in the left colon.

Barium enema

The cardinal feature of colorectal cancer on barium enema is a filling defect with irregular edges, often taking the form of an 'apple core' appearance (Figure 11.20). Over half of barium enemas are ordered solely on the basis of clinical symptoms, yet the correlation between symptoms and positive findings on barium enema is poor (Zarchy and Ershoff 1991; Johnson *et al.* 1996). Consequently, the overall diagnostic yield of routine barium enema for colorectal cancer is 5%, irrespective of the experience of the staff requesting the investigation (Vellacott and Virjee 1986; Smith 1997).

Single contrast barium enemas fail to detect 15% and double contrast enemas 7% of colorectal cancers (Figure 11.21). False negatives are mostly due to failure to recognize or misinterpretation of lesions in the rectosigmoid region. In revealing a polyp less than 5 mm, double contrast enemas have a sensitivity of 70%, compared with 80% in the detection of larger polyps (Rex *et al.* 1986). The overall sensitivity of double contrast barium enema compared with colonoscopy is about 70% (Markus *et al.* 1990). The sensitivity of barium enema can be increased to 80% if the films are read by two radiologists and to 90% if they are interpreted by three clinicians (Markus *et al.* 1990; Brady *et al.* 1994). However, this is accompanied by a decrease in specificity. The variable anatomy of the sigmoid colon, often with concomitant diverticular disease, can

result in lesions being missed in this region in one-quarter of cases. In symptomatic sigmoid diverticular disease, an associated carcinoma is found in 7% and adenomas in 27%, almost half of which are not detected by barium enema (Aldridge and Sim 1986).

Visualization of the sigmoid colon endoscopically reduces the time taken at X-ray in inspecting the sigmoid colon and increases the accuracy of the investigation. The combination of flexible sigmoidoscopy and double contrast barium enema is claimed to detect all cancers identified by colonoscopy (Hixson *et al.* 1989). However, one-third of benign polyps greater than 1 cm and two-thirds of those less than 1 cm are not detected by this combination of tests (Hixson *et al.* 1989). Up to 40% of tumours can be missed by either technique. Barium enema may fail to diagnose one-quarter of rectosigmoid polyps over 1 cm in diameter and endoscopy one-sixth. Rectosigmoidoscopy (60 cm) should therefore be used as a complement to double contrast enemas if this method is chosen for investigation of a patient with rectal bleeding. Provided that carbon dioxide is used instead of air, same-day flexible sigmoidoscopy and double contrast barium enema is claimed to diminish both cost and patient discomfort for colonic investigation without impairing quality (Brewster *et al.* 1994).

It is suggested that a barium enema should be performed in all cases of large-bowel obstruction, except when perforation is a possibility or when the caecum measures 10 cm or larger in diameter (Ericksen *et al.* 1990) (Figure 11.22). However, in such circumstances, barium enema is a poor predictor of malignancy, as two-thirds of suspected cancers turn out to be due to diverticular disease (King *et al.* 1990). In those with colonic stricture and an inconclusive barium enema it is possible to get a colonoscope, or paediatric gastroscope, above the stricture and obtain a pathological diagnosis in about half of cases (King *et al.* 1990). Combining colonoscopic biopsy with brush cytology can further aid diagnosis,

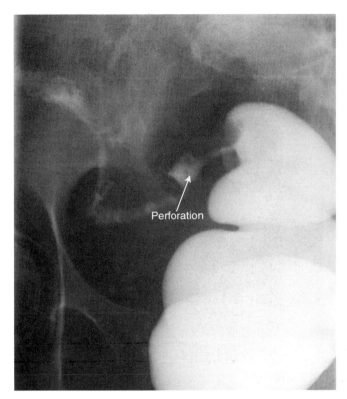

Figure 11.22 Water soluble enema in patient with perforated sigmoid colon tumour (arrowed).

detecting 85% of tumours. In future the ability to examine colonic effluents for K-*ras* oncogene mutations may provide a powerful and convenient source of sampling that may be adapted to population screening. Alternatively, if retrograde passage of barium on an enema is obstructed by a lesion in the left colon, additional diagnostic information can be obtained by giving the patient oral barium which will pass through the small bowel and identify the stenotic site in an average of 150 min without significant complications (Gotta *et al.* 1990).

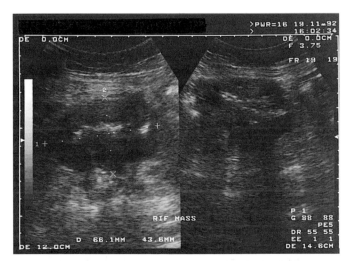

Figure 11.23 Ultrasound scan of right iliac fossa mass showing the 'pseudo-kidney' appearance (dark areas are the bowel wall, white areas intraluminal gas).

Other radiological investigations

Ultrasound may be useful in identifying colonic carcinoma (Figure 11.23). Features of colon cancer include irregularity and localized hypertrophy of the colonic wall to more than 10 mm (Uchida *et al.* 1993). The sensitivity of ultrasound in detecting colonic carcinomas is claimed to be 95% and the specificity almost 100% (Limberg 1990; Hernandez-Socorro *et al.* 1995). Others have reported that screening ultrasound detects between 50% and 75% of colon cancers, tumours over 4 cm having a high rate of detection (Uchida *et al.* 1993). Although polyps larger than 7 mm diameter can be identified in 90% of cases, smaller polyps may often be missed, so that colonoscopy is more accurate in these cases (Limberg 1990; Chui *et al.* 1994). Endorectal ultrasound is useful in staging rectal cancer, giving an accuracy of 67–90% in assessing the depth of wall invasion and 50–80% in predicting nodal involvement (Hildebrandt *et al.* 1994; Kaneko *et al.* 1996). The evaluation of lymph nodes is less accurate, (79%) and the accuracy of depth of invasion is almost halved if radiotherapy has been given. In a comparison of pre-operative endoluminal ultrasound (ELUS) and magnetic resonance imaging (MRI) in rectal carcinoma a comprehensive pre-operative staging (T + N) was made correctly in 68% by ELUS and in 48% by MRI (Thaler *et al.* 1994). In another series, since the introduction of endosonography, the proportion of abdominoperineal excisions dropped from 45% to 15% (Hildebrandt *et al.* 1994). Duplex colour Doppler sonography is claimed to be useful in detecting the subtle changes in liver perfusion that occur with otherwise undetected liver metastases (Leen *et al.* 1996). Using this technique, the Doppler perfusion index (DPI), defined as the ratio of hepatic arterial to total liver blood flow, can identify occult hepatic metastases and direct therapy accordingly (Leen *et al.* 1993). Colonoscopic ultrasound (endosonography) is useful in defining tumours which may be suitable for endoscopic treatment as it leads to a better selection of superficial cancers without lymph node metastases (Souquet *et al.* 1993; Hunerbein and Schlag 1997). Although it can distinguish colonic carcinoma from submucosal lipomas, it may fail to detect small metastatic glands.

Intra-operative assessment of tumour staging by surgeons is 66% accurate, with 17% of tumours being understaged and 17% overstaged (Loh *et al.* 1994; Meijer *et al.* 1995). Intra-operative ultrasonography is claimed to be able to improve tumour staging, detecting lesions not seen on computerized tomography (CT) in 20% and lesions not detected by bimanual palpation in 5% of patients. In another study occult hepatic metastases were detected by intra-operative ultrasound alone in 5% of patients (Stone *et al.* 1994). Restriction of intra-operative ultrasound (IOUS) imaging to patients with T3 or T4 lesions or recurrent cancers would have identified all metastases and increased the detection rate to 10%. The rate of false-negative findings on IOUS imaging was 13% overall, 0% for patients with T1 or T2 lesions, 3% for patients with node-negative findings and 7% for patients with T3, N0 lesions (Stone *et al.* 1994). The authors concluded that the small increment in the detection of occult metastases by IOUS liver imaging does not warrant its use in all patients with colorectal cancer, and that the procedure should be restricted to patients with T3, T4 lesions or recurrent cancers.

For evaluating primary colonic and rectal malignancies, CT and MRI are often complementary imaging methods which are useful in assessing patients suspected of having extensive disease and in deciding whether a patient will benefit from preoperative radiation (Scharling *et al.* 1996; Zerhouni *et al.* 1996). Conventional CT

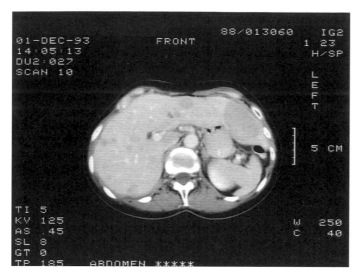

Figure 11.24 CT scan showing multiple low density liver metastases.

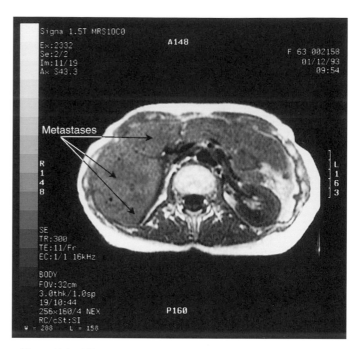

Figure 11.25 MR scan of liver metastases (same patient as Figure 11.24).

scanning is of limited value in detecting early disease but is claimed to improve the pre-operative staging for extensive or metastatic disease (Kerner *et al.* 1993; Thoeni and Rogalla 1995; Isbister and Al-Sanea 1996). Some believe it to be valuable in assessing the extent of spread having a sensitivity of 80%, specificity of 50%, positive predictive value of 70%, negative predictive value of 65% and overall accuracy of 68% (Pema *et al.* 1994). However, others report that pre-operative CT agrees with pathological staging in only one-third of cases, intra- and interobserver agreement being only 50% (Shank *et al.* 1990). The findings in one-third of cases are claimed to be clinically significant in that they allowed the surgeon to alter the proposed operative procedure or added additional technical information for consideration pre-operatively (Kerner *et al.* 1993). Some claim that the sensitivity of CT for detecting hepatic metastases is 100% with specificity 96% (Fisher *et al.* 1990). Although CT may reliably detect hepatic metastases, it only accurately demonstrates their number and location in 40% (Figure 11.24). Many of these cases could have been detected biochemically or at operation so that routine use of CT may be unnecessarily expensive (Fisher *et al.* 1990). In the rectum, CT can detect cancer from the localized thickening of the rectal wall, especially when air or water is injected into the lumen (Gazelle *et al.* 1995). It is also useful at identifying invasion of other organs and/or the pelvic wall, pelvic lymph nodes metastases and local recurrence. However, CT is of little use in screening or distinguishing malignant from benign rectal abnormalities because rectal mucosal pattern can not be imaged in detail. Contrast-enhanced CT, pre-operative intravenous urography or insertion of ureteric stents may be considered in the presence of urinary tract symptoms and large, fixed tumours of the rectosigmoid (Kerner *et al.* 1993). However, these procedures do not influence the incidence of peroperative urinary complications. Spiral CT scanning is of particular benefit in detecting bowel tumours in elderly patients in whom barium enema would be difficult or uncomfortable (Dixon *et al.* 1995; Amin *et al.* 1996; Thoeni 1997).

At present the applications of MR scanning are relatively limited, although it may be used to evaluate colon tumours, their recurrence, or hepatic metastases (Figure 11.25). MRI offers excellent tissue resolution which aids in distinguishing between localized colorectal disease and disease which invades muscle (Thoeni and Rogalla 1995). Also, MRI can add information with coronal views for determining whether a sphincter saving procedure can be performed, and

may be of benefit for assessing the subtle extent of tumour into muscle and bone. However, as with CT, MRI lacks the ability to assess depth of neoplastic involvement within bowel wall. This limitation is the major factor which, combined with the inability to diagnose metastatic tumour foci in normal sized nodes and microinvasion of perirectal fat, prevents optimal tumour staging. However, in rectosigmoid tumours magnetic resonance is claimed to give 90% sensitivity, 100% specificity, a positive predictive value of 100%, a negative predictive value of 90% with a 95% accuracy (McNicholas *et al.* 1994; Pema *et al.* 1994). Endorectal surface coil MR imaging also shows promise for staging rectal lesions (sensitivity 75%) (Schnall *et al.* 1994).

Because of the low accuracy for assessing early cancer stages, neither CT nor MRI are recommended for routine use in pre-operative staging. CT and MRI have a premier role in the assessment of recurrent colorectal neoplasms, with CT providing a

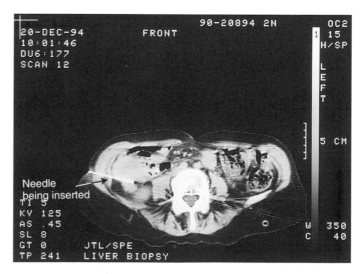

Figure 11.26 Percutaneous liver biopsy performed under CT control.

slightly better overall evaluation due to volume imaging, easy image reconstructions in different planes, and availability of excellent oral and intravenous contrast agents (Thoeni and Rogalla 1995). Cross-sectional imaging is the only method to evaluate fully patients with total anteroposterior resection, particularly male patients. Neither CT nor MRI can determine with certainty that a soft tissue density in the surgical bed following total AP resection represents recurrent tumour unless a clear mass is present which has increased in size over time. However, both methods surpass colonoscopy for detecting early tumour recurrence at the anastomotic site due to its extrinsic component and are useful for obtaining liver biopsies (Figure 11.26). In future Positron Emission Tomography (PET) may show promise (Falk *et al.* 1994; Tempero *et al.* 1995; Lai *et al.* 1996).

References

Adloff M, Arnaud JP, Bergamaschi R, Schloegel M. Synchronous carcinoma of the colon and rectum: prognostic and therapeutic implications. *Am. J. Surg.* 1989; 157: 299–302.

Aldridge MC, Sim AJW. Colonoscopy findings in symptomatic patients without X ray evidence of colonic neoplasms. *Lancet* 1986; ii: 833–4.

Amin Z, Boulos PB, Lees WR. Technical report: spiral CT pneumocolon for suspected colonic neoplasms. *Clin. Radiol.* 1996; 51: 56–61.

Astler VB, Coller FA. The prognostic significance of direct extension of carcinoma of the colon and rectum. *Ann. Surg.* 1954; 139: 846–52.

Barillari P, de Angelis R, Valabrega S, Indinnimeo M, Gozzo P, Ramacciato G, Fegiz G. Relationship of symptom duration and survival in patients with colorectal carcinoma. *Eur. J. Surg. Oncol.* 1989; 15: 441–5.

Barillari P, Ramacciato G, De Angelis R, Gozzo P, Indinnimeo M, Valabrega S, *et al.* Effect of preoperative colonoscopy on the incidence of synchronous and metachronous neoplasms. *Acta Chir. Scand.* 1990; 156: 163–6.

Beart RW, Steele GD Jr, Menck HR, Chmiel JS, Ocwieja KE, Winchester DP. Management and survival of patients with adenocarcinoma of the colon and rectum: a national survey of the Commission on Cancer. *J. Am. Coll. Surg.* 1995; 181: 225–36.

Bentzen SM, Balslev I, Pedersen M, Teglbjaerg PS, Hanberg Sorensen F, Bone J, *et al.* Blood transfusion and prognosis in Dukes' B and C colorectal cancer. *Eur. J. Cancer* 1990; 26: 457–63.

Blank M, Klussmann E, Kruger Krasagakes S, Schmitt Graff A, Stolte M, Bornhoeft G, *et al.* Expression of MUC2 mucin in colorectal adenomas and carcinomas of different histological types. *Int. J. Cancer* 1994; 59: 301–6.

Blenkinsopp W, Stewart-Brown S, Blesovsky L, Kearney G, Fielding LP. Histopathology reporting in large bowel cancer. *J. Clin. Pathol.* 1981; 34: 509–13.

Bonfanti G, Bombelli L, Bozzetti F, Doci R, Gennari L, Koukouras D. The role of CEA and liver function tests in the detection of hepatic metastases from colo rectal cancer. *HPB Surg.* 1990; 3: 29–36.

Bottger TC, Potratz D, Stockle M, Wellek S, Klupp J, Junginger T. Prognostic value of DNA analysis in colorectal carcinoma. *Cancer* 1993; 72: 3579–87.

Brady AP, Stevenson GW, Stevenson I. Colorectal cancer overlooked at barium enema examination and colonoscopy: a continuing perceptual problem. *Radiology* 1994; 192: 373–8.

Braverman DZ, Stankiewicz H, Goldstein R, Patz JK, Morali GA, Jacobsohn WZ. Ornithine decarboxylase: an unreliable marker for the identification of population groups at risk for colonic neoplasia. *Am. J. Gastroenterol.* 1990; 85: 723–6.

Brenna E, Skreden K, Waldum HL, Marvik R, Dybdahl JH, Kleveland PM, *et al.* The benefit of colonoscopy. *Scand. J. Gastroenterol.* 1990; 25: 81–8.

Brewster NT, Grieve DC, Saunders JH. Double contrast barium enema and flexible sigmoidoscopy for routine colonic investigation. *Br. J. Surg.* 1994; 81: 445–7.

Bryan NP, Jackson A, Raftery AT. Carcinoma of the sigmoid colon presenting as a scrotal swelling. *Postgrad. Med. J.* 1997; 73: 47–8.

Buchsbaum DJ, Khazaeli MB, Davis MA, Lawrence TS. Sensitization of radiolabeled monoclonal antibody therapy using bromodeoxyuridine. *Cancer* 1994; 73: 999–1005.

Busch OR, Marquet RL, Hop WC, Jeekel J. Colorectal cancer recurrence and perioperative blood transfusions: a critical reappraisal. *Semin. Surg. Oncol.* 1994; 10: 195–9.

Cali RL, Pitsch RM, Thorson AG, Watson P, Tapia P, Blatchford GJ, Christensen MA. Cumulative incidence of metachronous colorectal cancer. *Dis. Colon Rectum* 1993; 36: 388–93.

Carpelan-Holmstrom M, Haglund C, Lundin J, Jarvinen H, Roberts P. Preoperative serum levels of CA 242 and CEA predict outcome in colorectal cancer. *Eur. J. Cancer* 1996; 32: 1156–61.

Catalano MF, Levin B. Cancer of the colon and rectum. *Clin. Geriatr. Med.* 1991; 7: 331–46.

Chapuis PH, Newland RC, Dent OF, Bokey EL, Hinder JM. Current perspectives in staging large bowel cancer. *Aust. N.Z. J. Surg.* 1990; 60: 261–5.

Chui DW, Gooding GA, McQuaid KR, Griswold V, Grendell JH. Hydrocolonic ultrasonography in the detection of colonic polyps and tumors. *N. Engl. J. Med.* 1994; 331: 1685–8.

Cozart DT, Lang NP, Hauer Jensen M. Colorectal cancer in patients under 30 years of age. Contributors to the Southwestern Surgical Congress Unusual Case Registry. *Am. J. Surg.* 1993; 166: 764–7.

Cross SS, Bull AD, Smith JH. Is there any justification for the routine examination of bowel resection margins in colorectal adenocarcinoma? *J. Clin. Pathol.* 1989; 42: 1040–2.

Crucitti F, Sofo L, Doglietto GB, Bellantone R, Ratto C, Bossola M, Crucitti A. Prognostic factors in colorectal cancer: current status and new trends. *J. Surg. Oncol.* 1991; 2 (Suppl.): 76–82.

Cusack JC, Giacco GG, Cleary K, Davidson BS, Izzo F, Skibber J, Yen J, Curley SA. Survival factors in 186 patients younger than 40 years old with colorectal adenocarcinoma. *J. Am. Coll. Surg.* 1996; 183: 105–12.

Davidson BR, Sams VR, Styles J, Dean C, Boulos PB. Comparative study of carcinoembryonic antigen and epithelial membrane antigen expression in normal colon, adenomas and adenocarcinomas of the colon and rectum. *Gut* 1989; 30: 1260–5.

Dawson PM, Habib NA, Rees HC, *et al.* Influence of sialomucin at the resection margin on local tumour recurrence and survival of patients with colorectal cancer: a multivariate analysis. *Br. J. Surg.* 1987; 74: 366–9.

Dawson PM, Habib NA, Rees HC, Wood CB. Mucosal field change in colorectal cancer *Am. J. Surg.* 1987; 153: 281–3.

Deans GT, Parks TG, Rowlands BJ, Spence RA. Prognostic factors in colorectal cancer. *Br. J. Surg.* 1992; 79: 608–13.

Deans GT, Heatley M, Hamilton P, Williams K, Patterson C, Crockard A, *et al.* The role of flow cytometry in colorectal carcinoma. *Surg. Gynecol. Obstet.* 1993a; 177: 377–82.

Deans GT, Williamson K, Hamilton P, Heatley M, Arthurs K, Patterson CC, *et al.* DNA densitometry of colorectal cancer. *Gut* 1993b; 34: 1566–71.

Deans GT, Hamilton PW, Watt PCH, Heatley M, Williamson K, Patterson C, *et al.* Morphometric analysis of colorectal cancer. *Dis. Colon Rectum* 1993c; 36: 450–6.

Deans GT, Heatley M, Anderson N, Patterson C, Rowlands BJ, Parks TG, Spence RAJ. Jass' classification revisited. *J. Am. Coll. Surg.* 1994a; 179: 11–17.

Deans GT, Patterson CC, Parks TG, Spence RA, Heatley M, Moorehead RJ, Rowlands BJ. Colorectal carcinoma: importance of clinical and pathological factors in survival. *Ann. R. Coll. Surg. Engl.* 1994b; 76: 59–64.

Deguchi H, Tabuchi Y, Saitoh Y. CEA levels of draining venous blood and draining peripheral CEA gradient in colorectal cancer patients: correlation with postoperative survival. *Nippon Geka Gakkai Zasshi* 1990; 91: 575–80.

D'Eredita G, Serio G, Neri V, Polizzi RA, Barberio G, Losacco T. A survival regression analysis of prognostic factors in colorectal cancer. *Aust. NZ. J. Surg.* 1996; 66: 445–51.

Di Giorgio A, Tocchi A, Puntillo G, Botti C, Derme G, Basso L, *et al.* Age as a prognostic factor following excisional surgery for colorectal cancer. *Ann. Ital. Chir.* 1990; 61: 647–50.

DiSario JA, Burt RW, Kendrick ML, McWhorter WP. Colorectal cancers of rare histologic types compared with adenocarcinomas. *Dis. Colon Rectum* 1994; 37: 1277–80.

Dixon AK, Freeman AH, Coni NK. CT of the colon in frail elderly patients. *Semin. Ultrasound CT MR* 1995; 16: 165–72.

Donohue JH, Williams S, Cha S, Windschitl HE, Witzig TE, Nelson H, *et al.* Perioperative blood transfusions do not affect disease recurrence of patients undergoing curative resection of colorectal carcinoma: a Mayo North Central Cancer Treatment Group study. *J. Clin. Oncol.* 1995; 13: 1671–8.

Einspahr JG, Alberts DS, Gapstur SM, Bostick RM, Emerson SS, Gerner EW. Surrogate end-point biomarkers as measures of colon cancer risk and their use in cancer chemoprevention trials. *Cancer Epidemiol. Biomark. Prev.* 1997; 6: 37–48.

Ensley JF, Maciorowski Z, Hassan M, Pietraszkiewicz H, Sakr W, Heilbrun LK. Variations in DNA aneuploid cell content during tumor dissociation in human colon and head and neck cancers analyzed by flow cytometry. *Cytometry* 1993; 14: 550–8.

Ericksen AS, Krasna MJ, Mast BA, Nosher JL, Brolin RE. Use of gastrointestinal contrast studies in obstruction of the small and large bowel. *Dis. Colon Rectum* 1990; 33: 56–64.

Eyal A, Levin I, Segal S, Levi I, Klein B, Kuperman O. Variation of HLA ABC surface antigen expression on adenocarcinoma of the colon in correlation with the degree of differentiation. *Nat. Immun. Cell Growth Regul.* 1990; 9: 222–7.

Faenza A, Cunsolo A, Selleri S, Lucarelli S, Farneti PA, Gozzetti G. Correlation between plasma or blood transfusion and survival after curative surgery for colorectal cancer. *Int. J. Surg.* 1992; 77: 264–9.

Falk PM, Gupta NC, Thorson AG, Frick MP, Boman BM, Christensen MA, Blatchford GJ. Positron emission tomography for preoperative staging of colorectal carcinoma. *Dis. Colon Rectum* 1994; 37: 153–6.

Farrands PA, Hardcastle JD. Colorectal screening by self assessment questionnaire. *Gut* 1984; 25: 445–7.

Fisher ER, Robinsky B, Sass R, Fisher B. Relative prognostic value of the Dukes and the Jass systems in rectal cancer. Findings from the National Surgical Adjuvant Breast and Bowel Projects (Protocol R 01). *Dis. Colon Rectum* 1989; 32: 944–9.

Fisher KS, Zamboni WA, Ross DS. The efficacy of preoperative computed tomography in patients with colorectal carcinoma. *Am. Surg.* 1990; 56: 339–42.

Fitchett CW, Hoffman GC. Obstructing malignant lesions of the colon. *Surg. Clin. North Am.* 1986; 66: 807–20.

Garau I, Benito E, Bosch FX, Bargay J, Obrador A, Santamaria J, *et al.* Blood transfusion has no effect on colorectal cancer survival. A population based study. *Eur. J. Cancer* 1994; 30A: 759–64.

Garcia-Peche P, Vazquez Prado A, Fabra Ramis R, Trullenque Peris R. Factors of prognostic value in long term survival of colorectal cancer patients. *Hepatogastroenterology* 1991; 38: 438–43.

Gazelle GS, Gaa J, Saini S, Shellito P. Staging of colon carcinoma using water enema CT. *J. Comput. Assist. Tomogr.* 1995; 19: 87–91.

Giardiello FM, Hamilton SR, Hylind LM, Yang VW, Tamez P, Casero RA Jr. Ornithine decarboxylase and polyamines in familial adenomatous polyposis. *Cancer Res.* 1997; 57: 199–201.

Glick SN, Teplick SK, Balfe DM, Levine MS, Gasparaitis AE, Maglinte DD, *et al.* Large colonic neoplasms missed by endoscopy. *Am. J. Roentgenol.* 1989; 152: 513–7.

Goldberg EM, Simunovic LM, Drake SL, Mueller WF Jr, Verrill HL. Comparison of serum CA 19-9 and CEA levels in a population at high risk for colorectal cancer. *Hybridoma* 1989; 8: 569–75.

Gordon SR, Smith RE, Power GC. The role of endoscopy in the evaluation of iron deficiency anemia in patients over the age of 50. *Am. J. Gastroenterol.* 1994; 89: 1963–7.

Gotta C, Palau GA, Demos TC, Gonzalez Villaveiran R. Colonic stenoses: use of oral barium when retrograde flow is completely obstructed on barium enema studies. *Radiology* 1990; 177: 703–5.

Goulston KJ, Cook I, Dent OF. How important is rectal bleeding in the diagnosis of bowel cancer and polyps? *Lancet* 1986; ii: 261–5.

Green JB, Timmcke AE, Mitchell WT, Hicks TC, Gathright JB Jr, Ray JE. Mucinous carcinoma just another colon cancer? *Dis. Colon Rectum* 1993; 36: 49–54.

Griffioen G, Bosman FT, Verspaget HW, De Bruin PA, Biemond I, Lamers CB. Colorectal adenomas: clinical and morphological aspects. A review of 166 polyps from 124 Dutch patients. *AntiCancer Res.* 1989; 9: 1685–9.

Griffiths EK, Schapira DV. Serum ferritin and stool occult blood and colon cancer screening. *Cancer Detect. Prev.* 1991; 15: 303–5.

Grinberg M, Mansur AJ, Ferreira DO, Bellotti G, Pileggi F. Endocarditis caused by *Streptococcus bovis* and colorectal neoplasms. *Arq. Bras. Cardiol.* 1990; 54: 265–9.

Guthrie JA, Saifuddin A, Simpkins KC, deDombal FT. Is it worth doing barium enemas on patients with unexplained iron deficiency anaemia? *Clin. Radiol.* 1994; 49: 375–8.

Hall NR, Finan PJ, Stephenson BM, Purves DA, Cooper EH. The role of CA 242 and CEA in surveillance following curative resection for colorectal cancer. *Br. J. Cancer* 1994; 70: 549–53.

Halvorsen TB, Seim E. Degree of differentiation in colorectal adenocarcinomas: a multivariate analysis of the influence on survival. *J. Clin. Pathol.* 1988; 41: 532–7.

Heimann TM, Oh C, Aufses AH Jr. Clinical significance of rectal cancer in young patients. *Dis. Colon Rectum* 1989; 32: 473–6.

Heise RH, Van Winter JT, Wilson TO, Ogburn PL Jr. Colonic cancer during pregnancy: case report and review of the literature. *Mayo Clin. Proc.* 1992; 67: 1180–4.

Heiss MM, Mempel W, Delanoff C, Jauch KW, Gabka C, Mempel M, *et al.* Blood transfusion modulated tumor recurrence: first results of a randomized study of autologous versus allogeneic blood transfusion in colorectal cancer surgery. *J. Clin. Oncol.* 1994; 12: 1859–67.

Helfand M, Marton KI, Zimmer-Gembeck MJ, Sox HC Jr. History of visible rectal bleeding in a primary care population. Initial assessment and 10-year follow-up. *JAMA.* 1997; 277: 44–8.

Hemming AW, Davis NL, Kluftinger A, Robinson B, Quenville NF, Liseman B, LeRiche J. Prognostic markers of colorectal cancer: an evaluation of DNA content, epidermal growth factor receptor, and Ki 67. *J. Surg. Oncol..* 1992; 51: 147–52.

Heptner G, Domschke S, Domschke W. Comparison of CA 72-4 with CA 19-9 and carcinoembryonic antigen in the serodiagnostics of gastrointestinal malignancies. *Scand. J. Gastroenterol.* 1989; 24: 745–50.

Hermanek P Jr, Wiebelt H, Riedl S, Staimmer D, Hermanek P. Long term results of surgical therapy of colon cancer. Results of the Colorectal Cancer Study Group. *Chirurgie* 1994; 65: 287–97.

Hernandez-Socorro CR, Guerra C, Hernandez-Romero J, Rey A, Lopez-Facal P, Alvarez-Santullano V. Colorectal carcinomas: diagnosis and preoperative staging by hydrocolonic sonography. *Surgery* 1995; 117: 609–15.

Hewitt RE, Powe DG, Griffin NR, Turner DR. Relationships between epithelial basement membrane staining patterns in primary colorectal carcinomas and the extent of tumour spread. *Int. J. Cancer* 1991; 48: 855–60.

Heys SD, Sherif A, Bagley JS, Brittenden J, Smart C, Eremin O. Prognostic factors and survival of patients aged less than 45 years with colorectal cancer. *Br. J. Surg.* 1994; 81: 685–8.

Hildebrandt U, Schuder G, Feifel G. Preoperative staging of rectal and colonic cancer. *Endoscopy* 1994; 26: 810–2.

Hixson LJ, Sampliner RE, Chernin M, Amberg J, Kogan F. Limitations of combined flexible sigmoidoscopy and double contrast barium enema in patients with rectal bleeding. *Eur. J. Radiol.* 1989; 9: 254–7.

Hixson LJ, Fennerty MB, Sampliner RE, Garewal HS. Prospective blinded trial of colonoscopic miss rate of large colorectal polyps. *Gastrointest. Endosc.* 1991; 37: 125–7.

Hixson LJ, Garewal HS, McGee DL, Sloan D, Fennerty MB, Sampliner RE, Gerner EW. Ornithine decarboxylase and polyamines in colorectal neoplasia and mucosa. *Cancer Epidemiol. Biomarkers Prev.* 1993; 2: 369–74.

Hixson LJ, Emerson SS, Shassetz LR, Gerner EW. Sources of variability in estimating ornithine decarboxylase activity and polyamine contents in human colorectal mucosa. *Cancer Epidemiol. Biomarkers Prev.* 1994; 3: 317–23.

Houbiers JG, Brand A, van de Watering LM, Hermans J, Verwey PJ, Bijnen AB, *et al*. Randomised controlled trial comparing transfusion of leucocyte depleted or buffy coat depleted blood in surgery for colorectal cancer. *Lancet* 1994; 344: 573–8.

Hough DM, Malone DE, Rawlinson J, De Gara CJ, Moote DJ, Irvine EJ, *et al*. Colon cancer detection: an algorithm using endoscopy and barium enema. *Clin. Radiol.* 1994; 49: 170–5.

Isbister WH, al-Sanea O. The utility of pre-operative abdominal computerized tomography scanning in colorectal Surg. *J. Roy. Coll. Surg. Edin* 1996; 41: 232–4.

Imamura Y, Yasutake K, Yoshimura Y, Oya M, Matsushita K, Tokisue M, Sashikata T. Contents of tissue CEA and CA19-9 in colonic polyp and colorectal cancer, and their clinical significance. *Gastroenterol. Jpn.* 1990; 25: 186–92.

Irimura T, Matsushita Y, Hoff SD, Yamori T, Nakamori S, Frazier ML, *et al*. Ectopic expression of mucins in colorectal cancer metastasis. *Semin. Cancer Biol.* 1991; 2: 129–39.

Jakobsen EB, Eickhoff JH, Andersen J, Lundvall L, Stenderup JK. Perioperative blood transfusion and recurrence and death after resection for cancer of the colon and rectum. *Scand. J. Gastroenterol.* 1990; 25: 435–42.

James RD, Haboubi N, Schofield PF, Mellor M, Salhab N. Prognostic factors in colorectal carcinoma treated by preoperative radiotherapy and immediate surgery. *Dis. Colon Rectum* 1991; 34: 546–51.

Jass J, Love S, Northover J. A new prognostic classification for rectal cancer. *Lancet* 1987; i: 1333–5.

Jensen P, Krogsgaard MR, Christiansen J. Prognostic model for patients treated for colorectal adenomas with regard to development of recurrent adenomas and carcinoma. *Eur. J. Surg.* 1996; 162: 229–34.

Johnson CD, Ilstrup DM, Fish NM, Sauerwine SA, MacCarty RL, Stephens DH, Ward EM, Lantz EJ, Carlson HC. Barium enema: detection of colonic lesions in a community population. *Am. J. Roentgenol.* 1996; 167: 39–43.

Joyce WP, Fynes M, Moran KT, Gough DB, Dervan P, Gorey TF, Fitzpatrick JM. The prognostic value of nucleolar organiser regions in colorectal cancer: a 5 year follow up study. *Ann. R. Coll. Surg. Engl.* 1992; 74: 172–6.

Kaneko K, Boku N, Hosokawa K, Ohtsu A, Fujii T, Koba I, *et al*. Diagnostic utility of endoscopic ultrasonography for preoperative rectal cancer staging estimation. *Jpn. J. Clin. Oncol.* 1996; 26: 30 5.

Kasumi A, Kratzer GL. Fast growing cancer of the colon and rectum. *Am. Surg.* 1992; 58: 383–6.

Kato T, Kojima H, Hirai T, Sakamoto J, Yasui K, Yamamura Y, *et al*. The correlation between preoperative pathologic diagnosis of a biopsy specimen and postoperative pathologic diagnosis of a tissue specimen involving colorectal cancer patients. *Gan No Rinsho* 1989; 35: 1119–22.

Kawahara M, Terasaki PI, Chia D, *et al*. Use of four monoclonal antibodies to detect tumor markers. *Cancer* 1986; 58: 2008–12.

Kawasaki H, Tabuchi Y, Saitoh Y. Mitotic activity of cancer in the colorectum: correlation with histopathologic variables and survival. *Nippon Geka Gakkai Zasshi* 1990; 91: 837–43.

Kee F, Wilson RH, Gilliland R, Sloan JM, Rowlands BJ, Moorehead RJ. Changing site distribution of colorectal cancer. *Br. Med. J.* 1992; 305: 158.

Kerner BA, Oliver GC, Eisenstat TE, Rubin RJ, Salvati EP. Is preoperative computerized tomography useful in assessing patients with colorectal carcinoma? *Dis. Colon Rectum* 1993; 36: 1050–3.

Kim YJ, Ngoi SS, Godwin TA, DeCosse JJ, Staiano Coico L. Ploidy in invasive colorectal cancer. Implications for metastatic disease. *Cancer* 1991; 68: 638–41.

King DW, Lubowski DZ, Armstrong AS. Sigmoid stricture at colonoscopy an indication for surgery. *Int. J. Colorectal Dis.* 1990; 5: 161–3.

Laffer U, Jaggi P, Harder F, Metzger U, Egeli R, Weber W, *et al*. Blood transfusions and prognosis following curative resection of colorectal cancer: is there an association? *Helv. Chir. Acta* 1989; 56: 461–4.

Lai DT, Fulham M, Stephen MS, Chu KM, Solomon M, Thompson JF, Sheldon DM, Storey DW. The role of whole-body positron emission tomography with [18F]fluorodeoxyglucose in identifying operable colorectal cancermetastases to the liver. *Arch. Surg.* 1996; 131: 703–7.

LaMuraglia GM, Lacaine F, Malt RA. High ornithine decarboxylase activity and polyamine levels in human colorectal neoplasia. *Ann. Surg.* 1986; 204: 89–93.

Lee PY, Fletcher WS, Sullivan ES, Vetto JT. Colorectal cancer in young patients: characteristics and outcome. *Am. Surg.* 1994; 60: 607–12.

Leen E, Goldberg JA, Robertson J, Angerson WJ, Sutherland GR, Cooke TG, McArdle CS. Early detection of occult colorectal hepatic metastases using duplex colour Doppler sonography. *Br. J. Surg.* 1993; 80: 1249–51.

Leen E, Angerson WG, Cooke TG, McArdle CS. Prognostic power of Doppler perfusion index in colorectal cancer. Correlation with survival. *Ann. Surg.* 1996; 223: 199–203.

Leite JF, Granjo ME, Martins MI, Reis RC, Monteiro JC, Castro Sousa F. Effect of perioperative blood transfusions on survival of patients after radical surgery for colorectal cancer. *Int. J. Colorectal Dis.* 1993; 8: 129–33.

Levi F, La Vecchia C, Franceschi S, Te VC. Morphologic analysis of digestive cancers from the registry of Vaud, Switzerland. *Br. J. Cancer* 1991; 63: 567–72.

Lewis CT, Riley WE, Georgeson K, Warren JH. Carcinoma of the colon and rectum in patients less than 20 years of age. *South Med. J.* 1990; 83: 383–5.

Liewald F, Wirsching RP, Zulke C, Demmel N, Mempel W. Influence of blood transfusions on tumor recurrence and survival rate in colorectal carcinoma. *Eur. J. Cancer* 1990; 26: 327–35.

Limberg B. Diagnosis of large bowel tumours by colonic sonography. *Lancet* 1990; 335: 144–6.

Loh A, Jones D, Dickson GH. Accuracy of intraoperative staging in colorectal cancer. *J. R. Coll. Surg. Edinburgh* 1994; 39: 20–2.

Lorenz M, Baum RP, Oremek G, Inglis R, Reimann Kirkowa M, Hor G, *et al*. Tumor markers, liver function tests and symptoms in 115 patients with isolated colorectal liver metastases. *Int. J. Biol. Markers* 1989; 4: 18–26.

Love RR, Surawicz TS, Morrissey JF, Verma AK. Levels of colorectal ornithine decarboxylase activity in patients with colon cancer, a family history of nonpolyposis hereditary colorectal cancer, and adenomas. *Cancer Epidemiol. Biomarkers Prev.* 1992; 1: 195–8.

Markus JB, Somers S, O'Malley BP, Stevenson GW. Double contrast barium enema studies: effect of multiple reading on perception error. *Radiology* 1990; 175: 155–6.

Maxfield RG, Maxfield CM. Colonoscopy as a primary diagnostic procedure in chronic gastrointestinal tract bleeding. *Arch. Surg.* 1986; 121: 401–3.

McGahren ED 3rd, Mills SE, Wilhelm MC. Colorectal carcinoma in patients 30 years of age and younger. *Am. Surg.* 1995; 61: 78–82.

McIntyre AS, Long RG. Prospective survey of investigations in outpatients referred with iron deficiency anaemia. *Gut* 1993; 34: 1102–7.

McNicholas MM, Joyce WP, Dolan J, Gibney RG, MacErlaine DP, Hyland J. Magnetic resonance imaging of rectal carcinoma: a prospective study. *Br. J. Surg.* 1994; 81: 911–4.

Meijer S, Paul MA, Cuesta MA, Blomjous J. Intra-operative ultrasound in detection of liver metastases. *Eur. J. Cancer* 1995; 31A: 1210–1.

Mercer DW, Talamo TS. Multiple markers of malignancy in sera of patients with colorectal carcinoma: preliminary clinical studies. *Clin. Chem.* 1985; 31: 1824–8.

Metcalf JV, Smith J, Jones R, Record CO. Incidence and causes of rectal bleeding in general practice as detected by colonoscopy. *Brit. J. Gen. Pract.* 1996; 46: 161–4.

Milton JD, Eccleston D, Parker N, Raouf A, Cubbin C, Hoffman J, *et al*. Distribution of O acetylated sialomucin in the normal and diseased gastrointestinal tract shown by a new monoclonal antibody. *J. Clin. Pathol.* 1993; 46: 323–9.

Minsky BD, Mies C, Rich TA, Recht A. Lymphatic vessel invasion is an independent prognostic factor for survival in colorectal cancer. *Int. J. Radiat. Oncol. Biol. Phys.* 1989; 17: 311–8.

Modin S, Karlsson G, Wahlby L. Blood transfusion and recurrence of colorectal cancer. *Eur. J. Surg.* 1992; 158: 371–5.

Moertel CG, O'Fallon JR, Go VLW, et al. The preoperative carcinoembryonic antigen test in the diagnosis, staging, and prognosis of colorectal cancer. *Cancer* 1986; 58: 603–10.

Molland G, Dent OF, Chapuis PH, Bokey EL, Nicholls M, Newland RC. Transfusion does not influence patient survival after resection of colorectal cancer. *Aust. N.Z. J. Surg.* 1995; 65: 592–5.

Monreal M, Lafoz E, Casals A, Inaraja L, Montserrat E, Callejas JM, Martorell A. Occult cancer in patients with deep venous thrombosis. A systematic approach. *Cancer* 1991; 67: 541–5.

Moorehead RJ, Hoper M, McKelvey STD. Assessment of ornithine decarboxylase activity in rectal mucosa as a marker for colorectal adenomas and carcinomas. *Br. J. Surg.* 1987; 74: 364–5.

Mori M, Shimono R, Adachi Y, Matsuda H, Kuwano H, Sugimachi K, et al. Transitional mucosa in human colorectal lesions. *Dis. Colon Rectum* 1990; 33: 498–501.

Mulcahy HE, Patchett SE, Daly L, O'Donoghue DP. Prognosis of elderly patients with large bowel cancer. *Br. J. Surg.* 1994; 81: 736–8.

Nakagoe T, Fukushima K, Hirota M, Kusano H, Ayabe H, Tomita M, Kamihira S. An immunohistochemical study of the distribution of blood group substances and related antigens in primary colorectal carcinomas and metastatic lymph node and liver lesions, using monoclonal antibodies against A, B, H type 2, Le(a), and Le(x) antigens. *J. Gastroenterol.* 1994; 29: 265–75.

Ngoi SS, Staiano Coico L, Godwin TA, Wong RJ, DeCosse JJ. Abnormal DNA ploidy and proliferative patterns in superficial colonic epithelium adjacent to colorectal cancer. *Cancer* 1990; 66: 953–9.

Nicholls RJ, Dube S. The extent of examination by rigid sigmoidoscope. *Br. J. Surg.* 1982; 69: 438.

Nishioka K, Grossie VB, Chang TH, Ajani JA, Ota DM. Colorectal ornithine decarboxylase activity in human mucosa and tumors: elevation of enzymatic activity in distal mucosa. *J. Surg. Oncol.* 1991; 47: 117–20.

Norfleet RG, Ryan ME, Wyman JB, Rhodes RA, Nunez JF, Kirchner JP, Parent K. Barium enema versus colonoscopy for patients with polyps found during flexible sigmoidoscopy. *Gastrointest. Endosc.* 1991; 37: 531–4.

Nori D, Merimsky O, Samala E, Saw D, Cortes E, Chen E, Turner JW. Tumor ploidy as a risk factor for disease recurrence and short survival in surgically treated Dukes' B2 colon cancer patients. *J. Surg. Oncol.* 1995; 59: 239–42.

Northover J. The use of prognostic markers in surgery for colorectal cancer. *Eur. J. Cancer* 1995; 31A: 1207–9.

Norton SA, Armstrong CP. Lower gastrointestinal bleeding during anticoagulant therapy: a life-saving complication? *Ann. Roy. Coll. Surg. Engl.* 1997; 79: 38–9.

Nudelmann IL, Gutman H, Deutsch AA, Reiss R. Colon rectum cancer in patients above 70 years of age. *J. Exp. Clin. Cancer Res.* 1986; 5: 351–8.

Offerhaus GJ, Giardiello FM, Bruijn JA, Stijnen T, Molyvas EN, Fleuren GJ. The value of immunohistochemistry for collagen IV expression in colorectal carcinomas. *Cancer* 1991; 67: 99–105.

Ohuchi N, Takahashi K, Matoba N, Sato T, Taira Y, Sakai N, et al. Comparison of serum assays for TAG 72, CA19-9 and CEA in gastrointestinal carcinoma patients. *Jpn. J. Clin. Oncol.* 1989; 19: 242–8.

Onodera H, Maetani S, Nishikawa T, Tobe T. The reappraisal of prognostic classifications for colorectal cancer. *Dis. Colon Rectum* 1989; 32: 609–14.

Paganelli GM, Lalli E, Facchini A, Biasco G, Santucci R, Brandi G, Barbara L. Flow cytometry and *in vitro* triticated thymidine labeling in normal rectal mucosa of patients at high risk of colorectal cancer. *Am. J. Gastroenterol.* 1994; 89: 220–4.

Payne JE. International colorectal carcinoma staging and grading. *Dis. Colon Rectum* 1989; 32: 282–5.

Payne JE, Chapuis PH, Pheils MT. Surgery for large bowel cancer in people aged 75 years and older. *Dis. Colon Rectum* 1986; 29: 733–7.

Pema PJ, Bennett WF, Bova JG, Warman P. CT vs MRI in diagnosis of recurrent rectosigmoid carcinoma. *J. Comput. Assist. Tomogr.* 1994; 18: 256–61.

Phillips RW, Kikendall JW, Luk GD, Willis SM, Murphy JR, Maydonovitch C, et al. beta Carotene inhibits rectal mucosal ornithine

decarboxylase activity in colon cancer patients. *Cancer Res.* 1993; 53: 3723–5.

Plebani M, De Paoli M, Basso D, Roveroni G, Giacomini A, Galeotti F, Corsini A. Serum tumor markers in colorectal cancer staging, grading, and follow-up. *J. Surg. Oncol.* 1996; 62: 239–44.

Ponz de Leon M, Sant M, Micheli A, Sacchetti C, Di Gregorio C, Fante R, et al. Clinical and pathologic prognostic indicators in colorectal cancer. A population based study. *Cancer* 1992; 69: 626–35.

Qin Y, Willems G. Comparison of the classical autoradiographic and the immunohistochemical methods with BrdU for measuring proliferation parameters in colon cancer. *AntiCancer Res.* 1993; 13: 731–5.

Quirke P, Dixon MF. The prediction of local recurrence in rectal adenocarcinoma by histopathological examination. *Int. J. Colorectal Dis* 1988; 3: 127–31.

Rankin FW, Broders AC. Factors influencing prognosis in carcinoma of the rectum. *Surg. Gynecol. Obstet.* 1928; 46: 660–7.

Rayter Z, Surtees P, Tildsley G, Corbishley C. The prognostic value of argyrophil nucleolar organiser regions (AgNORs) in colorectal cancer. *Eur. J. Surg. Oncol.* 1992; 18: 37–40.

Recio P, Bussey HJR. The pathology and prognosis of carcinoma of the rectum in the young (Abridged). *Proc. R. Soc. Med.* 1965; 58: 789–90.

Rex DK, Lehman GA, Lappas JC, Miller RE. Sensitivity of double contrast barium study for left colon polyps. *Radiology* 1986; 158: 69–72.

Rockey DC, Cello JP. Evaluation of the gastrointestinal tract in patients with iron deficiency anemia. *N. Engl. J. Med.* 1993; 329: 1691–5.

Rowley S, Newbold KM, Gearty J, Keighley MR, Donovan IA, Neoptolemos JP. Comparison of deoxyribonucleic acid ploidy and nuclear expressed p62 c myc oncogene in the prognosis of colorectal cancer. *World J Surg.* 1990; 14: 545–50.

Scharling ES, Wolfman NT, Bechtold RE. Computed tomography evaluation of colorectal carcinoma. *Semin. Roentgenol.* 1996; 31: 142–53.

Schnall MD, Furth EE, Rosato EF, Kressel HY. Rectal tumor stage: correlation of endorectal MR imaging and pathologic findings. *Radiology* 1994; 190: 709–14.

Schwartz B, Bresalier RS, Kim YS. The role of mucin in colon cancer metastasis. *Int. J. Cancer* 1992; 52: 60–5.

Selby JV, Friedman GD, Collen MF. Sigmoidoscopy and mortality from colorectal cancer: The Kaiser Permanente multiphasic evaluation study. *J. Clin. Epidemiol.* 1988; 41: 427–34.

Shank B, Dershaw DD, Caravelli J et al. A prospective study of the accuracy of preoperative computed tomographic staging of patients with biopsy proven rectal carcinoma. *Dis. Colon Rectum* 1990; 33: 285–90.

Shepherd NA, Saraga EP, Love SB, Jass JR. Prognostic factors in colonic cancer. *Histopathology* 1989; 14: 613–20.

Shida H, Ban K, Matsumoto M, Masuda K, Imanari T, Machida T Yamamoto T. Prognostic significance of location of lymph node metastases in colorectal cancer. *Dis. Colon Rectum* 1992; 35: 1046–50.

Sibbering DM, Locker AP, Hardcastle JD, Armitage NC. Blood transfusion and survival in colorectal cancer. *Dis. Colon Rectum* 1994; 37: 358–63.

Sidoni A, Bufalari A, Alberti PF. Distal intramural spread in colorectal cancer: a reappraisal of the extent of distal clearance in fifty cases. *Tumori* 1991; 77: 514–7.

Siegert CE, Overbosch D. Carcinoma of the colon presenting as *Streptococcus sanguis* bacteremia. *Am. J. Gastroenterol.* 1995; 90: 1528–9.

Silman AJ, Mitchell P, Nicholls RJ, et al. Self reported dark red bleeding as a marker comparable with occult blood testing in screening for large bowel neoplasms. *Br. J. Surg.* 1983; 70: 721–4.

Slater G, Aufses AH Jr, Szporn A. Synchronous carcinoma of the colon and rectum. *Surg. Gynecol. Obstet.* 1990; 171: 283–7.

Slentz K, Senagore A, Hibbert J, Mazier WP, Talbott TM. Can preoperative and postoperative CEA predict survival after colon cancer resection? *Am. Surg.* 1994; 60: 528–31.

Smith C. Colorectal cancer. Radiological diagnosis. *Radiol. Clin. North Am.* 1997; 35: 439–56.

Souquet JC, Napoleon B, Pujol B, Ponchon T, Keriven O, Lambert R. Echoendoscopy prior to endoscopic tumor therapy more safety? *Endoscopy* 1993; 25: 475–8.

Speights VO, Johnson MW, Stoltenberg PH, Rappaport ES, Helbert B, Riggs M. Colorectal cancer: current trends in initial clinical manifestations. *South Med. J.* 1991; 84: 575–8.

Stebbing JF, Nash AG. Avoidable delay in the management of carcinoma of the right colon. *Ann. R. Coll. Surg. Engl.* 1995; 77: 21–3.

Stein W, Farina A, Gaffney K, Lundeen C, Wagner K, Wachtel T. Characteristics of colon cancer at time of presentation. *Fam. Pract. Res. J.* 1993; 13: 355–63.

Steine S, Stordahl A, Laerum F, Laerum E. Referrals for double contrast barium examination. Factors influencing the probability of finding polyps or cancer. *Scand. J. Gastroenterol.* 1994; 29: 260–4.

Steiner MG, Harlow SP, Colombo E, Bauer KD. Chromosomes 8, 12, and 17 copy number in Astler Coller stage C colon cancer in relation to proliferative activity and DNA ploidy. *Cancer Res.* 1993; 53: 681–6.

Stone MD, Kane R, Bothe A Jr, Jessup JM, Cady B, Steele GD Jr. Intraoperative ultrasound imaging of the liver at the time of colorectal cancer resection. *Arch. Surg.* 1994; 129: 431–5.

Stubbs RS, Nadkarni DM, Monsey HA. Faecal carcinoembryonic antigen in colorectal cancer patients. *Gut* 1986; 27: 901–5.

Talbot IC, Ritchie S, Leighton M, Hughes A, Bussey H, Morson B. The clinical significance of invasion of veins by rectal cancer. *Br. J. Surg.* 1980; 67: 439–42.

Tanaka M, Omura K, Watanabe Y, Oda Y, Nakanishi I. Prognostic factors of colorectal cancer: K ras mutation, overexpression of the p53 protein, and cell proliferative activity. *J. Surg. Oncol.* 1994; 57: 57 61.

Tartter PI. The association of perioperative blood transfusion with colorectal cancer recurrence. *Ann. Surg.* 1992; 216: 633–8.

Tate JJ, Rawlinson J, Royle G, Brunton F, Taylor I. Pre operative or post-operative colonic examination for synchronous lesions in colorectal cancer. *Br. J. Surg.* 1988; 75: 1016–18.

Tempero M, Brand R, Holdeman K, Matamoros A. New imaging techniques in colorectal cancer. *Semin. Oncol.* 1995; 22: 448–71.

Thaler W, Watzka S, Martin F, La Guardia G, Psenner K, Bonatti G, *et al.* Preoperative staging of rectal cancer by endoluminal ultrasound vs. magnetic resonance imaging. Preliminary results of a prospective, comparative study. *Dis. Colon Rectum* 1994; 37: 1189–93.

Thoeni RF, Rogalla P. CT for the evaluation of carcinomas in the colon and rectum. *Semin. Ultrasound CT MR* 1995; 16: 112–26.

Thoeni RF. Colorectal cancer. Radiologic staging. *Radiol. Clin. North Am.* 1997; 35: 457–85.

Thomas GD, Dixon MF, Smeeton NC, Williams N. Observer variation in the histological grading of rectal carcinomas. *J. Clin. Pathol.* 1983; 36: 385–91.

Tsioulias GJ, Triadafilopoulos G, Goldin E, Papavassiliou ED, Rizos S, Bassioukas P, Rigas B. Expression of HLA class I antigens in sporadic adenomas and histologically normal mucosa of the colon. *Cancer Res.* 1993; 53: 2374–8.

Uchida M, Sakoda J, Fujitoh H, Kumabe T, Oshibuchi M, Hayabuchi N, *et al.* Reappraisal of the clinical usefulness of transabdominal ultrasonography for advanced colon cancer a study of tumor detection. *Nippon Igaku Hoshasen Gakkai Zasshi* 1993; 53: 261–5.

Ueda T, Shimada E, Urakawa T. The clinicopathologic features of serum CA 19-9 positive colorectal cancers. *Surg. Today* 1994; 24: 518–25.

Vellacott KD, Virjee J. Audit on the use of the barium enema. *Gut* 1986; 27: 182–5.

Verazin G, Riley WM, Gregory J, Tautu C, Prorok JJ, Alhadeff JA. Serum sialic acid and carcinoembryonic levels in the detection and monitoring of colorectal cancer. *Dis. Colon Rectum* 1990; 33: 139–42.

Wang JY, Tang R, Chiang JM. Value of carcinoembryonic antigen in the management of colorectal cancer. *Dis. Colon Rectum* 1994; 37: 272–7.

Wang QA, Gao H, Wang YH, Chen YL. The clinical and biological significance of the transitional mucosa adjacent to colorectal cancer. *Jpn. J. Surg.* 1991; 21: 253–61.

Wherry DC, Thomas WM. The yield of flexible fiberoptic sigmoidoscopy in the detection of asymptomatic colorectal neoplasia. *Surg. Endosc.* 1994; 8: 393–5.

Wilking N, Petrelli N, Herrera Onnelas L, Walsh D, Mittelman A. A comparison of the rigid proctosigmoidoscope with the 65 cm flexible endoscope in the screening of patients for colorectal carcinoma. *Cancer* 1986; 57: 669–71.

Witzig TE, Loprinzi CL, Gonchoroff NJ, Reiman HM, Cha SS, Wieand HS, *et al.* DNA ploidy and cell kinetic measurements as predictors of recurrence and survival in stages B2 and C colorectal adenocarcinoma. *Cancer* 1991; 68: 879–88.

Xiang YY, Wang DY, Tanaka M, Suzuki M, Kiyokawa E, Igarashi H, Naito Y, Shen Q, Sugimura H. Expression of high-mobility group-1 mRNA in human gastrointestinal adenocarcinoma and corresponding non-cancerous mucosa. *Int. J. Cancer.* 1997; 74: 1–6.

Yamazoe Y, Maetani S, Nishikawa T, Onodera H, Tobe T, Imamura M. The prognostic role of the DNA ploidy pattern in colorectal cancer analysis using paraffin embedded tissue by an improved method. *Surg. Today* 1994; 24: 30–6.

Zarchy TM, Ershoff D. Which clinical variables predict an abnormal double contrast barium enema result? *Ann. Intern. Med.* 1991; 114: 137–41.

Zerhouni EA, Rutter C, Hamilton SR, Balfe DM, Megibow AJ, Francis IR, Moss AA, Heiken JP, Tempany CM, Aisen AM, Weinreb JC, Gatsonis C, McNeil BJ. CT and MR imaging in the staging of colorectal carcinoma: report of the Radiology Diagnostic Oncology Group II. *Radiol.* 1996; 200: 443–51.

12 Treatment of colorectal cancer

Tumours arising in polyps

Carcinoma *in situ* refers to malignant cells contained above the muscularis mucosae and occurs in 5% of endoscopically removed polyps (Stein and Coller 1993). Such lesions do not metastasise because lymphatics are absent above the muscularis mucosae so that complete excision, usually endoscopically results in cure (Stein and Coller 1993). Penetration of malignant cells through the muscularis mucosae constitutes invasive carcinoma and occurs in up to 5% of endoscopically removed polyps (Stein and Coller 1993). The incidence of invasive malignancy increases progressively from tubular through tubulovillous to villous adenomas. Lymph node involvement and recurrence in malignant polyps are closely related to the depth of invasion as classified by Haggit *et al.* (1985) (Table 12.1). Polyps without invasion of the stalk are not associated with recurrence or a poor prognosis even when composed entirely of cancer cells. The incidence of metastases or recurrence in level 3 or 4 lesions is 15% (Stein and Coller 1993). Malignant sessile polyps therefore tend to be more aggressive as any invasion represents a level 4 lesion (Haggit *et al.* 1985; Moore *et al.* 1994).

The size of the polyp does not correlate with either the risk of invasion or distant metastases, over half of all polyps demonstrating tumour invasion being under 2 cm. However, poorly differentiated and inadequately excised malignant polyps are associated with lymph node mestastases and recurrence (Cunningham *et al.* 1994; Hase *et al.* 1995). When the resection margins are involved, the risk of involved lymph nodes or recurrent disease is 50%, compared with 25% if tumour is close to the margin and 5% if the margins are clear (Stein and Coller 1993). However, there is a lack of consensus as to what constitutes an adequate resection margin, opinions varying from 1 to 10 mm (Cunningham *et al.* 1994).

Whether patients with invasive carcinoma in polyps should undergo surgery is also debatable. For each patient the risks of surgery (mortality rate 2% for those over 60 years) must be balanced against the risk of metastases or recurrence based on histolog-ical criteria and broad guidelines have been proposed. These suggest that all patients with level 4 lesions or those with level 3 lesions in the presence of poor tumour differentiation should undergo surgery. Patients with sessile polyps or involved resection margins should also undergo surgery. In those with clear margins, surgery may still be indicated as the 5% risk of metastatic or recurrent disease exceeds the mortality of surgical intervention. However, if the margins are clear and histological criteria are favourable, a 'watch and see' policy entails minimal risk of recurrence or metastasis of less than 2% (Stein and Coller 1993). Occasionally malignant polyps, usually of the caecum, cause an ileocolic intussusception which requires surgical intervention (Begos *et al.* 1997) (Figures 12.1 and 12.2a,b).

Invasive colonic cancers

In the absence of widespread metastases, resection of the tumour and its associated lymphatics should be performed. Mural clearance is usually easily achieved in colonic cancers and most authorities would attempt a 5 cm proximal and 5 cm distal clearance as nodal metastasis in a longitudinal direction is rare (Williams *et al.* 1983; Morikawa *et al.* 1994). As nodal excision requires resection of the arterial supply, margins are often much greater.

Turnbull and colleagues (1967) found the crude 5-year survival to be better when a no-touch technique was used. However, this has been criticized as being a non-randomized trial comparing several surgeons in which the survival advantage was limited to Dukes' C cases. More recent randomized trials do suggest a small survival ad-

Table 12.1 Classification of colorectal carcinoma arising in polyps	
Level 0	carcinoma *in situ*
Level 1	invasive carcinoma limited to the head of the polyp
Level 2	invasion of the neck
Level 3	invasion of the stalk
Level 4	invasion of the submucosa below the polyp

After Haggit *et al.* (1985)

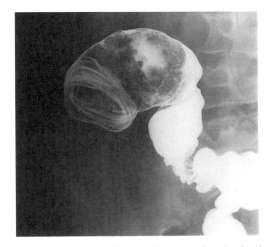

Figure 12.1 Barium enema in an ileocolic intussusception showing the classical 'coiled spring'.

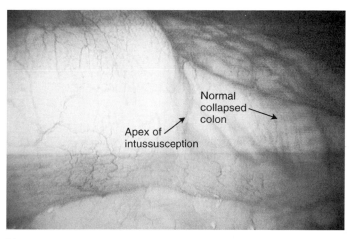

(a)

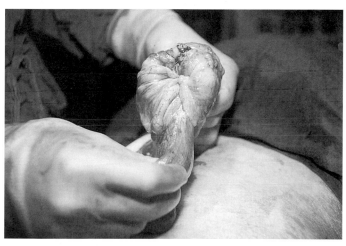

(b)

Figures 12.2 Ileocolic intussusception treated by laparoscopically assisted right hemicolectomy. (a) Laparoscopic view showing the apex of the intussusception (arrowed). (b) The exteriorized, almost reduced specimen.

vantage from the no-touch technique, especially for those with Duke's C tumours (Jeekal 1987), but many surgeons feel that the extent of local clearance is more important than a no-touch technique (MacFarlane *et al.* 1993).

Although early high ligation of the inferior mesenteric artery has long been advocated for excision of left-sided lesions, there is little evidence that this produces any improvement in survival (Staniunas and Schoetz 1993; Fengler and Pearl 1994). Similarly, there is no difference in survival between radical left hemicolectomy and segmental resection of the descending colon with preservation of the inferior mesenteric artery (Corder *et al.* 1992). Flush ligation of the inferior mesenteric vessel in left hemicolectomy abolishes the main blood supply to the rectum through the superior haemorrhoidal artery so that the distal colon and rectum are then supplied entirely by the inferior rectal branches of the pudendal arteries and the middle rectal branch of the internal iliac artery (Hall *et al.* 1995). Consequently, once the inferior mesenteric artery has been ligated flush with the aorta, the distal stump of bowel must not be too long (normally to the rectosigmoid junction) to ensure a good blood supply to the anastomosis. Alternatively, the mid-transverse colon may be anastomosed to the rectum or an ileorectal anastomosis per-

formed. A common sense approach on an individual patient basis is required that maximizes both tumour clearance and anastomotic blood supply.

In lesions of the distal sigmoid, the proximal line of resection is often through the mid-descending colon with sacrifice of the left colic and sigmoid branches or the inferior mesenteric artery. To ensure an adequate blood supply distally this often requires a high anterior resection anastomosing the mid-descending colon to the upper rectum. Subtotal or total colectomy is indicated for synchronous tumours of the right and left colon or in obstructed tumours with compromise of the caecum (Figure 12.3).

There is little difference in postoperative complications whether a colorectal anastomosis is performed by a stapling or suturing technique (Docherty *et al.* 1995; Fingerhut *et al.* 1995). In patients undergoing very low anterior resection, colonic J pouch reconstruction may be considered as an alternative to a straight coloanal anastomosis (Cavaliere *et al.* 1995; Mortensen *et al.* 1995; Hida *et al.* 1996; Ho *et al.* 1996).

Patients with apparent invasion of local viscera should undergo extensive radical excision if possible as long-term tumour control can be achieved (Cerdan *et al.* 1994; Fengler and Pearl 1994) (Figure 12.4). Almost half of apparently malignant adhesions represent a pathologically benign inflammatory response so that lymph node metastases is more closely related to survival and relapse rates than local infiltration (Cerdan *et al.* 1994).

Laparoscopic techniques may be used to mobilize the bowel and divide the principal blood supply; the resection and anastomosis usually being performed extracorporeally, with the use of a small

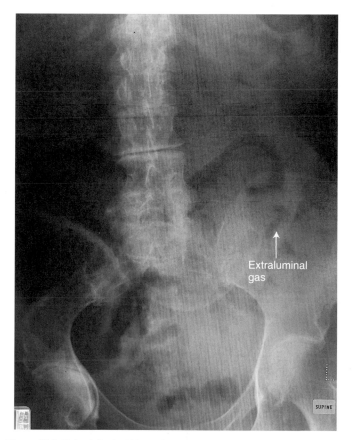

Figure 12.3 Plain abdominal X-ray of obstructing and perforated sigmoid carcinoma. Note the presence of gas on both sides of bowel wall and the absence of gas in the left colon.

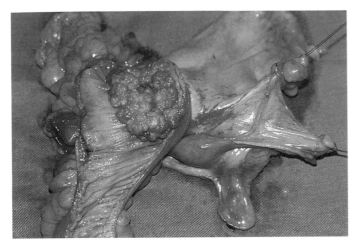

Figure 12.4 Specimen of a total pelvic clearance of rectum, bladder, and uterus.

incision (Schirmer 1996). Totally intracorporeal anastomosis is also possible (Sackier *et al.* 1993; Roe *et al.* 1994) (Figure 12.5). Analysis, using total operative time as an indication of learning, shows that approximately 11–15 completed laparoscopic colectomies are needed to learn this procedure comfortably (Simons *et al.* 1995). Laparoscopic colectomy is associated with similar morbidity and mortality rates to conventional open procedures with a shortened period of ileus, shorter hospital stay, and more rapid recovery (Elftmann *et al.* 1994; Vara-Thorbeck *et al.* 1994; Kwok *et al.* 1996). With experience operative times are similar to open procedures and the use of reusable equipment reduces the costs of the procedure (Monson *et al.* 1992). Concerns that the resection may be inadequate with respect to the amount of tissue and number of lymph nodes removed have not been confirmed (Gray *et al.* 1994; Vara-Thorbeck *et al.* 1994; Monson *et al.* 1995). However, the realization that tumour recurrence in the abdominal wall is a rare but highly significant complication of laparoscopic cancer surgery have cast doubt on the technique (Wexner 1995; Johnstone *et al.* 1996). Abdominal wall recurrence is generally confined to those with Dukes' C lesions. Recurrent cancer in minilaparotomy incisions may simply be due to local spread of cancerous cells. Remote port site recurrence may be due to the liberation of cancer cells throughout

the abdomen facilitated by intraperitoneal carbon dioxide insufflation during laparoscopy. This is supported by the finding of free malignant cells in peritoneal washings of colon cancers prior to resection which is compounded by tumour cells leaking out from lymphatics cut during the dissection (Leather *et al.* 1994). Many surgeons therefore are awaiting the results of controlled trials or restrict laparoscopic colectomy to those with advanced disease or benign conditions (Paik and Beart 1997; Stage *et al.* 1997).

Obstructed colonic lesions

Up to one-half of splenic flexure and one-quarter of left colon tumours present with obstruction (Figure 12.6). In contrast, only 6% of rectosigmoid lesions develop obstruction while the reported risk of obstruction in right colon tumours varies between 8% and 30% (Deans *et al.* 1994). Although right hemicolectomy is the established procedure for obstructed or perforated colon tumours extending as far as the splenic flexure, the optimum treatment for more distal tumours is uncertain (Figure 12.7).

Formerly, caecostomy was used to decompress the obstructed colon and allow later definitive surgery under more controlled conditions. The current applications of this technique are restricted due to its unreliability from frequent tube blockage and heavy demands on nursing care (Benacci and Wolff 1995). In one study only 62% of patients completed the therapeutic course, only a quarter of these

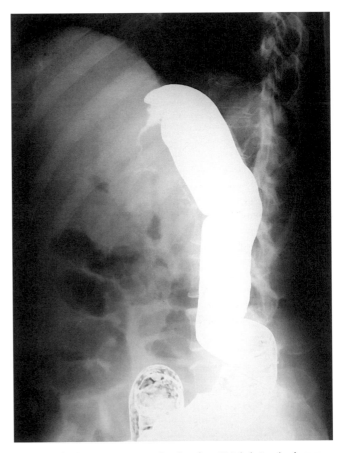

Figure 12.6 Single contrast enema showing almost total obstruction from a carcinoma of the splenic flexure.

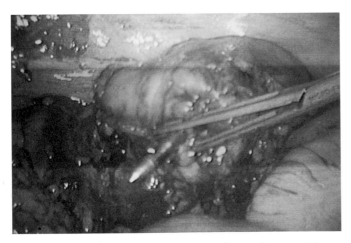

Figure 12.5 Total intracorporeal laparoscopic anterior resection for rectal carcinoma. The spike of the circular stapling device is projecting through the rectal stump and about to be attached to the proximal segment of bowel.

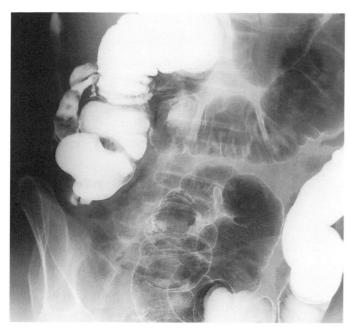

Figure 12.7 Barium study showing free leakage of contrast from a perforated caecal carcinoma.

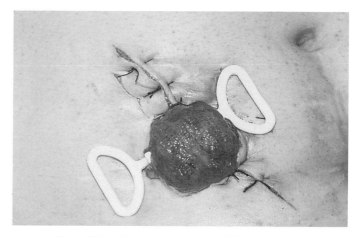

Figure 12.8 Initial defunctioning (sigmoid) loop colostomy.

without complications, the overall mortality being 24% (Kristiansen *et al.* 1990). Caecostomy can therefore only be recommended as an emergency measure for patients in such poor general condition that other forms of treatment are not possible. In such circumstances, the procedure may be performed under local anaesthesia or a drain inserted into the caecum under radiological control (Morrison *et al.* 1990). This is claimed to deflate the bowel effectively and permit colonic irrigation with early resection of the tumour, often within 48 h (Salim 1991). Alternatively a 'blow-hole' caecostomy may be performed with a low operative mortality (2%) and few stoma-related complications (Gurke *et al.* 1991).

The other, more preferred options for managing malignant obstruction of the left colon are the three-stage procedure, Hartmann's procedure, and a single stage, immediate resection with primary anastomosis.

Three-stage procedure

For many years, the standard treatment of the obstructed left colon was an initial defunctioning colostomy, subsequent resection of the tumour, followed by colostomy closure (Table 12.2). The efficacy of the loop colostomy as a defunctioning manoeuvre is questioned (Tuson and Everett 1990), although radiological studies suggest the distal limb is satisfactorily defunctioned (Morris and Rayburn 1991) (Figure 12.8).

About three-quarters of patients undergo tumour resection during the first hospital admission, with a mean hospital stay of 30–55 days (Deans *et al.* 1994). However, 25% of patients do not have the stoma closed to complete the planned third stage due to being unfit, or unwilling, to undergo a further operation (Deans *et al.* 1994). In addition, colostomy closure is associated with significant mortality (7%) and morbidity (20–40%) (Altomare *et al.* 1990).

Most reports show that the combined mortality of the three stages is similar to that of the procedure employing primary resection but that long-term survival is less (Sjodahl *et al.* 1992; Deans *et al.* 1994). The three-stage procedure therefore has a similar operative mortality, longer hospital stay and poorer long-term prognosis

than operations involving primary resection. When the cumulative morbidity and mortality of the three stages are taken into account, initial loop colostomy does not offer any survival advantage and has the distinct disadvantage of prolonging hospital stay and exposing patients to repeated operations (Kronborg 1995).

Hartmann's procedure

Primary tumour resection, closure of the rectal stump, and proximal end colostomy allows immediate, radical resection of the cancer while avoiding the risks of an anastomosis (Table 12.2). These advantages outweigh the disadvantage of a stoma, which should be temporary in most cases. Even if the stoma was to prove permanent, the terminal left iliac fossa colostomy is more easily managed than a loop colostomy.

The major reservations relating to Hartmann's procedure are the morbidity of colostomy closure and the high proportion of patients (about 40%) in whom the stoma proves permanent (Deans *et al.* 1994). Closure of the end colostomy takes longer than that of a loop colostomy, but the mortality (4%) and complication rates (15–30%) are similar (Mileski *et al.* 1990). Delaying colostomy closure for at least 6 months may reduce the morbidity and mortality associated with Hartmann's reversal (Pearce *et al.* 1992). However, one study reported no wound infections or anastomotic leaks from the colostomy reversal, regardless of the time lapse, which was as short as 10 days in some (Krukowski and Matheson 1988). The technical feasibility of laparoscopic reversal of Hartmann's is now established.

The overall mortality of an open Hartmann's procedure with colostomy closure is 10%, while that of the three-stage procedure is 7% (Deans *et al.* 1994). However, mean hospital stay is considerably shorter than the three-stage procedure, ranging from 17 to 30 days (Deans *et al.* 1994). Hartmann's procedure therefore combines primary resection of the tumour and relief of obstruction with an acceptable morbidity and mortality. It is particularly appropriate in perforation of the left colon or in the elderly, unfit patient and is a safer option for trainees and surgeons with limited experience of managing left colonic obstruction.

Primary resection with anastomosis

For many years surgeons were reluctant to perform a primary anastomosis on the obstructed, unprepared left colon for fear of anastomotic leakage (Biondo *et al.* 1997). Performing on-table colonic lavage permits primary anastomosis using a clean decompressed bowel but

Table 12.2 Comparison of staged procedures in the management of the obstructed left colon

Author	Year	No. patients	Number of deaths			Overall mortality (%)	Hospital stay (days)
			1st stage	2nd stage	3rd stage		
Three-stage							
Ambrosetti *et al.*	1989	8	0	1	0	12	41
de Almeida *et al.*	1991	20	NS	NS	NS	10	21
Gutman *et al.*	1989	71	6	0	0	9	NS
Malafosse *et al.*	1989	22	NS	NS	NS	7*	43
Sjodahl *et al.****	1992	48	3	4	0	15	41
Hartmann's							
Ambrosetti *et al.*	1989	36	4	0	--	11	44
Dixon *et al.*	1990	32	2	0	--	6	17**
Gandrup *et al.*	1992	43	4	0	--	9	19**
Koruth *et al.* ***	1985	29	1	0	--	6	26
Malafosse *et al.*	1989	14	NS	NS	--	7*	38
Pearce *et al.* ****	1992	145	12	3	—	12	NS
Sjodahl *et al.*	1992	11	1	0	—	10	NS
Primary anastomosis							
Ambrosetti *et al.*	1989	23	2	—	—	9	22
Amsterdam *et al.*	1985	25	1	—	—	4	NS
Brief *et al.*	1991	23	2	—	—	9	NS
de Almeida *et al.*	1991	11	1	—	—	9	9
Dorudi *et al.*	1990	18	0	—	—	0	11
Hong *et al.*	1989	8	0	—	—	0	NS
Koruth *et al.*	1985	47	4	—	—	8	13
Malafosse *et al.*	1989	6	NS	—	—	7*	14
Murray *et al.*	1991	21	0	—	—	0	NS
Sjodahl *et al.*	1992	18	1	—	—	6	19
Slors *et al.*	1989	14	1	—	—	7	NS
Wilson and Gollock	1989	18	2	—	—	11	NS
Yu	1989	24	1	—	—	4	NS

NS = not stated.
Hospital stay (median or mean) are for all stages combined unless otherwise stated.
*Mortality of entire series.
**Hospital stay of primary resection only.
***Includes operations on right and left colon.
****All Hartmann's procedures, not just for colon cancer. 80 had re-anastomosis with mortality of 8% and 4% for primary resection and re-anastomosis, respectively.
After Deans *et al.*, Br. J. Surg. 1994; 81: 1270–6.

can significantly prolong operating time (Radcliffe and Dudley 1983; Munro *et al.* 1995) (Figure 12.9). However, the importance of mechanical bowel preparation may be overstated, some reporting excellent results (one clinical leak and seven wound infections in 100 cases) from primary anastomosis without lavage (Duthie *et al.* 1990).

Operative mortality of primary anastomosis using on-table lavage is generally about 10% which compares favourably with that of the three-stage and Hartmann's procedures (Deans *et al.* 1994) (Table 12.2). Morbidity, principally anastomotic leakage (4%), and wound infection (25–60%) is also similar to that of other procedures but overall hospital stay (about 20 days) is considerably less (Ambrosetti *et al.* 1989; Deans *et al.* 1994). Crude 5-year survival is acceptable (40%), being greater than staged procedures but generally less than in those presenting without malignant obstruction (Sjodahl *et al.* 1992; Mulcahy *et al.* 1996). However, these good results may reflect primary anastomosis having been performed in a selected subset of low-risk patients.

Alternatively, all of the obstructed colon proximal to the tumour can be resected (subtotal colectomy) and a primary ileocolic anastomosis performed. This procedure relieves obstruction, resects the tumour, and restores continuity in a single stage while removing the grossly dilatated colon, traditionally considered a contraindication to primary anastomosis. In addition, synchronous tumours are removed and the risk of metachronous tumours greatly reduced.

Initial reports stressed the technical demands of this operation, but with care, good results can be obtained (Dorudi *et al.* 1990). Most studies, although reporting small numbers of cases, record an operative mortality of 3–11%, similar to that of other procedures (Deans *et al.* 1994). Morbidity is low (10%), anastomotic leakage occurring in 4% of cases with hospital stay generally 15–20 days (Stephenson *et al.* 1990; Deans *et al.* 1994). Subtotal colectomy carries a 20% risk of diarrhoea and/or faecal incontinence, particularly in elderly patients, but in time most patients pass two to three motions per day (Halevy *et al.* 1989; Stephenson *et al.* 1990; Papa *et al.* 1997).

Both methods of resection and primary anastomosis are therefore associated with similar morbidity and mortality, but with a shorter hospital stay and better 5-year survival than staged operations. However, avoidance of a stoma must be weighed against the risk of anastomotic leakage and the availability of a surgeon capable of undertaking a major colonic operation. The outcome of operations on obstructed colon lesions is not only related to the choice of operation but also surgical experience, the adequacy of assistance and out of hours operating (Chester and Britton 1989; Fielding *et al.* 1989). The low risk of

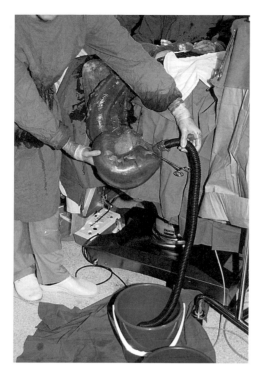

Figure 12.9 On-table lavage for obstructed sigmoid carcinoma. Note the splenic flexure has been fully mobilized to allow free flow of the irrigation fluid around the colon.

staged procedures in the hands of less experienced or specialized surgeons should be commended in the interests of minimizing the mortality rate at the expense of a greater hospital stay (Reinbach *et al.* 1994).

Non-operative treatments

In selected patients with obstructed left colon cancer non-operative treatment may be preferred to allow correction of medical problems. Deflation of the obstructed colon may be achieved with the introduction of a rectosigmoid stent using a flexible sigmoidoscope (Keen and Orsay 1992; Saida *et al.* 1996). Hydrostatic balloon dilatation is claimed to relieve two-thirds of obstructed malignant strictures after a single dilatation (Aston *et al.* 1989). It is suggested that endoscopic Nd–YAG laser recanalization is possible in over 80% of colon tumours after an average of three treatments, with low (2–5%) procedure-related morbidity and mortality (Loizou *et al.* 1990). In potentially resectable patients, it is claimed that this expensive technology permits preparation for surgery. The hospital stay and complication rates, however, are little different from immediate surgery and it is difficult to see any advantage from their routine use. In non-resectable cases, or where the prognosis is poor, they may obviate the need for general anaesthesia, improve symptoms, control haemorrhage, allow concomitant adjuvant therapy, and are therefore worth consideration.

Rectal tumours

The extent of tumour involvement is an important determinant of the metastatic potential of rectal cancer. Two-thirds of patients with tumours involving more than half the rectal circumference die from carcinoma compared with 10% when less than half the lumen is involved (Murray and Stahl 1993). Widespread metastatic spread is relatively rare, pulmonary, bony, or cerebral metastases occurring in

less than 10% of all cases (Cummings 1993; Murray and Stahl 1993; Farnell *et al.* 1996).

Tumours of the upper third of the rectum (9–13 cm) are best treated by anterior resection, while those of the lower third (less than 4 cm from the dentate line) require abdominoperineal resection. Treatment of middle third lesions (4–9 cm) may be by either of these procedures, depending on the size of the pelvis, and the build, age, and fitness of the patient (Heald and Karanjia 1993). Rectal cancers are rarely associated with distal intramural spread, so that the palpable and pathological lower border of the tumour are usually identical. Consequently a 2 cm clearance from the tumour on the distal margin is sufficient (Williams *et al.* 1983; Fengler and Pearl 1994; Morikawa *et al.* 1994). Total mesorectal excision is claimed to allow a 1 cm resection margin, thus reducing the incidence of abdominoperineal resection to 10% of all rectal cancers, without increasing local recurrence rates (3%) (Karanjia *et al.* 1990; Volpe *et al.* 1996). This technique employs sharp dissection of the avascular plane between visceral and somatic structures in the belief that tearing into tumour planes may compromise cancer clearance (Karanjia *et al.* 1994) (Figure 12.10). However, the high incidence of Dukes' A and B lesions may partly account for the low recurrence rate in some reports of mesorectal excision (Staniunas and Schoetz 1993), and the technique is questioned in upper third rectal tumours (Hainsworth *et al.* 1997).

In the event of failure of the stapling gun, a coloanal anastomosis may be performed per anum. A colonic 'J' pouch may reduce stool frequency, improve function, and fill in the emptied pelvis. The 'J' should not exceed 2 × 8 cm (Heald and Karanjia 1993). Anterior resection with extended pelvic lymphadenectomy appears to offer little improvement in local recurrence over total mesorectal excision, while increasing the risk of urinary (40% versus 10%) or sexual problems (75% versus 37%) (Hojo *et al.* 1989; Heald and Karanjia 1993). Some feel that total pelvic clearance procedures still have a place in selected patients with advanced rectal cancer as (despite major morbidity in up

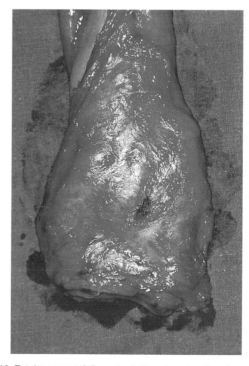

Figure 12.10 Total mesorectal dissection in the avascular plane in a specimen removed by low anterior resection. The glistening areolar tissue confirms the mesorectal plane has not been breached.

to 40% of cases) 5-year survival can be 35%, compared with a median survival of 10 months in those undergoing palliative procedures (Staniunas and Schoetz 1993; Volpe *et al.* 1996).

Local excision

Local excision of rectal lesions may be considered for early-stage rectal cancers that are too low to allow restorative resection or when age, infirmity, or presence of metastases precludes major resection (Minsky 1996) (Table 12.3). The tumour should preferably be mobile, small (<3 cm) and in the lower third of the rectum. It should not be poorly differentiated, as this indicates a high risk of developing lymph node metastases. The latter may be assessed using endorectal ultrasound (Minsky 1996). The procedure requires full-thickness excision of the rectal wall while allowing a 1–2 cm margin. A transanal approach is associated with a lower incidence of rectal fistula than the trans-sacral or transphincteric approaches (Heald and Karanjia 1993; Murray and Stahl 1993). Excision is successful in 70% of cases, 15% subsequently requiring a salvage abdominoperineal resection, resulting in an overall 5-year survival of 70% and cancer-specific 5-year survival of 90% (Murray and Stahl 1993; Saclardes 1997). The risk of local recurrence and cancer-specific death increase with depth of invasion (submucosa 5% and 1%, respectively; muscularis propria 18% and 8%, respectively; perirectal fat 22% and 20%, respectively) as well as with poorly differentiated tumours (Graham *et al.* 1990; Murray and Stahl 1993). In cases where there is doubt about relying solely on local excision, adjuvant radiotherapy may be used (Table 12.4). Transanal endoscopic microsurgery is a minimally invasive technique for local excision of tumours in the rectum and lower sigmoid colon (Brett and Hershman 1994; Frazee *et al.* 1995; Banerjee *et al.* 1996). It allows precise transanal dissection and suturing, and enables sphincter preserving local resection to be performed without an abdominal or perineal incision (Khanduja 1995; Petros *et al.* 1996; Thoresen *et al.* 1996). Long-term surveillance is required in all cases employing local excision. Monoclonal antibody therapy may reduce recuperance (Mentges *et al.* 1996).

Table 12.3 Surgical options for local excision of lesions of the rectum

Site	< 2 cm	2–3 cm Clinically benign	2–3 cm Clinically suspicious	>3 cm
Lower third	Endoscopic polypectomy	Per-anal submucous excision	Per-anal disc excision	Per-anal disc excision
Middle third				
Below 10 cm	Endoscopic polypectomy	Per-anal submucous excision	Per-anal disc excision or trans-anal microsurgery	Trans-sphincteric excision (Mason) or trans-anal microsurgery
Above 10 cm	Endoscopic polypectomy	Trans-sphincteric excision (Mason) or trans-anal microsurgery	Trans-anal microsurgery	Trans-anal microsurgery
Upper third	Endoscopic polypectomy	Abdominal submucous excision	Radical resection	Radical resection

Table 12.4 Outcome of local excision (LE) and irradiation (R) for colorectal cancer

Source	Treatment	Local control	Follow-up (median months)
Willet *et al.* 1989	LE; postoperative R 45 Gy/5 weeks ± boost	22/26	24
Rich *et al.* 1985	LE; postoperative R 40–60 Gy ± boost	16/17	18
McCready *et al.* 1989	Post parasacral approach; postoperative R 53 Gy/5 weeks	19/19	13
Otmezguine *et al.* 1989	Pre-operative R 35 Gy/3 weeks; LE; postoperative R 20 Gy	20/25	40
Marks *et al.* 1990	Pre-operative R 45 Gy/5 weeks; LE	11/14	31
Steele *et al.* 1991	LE; postoperative R 51 Gy/5 weeks with concurrent 5 FU	9/9	21
Bailey *et al.* 1992	LE, half received postop R 45-50 Gy	49/53	44 5-yr survival 74%
Coco *et al.* 1992	LE,. postop R 47 Gy if T2	33/36	68 5-yr survival 74%
Ota *et al.* 1992	LE, postop R 53 Gy, chemotherapy (5-FU) for T2 or T3	43/46	36 3-yr survival 93%
Rosenthal *et al.* 1992	Pre-operative R 5 Gy/1 day; LE; postoperative R 50.4 Gy/5 week	14/15	33 3-yr survival 94%
Rouanet *et al.* 1993	LE, postop R 37 Gy	16/18	61 5-yr survival 100%
Graham *et al.* 1994	LE, postop R 45 Gy, chemotherapy (5-FU/L)	18/18	18
Minsky *et al.* 1994	LE, postop R 53 Gy, chemotherapy (5-FU)	18/22	37 4-yr survival 79%
Bannon *et al.* 1995	Preop R (40-45 Gy), LE	38/44	40 5-yr survival 90%
Bleday *et al.* 1997	LE, postop R 54 Gy, chemotherapy (5-FU)	44/48	40.5

After: Cummings BJ. Radiation therapy for colorectal cancer. *Surg. Clin. North Am.* 1993; 73: 167–81, and Breen E, Bleday R. Preservation of the anus in the therapy of distal rectal cancers. *Surg. Clin. North Am.* 1997; 77: 71–83.

Electrocoagulation

This is successful either as curative or palliative treatment in tumours up to 8 cm diameter even if they involve the entire rectal circumference (Faivre *et al.* 1996). Postoperative mortality is 2%, complications (mainly delayed bleeding (10%) and stricture (5%)) occur in one-quarter of cases, and the mean number of treatments per patient is 3.5 (Murray and Stahl 1993). In those treated with curative intent, 60% do not develop metastatic or recurrent disease and 5-year survival is 70% (Murray and Stahl 1993). Survival is best in patients with papillary tumours under 3 cm diameter. Patients unfit for abdominoperineal resection who are treated by palliative electrocoagulation may have a 5-year survival up to 35%. The addition of adjuvant radiotherapy to electrocoagulation or local excision has not shown any significant increase in patient survival (Murray and Stahl 1993).

Radiotherapy

Radiation acts at a cellular level, highly charged electrons and free radicals interacting directly with DNA. This effectively kills tumour cells, but also causes a dose-dependent delay in wound and anastomotic healing due to tissue hypoxia and microvascular damage. In patients with radiation enteritis, anastomotic dehiscence rates of 50% are reported (Hatcher *et al.* 1984). The most severe retardation of healing occurs if radiation is given a few days before or after operation. Radiation given 2–3 weeks pre- or postoperatively lessens the detrimental effects on wound healing. There is no conclusive evidence that pre-operative radiotherapy increases surgical morbidity, provided a meticulous surgical technique is used (Fleshman and Myerson 1997).

Radiotherapy alone

Because of limited tissue tolerance for high-dose radiation exposure, external-beam irradiation has not proved effective for the curative treatment of carcinoma of the rectum. If curative radiotherapy is required, intracavitary radiation therapy is therefore preferable, similar selection criteria being employed as for local excision surgery (i.e. mobile T1/T2 tumours <3 cm diameter), with the addition that the lesion should be within 9 cm from the anal verge to provide access for the iridium implants (Table 12.5). Without anaesthesia, a modified sigmoidoscope is used to place a radiation probe in contact with the tumour to provide a total dose of about 100 Gy over a 4–6 week period (Papillon 1984). Ulcerated tumours may also require the introduction of radioactive needles into the rectal wall without risk of serious damage to adjacent structures or late radiation proctitis (Papillon 1984; Cummings 1993). The local failure rate is 10% and many of those in whom recurrence appears can be salvaged by surgery. Normal anal function is maintained in 95% of patients, disease-free survival being 75%, local recurrence 25%, and cancer-specific 5-year survival over 90% (Papillon 1984). Although non-randomized studies of pre-operative irradiation suggest that the number of regional lymph node metastases and pelvic recurrence are reduced when used as an adjuvant to conventional surgery, there is no definite evidence that radiation can eradicate unresected lymph node metastases (Cummings 1993). Some therefore consider that combining radiotherapy with local excision may result in little benefit, although this may be improved with the addition of chemotherapy.

Adjuvant radiotherapy

Pre-operative radiotherapy

For colonic tumours, radiotherapy alone is not as effective as surgery in those who would normally be treated by major colonic resection and surgeon-related variation is the most important determinant of outcome (Aleman *et al.* 1995; Holm *et al.* 1997). Two uncontrolled trials of adjuvant radiotherapy for Dukes' B and C tumours showed a slight improvement in survival, but the evidence supporting adding radiotherapy to surgery for colon cancer is sparse (Douglass 1991). Adjuvant radiotherapy for colon cancer is therefore normally reserved for those unfit for, or who refuse, surgical treatment. In such circumstances, about one-third of mobile or partially fixed tumours can respond to doses of 50 Gy in 20 fractions over 4 weeks (Cummings 1993).

Despite apparently curative resection, up to one-third of patients with rectal carcinoma develop pelvic recurrence after a median of 12 months. For rectal cancer pre-operative radiotherapy has theoretical advantages of increased radiosensitivity of tumour cells that are well oxygenated, a low incidence of small bowel enteritis and reduction in the shedding of tumour cells when the tumour is manipulated during surgery (Aleman *et al.* 1995). The problem with pre-operative radiotherapy is that patients with Dukes' A lesions do not require adjuvant therapy because of their high cure rate by surgery alone whereas patients with metastases outside the radiation field (Dukes' D) are not benefited because the distant disease usually becomes life-threatening before pelvic recurrences appear. Consequently, evidence supporting pre-operative radiotherapy in rectal carcinoma is inconclusive (Table 12.6).

Early trials of single low-dose pre-operative radiotherapy failed to detect any improvement in survival in those receiving adjuvant therapy. In the original Veterans Administration Surgical Adjuvant Group (VASAG) trial, 700 patients were randomized to surgery alone or low-dose (25 Gy) pre-operative irradiation, including a perineal boost for patients with low-lying tumours (Higgins *et al.* 1976). Five-year survival of the surgical group was 28% compared with 41% in those receiving adjuvant radiotherapy, radiation also reducing the number of involved lymph glands in the resected specimen and subsequent pelvic recurrence. A second Veterans Administration trial of pre-operative intermediate dose (31.5 Gy) radiotherapy with surgery alone in patients undergoing abdominoperineal resection failed to

Table 12.5 Outcome of intrarectal irradiation used as sole treatment for cure of rectal cancer

Source	No. patients	Local recurrence (%)	Cancer deaths (%)	5-year survival (%)
Papillon 1990	158 polypoid	4	10	73 crude
	49 ulcerated	10	12	69 crude
Lavery *et al.* 1987	62	18	10	—
Sischy *et al.* 1988	192	5	2	—
Roth *et al.* 1988	72	22	13	66

After: Cummings BJ. Radiation therapy for colorectal cancer. *Surg. Clin. North Am.* 1993; 73: 167–81.

Table 12.6 Trials of pre-operative and postoperative adjuvant radiotherapy for rectal cancer

Source	No. patients	Radiation dose (Gy/fraction/ days) Surg. alone (%)	5-year survival; (%)	5-year Radio + Surg Surg. alone (%)	Local recurrence Radio + Surg (%)	Local recurrence Surg. alone (%)	Extrapelvic recurrence Radio + Surg (%)	Extrapelvic recurrence (%)
Pre-operative								
MRC (1984)	850	5/1/1	47	50	43	45	50	48
		20/10/14	46	—	47	—	49	—
VASOG II (Higgins *et al.*, 1986)	314	31.5/18/24	50	50	NS	NS	NS	NS
Dahl *et al.* 1990	259	31.5/18/24	64	61	21	14	16	17
EORTC (Gerard *et al.* 1988)	341	34.5/15/19	59	69	35 (p < 0.05)	15 (p < 0.05)	22	23
Stockholm Rectal Cancer Group (1990)	679	25/5/7	50	55	25 (p < 0.05)	11 (p < 0.05)	23	17
Stockholm Rectal Cancer Group (1996)	557	25/5/7	50 (*P* < 0.02)	55 (*P* < 0.02)	21 (*P* < 0.01)	10 (*P* < 0.01)	19 (*P* < 0.02)	26 (*P* < 0.02)
Swedish Rectal Cancer Trial 1997	1168	25/5/7	58 (*P* < 0.004)	48 (*P* < 0.004)	11 (*P* < 0.001)	27 (*P* < 0.001)	NS	NS
Postoperative								
GITSG (1985)	108	45/24/35	43	52	24	20	34	30
NSABP (Fisher *et al.* 1988)	368	50/28/36	43	40	25	16	26	31
Denmark (Balslev *et al.* 1986)	494	50/25/49	No difference	No difference	18	16	24	26
Netherlands (Treurniet- Donker *et al.* 1991)	174	50/25/35	55	45	33	24	27	39
EORTC (Arnaud *et al.* 1997)	172	46/25/38	No difference	No difference	No difference	No difference	No difference	No difference

show any significant difference in either survival or lymph node metastases in those receiving adjuvant radiotherapy (Higgins *et al.* 1986). The European (EORTC) and Stockholm trials both confirm the absence of a survival advantage from pre-operative radiotherapy, but suggest a reduction in pelvic recurrence (Gerard *et al.* 1988; Stockholm Rectal Cancer Study Group 1990). In the EORTC trial those who did develop recurrence had a longer period before these recurrences became apparent ('prolonged disease-free interval').

In patients with fixed or inoperable tumours, high-dose, pre-operative radiotherapy is claimed to render up to 80% of these tumours operable, with the tumour becoming pathologically un-detectable in 5% (Marks *et al.* 1990). There appears to be no adverse effect on subsequent surgery or anastomotic healing, although local recurrence rates may be high (up to 50%)(Cummings 1993).

Postoperative radiotherapy

In contrast to pre-operative radiotherapy, postoperative radiotherapy results in significant morbidity from small bowel irradiation, requires prolonged treatment (4–5 weeks) and may need to be delayed by surgical complications. However, it has the advantage that, because the pathology is known, it may be restricted to those with more advanced tumours. There are three trials of postoperative radiotherapy (5000

rads in 4–5 weeks) in Dukes' B and C patients (Table 12.6) The Gastrointestinal Tumor Study Group (GITSG) trial (1985) was prematurely terminated when preliminary analysis suggested a survival advantage from adjuvant therapy, although this was not confirmed on more detailed analysis. In the Danish study (Balslev *et al.* 1986) there was also no significant improvement in overall survival, although local recurrence was reduced for Dukes' C patients only. The NSABP study revealed no difference in survival but a 10% reduction in local recurrence in those receiving radiotherapy (Fisher *et al.* 1988). A meta-analysis of the randomized trials of pre-and postoperative radiotherapy suggested that radiotherapy might reduce the odds of death by 10%, corresponding to an improvement in 5-year survival of only 2%, the improvement in survival being better (4%) for those undergoing curative resection (Buyse *et al.* 1988).

Adjuvant radiotherapy, given pre-operatively or postoperatively, therefore reduces the risk of pelvic recurrence but without influencing survival rates or the risk of extrapelvic metastases (Cummings 1993; Arnaud *et al.* 1997). This is partly related to differences in dose schedules among trials, most series using moderately low doses of radiation. With such doses, neither the postoperative anastomotic leakage rate nor the incidence of late small bowel enteritis is increased (Cummings 1993).

Table 12.7 Randomized trials of adjuvant chemotherapy for colon cancer

Source	Regimen	No. patients	Statistically significant benefit from chemotherapy
GITSG (1984)	5-FU/semustine versus BCG versus 5-FU/semustine/BCG versus no treatment	621	None
SWOG (Panettiere et al. 1988)	5-FU/semustine versus 5-FU/semustine/BCG versus no treatment	309/317	None
VASAG (Higgins et al. 1984)	5-FU daily X 5, and again at 6 weeks versus no treatment	338	Overall survival
COG (Grage and Moss 1981)	5-FU for 1 year versus no treatment	223	Disease free survival
NSABP (Wolmark et al. 1988)	Semustine/vincristine/5-FU versus BCG versus no treatment	1166	Overall survival
Windle et al. 1987	Levamisole/5-FU for 1 year versus 5-FU versus no treatment	141	Overall survival (levamisole/5-FU)
NCCTG (Laurie et al. 1989)	Levamisole/5-FU for 1 year versus levamisole alone versus no treatment	401	Overall survival (Dukes' C only) (levamisole/5-FU)
Intergroup (Moertel et al. 1990)	Levamisole/5-FU for 1 year versus no treatment	1296	Overall survival
Taylor et al. (1985)	Postoperative 5-FU portal vein infusion X 7 days versus no treatment	244	Overall survival
IMPACT (1995)	Postoperative 5-FU + folinic acid versus surgery alone for 6 months	1526 Dukes B+C	Overall survival Recurrence
NSABP (Wolmark et al. 1990)	Postoperative 5-FU portal vein infusion X 7 days versus no treatment	1158	Overall survival
SAKK 1996	Postoperative portal mitomycin C + 5-FU vs surgery alone	533	Overall survival Recurrence
CCCSGJ (1995)	Postoperative mitomycin C +/- 5-FU for 6 months versus surgery alone	1805	Colon cancer: Dukes' C only Rectal cancer: Overall survival
Moertel et al. 1995	Levamisole +/- 5-FU for 48 weeks	929 Dukes'C	Overall survival
Hellenic Oncology Group (Kosmidis et al. 1996)	5-FU and levamisole +/- alpha interferon	106 Dukes C	Interferon no benefit
Recchia et al. 1996	5-FU and levamisole +/- alpha interferon (low dose)	100 Dukes'C	Interferon no benefit
MRC (Seymour et al. 1996)	5-FU and levamisole +/- alpha interferon	260 Dukes'C	Interferon no benefit
Advanced disease			
Kohne et al. 1997	5-FU + levamisole +/– interferon	77	Interferon no benefit
Cunningham et al. 1995	Tomudex vs 5-FU and levamisole	439 Dukes D	Tomudex fewer side effects and better response rates
Zaleberg et al. 1996	Tomudex vs no treatment of liver metastases	117 Dukes D	Tomudex response rate 26%
Rougier et al. 1997	Irinotecan +/– 5-FU	213 Dukes C + D	Irinotecan effective if resistant to 5-FU

Table 12.8 Randomized trials of adjuvant chemotherapy for rectal cancer

Source	Regimen	No. patients	Statistically significant benefit from chemotherapy
GITSG (1985)	Semustine/5-FU versus radiotherapy versus semustine/5-FU	227	Overall survival benefit for combined versus no treatment
NSABP (Fisher et al. 1988)	Semustine/vincristine/5-FU versus radiotherapy versus no treatment	555	Overall survival benefit for chemotherapy versus no treatment
NCCTG (Krook et al. 1991)	Semustine/5-FU/radiotherapy versus radiotherapy	204	Overall survival benefit for combined treatment

Chemotherapy

Intravenous boluses of 5-fluorouracil (5-FU) or floxuridine (FUDR) give response rates of up to 20% resulting in symptomatic improve-ment (Levithan 1993; Bleiberg 1996; Diaz-Canton and Pazdur 1997). Response rates can be increased to 30% by continuous infu-sion regimens, but this requires hospital admission (Levithan 1993; Sobrero et al. 1997). The side-effects of 5 FU (fatigue, mild nausea, diarrhoea, mucositis, or myelosuppression) are usually well tolerated (Steele 1995). There is no evidence that single-agent treatment with these drugs prolong survival so that treatment is normally delayed until patients are symptomatic (Levithan 1993; Bleiberg 1996). The potency of 5-FU can be enhanced by the administration of reduced folates (leucovorin) (Sinicrope and Sugarman 1995; Erlichman *et al.* 1996). Randomized trials show that the addition of leucovorin to 5-FU increases response rates from 10% to 48% and median survival from 9.6 to 26 months (Doroshow *et al.* 1990; Kemeny *et al.* 1990; Erlichman *et al.* 1996). The side-effects are similar, although often more severe, than with 5-FU alone and may delay treatment or require hospitalization (Sobrero *et al.* 1997).

The combination of 5-FU with alpha-interferon is claimed to give a 75% response rate, but side-effects are sufficiently common that it is generally used as second- or third-line treatment in those with symptomatic metastatic disease (Wadler *et al.* 1989; Seymour *et al.* 1996). The combination of 5-FU with other agents, such as methyl-CCNU, vincristine, streptozocin, or cis-platinum, results in only slightly better response rate than those of 5-FU alone, at the expense of greatly increased toxicity (Levithan 1993; Rustum *et al.* 1997).

Several trials of adjuvant chemotherapy in addition to surgery for colorectal cancer have been performed and produced contradictory results due to differences in study design (Tables 12.7 and 12.8) (Steele 1995). The Gastrointestinal Tumor Study Group (GITSG) trial of Dukes' B and C colonic cancers revealed no significant difference in disease-free or overall survival between controls, chemotherapy with 5-FU and methyl-CCNU, immunostimulation with BCG or a combination of immuno- and chemotherapy, but leukaemia developed in seven patients receiving chemotherapy (GITSG 1984). In rectal cancer, however, patients who received radiotherapy and chemotherapy had lower recurrence rates and a trend to better survival than the surgery only group, although non-haematological side-effects occurred in 35% (GITSG 1985). In the first Veterans Administration study (VASOG) an improvement in survival was only apparent in Dukes' C patients receiving 5-FU and methyl-CCNU (Higgins *et al.* 1984). In the second study there was no survival advantage from 5-FU, methyl-CCNU, and immunotherapy in those with incomplete resection. In contrast, the NSABP studies have shown significant reductions in mortality in the chemotherapy-treated groups, but at the cost of substantial toxicity (Fisher *et al.* 1988; Wolmark *et al.* 1988). A pooled analysis of three multicentre trials in Dukes' B and C tumours revealed that fluorouracil with folinic acid significantly reduced mortality by 22% and recurrence by 35%, increasing 3-year disease-free survival

from 62% to 71% and overall survival from 78% to 83% (IMPACT 1995). Compliance with treatment was good; more than 80% of patients completed the planned treatment with severe toxic effects occurring in fewer than 3% of cases. Very similar results were obtained for Dukes' C lesions in the trial by Moertel *et al.* (1995). The Japanese experience suggests that survival in rectal cancer and in Duke's C colon cancer is improved by the addition of 5-FU and mitomycin C (CCCSGJ 1995). For patients refractory to flurouraine, irinotecan or tomudex can prove effective second line treatment (Diaz-Canton and Pazdur 1997). Although more studies are required, the evidence suggests that patients with Duke's C tumours, and possibly some with Duke's B lesions, benefit from adjuvant chemotherapy. A summary of trials combining adjuvant radio- and chemotherapy is shown in Table 12.9.

Hepatic artery and portal vein perfusion

Normal hepatocytes derive 75% of their blood supply from the portal vein, whereas liver metastases obtain 90% of their blood from the hepatic artery. This differential blood supply has been utilized in trials of regional chemotherapy for metastatic disease (Laffer and Metzger 1995; Vautley *et al.* 1996a). Catheters inserted into the hepatic artery are associated with response rates of 60%, although there is no definite improvement in survival (Chang *et al.* 1987) liver infusion group 1997. However, the Swiss experience suggests that at a median follow up of 8 years, adjuvant therapy reduced the risk of recurrence by 20% and the risk of death by 25% (SAKK 1995). Problems include the anatomical variation of the hepatic artery, catheter displacement, chemical hepatitis, or acalculous cholecystitis as well as gastroduodenal ulcers if the vessels supplying the stomach and duodenum are not ligated (Levithan 1993; Penna and Nordlinger 1996). In up to one-half of cases the pump becomes dislodged or minor local complications such as thrombosis occur (Tuchmann *et al.* 1990). Toxic effects could be managed by reducing the dose. Response rates of over 40% are recorded with mean survival time of about 12 months and mean interval until relapse of 10 months (Tuchmann *et al.* 1990; Cohen *et al.* 1996)).

Taylor *et al.* (1985) randomized 244 patients undergoing 'curative' resection to no further treatment or a continuous infusion of 5-FU through the portal vein for 1 week. The perfusion group had fewer

Table 12.9 Summary of trials of adjuvant radio- and chemotherapy for the treatment of rectal cancer

Source	No. patients	Radiation dose (Gy/fraction/ days)	5 year survival R + S	5 year survival S + R + C	Local recurrence S + R	Local recurrence S + R + C	Extrapelvic recurrence S + R	Extrapelvic recurrence S + R + C
Pre-operative								
EORTC (Gerard *et al.* 1988) (Dukes' A–C)	247	34.5/15/19 + 5FU	59	46	15	15	No difference	No difference
Postoperative								
GITSG (1985)	202	45/25/35	52	59 (*P* < 0.05)	20	11	30	26
ECOG (Mansour *et al.* 1991)	237	47/27/37	46	50	NS	NS	NS	NS
NCCTG (Krook *et al.* 1991)	204	50/28/38	47	58 (*P* < 0.05)	25	14 (*P* < 0.05)	46	29 (*P* < 0.05)

S, surgery; R, radiotherapy; C, chemotherapy.
After: Cummings BJ. Radiation therapy for colorectal cancer. *Surg. Clin. North Am.* 1993; 73: 167–81.

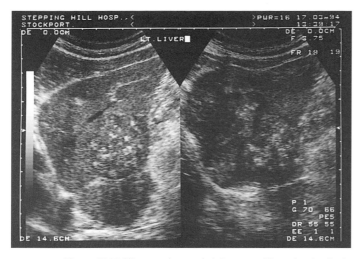
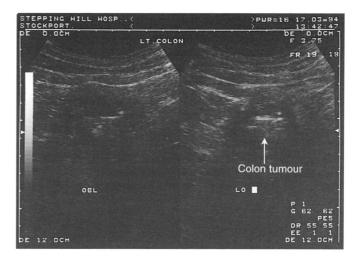

Figure 12.11 Ultrasound scan of abdomen and liver, showing the 'pseudo-kidney' appearance of a colonic neoplasm, with liver metastases.

deaths (26 versus 54) and liver metastases (five versus 22), although the benefit was limited to those with Dukes' B tumours. However, the overall advantage of 5-FU delivered via the portal vein remains to be determined (Levithan 1993; Penna and Nordlinger 1996).

Hepatic metastases

Despite apparently curative resection for colorectal cancer 40% of patients die within 5 years and 80% of these die within 3 years from predominantly liver metastases (Fong *et al.* 1996; Taylor 1996). At the time of initial surgery for colorectal cancer 15% of patients will have obvious liver involvement and intra-operative ultrasound will detect occult metastases in a further 10% (McMaster *et al.* 1989) (Figure 12.11). This may be an underestimate as autopsy studies reveal that two-thirds of patients who die of colorectal cancer have hepatic involvement (Asbun and Hughes 1993). The majority of metastases develop within 2–3 years of the original colonic resection. Metastatic liver disease is the primary determinant of patient survival in colorectal carcinoma. The median survival from the time of diagnosis of metastatic liver disease is 4–12 months for unselected groups, whereas 45% of patients with a solitary metastatic lesion may be alive at 2 years and 12% alive at 3 years (Ashbun and Hughes 1993; Burke and Allen-Mersh 1996). In the absence of resection 5-year survival is rare (Blumgart and Fong 1995).

Survival in those with liver metastases and no treatment depends on the tumour load in the liver resulting in 1-year survival varying from 15% to 40% (McMaster *et al.* 1989; Adloff *et al.* 1990) (Figure 12.12). Median survival is 17 months in those with under 25% of the liver replaced compared with 3 months if over 75% of the liver is replaced or there are more than four metastases (McMaster *et al.* 1989). The stage of the original tumour is also important—5-year survival following hepatic resection for those originally thought to have Dukes' B tumours is 50% compared with 20% for Dukes' C lesions (McMaster *et al.* 1989). In a study using multivariate analysis, the presence of satellite metastases, primary tumour grade, the time of metastasis diagnosis, diameter of the largest metastasis, anatomic versus non-anatomical approach, year of resection, and mesenteric lymph node involvement each independently affected both crude and tumour-free survival (Scheele *et al.* 1995). Computerized tomography (CT) portograms

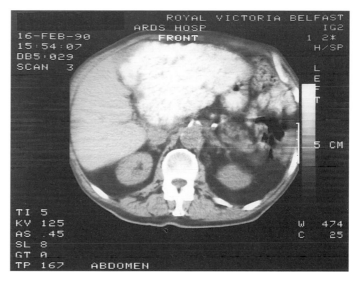

Figure 12.12 CT scan showing extensive liver replacement by a calcified mucinous metastasis.

are claimed to be only second to intra-operative ultrasound at detecting occult liver metastases with an accuracy of over 90% (Figure 12.13). Dynamic hepatic scintigraphy enhances the diagnostic accuracy of isotope liver scans above the standard 80% by providing an hepatic perfusion index (McArdle 1989).

Only a small subset of patients with metastatic colorectal cancer will benefit from hepatic resection or cryotherapy (Adam *et al.* 1997a; Korpan 1997). In the GITSG study, only 46% of those considered to have potentially resectable lesions on pre-operative investigations underwent curative resection (Steele *et al.* 1991). Overall 30-day mortality was 3% and morbidity 15% (20% for hepatic resection, 5% for second look laparotomy) (Adloff *et al.* 1990). As there is no survival advantage in performing liver resection at the same time as the initial colonic resection, many authors prefer delaying resection for 2–3 months except in the presence of a solitary, easily resectable metastasis. The only absolute contraindication to hepatic resection is the inability to obtain a cure because of involvement of lymph nodes or an inadequate hepatic resection margin (Figure 12.14). After liver resection, recurrent liver metastases occur in 60% of patients, usually representing occult disease undetected at the time of the original hepatic resection. The principal poor prognostic factors related to hepatic resection are a short disease-free interval between resection

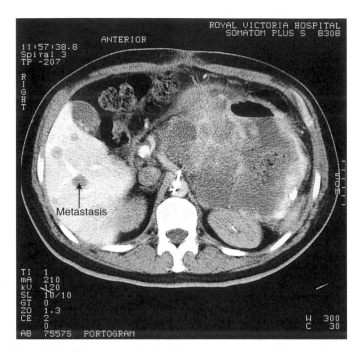

Figure 12.13 CT portogram showing a huge colonic primary with multiple liver metastases (arrowed).

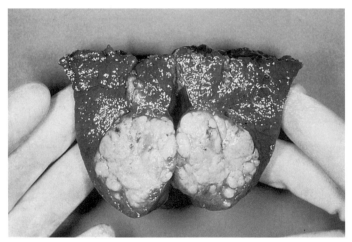

Figure 12.14 Liver resection showing margins well clear of tumour.

of colonic and hepatic tumours, multiple liver metastases, advanced Dukes' stage, tumour within 1 cm of the resection margin, and involvement of hepatic or coeliac lymph nodes (Asbun and Hughes 1993). The overall cumulative survival rates were 82%, 63%, and 32% at 1, 2, and 3 years, respectively. The significant factor affecting prognosis was only whether the secondary tumours were encapsulated or not (Morino *et al.* 1991). Chemotherapy appears to offer little reduction in the recurrence rate following hepatic resection (Bismuth *et al.* 1996). Repeated liver resections can be accomplished with a low morbidity and operative mortality under 10% (Asbun and Hughes 1993; Neeleman and Andersson 1996; Wanebo *et al.* 1996; Adam *et al.* 1997*b*). Median survival after second liver resection is 18 months with a long-term disease-free survival of 35% in selected patients.

Metastases to other sites

Pulmonary metastases occur in 10% of patients with colorectal carcinoma, usually in association with metastases to other organs (Figures 12.15 and 12.16). Long-term survival is exceptional without surgical treatment (Girard *et al.* 1996). Pulmonary resection should be considered in the 10% of patients with solitary lung metastasis as survival can be 70% at 2 years and 30% at 5 years (Brister *et al.* 1988;

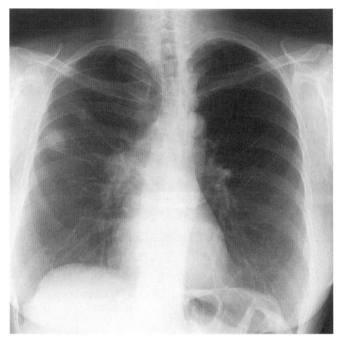

Figure 12.15 Chest X-ray showing lung and hilar secondaries from carcinoma of the caecum.

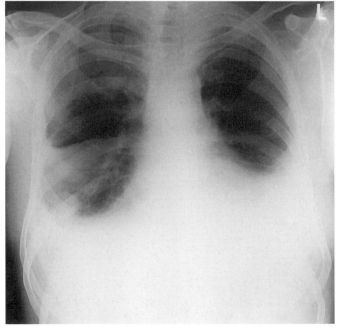

Figure 12.16 Chest X-ray showing pleural secondaries from a colonic primary.

Vigneswaran 1996). The rare patients with cerebral metastases may also obtain palliative relief of neurological symptoms from surgery, while radiotherapy is indicated to relieve the pain of bony metastases (Hammond *et al.* 1996). Penile metastases from retrograde venous or lymphatic invasion are rare and associated with a poor prognosis despite surgical or chemotherapeutic intervention (Asbun and Hughes 1993).

The ovary is the site of metastatic disease in 3–8% of women with colorectal cancer (Nogueras and Jagelman 1993). Oophorectomy at the time of bowel resection will prevent repeat laparotomy to resect an ovarian mass in the 2% of women who develop meta-chronous ovarian deposits. Metachronous ovarian metastases cause considerable morbidity and are associated with poor survival, so that bilateral oophorectomy is suggested even in those with unilateral disease (Asbun and Hughes 1993). Some even recommend pro-phylactic oophorectomy in premenopausal females with advanced disease (peritoneal implants) and in all postmenopausal females (Nogueras and Jagelman 1993). Patients with peritoneal seedlings

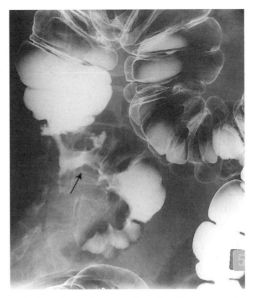

Figure 12.19 Barium enema demonstrating extensive compression of the colon by a secondary hypernephroma of the kidney (arrowed).

rarely do well. However, in highly selected patients Sugarbaker (1995) has advocated a combination of cytoreductive surgery and intraperi-toneal chemotherapy. Selection factors that correlate with long-term benefit of this treatment are: (i) low grade of malignancy; (ii) lack of lymph node or liver metastases; and (iii) treatment of low volume disease. For patients with moderate or high-grade colorectal cancer, only a low volume of disease can be treated successfully. For patients with low-grade cancer, peritonectomy procedures are used to achieve minimal residual disease before initiating the intraperitoneal chemotherapy. In properly selected patients, peritoneal carcinomatosis from colorectal and appendiceal cancer is a treatable condition that may result in long-term disease-free survival (Cintron and Pearl 1996).

The colon or rectum may also be a site of secondary tumour de-posits from primary tumours elsewhere, such as the breast (Figure 12.17), prostate (Figure 12.18), kidney (Figure 12.19), or ovary.

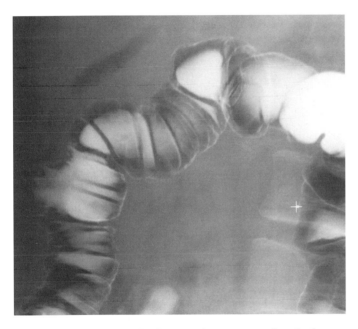

Figure 12.17 Barium enema showing serosal metastases on the colon from a breast primary (arrowed).

Postoperative follow-up

Colonoscopic surveillance after resection for colorectal cancer has been advocated to improve detection of anastomotic recurrence, and of synchronous and metachronous tumours. The benefit provided by colonoscopy remains unproven, and the best timing of examina-tion is unclear (Ohlsson *et al.* 1995; Richert-Boe 1995). Meta-chronous colon cancers arise in 3–6% and polyps in about 10% of those who have undergone resection for colorectal cancer (Patchett *et al.* 1993). The calculated annual incidence for metachronous tumours is 0.3% per year, corresponding to a cumulative incidence at 18 years of 6% (Cali *et al.* 1993). Of patients with colorectal cancer under 40 years of age, 10% will develop a metachronous col-orectal carcinoma which rises to a cumulative risk of 30% after 40 years of follow-up (Bruckstein 1989). Almost half of metachronous lesions occur within 2 years of operation, the interval yield for polyps being 3% per year (Kiefer *et al.* 1986; Iominaga *et al.* 1996). The risk of metachronous cancers is greatest in those who presented initially with synchronous neoplastic lesions. Over half of these patients develop metachronous adenomas compared with 10% of

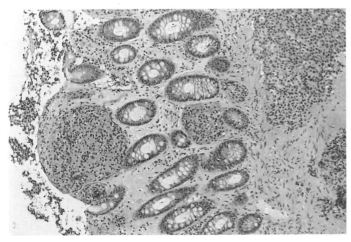

Figure 12.18 Prostatic carcinoma invading the rectum. H&E×100.

those with no polyps initially (Dasmahapatra *et al.* 1989). If the minimum length of the polyp–cancer sequence is 3–5 years, this suggests a failure of traditional pre-operative evaluation (Kiefer *et al.* 1986). The principal benefit of follow-up colonoscopy is in detecting polyps and second carcinomas rather than anastomotic recurrence (Kiefer *et al.* 1986; Patchett *et al.* 1993). Most suture line recurrences occur within 2 years, local or metastatic progression occurring in 15% of patients, despite normal colonoscopic findings (Michael *et al.* 1989). In a study of over 250 follow-up colonoscopies eight anastomotic recurrences were detected, six of which were clinically suspected and only one of which was potentially curative (Aubert *et al.* 1989). In one study regular colonoscopic postoperative surveillance identified intraluminal recurrence without evidence of extraluminal spread in 5% of cases (Patchett *et al.* 1993). Three-quarters of these recurrences were at the site of the anastomosis, the remainder representing metachronous tumour development. All of these patients were symptomatic at the time of diagnosis and the authors suggest that colonoscopic surveillance will rarely allow early detection of asymptomatic intraluminal bowel recurrence (Patchett *et al.* 1993). The limited prognostic value of colonoscopy in detecting recurrence is because suture line recurrence is usually associated with extensive local disease while mucosal recurrence often develops from existing local lymphatic invasion (Ohlsson *et al.* 1995). Against this, some claim that in asymptomatic patients, resection for potential cure can be achieved in up to half of anastomotic recurrences discovered by surveillance. The greatest benefit of colonoscopy is therefore in detecting metachronous lesions as, the cumulative survival rate after operation for a metachronous colorectal carcinoma is 41% after 20 years of observation (Bruckstein 1989).

Only patients who have undergone curative resection should enter colonoscopic surveillance programmes, but the recommended intervals are variable (Sugarbaker 1995). Some claim that a follow-up regimen of clinical examination, liver function tests, carcinoembryonic antigen (CEA), and chest X-ray every 3 monthly for the first 2 years postoperatively and every 6 months thereafter, with colonoscopy or barium enema and proctoscopy every 6 months for the first 2 years postoperatively and every year thereafter is required to detect recurrence (Aubert *et al.* 1989; Bruckstein 1989; Rocklin *et al.* 1990). Some recommend that annual colonoscopy for at least the first 4 years after curative resection will detect both recurrence and metachronous lesions (Kiefer *et al.* 1986; Juhl *et al.* 1990).

Others believe that frequent surveillance is not justified in the early postoperative years and colonoscopy should be confined to a single procedure to exclude synchronous lesions. They suggest that colonoscopic follow-up can be delayed until 2–4 years, earlier follow-up being reserved for patients with numerous polyps or with a polyp which had been removed piecemeal (Bruckstein 1989; Winawer *et al.* 1993). These authors believe that local recurrence which is curable is unlikely to be influenced by more frequent examinations and the area of most common recurrence, the rectum can be seen on rigid sigmoidoscopy. However, rigid sigmoidoscopic surveillance at 1 year adds little to the diagnostic yield of colon cancer screening, adenomas being found in only 1% of patients (Brint *et al.* 1993). However, patients with synchronous tumours, or those who developed colorectal cancer under the age of 40 years, should undergo life-long surveillance (Adloff *et al.* 1989; Bruckstein *et al.* 1989).

Recurrent colorectal cancer

Follow-up studies of patients undergoing potentially curative operations for colorectal cancer reveal a recurrence rate of about 25%

Table 12.10 Comparison of various tests in detecting recurrent colorectal cancer

Test	Comments	
Clinical examination	Sensitivity (overall)	45%
Colonoscopy	Sensitivity (overall)	45%
	Sensitivity (anastomotic recurrence)	90%
CT scan	Sensitivity (overall)	40–85%
	Sensitivity (Liver metastases)	60–90%
	Sensitivity (abdominal excluding liver)	40–70%
	Sensitivity (pelvic recurrence)	25%
	Specificity (overall)	95%
Barium enema	Sensitivity (overall)	55%
	Sensitivity (anastomotic recurrence)	88%
Ultrasound scan	Sensitivity (overall)	60%
Faecal occult bloods	Sensitivity (overall)	25–40%
Tumour markers		
CEA	Sensitivity (overall)	70–90%
	Specificity (overall)	80%
	Predictive value of normal result	90%
	Predictive value of test > 5 ng/ml	80%
CA19-9	Sensitivity (overall)	20–40%
	Specificity (overall)	95%
Radio-immunoscintigraphy	Sensitivity (overall)	70–90%
	Specificity (overall)	90%
	Accuracy (abdomen excluding liver)	65%
	Accuracy (liver)	55%

(Fantini and DeCosse 1990; Juhl *et al.* 1990; Rocklin *et al.* 1990). About one-quarter of these recurrences develop within 1 year, two-thirds within 2 years, 80% within 3 years, and 95% within 4 years of resection (Soreide and Norstein 1997). Immunohistochemical staining suggests that loco-regional recurrences develop from remnant cells of the primary tumour left behind at surgery rather than *de novo* mucosal changes at the anastomosis (Hohenberger *et al.* 1990). Consequently, anastomotic recurrence occurs in only 5% of colorectal cancers within 30 months (Juhl *et al.* 1990). Multivariate analysis reveals risk factors for loco-regional recurrence to be tumour size, perineural and venous invasion, a tumour located less than 10 cm from the anal verge and a patient aged over 70 years (Bentzen *et al.* 1992).

Clinical examination and endoscopy both have an overall sensitivity of 45% for detecting recurrence (Wanebo *et al.* 1989) (Table 12.10). The liver is the most common site of metastases so that CT scanning but not liver function tests is often beneficial (Sardi *et al.* 1989; Fantini and DeCosse 1990; Carter *et al.* 1996). However, for detecting anastomotic recurrence, barium enema has a sensitivity of 88%, compared with 70% for CT (Chen *et al.* 1987). Magnetic resonance imaging, ultrasonography, and endorectal ultrasound have also shown some promise in detection of recurrence without exposing patients to ionizing radiation (Dresing and Stock 1990; Fantini and DeCosse 1990) (Figures 12.20–12.22). In contrast to screening for primary tumours, faecal occult blood testing is insufficiently sensitive (25–40%) for detecting recurrent colorectal cancer, with patient compliance rates of 80% (Crowson *et al.* 1991; Jahn *et al.* 1992). Faecal occult blood testing, barium enema, and colonoscopy are therefore more useful for detecting metachronous primary carcinomas than tumour recurrence (Fantini and DeCosse 1990; Kjeldsen

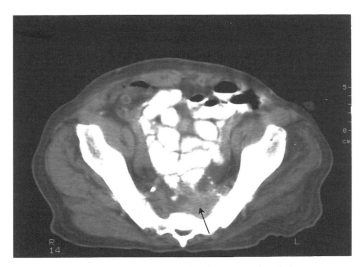

Figure 12.20 Magnetic resonance scan showing eccenteric soft tissue mass. Destruction of the sacrum confirms the mass to be recurrent tumour (arrowed).

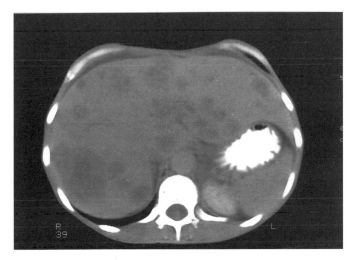

Figure 12.21 Magnetic resonance scan showing multiple liver metastases which were associated with a rise in CEA.

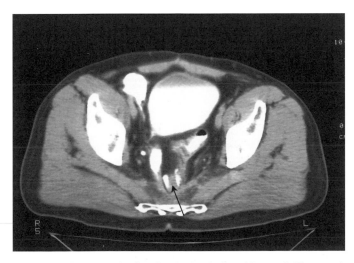

Figure 12.22 Post-operative fibrosis tethering the bowel (arrowed). The mass is in the mid-line and remained unchanged on serial follow-up.

et al. 1997). In patients who have had a Hartmann's procedure, regular endoscopy of the rectal stump is recommended as recurrent tumour at this site may be asymptomatic (Haas *et al.* 1990).

One half of recurrences are detected by serial CEA levels, one-third by chest X-ray and one-fifth by endoscopy (Sardi *et al.* 1989; Quentmeier *et al.* 1990; Rocklin *et al.* 1990). In 60% of patients an increased CEA level precedes the recognition of recurrence, while in 15% the diagnosis can be confirmed only by a second-look operation (Quentmeier *et al.* 1990). A rising CEA value is the best predictor of recurrence (Barillari *et al.* 1989; Sardi *et al.* 1989; Vauthey *et al.* 1996b) (Table 12.10). A rise in CEA levels of over 5% per month identifies those at risk of recurrence with an accuracy of 80%, sensitivity rate for recurrence of 85%, and specificity rate for no relapse of 75% (Sardi *et al.* 1989). A serum CEA within the normal range is 90% predictive that the patient is disease-free or in remission while over 80% of the patients with recurrence demonstrate an elevated CEA level greater than 5 ng/ml at the time of diagnosis (Barillari *et al.* 1989; Quentmeier *et al.* 1990). When CEA levels rise and other methods of imaging cannot account for the change, a second-look operation is generally appropriate (Fantini and DeCosse 1990; Einspahr *et al.* 1997).

Radioimmunoscintigraphy is particularly useful in detecting recurrent disease in patients with a rising serum CEA level but negative findings for CT scans of the abdomen and pelvis, chest radiograph, and colonoscopy or barium enema (Patt *et al.* 1990; Lane *et al.* 1994). This technique, combined with planar and single-photon emission CT (SPECT) scans at 72 and 144 h, is claimed to be about 90% accurate in correctly locating histologically proven tumour recurrence (Duda *et al.* 1990; Patt *et al.* 1990). The reported sensitivity of immunoscintigraphy for extrahepatic recurrence is 70–90% (Holting *et al.* 1990; Patt *et al.* 1990; Rutgers 1995). In a multicentre trial, the sensitivity of immunoscintigraphy for all recurrence, including hepatic, was 82% and specificity 91%, which compared favourably with 52% and 95%, respectively for CT and 59% and 100% for ultrasonography (Chetanneau *et al.* 1990). In addition, recurrent tumours tend to be detected earlier byimmunoscintigraphy than by conventional methods. Radioimmunoguided surgery (RIGS system) is performed using a hand-held gamma detector intra-operatively and externally after injection of radiolabelled (^{125}I) monoclonal antibody (Delaloye and Delaloye 1995). Advocates of the technique claim that major abdominal operations can be avoided in one-third of patients, modified in a further third, and selective chemotherapy or radiotherapy advised based on findings of the RIGS system (Nieroda *et al.* 1989; Aftab *et al.* 1996).

Many feel that second-look laparotomy for early detection of recurrent tumour is rarely indicated because of the advance in the above diagnostic techniques. However, the primary aim of post-operative surveillance of patients with carcinoma of the colon and rectum is to detect recurrent tumour when cure is still possible (Fantini and DeCosse 1990). In patients with recurrent disease re-intervention can offer a substantial chance of complete cancer clearance (Yamamoto *et al.* 1996; Soreide and Norstein 1997). Selected second-look surgery based on demonstrated recurrences results in a resectability rate of 60% for local disease, 20% in metachronous liver metastases, and 15% in other abdominal intracavitary relapse or pulmonary secondaries (Quentmeier *et al.* 1990). Successful resection is significantly less common in patients with symptomatic recurrent disease (35%) compared with asymptomatic patients with CEA-directed positive imaging (60%) and second-look patients (65%). In one study of 45 patients undergoing re-exploration based on rising CEA titres, recurrence was found in 42, of whom 23 had resectable disease (Wanebo *et al.* 1989). The median survival time was 43 months and the estimated 5-year survival rate was 38%

(Wanebo *et al.* 1989). In another study, the excisional rate of liver metastases was 57%, with a salvage rate of 75%, and the excisional rate of metastatic lymph nodes was 50%, with a salvage rate of 100% (Shindo *et al.* 1989). Others confirm that 5-year survival after complete re-resection approaches 40% irrespective of the site of recurrent disease, compared with a median survival of 9 months in patients not operated or undergoing incomplete resection (Secco *et al.* 1989). Second-look laparotomy therefore still has a place in some cases of asymptomatic patients with rising CEA titres, cases of undeterminable signs or those with post-chemotherapeutic or post-irradiation improvement (Shindo *et al.* 1989). In such selected patients, reoperation may improve survival (Wanebo *et al.* 1989). If this is considered pre-operative chemoradiation may increase resectability and enable sphincter preserving surgery in patients with locally advanced pelvic recurrence (Lowy *et al.* 1996).

References

Adam R, *et al.* Place of cryosurgery in the treatment of malignant liver tumors. *Ann. Surg.* 1997a; 225: 39–50.

Adam R, *et al.* Repeat hepatectomy for colorectal liver metastases. *Ann. Surg.* 1997b; 225: 51–62.

Adloff M, *et al.* Synchronous carcinoma of the colon and rectum: prognostic and therapeutic implications. *Am. J. Surg.* 1989; 157: 299–302.

Adloff M, *et al.* Hepatic metastasis of colorectal cancer. Should it be surgically treated? Report of 55 cases. *Chirurgie* 1990; 116: 144–9.

Aftab F, *et al.* Radioimmunoguided surgery and colorectal cancer. *Eur. J. Surg. Oncol.* 1996; 22: 381–8.

Aleman BM, *et al.* The current role of radiotherapy in colorectal cancer. *Eur. J. Cancer* 1995; 31A: 1333–9.

Altomare DF, *et al.* Protective colostomy closure: the hazards of a 'minor' operation. *Int. J. Colorect. Dis.* 1990; 5: 73–8.

Ambrosetti P, *et al.* Single stage excision anastomosis of left colonic obstruction excision treated as an emergency. *Chirurgie* 1989; 115 (Suppl. 2): I–VII.

Amsterdam E, Krispin M. Primary resection with colocolostomy for obstructive carcinoma of the left side of the colon. *Am. J. Surg.* 1985; 150: 558–60.

Arnaud J, *et al.* Radical surgery and postoperative radiotherapy as combined treatment in rectal cancer. Final results of a phase III study of the European Organization for Research and Treatment of Cancer. *Br. J. Surg.* 1997; 84: 352–8.

Asbun HJ, Hughes KS. Management of recurrent and metastatic colorectal carcinoma. *Surg. Clin. North Am.* 1993; 73: 145–66.

Aston NO, *et al.* Endoscopic balloon dilatation of colonic anastomotic strictures. *Br. J. Surg.* 1989; 76: 780–2.

Aubert A, *et al.* Colonoscopic surveillance of patients operated on in colorectal cancer. Retrospective evaluation of 269 tests in 125 patients. *J. Chir.* 1989; 126: 225–8.

Balslev I, *et al.* Postoperative radiotherapy in Dukes B and C carcinoma of the rectum and rectosigmoid. *Cancer* 1986; 58: 22–6.

Banerjee AK, *et al.* Prospective study of the proctographic and functional consequences of transanal endoscopic microsurgery. *Brit. J. Surg.* 1996; 83: 211–3.

Bailey HR, Huval WV, Max E. Local excision of carcinoma of the rectum for cure. *Surgery* 1992; 111: 555–61.

Bannon JP, *et al.* Radical and local excisional methods of sphincter-sparing surgery after high-dose radiation for cancer of the distal 3 cm of the rectum. *Ann. Surg. Oncol.* 1995; 2: 221–7.

Barillari P, *et al.* Relationship of symptom duration and survival in patients with colorectal carcinoma. *Eur. J. Surg. Oncol.* 1989; 15: 441–5.

Begos DG, *et al.* The diagnosis and management of adult intussusception. *Am. J. Surg.* 1997; 173: 88–94.

Benacci JC, Wolff BG. Cecostomy. Therapeutic indications and results. *Dis. Colon Rectum* 1995; 38: 530–4.

Bentzen SM, *et al.* Time to loco-regional recurrence after resection of Dukes' B and C colorectal cancer with or without adjuvant postoperative radiotherapy. A multivariate regression analysis. *Br. J. Cancer* 1992; 65: 102–7.

Biondo S, *et al.* Intraoperative colonic lavage and primary anastomosis in peritonitis and obstruction. *Br. J. Surg.* 1997; 84: 222–5.

Bismuth H, *et al.* Resection of nonresectable liver metastases from colorectal cancer after neoadjuvant chemotherapy. *Ann. Surg.* 1996; 224: 509–20.

Bleday R, *et al.* Prospective evaluation of local excision for small rectal cancers. *Dis. Colon Rectum* 1997; 40: 388–92.

Bleiberg H. Role of chemotherapy for advanced colorectal cancer: new opportunities. *Semin. Oncol.* 1996; 23: 42–50.

Blumgart LH, Fong Y. Surgical options in the treatment of hepatic metastasis from colorectal cancer. *Curr. Probl. Surg.* 1995; 32: 333–421.

Breen E, Bleday R. Preservation of the anus in the therapy of distal rectal cancers. *Surg. Clin. North Am.* 1997; 77: 71–83.

Brett M, Hershman M. Transanal endoscopic microsurgery. *Br. J. Hosp. Med.* 1994; 52: 386–9.

Brief DK, *et al.* Defining the role of subtotal colectomy in the treatment of carcinoma of the colon. *Ann. Surg.* 1991; 213: 248–52.

Brint SL, *et al.* Colorectal cancer screening: is one year surveillance sigmoidoscopy necessary? *Am. J. Gastroenterol.* 1993; 88: 2019–21.

Brister SJ, *et al.* Contemporary operative management of pulmonary metastases of colorectal origin. *Dis. Colon Rectum* 1988; 31: 786–92.

Bruckstein AH. Update on colorectal cancer. Risk factors, diagnosis, and treatment. *Postgrad. Med.* 1989; 86: 83–5.

Burke D, Allen-Mersh TG. Colorectal liver metastases. *Postgrad. Med. J.* 1996; 72: 464–9.

Buyse M, *et al.* Adjuvant therapy for colorectal cancer: why we still don't know. *JAMA* 1988; 259: 3571–3.

Cali RL, *et al.* Cumulative incidence of metachronous colorectal cancer. *Dis. Colon Rectum* 1993; 36: 388–93.

Carter R, *et al.* A prospective study of six methods for detection of hepatic colorectal metastases. *Ann. Roy. Coll. Surg. Eng.* 1996; 78: 27–30.

Cavaliere F, *et al.* Coloanal anastomosis for rectal cancer. Long term results at the Mayo and Cleveland Clinics. *Dis. Colon Rectum* 1995; 38: 807–12.

Cerdan FJ, *et al.* The results after extensive radical resection of locally advanced colorectal carcinoma. *Rev. Esp. Enferm. Dig.* 1994; 85: 435–9.

Chang AE, *et al.* A prospective randomized trial of regional versus systemic continuous 5 fluorodeoxyuridine chemotherapy in the treatment of colorectal liver metastases. *Ann. Surg.* 1987; 206: 685–90.

Chen YM, *et al.* Recurrent colorectal carcinoma: evaluation with barium enema examination and CT. *Radiology* 1987; 163: 307–10.

Chester J, Britton D. Elective and emergency surgery for colorectal cancer in a district general hospital: impact of surgical training on patient survival. *Ann. R. Coll. Surg. Engl.* 1989; 71, 370–4.

Chetanneau A, *et al.* Multi centre immunoscintigraphic study using indium 111 labelled CEA specific andor 19-9 monoclonal antibody F(ab['])2 fragments. *Eur. J. Nuclear Med.* 1990; 17: 223–9.

Cintron JR, Pearl RK. Colorectal cancer and peritoneal carcinomatosis. *Semin. Surg. Oncol.* 1996; 12: 267–78.

Coco C, *et al.* Conservative surgery for early cancer of the distal rectum. *Dis. Colon Rectum* 1992; 35: 131–6.

Colorectal Cancer Chemotherapy Study Group of Japan (CCCSGJ). Five year results of a randomized controlled trial of adjuvant chemotherapy for curatively resected colorectal carcinoma. *Jpn. J. Clin. Oncol.* 1995; 25: 91–103.

Corder AP, *et al.* Flush aortic tie versus selective preservation of the ascending left colic artery in low anterior resection for rectal carcinoma. *Br. J. Surg.* 1992; 79: 680–2.

Crowson MC, *et al.* Haemoccult testing as an indicator of recurrent colorectal cancer: a 5-year prospective study. *Eur. J. Surg. Oncol.* 1991; 17: 281–4.

Cummings BJ. Radiation therapy for colorectal cancer. *Surg. Clin. North Am.* 1993; 73: 167–81.

Cunningham KN, *et al.* Long term prognosis of well differentiated adenocarcinoma in endoscopically removed colorectal adenomas. *Dig. Dis. Sci.* 1994; 39: 2034–7.

Cunningham D, *et al.* 'Tomudex' (ZD1694): results of a randomised trial in advanced colorectal cancer demonstrate efficacy and reduced mucositis and leucopenia. The 'Tomudex' Colorectal Cancer Study Group. *Eur. J. Cancer* 1995; 31A(12): 1945–54.

Dahl O, *et al.* Low dose preoperative radiation postpones recurrences in operable rectal cancer. *Cancer* 1990; 66: 2286–90.

Dasmahapatra KS, Lopyan K. Rationale for aggressive colonoscopy in patients with colorectal neoplasia. *Arch. Surg.* 1989; 124: 63–6.

de Almeida AM, *et al.* Surgical management of acute, malignant obstruction of the left colon with colostomy. *Acta. Med. Port.* 1991; 4: 257–62.

Deans GT, *et al.* The modern management of malignant obstruction of the left colon. *Br. J. Surg.* 1994; 81: 1270–6.

Delaloye AB, Delaloye B. Radiolabelled monoclonal antibodies in tumour imaging and therapy: out of fashion? *Eur. J. Nuclear Med.* 1995; 22: 571–80.

Dixon AR, Holmes JT. Hartmann's procedure for carcinoma of rectum and distal sigmoid colon: 5-year audit. *J. Roy. Coll. Surg. Edinb.* 1990; 35: 166–8.

Docherty JG, et al. Comparison of manually constructed and stapled anastomoses in colorectal surgery. West of Scotland and Highland Anastomosis Study Group. Ann. Surg. 1995; 221: 176–84.

Doroshow JH, et al. Prospective randomized comparison of fluorouracil versus fluorouracil and high dose continuous infusion leucovorin calcium for the treatment of advanced measurable colorectal cancer in patients previously unexposed to chemotherapy. J. Clin. Oncol. 1990; 8: 491–501.

Dorudi S, et al. Primary restorative colectomy in malignant left sided large bowel obstruction. Ann. R. Coll. Surg. Engl. 1990; 72: 393–5.

Douglass HO. Adjuvant therapy for colon cancer. In: Moossa AR, Schimpff SC, Robson MC, eds. Comprehensive textbook of oncology, 2nd edn. Baltimore: Williams and Wilkins, 1991: 934–41.

Dresing K, Stock W. Ultrasonic endoluminal examination in the follow up of colorectal cancer. Initial experience and results. Int. J. Colorect. Dis. 1990; 5: 188–94.

Duda RB, et al. Radioimmune localization of occult carcinoma. Arch. Surg. 1990; 125: 866–70.

Duthie GS, et al. Bowel preparation or not for elective colorectal surgery. J. R. Coll. Surg. Edinburgh 1990: 35; 169–71.

Einspahr JG, et al. Surrogate end-point biomarkers as measures of colon cancer risk and their use in cancer chemoprevention trials. Cancer Epidemiol. Biomark. Prev. 1997; 6: 37–48.

Elftmann TD, et al. Laparoscopic assisted segmental colectomy: surgical techniques. Mayo Clin. Proc. 1994; 69: 825–33.

Erlichman C, et al. A phase II trial of 5 fluorouracil and 1 leucovorin in patients with metastatic colorectal cancer. Am. J. Clin. Oncol. 1996; 19: 26–31.

Faivre J, et al. Transanal electroresection of small rectal cancer: a sole treatment? Dis. Colon Rectum 1996; 39: 270–8.

Famell GF, et al. Brain metastases from colorectal carcinoma. The long term survivors. Cancer 1996; 78· 711–15

Fantini GA, DeCosse JJ. Surveillance strategies after resection of carcinoma of the colon and rectum. Surg. Gynecol. Obstet. 1990; 171: 267–73.

Fengler SA, Pearl RK. Technical considerations in the surgical treatment of colon and rectal cancer. Semin. Surg. Oncol. 1994; 10: 200 7.

Fielding LP, et al. Factors influencing mortality after curative resection for large bowel cancer in elderly patients. Lancet 1989; i: 595–7.

Fingerhut A, et al. Supraperitoneal colorectal anastomosis: hand sewn versus circular staples a controlled clinical trial. French Associations for Surgical Research. Surgery 1995; 118: 479–85.

Fisher B, et al. Postoperative adjuvant chemotherapy or radiation therapy for rectal cancer: Results from NSABP protocol R 01. J. Natl Cancer Inst. 1988; 80: 21–6.

Frazee RC, et al. Transanal excision of rectal carcinoma. Am. Surg. 1995; 61: 714–7.

Gandrup P, Lund L, Balslev I. Surgical treatment of acute malignant large bowel obstruction. Eur. J. Surg. 1992; 158: 427–30.

Gastrointestinal Tumor Study Group (GITSG). Adjuvant therapy of colon cancer results of a prospectively randomised trial. N. Engl. J. Med. 1984; 310: 737–43

Gastrointestinal Tumor Study Group (GITSG). Prolongation of the disease free interval in surgically treated rectal carcinoma. N. Engl. J. Med. 1985; 312: 1465–70.

Gerard A, et al. Preoperative radiotherapy as adjuvant treatment in rectal cancer. Ann. Surg. 1988; 208: 606–12.

Girard P, et al. Surgery for lung metastases from colorectal cancer: analysis of prognostic factors. J. Clin. Oncol. 1996; 14: 2047–53.

Graham RA, et al. Local excision of rectal carcinoma. Am. J. Surg. 1990; 160: 306–12.

Graham RA, et al. Local excision of rectal carcinoma: Early results with combined chemoradiation therapy using 5-fluorouracil and leucovorin. Dis. Colon Rectum 1994; 37: 308–12.

Grage TB, Moss SE. Adjuvant chemotherapy in cancer of the colon and rectum: Demonstration of effectiveness of prolonged 5-FL chemotherapy in a prospectively randomized trial. Surg. Clin. North Am. 1981; 61: 1321–8.

Graham RA, et al. Local excision of rectal carcinoma. Early results with combined chemoradiation therapy using 5-fluorouracil and leucovorin. Dis. Colon Rectum 1994; 37: 308–12.

Gray D, et al. Adequacy of lymphadenectomy in laparoscopic assisted colectomy for colorectal cancer: a preliminary report. J. Surg. Oncol. 1994; 57: 8–10.

Gurke L, et al. Is cecostomy still current for emergency relief of the colon? Helv. Chir. Acta 1991; 57: 961–4.

Gutman M, et al. Proximal colostomy: still an effective emergency measure in obstructing carcinoma of the large bowel. J. Surg. Oncol. 1989; 41: 210–12.

Haas PA, et al. Endoscopic examination of the colon and rectum distal to a colostomy. Am. J. Gastroenterol. 1990; 85: 850–4.

Haggit RC, et al. Prognostic factors in colorectal carcinomas arising in adenomas: Implications for lesions removed by endoscopic polypectomy. Gastroenterology 1985; 89: 328–36.

Hainsworth P, et al. Evaluation of a policy of total mesorectal excision for rectal and rectosigmoid cancers. Br. J. Surg. 1997; 84: 652–6.

Halevy A, et al. Emergency subtotal colectomy. A new trend for treatment of obstructing carcinoma of the left colon. Ann. Surg. 1989; 210: 220–3.

Hall NR, et al. High tie of the inferior mesenteric artery in distal colorectal resections a safe vascular procedure. Int. J. Colorect. Dis. 1995; 10: 29–32.

Hammond MA, et al. Colorectal carcinoma and brain metastasis: distribution, treatment, and survival. Ann. Surgical Oncol. 1996; 3: 453–63.

Hase K, et al. Long term results of curative resection of 'minimally invasive' colorectal cancer. Dis. Colon Rectum 1995; 38: 19–26.

Hatcher PA, et al. Surgical aspects of intestinal injury due to pelvic radiotherapy. Ann. Surg. 1984; 201: 470–5.

Heald RJ, Karanjia ND. The management of colorectal cancer. Curr. Pract. Surg. 1993; 5: 195–201.

Hida J, et al. Functional outcome after low anterior resection with low anastomosis for rectal cancer using the colonic J-pouch. Prospective randomized study for determination of optimum pouch size. Dis. Colon Rectum 1996; 39: 986–91.

Higgins GA, et al. Adjuvant chemotherapy in the surgical treatment of large bowel cancer. Cancer 1976; 38: 1461–7.

Higgins GA, et al. Efficacy of prolonged intermittent therapy with combined 5-fluorouracil and methyl CCNU following resection for carcinoma of the large bowel. A Veterans Administration Surgical Oncology Group report. Cancer 1984; 53: 1–8.

Higgins GA, et al. Preoperative radiation and surgery for cancer of the rectum: Veterans Administration Surgical Oncology Group Trial II. Cancer 1986; 58: 352–60.

Ho YH, et al. Prospective randomized controlled study of clinical function and anorectal physiology after low anterior resection: comparison of straight and colonic J pouch anastomoses. Brit. J. Surg. 1996; 83: 978–80.

Hohenberger P, et al. Tumor recurrence and options for further treatment after resection of liver metastases in patients with colorectal cancer. J. Surg. Oncol. 1990; 44: 245–51.

Hojo K, et al. An analysis of survival, voiding and sexual function after wide iliopelvic lymphadenectomy in patients with carcinoma of the rectum, compared with conventional lymphadenectomy. Dis. Colon Rectum 1989; 32: 128–33.

Holm T, et al. Influence of hospital- and surgeon-related factors on outcome after treatment of rectal cancer with or without preoperative radiotherapy. Br. J. Surg. 1997; 84: 657–63.

Holting T, et al. Current status of immunoscintigraphy in colorectal cancer—results of 5 years' clinical experiences. Eur. J. Surg. Oncol. 1990; 16: 312–8.

Hong JC, Hwang DM, Wang YH. Intraoperative colon irrigation in the management of obstructing left-sided colon cancer. Kao Hsiung I Hsueh Ko Hsueh Tsa Chih 1989; 5: 309–13.

International Multicentre Pooled Analysis of Colon Cancer Trials (IMPACT) investigators. Efficacy of adjuvant fluorouracil and folinic acid in colon cancer. Lancet. 1995; 345: 939–44.

Jahn H, et al. Can Hemoccult II replace colonoscopy in surveillance after radical surgery for colorectal cancer and after polypectomy? Dis. Colon Rectum 1992; 35: 253–6.

Jeekal J. Can radical surgery improve survival in colorectal cancer? World J. Surg. 1987; 11: 412–17.

Johnstone PA, et al. Port site recurrences after laparoscopic and thoracoscopic procedures inmalignancy. J. Clin. Oncol. 1996; 14: 1950–6.

Juhl G, et al. Six year results of annual colonoscopy after resection of colorectal cancer. World J. Surg. 1990; 14: 255–60.

Karanjia ND, et al. The close shave in anterior resection. Br. J. Surg. 1990; 77: 510–12.

Karanjia ND, et al. Leakage from stapled low anastomosis after total mesorectal excision for carcinoma of the rectum. Br. J. Surg. 1994; 81: 1224–6.

Keen RR, Orsay CP. Rectosigmoid stent for obstructing colonic neoplasms. Dis. Colon Rectum 1992; 35: 912–3.

Kemeny N, et al. Continuous intrahepatic infusion of floxuridine and leucovorin through an implantable pump for the treatment of hepatic metastases from colorectal carcinoma. Cancer 1990; 65: 2446–50.

Khanduja KS. Transanal endoscopic microsurgery. Results of the initial ten cases. Surg. Endosc. 1995; 9: 56–60.

Kiefer PJ, et al. Metachronous colorectal cancer. Time interval to presentation of a metachronous cancer. Dis. Colon Rectum 1986; 29: 378–82.

Kjeldsen B, et al. A prospective randomized study of follow-up after radical surgery for colorectal cancer. Br. J. Surg. 1997; 84: 666–9.

Kohne CH, et al. Phase II evaluation of 5-fluourouracil plus folinic acid and alpha 2b-interferon in metastatic colorectal cancer. Oncol. 1997; 54: 96–101.

Korpan N. Hepatic cryosurgery for liver metastases: Long-term follow-up. *Am. Surg.* 1997; 225: 193–201.

Kosmidis PA, *et al.* Fluorouracil and leucovorin with or without interferon alfa-2b in advanced colorectal cancer: analysis of a prospective randomized phase III trial. Hellenic Cooperative Oncology Group. *J. Clin. Oncol.* 1996; 14: 2682–7.

Koruth NM, *et al.* Immediate resection in emergency large bowel surgery: a 7 year audit. *Br. J. Surg.* 1985; 72: 703–7.

Kristiansen VB, *et al.* Cecostomy can not be recommended as a routine method in the treatment of acute left sided obstructive colon cancer. *Ugeskrift Laeger* 1990; 152: 101–3.

Kronborg O. Acute obstruction from tumour in the left colon without spread. A randomized trial of emergency colostomy versus resection. *Int. J. Colorect. Dis.* 1995; 10: 1–5.

Krook JE, *et al.* Effective surgical adjuvant therapy for high-risk rectal carcinoma. *N. Engl. J. Med.* 1991; 324: 709.

Krukowski ZH, Matheson NA. A ten year computerised audit of infection after abdominal surgery. *Br. J. Surg.* 1988; 75; 857–61.

Kwok SP, *et al.* Prospective evaluation of laparoscopic assisted large bowel excision for cancer. *Ann. Surg.* 1996; 223: 170–6.

Laffer UT, Metzger U. Intraportal chemotherapy for colorectal hepatic metastases. *World J. Surg.* 1995; 19: 246–51.

Lane DM, *et al.* Radioimmunotherapy of metastatic colorectal tumours with iodine 131 labelled antibody to carcinoembryonic antigen: phase III study with comparative biodistribution of intact and F(ab[']))2 antibodies. *Br. J. Cancer* 1994; 70: 521–5.

Lavery IC, *et al.* Definitive management of rectal cancer by contact (endocavitary) irradiation. *Dis. Colon Rectum* 1987; 30: 835–9.

Laurie JA, *et al.* Surgical adjuvant therapy of large-bowel carcinoma: An evaluation of levamisole and the combination of levamisole and fluorouracil. *J. Clin. Oncol.* 1989; 7: 1447–51.

Leather AJ, *et al.* Detection of free malignant cells in the peritoneal cavity before and after resection of colorectal cancer. *Dis. Colon Rectum* 1994; 37: 814–9.

Levithan N. Chemotherapy in colorectal cancer. *Surg. Clin. North Am.* 1993; 73: 183–98.

Loizou LA, *et al.* Endoscopic Nd[:]YAG laser treatment of rectosigmoid cancer. *Gut* 1990; 31: 812–6.

Lowy AM, *et al.* Preoperative infusional chemoradiation, selective intraoperative radiation, and resection for locally advanced pelvic recurrence of colorectal adenocarcinoma. *Ann. Surg.* 1996; 223: 177–85.

MacFarlane JK, *et al.* Mesorectal excision for rectal cancer. *Lancet* 1993; 341: 457–60.

Malafosse M, *et al.* Traitement des occlusions aigues par cancer du colon gauche. *Chirurgie* 1989; 115(Suppl 2): 123–5.

Mansour EG, *et al.* A comparison of postoperative adjuvant chemotherapy, radiotherapy or combination therapy in potentially curable resectable rectal carcinoma [abstract]. *Proc. Am. Soc. Clin. Oncol.* 1991; 10: 154.

Marks G, *et al.* High dose preoperative radiation and full thickness local excision. *Dis. Colon Rectum* 1990; 33: 735–9.

McArdle CS. Hepatic colorectal metastases. Detection and follow up. *Curr. Pract. Surg.* 1989; 1: 76–80.

McCready DR. Prospective phase I trial of conservative management of low rectal lesions. *Arch. Surg.* 1989; 124: 67–74.

McMaster P, Buist L. Hepatic colorectal metastases. Selection of patients for surgery. *Curr. Pract. Surg.* 1989; 1: 73–5.

Mentges B, *et al.* Indications and results of local treatment of rectal cancer. *Br. J. Surg.* 1997; 84: 348–51.

Michael Z, *et al.* Colonoscopic surveillance after diagnosis of carcinoma of the colon and rectum. *Ann. Chir.* 1989; 43: 568–9.

Mileski WJ, *et al.* Rates of morbidity and mortality after closure of loop and end colostomy. *Surg. Gynecol. Obstet.* 1990; 171: 17–21.

Minsky BD, *et al.* Local excision and postoperative radiation therapy for rectal cancer. *Am. J. Clin. Oncol.* 1994; 77: 411–16.

Minsky BD. Conservative management of early rectal cancer. *Int. J. Radiat. Oncol. Biol. Phys.* 1996; 34: 961–2.

Moertel CG, *et al.* Levamisole and fluorouracil for adjuvant therapy of resected colon carcinoma. *N. Engl. J. Med.* 1990; 322: 352–4.

Moertel CG, *et al.* Fluorouracil plus levamisole as effective adjuvant therapy after resection of stage III colon carcinoma: a final report. *Ann. Intern Med.* 1995; 122: 321–6.

Moertel CC, *et al.* Intergroup study of fluorouracil plus levamisole as adjuvant therapy for stage II/Dukes' B2 colon cancer. *J. Clin. Oncol.* 1995; 13: 2936–40.

Monson JR, *et al.* Prospective evaluation of laparoscopic assisted colectomy in an unselected group of patients. *Lancet* 1992; 340: 831–3.

Monson JR, *et al.* Laparoscopic colonic surgery. *Br. J. Surg.* 1995; 82: 150–7.

Moore JW, *et al.* Management of the malignant colorectal polyp: the importance of clinicopathological correlation. *Aust. N.Z. J. Surg.* 1994; 64: 242–6.

Morikawa E, *et al.* Distribution of metastatic lymph nodes in colorectal cancer by the modified clearing method. *Dis. Colon Rectum* 1994; 37: 219–23.

Morino T, *et al.* Clinico pathological features of liver metastases from colorectal cancer in relation to prognosis. *Nippon Geka Hokan* 1991; 60: 154–64.

Morris DM, Rayburn D. Loop colostomies are totally diverting in adults. *Am. J. Surg.* 1991; 161: 668–71.

Morrison MC, *et al.* Percutaneous cecostomy: controlled transperitoneal approach. *Radiology* 1990; 176: 574–6.

Mortensen NJ, *et al.* Colonic J pouch anal anastomosis after rectal excision for carcinoma: functional outcome. *Br. J. Surg.* 1995; 82: 611–3.

MRC: Second Report of an MRC Working Party. The evaluation of low dose preoperative X-ray therapy in the management of operable rectal cancer: Results of a randomly controlled trial. *Br. J. Surg.* 1984; 71: 21–4.

Mulcahy HE, *et al.* Long-term outcome following curative surgery for malignant large bowel obstruction. *Brit. J. Surg.* 1996; 83: 46–50.

Munro A, *et al.* Total colonic mobilization and exteriorization facilitates intra operative colonic irrigation. *J. R. Coll. Surg. Edinburgh* 1995; 40: 171–2.

Murray JJ, *et al.* Intraoperative colonic lavage and primary anastomosis in nonelective colon resection. *Dis. Colon Rectum* 1991; 34: 527–31.

Murray JJ, Stahl TJ. Sphincter saving alternatives for treatment of adenocarcinoma involving distal rectum. *Surg. Clin. North Am.* 1993; 73: 131–44.

Neeleman N, Andersson R. Repeated liver resection for recurrent liver cancer. *Brit. J. Surg.* 1996; 83: 893–901.

Nieroda CA, *et al.* The impact of radioimmunoguided surgery (RIGS) on surgical decision making in colorectal cancer. *Dis. Colon Rectum* 1989; 32: 927–32.

Nogueras JJ, Jagelman DG. Principles of surgical resection. Influence of surgical technique on treatment outcome. *Surg. Clin. North Am.* 1993; 73: 103–16.

Ohlsson B, *et al.* Follow up after curative surgery for colorectal carcinoma. Randomized comparison with no follow up. *Dis. Colon Rectum* 1995; 38: 619–26.

Ota DM, Skibber J, Rich TA. M.D. Anderson cancer center experience with local excision and multimodality therapy for rectal cancer. *Surg. Oncol. Clin. North Am.* 1992; 1: 147–52.

Otmezguine Y, *et al.* A new combined approach in the conservative management of rectal cancer. *Int. J. Radiat. Oncol. Biol. Phys.* 1989; 17: 539–44.

Paik PS, Beart RW Jr. Laparoscopic colectomy. *Surg. Clin. North Am.* 1997; 97: 1–13.

Panettiere FJ, *et al.* Adjuvant therapy in large bowel adenocarcinoma: Long-term results of a Southwest Oncology Group study. *J. Clin. Oncol.* 1988; 6: 947–9.

Papillon J. New prospects in the conservative treatment of rectal cancer. *Dis. Colon Rectum* 1984; 27: 695–700.

Papillon J. Present status of irradiation therapy in the conservative management of rectal cancer. *Radiother. Oncol.* 1990; 17: 275–82.

Patchett SE, *et al.* Colonoscopic surveillance after curative resection for colorectal cancer. *Br. J. Surg.* 1993; 80: 1330–2.

Patt YZ, *et al.* Imaging with indium 111 labeled anticarcinoembryonic antigen monoclonal antibody ZCE 025 of recurrent colorectal or carcinoembryonic antigen producing cancer in patiewelcome datacompnts with rising serum carcinoembryonic antigen levels and occult metastases. *J. Clin. Oncol.* 1990; 8: 1246–54.

Pearce NW, *et al.* Timing and method of reversal of Hartmann's procedure. *Br. J. Surg.* 1992; 79: 839–41.

Penna C. Nordlinger B. Locoregional chemotherapy for adjuvant treatment of colorectal adenocrrcinoma. *Eur. J. Cancer* 1996; 32: 1117–22.

Petros JG, *et al.* Retroperitoneal and abdominal wall emphysema after transanal excision of a rectal carcinoma. *Am. Surg.* 1996; 62: 759–61.

Quentmeier A, *et al.* Reoperation for recurrent colorectal cancer: the importance of early diagnosis for resectability and survival. *Eur. J. Surg. Oncol.* 1990; 16: 319–25.

Radcliffe AG, Dudley HAF. Intraoperative antegrade irrigation for the large intestine. *Surg. Gynecol. Obstet.* 1983: 156; 721–3.

Recchia F, *et al.* Randomized trial of 5-fluorouracil and high-dose folinic acid with or without alpha-2B interferon in advanced colorectal cancer. *Am. J. Clin. Oncol.* 1996; 19: 301–4.

Reinbach DH, *et al.* Effect of the surgeon's specialty interest on the type of resection performed for colorectal cancer. *Dis. Colon Rectum* 1994; 37: 1020–3.

Rich TA, *et al.* Definitive treatment of low rectal cancer with sphincter preservation by radiation therapy with or without local excision of fulguration. *Radiology* 1985; 156: 527–33.

Richert-Boe KE. Heterogeneity of cancer surveillance practices among medical oncologists in Washington and Oregon. *Cancer* 1995; 75: 2605–12.

Rocklin MS, *et al.* Postoperative surveillance of patients with carcinoma of the colon and rectum. *Am. Surg.* 1990; 56: 22–7.

Roe AM, *et al.* Indications for laparoscopic formation of intestinal stomas. *Surg. Laparosc. Endosc.* 1994; 4: 345–7.

Rosenthal SA, et al. Conservative management of extensive low-lying rectal carcinomas with transanal local excision and combined preoperative and postoperative radiation therapy. Cancer 1992; 69: 335–41.

Roth SL, et al. Results of endocavitary irradiation of early rectal tumors. Acta Oncol. 1988; 27: 825–29.

Rouanet P, et al. Conservative treatment for low rectal carcinoma by local excision with or without radiotherapy. Br. J. Surg. 1993; 80: 1452–6.

Rougier P, et al. Phase II study of irinotecan in the treatment of advanced colorectal cancer in chemotherapy-naive patients and patients pretreated with fluorouracil-based chemotherapy. J. Clin. Oncol. 1997; 15: 251–60.

Rustum YM, et al. Thymidylate synthase inhibitors in cancer therapy: direct and indirect inhibitors. J. Clin. Oncol. 1997; 15: 389–400.

Rutgers EJ. Radio immunotargeting in colorectal carcinoma. Eur. J. Cancer 1995; 31A: 1243–7.

Sackier JM, et al. Laparoscopic endocorporeal mobilization followed by extracorporeal sutureless anastomosis for the treatment of carcinoma of the left colon. Dis. Colon Rectum 1993; 36: 610–2.

Saida Y, et al. Stent endoprosthesis for obstructing colorectal cancers. Dis. Colon Rectum 1996; 39: 552–5.

Salim AS. Percutaneous decompression and irrigation for large bowel obstruction. New approach. Dis. Colon Rectum 1991; 34: 973–80.

Sardi A, et al. Radioimmunoguided surgery in recurrent colorectal cancer: the role of carcinoembryonic antigen, computerized tomography, and physical examination. South Med. J. 1989; 82: 1235–44.

Scheele J, et al. Resection of colorectal liver metastases. World J. Surg. 1995; 19: 59–71.

Schirmer BD. Laparoscopic colon resection. Surg. Clin. North Am. 1996; 76: 571–83.

Secco GB, et al. Colorectal cancer: prognosis after curative surgical treatment without extended elective lymphadenectomy in patients in Dukes C stage G. Chirurgie 1989; 10: 557–61.

Seymour MT, et al. Randomized trial assessing the addition of interferon alpha-2a tofluorouracil and leucovorin in advanced colorectal cancer. Colorectal Cancer Working Party of the United Kingdom Medical Research Council. J. Clin. Oncol. 1996; 14: 2280–8.

Shindo K, et al. Clinical evaluation of second look operations in colorectal cancer. Gan To Kagaku Ryoho 1989; 16: 1283–8.

Simons AJ, et al. Laparoscopic assisted colectomy learning curve. Dis. Colon Rectum 1995; 38: 600–3.

Sinicrope FA, Sugarman SM. Role of adjuvant therapy in surgically resected colorectal carcinoma. Gastroenterology 1995; 109: 984–93.

Sischy B, Hinson EJ Wilkinson DR. Definitive radiation therapy for selected cancers of the rectum. Br. J. Surg. 1988; 75: 901–3.

Sjodahl R, et al. Primary versus staged resection for acute obstructing colorectal carcinoma. Br. J. Surg. 1992; 79: 685–8.

Slors JF, et al. One-stage colectomy and ileorectal anastomosis for complete left-sided obstruction of the colon. Neth. J Surg 1989; 41: 1–4.

Sobrero AF, et al. Fluorouracil in colorectal cancer—a tale of two drugs: implications for biochemical modulation. J. Clin. Oncol. 1997; 15: 368–81.

Soreide O, Norstein J. Local recurrence after operative treatment of rectal carcinoma: a strategy for change. J. Am. Coll. Surg. 1997; 184: 84–92.

Stage JG, et al. Prospective randomized study of laparoscopic versus open colonic resection of adenocarcinoma. Br. J. Surg. 1997; 84: 391–6.

Staniunas RJ, Schoetz DJ Jr. Extended resection for carcinoma of colon and rectum. Surg. Clin. North Am.. 1993; 73: 117–29.

Steele G, et al. A pilot study of sphincter-sparing management of adenocarcinoma of the rectum. Arch. Surg. 1991; 126: 696–700.

Steele G Jr. Adjuvant therapy for patients with colorectal cancer. World J Surg. 1995; 19: 241–5.

Steele G, et al. A prospective evaluation of hepatic resection for colorectal carcinoma metastases to the liver: Gastrointestinal Tumour Study Group protocol 6584. J. Clin. Oncol. 1991; 9: 1105–12.

Stein BL, Coller JA. Management of malignant colorectal polyps. Surg. Clin. North Am. 1993; 73: 47–66.

Stephenson BM, et al. Malignant left sided large bowel obstruction managed by subtotal/total colectomy. Br. J. Surg. 1990; 77: 1098–102.

Stockholm Rectal Cancer Study Group. Preoperative short term radiation therapy in operable rectal cancer. Cancer 1990; 66: 49–55.

Stockholm Colorectal cancer Study Group. Randomized study on preoperative radiotherapy in rectal carcinoma. Ann. Surgical Oncol. 1996; 3: 423–30.

Sugarbaker PH. Follow up of colorectal cancer. Tumori 1995a; 81 (Suppl. 3): 126–34.

Sugarbaker PH. Patient selection and treatment of peritoneal carcinomatosis from colorectal and appendiceal cancer. World J. Surg. 1995b; 19: 235–40.

Swedish Rectal Cancer Trial. Improved survival with preoperative radiotherapy in resectable rectal cancer. N. Engl. J. Med. 1997; 336: 980–7.

Swiss Group for Clinical Cancer Research (SAKK). Long term results of single course of adjuvant intraportal chemotherapy for colorectal cancer. Lancet 1995; 345: 349–53.

Taylor I, et al. A randomized controlled trial of adjuvant portal vein cytotoxic perfusion in colorectal cancer. Br. J. Surg. 1985; 72: 359–62.

Taylor I, Liver metastases from colorectal cancer: lessons from past and present clinical studies. Brit. J. Surg. 1996; 83: 456–60.

Thoresen JE, et al. Transanal endoscopic microsurgery. Tidsskr Nor Laegeforen 1996; 116: 52–3.

Tominaga T, et al. Prognostic factors for patients with colon or rectal carcinoma treated with resection only. Five-year follow-up report. Cancer 1996; 78: 403–8.

Treurniet-Donker AD, et al. Postoperative radiation therapy for rectal cancer: An interim analysis of a prospective, randomized multicenter trial in the Netherlands. Cancer 1991; 67: 2042–5.

Tuchmann A, et al. Hepatic artery infusion chemotherapy. HPB Surg. 1990; 2: 21–8.

Turnbull RB Jr, et al. Cancer of the colon: the influence of the no touch isolation technique on survival rates. Ann. Surg. 1967; 166: 420–7.

Tuson JR, Everett WG. A retrospective study of colostomies, leaks and strictures after colorectal anastomosis. Int. J. Colorect. Dis. 1990; 5: 44–8.

Vara Thorbeck C, et al. Indications and advantages of laparoscopy assisted colon resection for carcinoma in elderly patients. Surg Laparosc Endosc. 1994; 4(2): 110–8.

Vauthey JN, et al. Management of recurrent colorectal cancer: another look at carcinoembryonic antigen-detected recurrence. Dig. Dis. 1996b; 14: 5–13.

Vauthy JN, et al. Arterial therapy of hepatic colorectal metastases. Brit. J. Surg. 1996a; 83: 447–55.

Vigneswaran WT. Management of pulmonary metastases from colorectal cancer. Semin. Surg. Oncol. 1996; 12: 264–6.

Volpe C, et al. Wide perineal dissection and its effect on local recurrence following potentially curative abdominoperineal resection for rectal adenocarcinoma. Cancer Invest. 1996; 14: 1–5.

Wadler S, et al. Fluorouracil and recombinant alpha 2a interferon: an active regimen against advanced colorectal carcinoma. J. Clin. Oncol. 1989; 7: 1769–74.

Wanebo HJ, et al. Prospective monitoring trial for carcinoma of colon and rectum after surgical resection. Surg. Gynecol. Obstet. 1989; 169: 479–87.

Wanebo HJ, et al. Current perspectives on repeat hepatic resection for colorectal carcinoma: a review. Surg. 1996; 119: 361–71.

Williams NS, et al. Reappraisal of the 5 cm rule of distal excision for carcinoma of the rectum: a study of distal intramural spread and of patients survival. Br. J. Surg. 1983; 70: 150–4.

Wilson RG, Gollock JM. Obstructing carcinoma of the left colon managed by subtotal colectomy. J. Roy. Coll. Surg. Edinb. 1989; 34: 25–6.

Willett CG, et al. Patterns of failure following local excision and postoperative radiation therapy for invasive rectal adenocarcinoma. J. Clin. Oncol. 1989; 7: 1003–10.

Windle R, Bell PRF, Shaw D. Five year results of a randomised trial of adjuvant 5-fluorouracil and levamisole in colorectal cancer. Br. J. Surg. 1987; 74: 569–72.

Winawer SJ, et al. Prevention of colorectal cancer by colonoscopic polypectomy. The National Polyp Study Workgroup. N. Engl. J. Med. 1993; 329: 1977–81.

Wolmark N, et al. Postoperative adjuvant chemotherapy or BCG for colon cancer: results from NSABP protocol C 01. J. Natl Cancer Inst. 1988; 80: 30–6.

Wolmark N, et al. Adjuvant therapy of Dukes' A, B, and C adenocarcinoma of the colon with portal-vein fluorouracil hepatic influsion: Preliminary resutls of National Surgical Adjuvant Breast and Bowel Project protocol C-02. J. Clin. Oncol. 1990; 8: 1466–70.

Yamamato Y, et al. Surgical treatment for the recurrence of colorectal cancer. Surg. Today 1996; 26: 164–8.

Yu BM. Surgical treatment of acute intestinal obstruction caused by large bowel carcinoma. Chung Hua Wai Ko Tsa Chih 1989; 27: 285–6.

Zaleberg JR, et al. ZD1694. A novel thymidylate synthase inhibitor with substantial activity in the treatment of patients with advanced colorectal cancer. Tomudex Colorectal Study Group. J. Clin. Oncol. 1996; 14: 716–21.

13 Disorders of motility and the muscle wall

Constipation

Constipation is a common complaint with a reported prevalence varying between 2% and 20% of the population (Sonnenberg and Koch 1989; Talley *et al.* 1993; Harari *et al.* 1996). It is often defined as the passage of fewer than three bowel movements per week but the term may also refer to straining at stool, a sensation of incomplete evacuation, or a need for laxatives (Whitehead *et al.* 1989). In a recent study on constipation, a working party took note of the following: (i) straining at stool; (ii) feeling of incomplete evacuation; (iii) passage of hard stools; and (iv) passage of fewer than three stools per week. A diagnosis of constipation was accepted on the basis of a combination of two of the above being present 25% of the time during the previous year. The passage of fewer than two stools per week on average was also regarded as diagnostic by itself (Drossman *et al.* 1990; Talley *et al.* 1993). Other authors suggest that the passage of less than five stools per week should be regarded as abnormal (Devroede 1993; Ashraf *et al.* 1996). Regardless of the exact definition, constipation leads to a billion pound per annum business with over-the-counter laxative sales accounting for four million dollars in the USA alone (Tedesco and DiPiro 1985). In assessing patients presenting with constipation a thorough history is essential, in particular defining exactly what the patient means by the term (Talley *et al.* 1996). Enquiries should be made concerning the age at onset of symptoms and their duration, the average length of time spent straining at stool, the use of laxatives, and the role of any digital techniques to facilitate evacuation. Drug ingestion, past medical history, and details of previous surgery may shed light on the cause of the constipation. Among those patients with no obvious cause for their constipation, the important aetiological role of psychological factors must be recognized and gentle probing carried out in a search for evidence of previous psychosocial trauma, especially childhood sexual or physical abuse (Arnold *et al.* 1990; Drossman *et al.* 1990; Brook 1991). Evidence of systemic disease may be uncovered by either the history or the general examination. Physical examination must include digital examination of the rectum. Whether presenting with a change of bowel habit and recent-onset constipation or long-standing symptoms, a colonoscopy or barium enema and sigmoidoscopy should be carried out. On the basis of history, examination, colonoscopy/barium enema and the appropriate use of blood tests the majority of causes other than the 'idiopathic' colonic group can be excluded (Table 13.1).

Idiopathic constipation

At this stage all patients should be given a trial in which conservative measures are adopted. These include reassurance, increasing the

Table 13.1 Causes of constipation

Constitutional	Diet
	Pregnancy
	Old age
	Immobility
Pharmacological agents	Analgesics
	Aluminium-containing antacids
	Anticholinergics
	Antidepressants
	Diuretics
Metabolic/endocrine	Hypothyroidism
	Hypercalcaemia
	Uraemia
	Hypokalaemia
	Amyloidosis
Neurological	CNS/spinal cord disease
	Myotonia dystrophica
	Autonomic neuropathy
Psychological	Anorexia nervosa
	Depression
Colonic (organic)	Tumour
	Inflammation
	Chronic infection, e.g. tuberculosis/ lymphogranuloma venereum
	Hirschsprung's disease
	Chagas' disease
	Acquired megarectum
	Diverticular disease
	Ischaemic stricture
	Intestinal pseudo-obstruction
Colonic ('idiopathic')	Irritable bowel syndrome
	Colonic inertia (slow transit)
	Obstructed defecation
Anal disease	Tumour
	Fissure
	Stenosis

fluid and fibre content in the diet and the use of bulking agents such as ispaghula, or methyl cellulose or saline cathartics such as magnesium sulphate. The introduction of these measures along with a daily stool chart for 1 month should confirm a symptomatic improvement in the majority of patients. Patients who fail to respond satisfactorily to defined and regular regimen merit further investigation to delineate the nature of their 'idiopathic' constipation. Transit studies and anorectal physiological testing are the two main methods of investigation (Karasick and Ehrlich 1996). There are a multitude of methodologies and formulae for assessing colonic transit. One of the simplest measures of transit rate is to assess the proportion of radio-opaque markers passed in a given time (Figure 13.1).

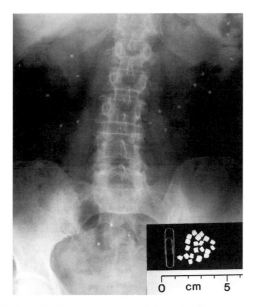

Figure 13.1 X-ray showing radio-opaque pellets used in the measurement of intestinal transit rate.

Normally some of the ingested markers will be passed per rectum within 3 days and 80% of them within 5 days (Hinton *et al.* 1969; Devroede and Soffie 1973; Fleshman *et al.* 1992). It has also been suggested that determination of the site within the large bowel where the markers preferentially lodge can help distinguish between slow transit and so-called 'outlet obstruction'. In obstructed defecation 80% of the markers will have reached the rectum within 3 days as in normal individuals but they will be retained there even after the fifth day (Fleshman *et al.* 1992).

Facilities within an anorectal laboratory include manometry, assessment of rectal balloon expulsion, electromyography (EMG), and

defecography (Parks 1992). Anorectal manometry is helpful in the diagnosis of an adult presenting with Hirschsprung's disease by revealing an absence of the recto-anal inhibitory reflex. In a normal subject, the internal anal sphincter relaxes in response to distension of the rectum by a balloon, the reflex being mediated through local visceral nerve plexuses in the submucosal and mesenteric layers (Figure 13.2). This does not occur in Hirschsprung's disease in contrast to chronic idiopathic constipation where the recto-anal inhibitory reflex is usually demonstrable. Some cases of megarectum may require large balloon volumes to induce the recto-anal inhibitory reflex (Verduron *et al.* 1988) The reflex may be absent in some patients with stool in the rectum who do not suffer from Hirschsprung's disease (Devroede 1993). Diagnosis of the latter must therefore be confirmed by demonstrating aganglionosis on rectal biopsy (Whitehouse and Kernohan 1948).

The ability to expel a balloon from the rectum is regarded by many as an important test, which helps to distinguish those with obstructed defecation from those with slow transit constipation (Parks 1992). For this test a balloon attached to a catheter is inflated in the rectum with 50 ml of water at body temperature. If the patient finds it impossible to expel the balloon further weights in 50 g increments can be added to the catheter which is passed over a pulley (Figure 13.3). Normal subjects can expel balloon containing 50 ml of water without the addition of weights (Heine *et al.* 1993).

Electromyography has been proposed as a method of diagnosing inappropriate activity, within the puborectalis or external anal sphincter muscles during straining at stool when the muscles should be relaxing (Turnbull *et al.* 1986). However, inappropriate muscle activity has also been found in some patients with pelvic pain (Jones *et al.* 1987*a*) and in some asymptomatic individuals (Barnes and Lennard-Jones 1988). A recent study using ambulatory electromyographic recordings suggests that laboratory testing overestimates the frequency of the problem (Duthie *et al.* 1991). Defecating proctography allows visualization of the pelvic floor and anorectal movements during the act of defecation. Video recording of the radiological images facilitates assessment of the changes in rectal configuration which occur during evacuation (Figure 13.4). In particular, occult prolapse of the rectum is most easily visualized using this technique (Kuijpers and Strijk 1984). It also allows measurement of the anorectal angle and pelvic floor descent to be made (Mackle *et al.* 1990).

Depending on the normality/abnormality of the colonic transit time and pelvic floor anorectal function, idiopathic constipation may

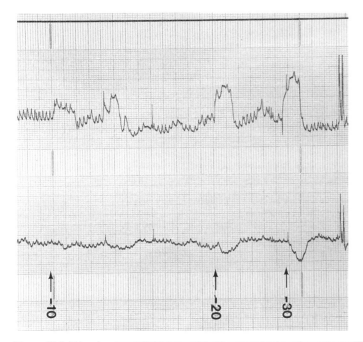

Figure 13.2 Normal recto-anal inhibitory reflex. Upper tracing from the rectum, lower tracing from anal canal. The anal sphincter is seen to relax in response to rectal distension by the volume indicated.

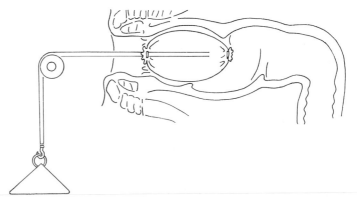

Figure 13.3 Illustration of technique used in balloon expulsion test. If required, weights may be added in 50 g increments.

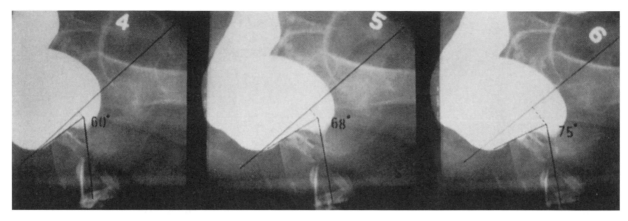

Figure 13.4 Proctogram demonstrating non-relaxing puborectalis. (a) At rest; (b) during contraction; (c) during straining. There is little change in the anorectal angle. From J.M.N. Jorge *et al. Dis. Colon Rectum* 1994; 37: 927–31 courtesy of publishers.

Table 13.2 Treatment of types of constipation

Obstructed defecation	Slow transit Absent	Present
Absent	Conservative* measures	Conservative measures
	Surgery	Suppositories/enemas
Present	Conservative measures	Conservative measures
	Avoid straining	Suppositories/enemas
	Biofeedback	Obstructed defecation measures
	?Psychotherapy	Slow transit surgery

*Conservative measures in the treatment of constipation
  Increase fluid intake
  Increase fibre intake (> 30 g/day)
  Exercise
  Respond to urge to pass stool
  Reassurance

be divided into four groups warranting differing degrees of intervention (Table 13.2).

Patients with normal colonic transit and normal defecation

Patients in this category will often have a variable frequency of defecation, alternating between constipation and diarrhoea. Additional symptoms in keeping with the irritable bowel syndrome such as abdominal distension and pain are not uncommon (Drossman *et al.* 1990*b*). Treatment of such patients rests with conservative measures. These include increasing reassurance, the consumption of fluid, ensuring a daily intake of at least 30 g dietary fibre and laxatives as required (Table 13.2). For long-term usage, bulking agents are preferable but a large part of the efficacy of all laxative agents may be placebo-related (Lasagna *et al.* 1951; Hodgson 1977). Where a history of psychological trauma has been obtained, the involvement of colleagues trained in psychology is appropriate. To date the use of behavioural therapy or psychotherapy have largely been confined to irritable bowel syndrome-type patients (Latimer 1983; Blanchard *et al.* 1988).

Patients with delayed transit but normal defecation

Patients in this group fall into the category of 'colonic inertia'. Despite being regarded as a 'functional' or 'idiopathic' condition,

specific pathophysiological abnormalities can be demonstrated. Those whose symptoms develop before the age of 10 years may have a genetic component to their condition as a specific fingerprint pattern occurs more frequently than in the normal population (Gottlieb and Schuster 1986). Silver staining and immunohistochemistry have revealed that apparently normal axon bundles in the myenteric plexus stain much less than normal or fail to stain at all with the monoclonal antibody suggesting a visceral neuropathy (Krishnamurthy *et al.* 1985; Schouten *et al.* 1993). The peristaltic mass movements responsible for colonic transit are reduced in duration by over 40% and reduced in frequency by almost 60% when compared with controls (Bassotti *et al.* 1988). Gastrointestinal neurotransmitter levels are altered with lowered levels of vasoactive intestinal polypeptide (Milner *et al.* 1990) and elevated serotonin (Lincoln *et al.* 1990).

Treatment of these patients like those with normal transit rates begins with conservative measures. Where these fail, a more aggressive use of rectally delivered laxatives may help to keep the bowel empty. Bisacodyl suppositories may be effective or it may be necessary to resort to disposable phosphate enemas to achieve evacuation. Studies have shown cisapride, the prokinetic agent, when taken orally to be effective in some cases of slow transit constipation, increasing stool frequency, and reducing laxative usage (Hernandez *et al.* 1988). Only when all medical therapy has failed and the symptoms dominate the patient's life should surgery be considered (Kamm *et al.* 1988*a*). The possibility of any underlying psychosocial factor to explain the constipation should again be explored. Full investigation must be performed to ensure that there is slow colonic transit, that there is no anorectal dysfunction and no other organic cause for the constipation.

Only when these conditions are met should surgery be contemplated. The operation of choice is colectomy and ileorectal anastomosis which nowadays may be associated with a mortality rate of 1–2%. This operation was first carried out in 1908 with an 80% success rate (Lane 1908). More up-to-date series have reported very similar outcomes (Vasilevsky *et al.* 1988; Yoshioka and Keighley 1989). In addition to those whose constipation fails to improve as many as 22% may experience diarrhoea, 11% faecal incontinence, and 24% develop small bowel obstruction (Devroede 1993). In view of these complications, priority must be given to identify and exclude patients with outlet obstruction in an effort to predict those who can expect a good response to surgery. One recent series of appropriately assessed patients reported a 100% success rate with no incontinence but 11% of patients developed a small bowel obstruction (Pemberton *et al.* 1991). Other operations such as limited colonic resection (Fasth *et al.* 1983; Todd 1985) and anorectal myomectomy yield unacceptably poor results (Pinho *et al.* 1990).

In a small series of 13 patients who had had previous colonic resection and whose constipation persisted, proctectomy and ileal pouch anastomosis was undertaken. This procedure was associated with an 85% complication rate in this group, a mean frequency of defecation of 4.8 times during the day and 1.2 times during the night, and half the patients had night-time soiling. Two patients ultimately had to have the pouches excised and ileostomies established (Hosie *et al.* 1990).

Patients with obstructed defecation and normal colonic transit

In 1985, Preston and Lennard-Jones reported that many patients with severe constipation were unable to relax the pelvic floor muscles appropriately. Using EMG they demonstrated a paradoxical increase in puborectalis and external anal sphincter activity instead of the expected inhibition of motor activity during straining (Preston *et al.* 1985). They referred to this condition as anismus. Other studies have questioned the specificity of this condition, identifying it in 33% of patients with pelvic pain but no difficulty in defacation (Jones *et al.* 1987a). As the initial description of anismus, a number of tests have been used to facilitate in making a diagnosis (Wexner *et al.* 1992; Jorge *et al.* 1993). These tests include anorectal manometry, balloon expulsion studies, defecating proctography, and EMG. Difficulties and confusion have arisen when investigators sought to use any one specific test as diagnostic (Thirlby 1992; Duthie and Bartolo 1992). As argued by Pemberton, it is the interpretation of the combination of tests by an experienced clinician that is important (Pemberton 1992). This approach is supported by the good results from surgery in appropriately selected patients with constipation (Pemberton *et al.* 1991).

In treating patients with anismus, initial management again involves conservative measures with the additional advice that patients should avoid straining at stool. In the past, surgical division of puborectalis and the external anal sphincter muscles, or anorectal myectomy was attempted (Wallace and Madden 1969; Barnes *et al.* 1985; Kuijpers *et al.* 1986; Kamm *et al.* 1988b; Pinho *et al.* 1989). Injection of botulinum toxin into the puborectalis to cause partial paralysis in cases of anismus with intractable constipation has also been tried (Hallan *et al.* 1988). All these interventions carry a significant risk of faecal incontinence and are generally not recommended. Biofeedback relaxation techniques have been applied to this condition with initial success rate ranging from 56% to 80% but unfortunately the improvement is not always maintained. However, this is now the management of choice for anismus is a number of centres especially as surgery has little to offer these patients. Results of biofeedback retraining in children are disappointing in the long-term with only about one-third of patients continuing to benefit at 2-year follow-up (Kawimbe *et al.* 1991; Lestar *et al.* 1991; Wexner *et al.* 1991; Loening-Baucke 1996).

Patients with obstructed defecation and abnormal colonic transit

These patients should have their obstructed defecation treated and preferably cured before surgery for delayed transit is considered (Fasth *et al.* 1983; Heine *et al.* 1993). One group debates this approach and advocate performing the surgery required for slow transit constipation regardless of the presence of anismus (Duthie and Bartolo 1992).

Summary

Constipation is a common problem. The vast majority of sufferers manage the condition themselves. Those presenting to hospital for assessment represent only the tip of the iceberg. In one recent study of 277 such patients, only 15% were deemed suitable for surgery (Todd 1985). However, while a surgical solution is applicable only to the minority, appropriate use of general measures and medication may benefit the majority with biofeedback being reserved for a selected group.

Idiopathic megarectum and megacolon

The combination of constipation with a dilated colon must be differentiated from constipation in the presence of a normal diameter colon (idiopathic constipation). When the colon is dilated, assessment of the rest of the intestinal tract by small bowel series must be performed to exclude chronic idiopathic intestinal pseudo-obstruction. If the disease is confined to the large bowel, Hirschsprung's disease, and other causes of secondary dilatation such as Chagas' disease, hypothyroidism, or systemic sclerosis must be excluded. The remainder of patients with a dilated large bowel are diagnosed as having idiopathic megarectum and megacolon.

The aetiology of the condition is unknown. It may appear at birth, in childhood or in adulthood (Barnes *et al.* 1986). Histological examination of both nerves and muscle is normal (Stabile and Kamm 1991).

Clinical features

Idiopathic megarectum and megacolon is predominantly a disease of young people, the average age of patients coming to surgery being 19–40 years (Stabile *et al.* 1991, 1992a, b). Males and females are affected equally and a quarter of patients have some degree of mental handicap (Lane and Todd 1977; Kamm and Stabile 1991). Presenting clinical features are typically constipation (100%), laxative usage (90%), and abdominal pain (80–90%). Features of obstructed defecation are present in half the patients and up to 60% may have faecal incontinence.

Diagnosis is arbitrarily made when the rectal diameter is greater than 6.5 cm at the pelvic brim on lateral X-ray (Wexner *et al.* 1992). Further investigation involves a barium enema (Figure 13.5) to determine the approximate extent of the dilatation, a small bowel series to exclude generalized gastrointestinal dilatation in keeping with chronic idiopathic intestinal pseudo-obstruction and anal manometry/rectal biopsy to exclude Hirschsprung's disease.

Treatment

The majority of patients can be managed by conservative measures. Oral lactulose in sufficient quantity combined with an adequate fluid intake may be all that is required to prevent faecal impaction. Other patients whose constipation is obstinate may require enemas on a regular basis. Approximately half of those referred to a surgical clinic because of the condition will have a successful outcome with these measures (Lane and Todd 1977). When these measures fail

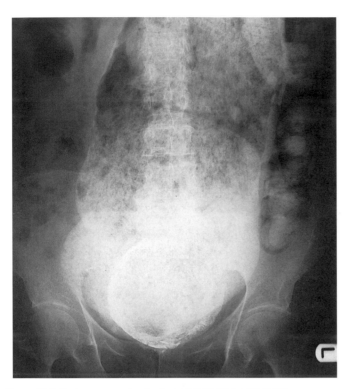

Figure 13.5 Barium enema showing huge faecaloma in patient with megarectum and megacolon.

and the patient's quality of life is poor, surgery may be contemplated. The options open to the surgeon include local sigmoid resection, partial colectomy and colo-anal anastomosis, colectomy and ileorectal anastomosis, colectomy and restorative procedures, e.g. the Duhamel procedure, and finally stoma formation. The Duhamel technique, originally described for Hirschprung's disease, involves resecting the upper rectum and dilated portion of colon, and bringing normal colon down retrorectally to anastomose to the posterior wall at the junction of the rectum with the anal canal. The posterior rectal wall and anterior colonic wall higher up are divided and sutured together either manually or by a linear stapler to enlarge the cavity (Duhamel 1964) (Figure 13.6). The currently recommended operation of choice for those with a rectum that is not grossly distended is colectomy and ileorectal anastomosis (Stabile and Kamm

1991; Stabile *et al.* 1991). However, it must be borne in mind that even from among advocates of the operation, the reported incidence of faecal incontinence is higher than for other operative procedures (Stabile *et al.* 1991). When the rectum is too dilated to be anastomosed to bowel of normal calibre, the Duhamel procedure is a reasonable but less successful alternative (Stabile and Kamm 1991). If previous surgery has been unsuccessful and the patient is willing to contemplate a stoma then either colostomy or ileostomy may be the best long-term acceptable option (Stabile *et al.* 1992*a*).

For all these operations it is important to emphasize to the patient that although the surgery may improve bowel frequency and reduce the need for laxatives, its effect on abdominal pain and distension is less certain. Such counselling may avoid unsatisfactory surgical results and disenchanted patients (Stabile *et al.* 1991).

Pelvic floor disorders

The individual disorders discussed in this section, solitary rectal ulcer syndrome, rectal prolapse, and faecal incontinence, are all well recognized and documented entities. However, in many patients, the pathophysiology underlying their presentation is poorly understood (Mackle and Parks 1986). The present incomplete knowledge of these conditions has led to speculation over links between them (du Boulay *et al.* 1983). The common finding of a solitary rectal ulcer with either mucosal prolapse, rectal intussusception, or rectal prolapse does point to some degree of association (Mackle *et al.* 1990; Binnie *et al.* 1992). One proposed unifying mechanism is outlined below. The suggested initiating problem is that of difficulty in defecation leading to excessive straining at stool. The obstructed defecation may relate to inappropriate contraction of either the puborectalis muscle (Rutter and Riddell 1975; Lane 1975; Snooks *et al.* 1985*b*), the external sphincter (Barnes and Lennard-Jones 1988; Kuijpers and Bleijenberg 1985), or both (Womack *et al.* 1987). As a result of straining, rectal prolapse (either mucosal or complete) may occur. Mucosal prolapse, especially of the anterior rectal wall, often precedes rectal intussusception and complete rectal prolapse (Broden and Snellman 1968; Allen-Mersh *et al.* 1987). In addition to straining, other factors are believed to be important in the development of prolapse. Excessive perineal descent may be obvious clinically (Figure 13.7). It may be measured using a perineometer as

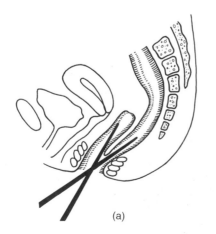
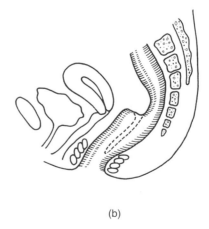

(a)   (b)

Figure 13.6 Diagram illustrating the Duhamel procedure.

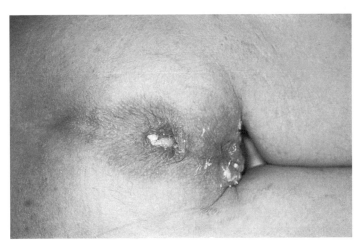

Figure 13.7 Descending perineum syndrome with patient straining in left lateral position.

illustrated in Figure 13.8. Excessive perineal descent leads to effacement of the anorectal angle favouring of anterior mucosal prolapse (Parks *et al.* 1966). This in turn has been found to be a manifestation of pudendal nerve damage due to stretching nerve damage and muscle weakness (Jones *et al.* 1987*b*), often on a basis of prolonged constipation (Kiff *et al.* 1984) or vaginal delivery (Snooks *et al.* 1984).

Some degree of prolapse is demonstrated in up to 100% of patients with solitary rectal ulcer syndrome in some series (Binnie *et al.* 1992). However, prolapse by itself is not sufficient to explain the occurrence of ulceration as the majority of patients with rectal prolapse do not develop ulceration (Lam *et al.* 1992). Various additional factors have been suggested for the progression from prolapse to the mucosal changes of solitary rectal ulceration. These include prolapse on to the inappropriately contracting puborectalis or external anal sphincter muscles (Rutter 1974; Rutter and Riddell 1975), a marked perineal descent (Snooks *et al.* 1985*b*; Mackle *et al.* 1990), and a high rectal voiding pressure compressing the mucosa and resulting in venous congestion and damage (Womack *et al.* 1987). One follow-up study of 250 patients with mucosal prolapse has demonstrated progression in some patients to both solitary rectal ulcer and complete rectal prolapse. The risk of developing perineal descent within 5 years of presentation was less than 10%. However, those

who already had perineal descent had a 30% chance of developing sphincter laxity during a 5-year period. Complete rectal prolapse occurred in three of 15 (20%) patients with clinical perineal descent and lax sphincters but was not encountered in the absence of these signs (Allen-Mersh *et al.* 1987).

Solitary rectal ulcer syndrome

Interest in the condition known as the solitary rectal ulcer syndrome can be traced back to Madigan 30 years ago (Madigan 1964). However, in 1842, Cruveilheir described four cases of chronic ulceration of the rectum which probably represent the first report of this condition (Cruveiheir 1842). It is predominantly a disease of youth and middle-age, 80% presenting before the age of 50 years with an approximately equal sex distribution, although in some series a somewhat higher proportion of females were affected (Devroede and Soffie 1973; Martin *et al.* 1981; Tjandra *et al.* 1992).

The condition is inappropriately named considering a solitary ulcer is only found in approximately 40% of patients, a further 20% having multiple ulcers. The remainder have polypoid lesions or oedematous, hyperaemic mucosa (Martin *et al.* 1981). Biopsy of the lesion, or the adjacent tissue if frank ulceration is present, reveals typical histological changes (Bogomoletz 1992). The early findings are those of hypertrophy of the muscularis mucosae, fibromuscular obliteration of the lamina propria, and crypt hyperplasia (Figure 13.9). Progression to the ulcerative stage will reveal superficial erosions, ulceration, fibrosis, haemorrhage, and deep cyst formation. The cyst formation is due to mucus-secreting columnar epithelium migrating into the submucosa. The histological patterns encountered have led in the past to the use of the various synonyms for solitary rectal ulcer syndrome such as localized colitis cystica profunda and hamartomatous inverted polyp (Epstein *et al.* 1966).

Clinical features

The majority of patients present with a history of passing bright red blood or mucus per rectum and of an alteration in bowel habit (Binnie *et al.* 1992; Tjandra *et al.* 1992). On questioning, almost all will admit to difficulty in defecation (Mackle *et al.* 1990; Binnie *et al.* 1992).

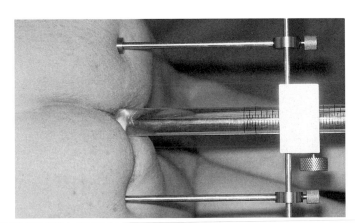

Figure 13.8 Clinical measurement of perineal descent using a perineometer. The feet of the horizontal limbs are placed over the ischial tuberosities. Movement of the graduated central perspex rod is measured while straining.

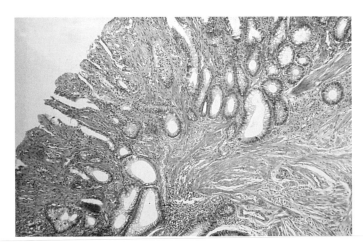

Figure 13.9 Photomicrograph of solitary rectal ulcer syndrome showing hypertrophy of the muscularis mucosae and streaming of fibromuscular tissue between the crypts. H&E×100.

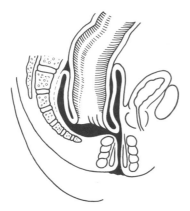

Figure 13.10 Diagrammatic representation of how the mucosa may be traumatised during mid-rectal intussusception.

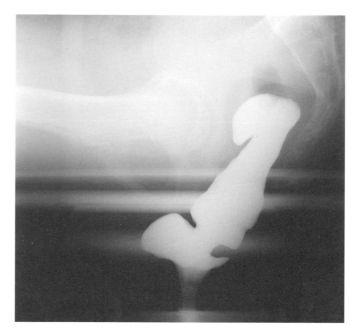

Figure 13.12 Proctogram showing gross perineal descent, increased anorectal angle and rectal intussusception.

Examination of the perineum, especially on straining, may sometimes demonstrate complete rectal prolapse. During digital examination of the rectum it may be possible to feel a flap of mucosal prolapse. The leading edge of mid-rectal intussusception may be traumatized by the contracting sphincter mechanism and be a factor in the causation of the solitary rectal ulcer syndrome (Figure 13.10). At proctoscopy/sigmoidoscopy, the lesion is anterior or anterolateral in over 75% of cases (Tjandra *et al.* 1992). The macroscopic appearance maybe that of well circumscribed superficial ulceration with surrounding proctitis, granular and hyperaemic mucosa without ulceration or polypoid lesions (Figure 13.11).

Further specialized tests may be carried out, especially if surgery is contemplated. Investigation is directed towards delineating the extent of rectal intussusception. The most effective means of demonstrating this is by defecating proctogram (Figure 13.12).

Treatment

The initial management of patients with solitary rectal ulceration is conservative. The general measures applied in the treatment of constipation (Table 13.2) along with the avoidance of straining at stool should be recommended. Further treatment may then be aimed at the local lesion or the supposed underlying problem. Various topical agents have been used in the past with little success, for example, corticosteroids, carbenoxolone (Madigan and Morson 1969) and sul-

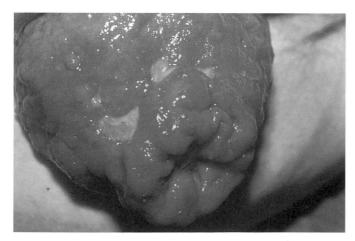

Figure 13.11 Prolapsing rectum with discrete, well demarcated areas of solitary rectal ulceration.

phasalazine (Kennedy *et al.* 1977). More recently, claims have been made for symptomatic improvement from the use of sucralfate retention enemas in six patients, at least in the short term (Zargar *et al.* 1991). Macroscopic appearances also improved but histological abnormalities were not appreciably altered. The application of a human fibrin sealant (Ederle *et al.* 1992) has also been advocated on the premise that it stimulates fibroblast and vascular proliferation with tissue regeneration in addition to its haemostatic and sealing effect (Ederle *et al.* 1992). Solitary rectal ulcers in six patients treated with fibrin sealant were said to heal within 14 days and remain healed at 1 year, although the typical histological findings of the syndrome persisted. Local surgical treatment of the lesion, generally by excision has met with limited success (Tjandra *et al.* 1992) and is not generally recommended (Lam *et al.* 1992).

In view of the fact that a solitary rectal ulcer is not infrequently associated with either occult mid-rectal intussusception or overt rectal prolapse a modified form of abdominal rectopexy has been advocated whereby both the anterior and posterior aspects of the rectum are given support. Of 14 patients with the solitary rectal ulcer syndrome without overt rectal prolapse symptomatic improvement was achieved in 12 instances with respect to tenesmus, bleeding, and passage of mucus (Nicholls and Simson 1986).

In the wider treatment of the condition, anteroposterior rectopexy has been advocated for ulceration associated with internal intussusception (Nicholls and Simson 1986; Costalat *et al.* 1990). However, the results of surgery are not uniformly good. Other surgical techniques have included the Ripstein procedure (Ihre and Selison 1975), posterior rectopexy, anterior resection (Cruveiheir 1842) and diversion (Tjandra *et al.* 1992) with variable and sometimes disappointing outcome. Based on the common association with obstructed defecation, biofeedback techniques have been used either alone or in conjunction with surgery. 'Anismus', i.e. anorectal outlet obstruction due to inappropriate contraction of the puborectalis muscle has been successfully treated in some cases by EMG biofeedback. Binnie and colleagues reported that among 17 patients with solitary rectal ulceration treated by biofeedback there was a total of four recurrences compared with 15 episodes of recurrence in 14 patients in the non-biofeedback group (Binnie *et al.* 1992).

Even in the studies which demonstrated macroscopic ulcer healing, other histological findings persisted, suggesting that the underlying pathological mechanism had been unaffected (Zargar *et al.* 1991; Ederle *et al.* 1992). In a group of 80 cases of solitary rectal ulceration managed at the Cleveland Clinic, Ohio, there were 21 patients who were asymptomatic and in whom incidental diagnosis was made (Tjandra *et al.* 1992). These patients were managed expectantly with or without dietary advice and bulk laxatives. They remained asymptomatic during the follow-up period.

Rectal prolapse

Rectal prolapse may be complete, involving the full thickness of the rectum, or partial, involving only the mucosa and submucosa. Prolapse may be overt, appearing through the anus or concealed, being confined to the intussusception of the mid-rectum into the lower rectum/anal canal.

Rectal prolapse may present at any age but tends to occur more often at the extremes of life. In childhood rectal prolapse which tends to be related to constipation and straining at stool is usually confined to the mucosa. Occasionally, children develop a complete prolapse and in this instance cystic fibrosis should be excluded.

In adults, mucosal prolapse may present in the third and fourth decade, associated with haemorrhoids and other pelvic floor disorders. By contrast, complete prolapse is usually a disease of middle-aged to elderly females, reportedly affecting women six times more commonly than men (Kupfer and Goligher 1970; Rutter and Riddell 1975; Schrock 1993).

While controversy still exists concerning the pathogenesis of rectal prolapse, attention has focused on two main mechanisms, namely: (i) sliding herniation and (ii) rectal intussusception (Figure 13.10). In fact, it may be that both mechanisms are involved. Numerous factors have been considered to be relevant in the aetiology of rectal prolapse and these include, raised intra-abdominal and intrapelvic pressure as a consequence of poor bowel habit or chronic cough, redundancy of the rectosigmoid colon, deep peritoneal pelvic pouch, long mesorectum or poor fascial attachment of the rectum to surrounding structures, pelvic floor defect with separation of levator muscles, weak external sphincter muscles, obstetric injuries, and neurological disease. While it is evident that patients with complete rectal prolapse have a pelvic floor defect and stretched anal musculature it may be unclear whether these abnormalities are the cause or the effect of the prolapse.

Clinical features

Patients with complete rectal prolapse typically complain of a mass protruding through the anus on defecation (Figure 13.11). In the early stages it may reduce spontaneously but later may require manual replacement. On questioning, 40% of patients have some degree of incontinence for solid stool and 60% will also admit to incontinence for liquid stool or flatus (Penfold and Hawley 1972). Other symptoms include mucus discharge and bleeding due to trauma to the mucosa.

On inspection of the anus it may appear patulous (Figure 13.13) with evidence of soiling on the perineum. There may be no evidence of a prolapse even after requesting the patient to strain, espe-

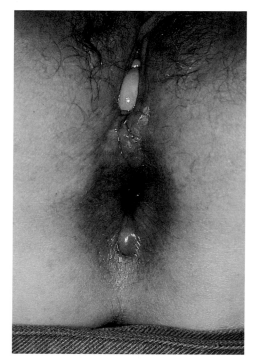

Figure 13.13 Patulous anus in a patient suffering from prolapse of rectum.

cially if the patient is in the left lateral position on the examination couch. It may take several minutes for the prolapse to appear, even in the squatting position. Rectal examination reveals poor anal tone with a defective squeeze pressure. When overt prolapse is not demonstrable, it may be possible to feel the flap of concealed mucosal prolapse between two fingers inserted through a patulous anus. Sigmoidoscopy may be normal or may reveal mild proctitis related to the movement of the prolapse. However, if during sigmoidoscopy the patient is asked to strain down, the rectal wall may bulge into the end of the scope and tend to follow it downwards as the instrument is withdrawn.

Treatment

In children, prolapse responds well to relief of constipation and adequate training of bowel habit. The condition tends to be self-limiting in children and usually resolves as the child grows and the sacral concavity develops. If the use of stool softeners and strapping of the buttocks prove inadequate then injection sclerotherapy is advised. Sclerosis may be achieved using 70% alcohol or 5% phenol in oil. Over 80% cure rate can be achieved by one therapeutic session and the remainder are usually controlled by repeated injections. Using a technique of linear cautery of the anorectum a success rate of 97% was reached by Hight *et al.* (1982).

In adults with mucosal prolapse, attention to consistency of stools and avoidance of straining need to be stressed. For further treatment a number of options are available. Rubber band ligation or injection sclerotherapy will lead to symptomatic improvement in three-quarters of the patients. Where there is considerable mucosal redundancy this may be dealt with satisfactorily by mucosal haemorrhoidectomy. However, if in an elderly patient the sphincter tone is deficient the result of surgical intervention may be suboptimal in terms of continence even though the prolapse has been corrected.

Once complete prolapse has occurred, conservative measures on their own will not resolve the problem. Although surgery does offer the opportunity for curing the condition, the age and frailty of many of these patients must be borne in mind when considering the many surgical options. More than 200 different operations have been tried for the treatment of this condition indicating that there is no ideal solution (Kuijpers 1992). In determining which treatment is most appropriate for the individual patient, factors to be considered must include: (i) its success/relapse rate; (ii) its side-effects, such as constipation; and (iii) the operative risk inherent in the procedure.

Perineal approach

The Délorme's operation although described in 1900 has gained increasing popularity recently particularly as it avoids abdominal

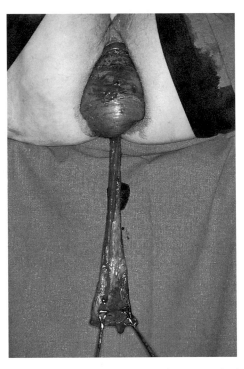

Figure 13.14 Delorme's operation. The long tube of mucosa and submucosa has been stripped from the prolapsed rectal muscle.

surgery and has a distinct appeal for the elderly and frail (Délorme 1900; Monson et al. 1986). In this procedure a long tube of redundant rectal mucosa is stripped from the underlying bowel wall (Figure 13.14), the muscle is plicated and the mobilized mucosa excised (Figure 13.15). The prolapsed rectum is then returned to the pelvis, the previously placed sutures are tightened to bunch up the muscle and achieve mucosa to mucosa approximation. Finally, each interrupted suture is tied intraluminally. Morbidity and mortality rates are extremely low. In fact the mortality has been zero in several sizeable series. Although recurrence has been reported in up to one-quarter of patients an overall relapse rate of the order of 5–15% over the next 2–10 years is more likely (Swinton and Palmer 1960). Should failure occur a repeat Délorme's procedure can be undertaken without difficulty. Other perineal operations using encircling materials such as wire, nylon, or sialastic rings to control complete prolapse have now been largely abandoned on account of the high risk of relapse and of complications related to the procedures (Wassef et al. 1986; Dietzen and Pemberton 1989; Sainio et al. 1991).

Abdominal approach

The gold standard in terms of curing rectal prolapse is abdominal rectopexy (with or without sigmoid resection) (Keighley et al. 1983). Different suspension-fixation types of procedure have their advocates. In Great Britain and Ireland abdominal posterior rectopexy using polyvinyl alcohol sponge (Ivalon) is widely practised (Figure 13.16a). The mortality rate is less than 1%, operative morbidity is low, and recurrent prolapse rate is approximately 3% overall (Wassef et al. 1986). The major drawback is the high incidence of constipation following surgery which occurs in approximately one-third of patients (Penfold and Hawley 1972; Holmstrom et al. 1986; Mann and Hoffman 1988; McCue and Thomson 1991; Pemberton et al. 1991; Tjandra et al. 1993). This would appear to relate to perirectal fibrosis and impaired contractility in the fixed rectum (Siproudhis et al. 1993).

Anterior rectopexy (Ripstein) whereby a sling of synthetic material is passed around the front and sides of the rectum and is fixed to the sacrum posteriorly (Figure 13.16b) may also lead to constipation and is even more liable to cause constriction and obstruction than

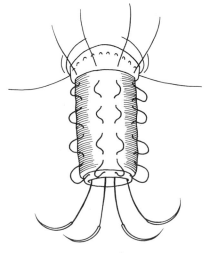

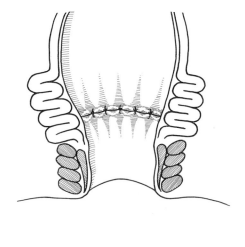

Figure 13.15 Delorme's operation. (a) Interrupted plication sutures are inserted and left untied; (b) the prolapse is reduced, sutures are tightened to concertina the muscle and approximate mucosa to mucosa. Finally, the sutures are tied intraluminally.

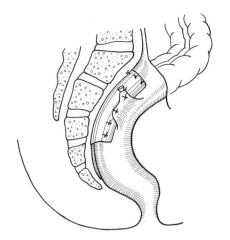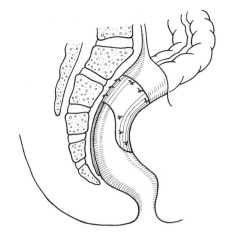

Figure 13.16 Diagram illustrating abdominal rectopexy. (a) Ivalon sponge (polyvinyl alcohol) procedure; (b) anterior (Ripstein) rectopexy.

posterior rectopexy. The recurrence rate is comparable to the Ivalon sponge procedure. Recently, there has been a trend to avoid the use of synthetic mesh and fix the mesorectum to the presacral fascia by direct suture in an effort to reduce the incidence of constipation and other complications.

Other surgeons have advocated a policy of sigmoid colectomy with anastomosis of the descending colon to the upper rectum (Frykman and Goldberg 1969; Deen *et al.* 1994). This procedure does add to the risk of operative complications because a colorectal anastomosis has been made (Kuijpers 1992). However, results from this procedure have been good and it is reasonable to consider resection plus sutured rectopexy in young fit patients suffering from slow transit constipation. Where the operations have been undertaken in well selected cases in dedicated units the mortality has been about 1–2% and better functional results have been achieved. Recurrence rates range from 0 to 4% with a mean of about 2%. In older patients and particularly if there is a tendency to loose motions, post resection incontinence may become more problematic because of poor anal tone in this age group.

In a controlled trial in which abdominal resection rectopexy (with pelvic floor repair) was compared to perineal rectosigmoidectomy (with pelvic floor repair) the results of the former procedure were superior both physiologically and functionally. In particular the authors emphasized the importance of preserving the anorectal reservoir (Deen *et al.* 1994).

In the past few years abdominal laparoscopic procedures have emerged as a surgical option in the treatment of complete rectal prolapse. Minimally invasive techniques have been used to achieve fixation of the rectum to the sacrum either by direct suture or by using Marlex or Teflon mesh. Even resection rectopexy can be undertaken laparoscopically. These techniques may well play a greater part in the future but it will take several years before it is clear how they compare with well established techniques in terms of mortality, morbidity, and functional outcome.

Faecal incontinence

Continence requires the complex interaction of sensory and motor neurones and muscle groups. The chief muscles responsible for control of defecation are the internal anal sphincter (IAS), the external anal sphincter (EAS), and puborectalis. The IAS is largely responsible for the resting anal tone and is under autonomic control (Frenckner and Euler 1975; Schweiger 1979; Lestar *et al.* 1989). Analogous to the lower oesophageal sphincter, both low basal tone and spontaneous relaxation are causes of incontinence (Sun *et al.* 1989, 1990). When the IAS relaxes the EAS, which is under voluntary control, contracts to preserve continence. However, the striated muscle fatigues readily and maximal voluntary contraction can only be maintained for less than a minute (Schuster *et al.* 1965). Puborectalis acts together with the EAS for the preservation of continence (Shafik 1975). It has been hypothesized that one of its main actions is to preserve an acute angle between the rectum and anus, possibly tending to occlude the lumen by a flap valve mechanism (Parks *et al.* 1966). Although the flap valve theory is now in doubt, the importance of the puborectalis muscle remains (Bartolo *et al.* 1986).

The recto-anal sensory mechanism is another element in the preservation of continence. Reduced sensation in the rectum has been noted in patients with idiopathic incontinence (Lubowski and Nicholls 1988). It also contributes to the incontinence noted in patients with reduced levels of consciousness or diabetes (Wald and Tunuguntla 1984).

During the reflex relaxation of the IAS in response to rectal distension, the upper anal canal is exposed to rectal contents (Duthie and Bennett 1963). The rich innervation of this area may be important in discriminating between faeces and flatus. This 'sampling' is absent in a significant number of incontinent patients (Miller *et al.* 1988).

Other factors contributing to the maintenance of continence include the intraluminal volume of liquid stool, the rectal capacity, and the rectal compliance, which may be relevant, for example, in inflammatory bowel disease incontinence (Rao *et al.* 1987).

Aetiology (Table 13.3)

Copious diarrhoea, regardless of the origin may result in incontinence. In the elderly, faecal impaction with overflow incontinence may be the chief mechanism, especially in the institutionalized patient (Barrett *et al.* 1989; Romero *et al.* 1996).

Abnormalities of the nervous system, regardless of the level, may cause incontinence. In diabetes, the incontinence stems from a combination of sensory and motor neuropathy which may involve both

Table 13.3 Causes of faecal incontinence

Diarrhoea	Faecal impaction with overflow
Neurological	Dementia/cardiovascular accident
	Multiple sclerosis
	Neoplasms of the central nervous system
	Trauma to the central nervous system
	Neuropathy, e.g. diabetes
Abnormal rectum	Inflammatory bowel disease
	Rectal surgery
	Neoplasms
Direct sphincter damage	Accidental trauma
	Obstetric injury
	Anorectal surgery
Local nerve damage	Vaginal delivery
	Chronic straining
	Pelvic floor disorder

Table 13.4 History taking in faecal incontinence

Severity	to flatus/liquid/solid
	frequency
	use of pads
	life-style alteration
	previous anorectal surgery
Medical history	change in bowel habit
	associated diseases (e.g. diabetes)
	medication
	anorectal surgery
Obstetric history	vaginal delivery
	prolonged labour
	assisted labour
	episiotomy/tear

Table 13.5 Physical examination in faecal incontinence

Perineal inspection	Soiling
	Episiotomy scar
	Fistula/fistula scars
	Lax anus
	Prolapse
Rectal examination	Resting and squeeze tone
	Masses
	Faecal 'boulders'
Proctosigmoidoscopy	Haemorrhoids
	Proctitis
	Solitary rectal ulcer
	Neoplasia

autonomic and somatic components. In addition to this, the diarrhoea that such patients tend to experience adds to the difficulties in maintaining continence.

A relatively common surgically correctable cause for faecal incontinence is a localized sphincter defect resulting from trauma, obstetric manipulation or previous surgical procedure (Stricker *et al.* 1988). The surgical procedures most often associated with faecal incontinence are those for the treatment of anal fistula. However, incontinence has also been reported after poorly executed haemorrhoidectomy (Read *et al.* 1982) or manual anal dilatation (MacIntyre and Balfour 1972). In this latter instance repair procedures have little to offer in view of the diffuse nature of the lesion and hence the Lord procedure of manual anal dilatation is best avoided. Vaginal delivery may result in faecal incontinence due to a combination of both direct sphincter damage and nerve injury (Snooks *et al.* 1985*a*).

Rectal prolapse results in faecal incontinence in two-thirds of patients, and for reasons discussed in the section on pelvic floor disorders, pudendal nerve damage as well as dilatation of the anal sphincteric musculature resulting from the repeatedly prolapsing rectum are aetiologically important. After correction of the prolapse by operation the tone in the sphincters will generally improve because stretching of the sphincters and reflex inhibition of the sphincteric mechanism by the descending rectum are no longer occurring.

Clinical features

The chief aspects of history taking in faecal incontinence are listed in Table 13.4. In particular it is important to establish the severity of the incontinence and the impact it is having on the individual's life-style. A full physical examination must include examination of the rectum, both digitally and sigmoidoscopically. Examination may provide a clue to the aetiology of the condition (Table 13.5).

Investigation

Where there is an unexplained change in bowel habit or additional colonic symptoms, such as the passage of altered blood, colonoscopy or barium enema is indicated. Anorectal manometry assesses anal tone both at rest and during maximal squeeze. Both of these parameters are reduced in incontinent patients (Felt-Bersma *et al.* 1990). Approximately 85% of the resting tone is contributed by the inter-

nal anal sphincter and manometric studies reveal that two-thirds of patients with idiopathic faecal incontinence have reduced resting anal canal pressure. Use of unidirectional sensors or water-perfused ports facilitates the mapping of a sphincter profile (Perry *et al.* 1990). Sensation both in the rectum and at the anal margin may be assessed. By inflating a balloon in the rectum an assessment is made of the volume required to induce sensation. This volume is higher in patients with incontinence (Lubowski and Nicholls 1988). Rectal sensation may also be assessed by determining the magnitude of electric current applied to the mucosa that is required before being felt by the patient (Rogers 1992). However, temperature sensation may well be the key mechanism to discriminating faeces from flatus. It is abnormal in incontinent patients (Miller *et al.* 1987). Electromyography can help to identify the position of the deficit in the sphincter mechanism. Smooth muscle activity can be measured using either surface electrodes in the anal canal or bipolar fine hooked wire electrodes inserted directly into the muscle from the perineum. Electromyography may also highlight the sphincter reinnervation typically seen in pelvic neuropathy (Bartolo *et al.* 1983). Pudendal nerve terminal motor latency may be measured using a glove-mounted electrode passed via the anal canal (Figures 13.17 and 13.18). The St Mark's disposable transrectal pudendal nerve stimulating device consists of two stimulating electrodes near the tip. Localization of the stimulus is improved by having the cathode of the stimulating electrode smaller than the anode. Two recording electrodes are sited 3–4 cm more proximally to detect the evoked contraction of the external anal sphincter muscles. Pudendal nerve

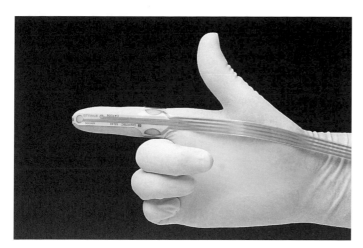

Figure 13.17 St Mark's disposable transrectal pudendal electrode, manufactured by Dantec Electronics, Denmark.

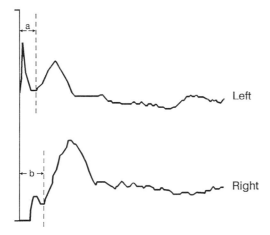

Figure 13.18 Assessment of pudendal nerve terminal motor latency. The latent period between nerve stimulation and electromechanical response of anal sphincter is recorded using an oscilloscope. (a) Left pudendal nerve—2.8 ms; (b) right pudendal nerve 3.5 ms (normal value—up to 2.2 ms).

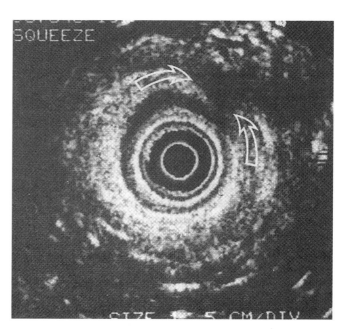

Figure 13.19 Ultrasound of anal sphincter demonstrating an anterior muscle defect. From A.H. Sultan *et al. N. Engl. J. Med.* 1993; 329: 1905–11, courtesy of publishers.

terminal motor latency is the best predictor as to whether or not a good outcome will be achieved after sphincter repair (Wexner *et al.* 1991).

Defecating proctography has been described earlier, static and dynamic residual images contributing most to the assessment. Anal ultrasound is increasingly being used to locate sphincter defects and correlates well with EMG results (Cuesta *et al.* 1992) (Figure 13.19).

Treatment

Management must be tailored to the individual, taking into account the severity of the incontinence and its attendant social disability, the nature of the cause, and the general health/frailty of the patient.

Conservative measures are sufficient to provide an acceptable lifestyle for many patients. Such measures include the use of bulking agents and antidiarrhoeal medication such as loperamide. Underlying faecal impaction must also be treated. For the young, fit patient with neurological faecal incontinence, e.g. spina bifida or spinal trauma, antidiarrhoeal agents can be used to help achieve as near normal social function as possible during the day, with laxa-

tives and enemas used once or twice a week in the evening to avoid faecal impaction.

Biofeedback training is of considerable benefit for selected patients in whom conservative therapy is insufficient (Figure 13.20). While biofeedback proved to be disappointing in the treatment of constipation associated with paradoxical external sphincter contraction it helped 73% of patients with incontinence and its use was recommended regardless of the causes or severity of the incontinence or the findings on anorectal manometry. Best results are obtained in the motivated, intelligent patient with some degree of rectal sensation and the ability to contract the EAS voluntarily (Madoff *et al.* 1992). The technique involves training the patient to perceive ever decreasing sizes of balloons inflated in the rectum. In addition to enhancing their perception, the patient is also taught to contract the EAS voluntarily in response to the distension. A visual

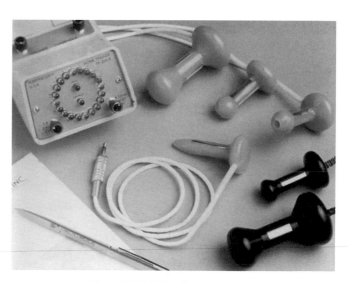

Figure 13.20 Biofeedback apparatus.

representation of the EAS contraction, usually detected by an anal plug electrode, is watched by the patient on a monitor and training is undertaken to reinforce the correct muscle action. Successful treatment, measured by a 90% reduction in the episodes of incontinence, has been reported in two-thirds of cases (MacLeod 1987).

Surgical treatment

Where there is evidence of a defect in the sphincter mechanism, the operation of choice is direct repair of the overlapped mobilized ends. An acceptable degree of continence is achieved in 80–90% of patients (Miller *et al.* 1989; Fleshman *et al.* 1991). A recent study suggests that end to end suturing with preservation of fibrous tissue at both ends may be equally effective (Arnaud *et al.* 1991). Where there is associated pudendal nerve damage, the outcome is poor (Laurberg *et al.* 1988).

Obstetric tears should be repaired immediately post-partum. Where this fails, a second attempt may be delayed for 3 months or performed straight away (Christiansen 1992). In the absence of an anatomical defect in the sphincter, surgical management of faecal incontinence is less straightforward. Depending on the circumstances some of the surgical options listed in Table 13.6 may be applicable to an individual patient. The post-anal repair, which involves plicating the levator ani, puborectalis and EAS muscles posteriorly, was designed to address this issue (Parks 1975). Although theoretically designed to increase the anorectal angle, im-

Table 13.6 Surgical techniques used in management of faecal incontinence

Overlapping anterior anal sphincter repair
Post anal repair
Anterior sphincteroplasty and levatoplasty
Total pelvic floor repair (combined anterior and posterior repair)
Gracilis or gluteus maximus muscle transposition
Artificial anal sphincter implant
Pudendal nerve stimulator implant
Left iliac fossa end colostomy

proved faecal continence does not seem to depend upon this and symptomatic benefit may result from post-anal repair even though significant alteration of the anorectal angle has not been achieved (Womack *et al.* 1988). Initial improvement is seen in 60–80% of patients (Womack *et al.* 1988; Orrom *et al.* 1991) but a prolonged follow-up suggests that 50% still wear pads (Pemberton *et al.* 1991). As with direct sphincter repair, evidence of coexisting pudendal neuropathy reduces the chances of a successful result (Rainey *et al.* 1990). Recently, total pelvic floor repair (post-anal repair plus anterior levatorplasty and EAS plication) was significantly better than either of the two operations alone, with eight of 12 patients being completely continent on follow-up of 2 years (Deen *et al.* 1993).

Attention has recently been focused on surgery for faecal incontinence due to primary neurological diseases such as spinal trauma and cauda equina lesions. Experience with muscle transfer operations and implantable artificial sphincters is growing and the techniques can be applied to other forms of faecal incontinence where there is significant sphincter loss precluding repair or plication. Such operations may be appropriate upon failure of other methods in selected cases.

Gracilis and gluteus maximus are the two commonest muscles used for transposition and encirclement of the anus (Christiansen *et al.* 1990; Pearl *et al.* 1991) (Figure 13.21). The chief drawback in this technique has been the inability of the transposed muscle to emulate the prolonged contraction of the sphincter without fatigue (Williams *et al.* 1991). By electrical stimulation the predominantly Type II fast twitch gracilis may be converted into a slow twitch, fatigue-resistant muscle (Williams *et al.* 1992). This can now be achieved using an implantable long-term stimulator, resulting in complete continence in up to 65% of patients (Konsten *et al.* 1993).

An alternative approach in patients with neuromuscular disorders has been to implant an artificial anal sphincter (Figure 13.22). Although initial procedures were associated with a high incidence of mechanical failures and need for revisional surgery, subsequent modifications have led to improved results. Among 10 patients in whom the system has been functioning for more than 6 months, the outcome was considered excellent in five instances with only occasional leakage of flatus, good in three and acceptable in two in whom the cuff lead to obstructed defecation (Christiansen and

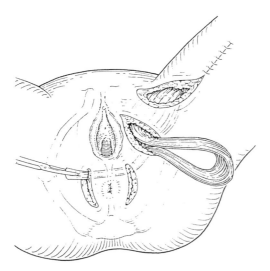
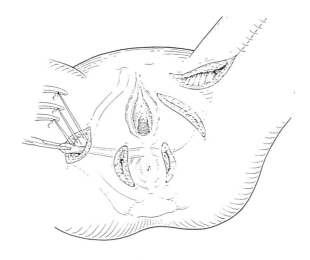

Figure 13.21 Diagrammatic representation of the gracilis muscle transposition. The mobilized muscle encircles the anal canal and is attached to the contralateral ischium. From M.R.B. Keighley and N.S. Williams. *Surgery of the anus, rectum and colon.* London: WB Saunders, 1993: 558.

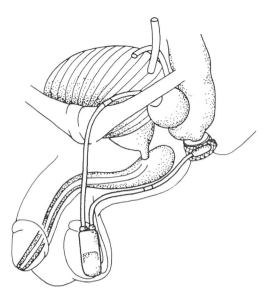

Figure 13.22 Illustration of the artificial anal sphincter apparatus *in situ*. From J. Christiansen and B. Sparso, *Ann. Surg.* 1992; 215: 383–6, courtesy of publishers.

Sparso 1992). It is also possible to implant a pudendal nerve stimulator, with electrical stimulation only being stopped during micturition or defecation (Schmidt *et al.* 1990).

Colostomy is the final surgical option when other approaches to the management of incontinence have failed or are not applicable. Providing the patient with a manageable, accessible, sealed bag is a preferable alternative to what amounts to a perineal stoma. In conclusion, the last 15 years has witnessed the development of several new techniques and operations some of which are still in the early stages of evolution as well as the continued application of established techniques (Table 13.6). For the individual patient it is necessary to determine which offers the best long-term alternative.

Intussusception

Intussusception involves the invagination of a proximal portion of bowel (intussusceptum) into a distal section (intussusceptiens) (Figure 13.23). It may be either primary (no focal cause) or sec-

ondary (a precipitating focus or 'lead point' is present). In children it is the commonest cause of intestinal obstruction and there is rarely a distinct precipitating 'lead lesion' (Skipper *et al.* 1990). It is a much rarer disease in adults, only 5–16% of cases being reported in adults (Stubenbord and Thorbjarnarson 1970; Agha 1986). However, there is considerable regional variation and in one Nigerian series, 42% of the cases occurred in adults (Elebute and Adesola 1964). In this series 92% of the intussusceptions were idiopathic and may relate to endemic enteric infections. Three-quarters of adult intussusceptions have an explanatory cause, more than half being due to tumour (Gordon *et al.* 1991). In general, benign tumours are more common precipitants than malignant tumours, but this ratio is reversed in the case of colonic lesions. Other causes include Meckel's diverticulum and adhesions.

Clinical features

Children classically present with episodes of severe colicky abdominal pain and the passage of 'currant-jelly' stools. There is characteristically a sausage-shaped mass palpable in the colon.

Crampy abdominal pain will be present in three-quarters of patients, nausea and vomiting in 70%, abdominal tenderness or distension in 60%, and an abdominal mass in 50% (Felix *et al.* 1976). Less than 20% of cases present acutely for the first time and more than half will have had symptoms for at least 1 month (Stubenbord and Thorbjarnarson 1970). Routine blood tests including white cell count are unhelpful and do not discriminate those with necrotic bowel (Cotler and Cohn 1961).

A high index of suspicion and evidence of bowel obstruction on plain abdominal X-ray may point towards the diagnosis. Barium enema will confirm the diagnosis of colonic intussusception, demonstrating the 'claw sign' of distal barium spreading its 'claws' around the negative image of the proximal intussusceptum (Figure 13.24). CT is increasingly helpful in making the diagnosis in cases under investigation of an abdominal mass or long-standing, non-specific symptoms (Lorigan and DuBrow 1990; Bar-Ziv and Solomon 1991). The characteristic image is of bowel thickened by the double/triple

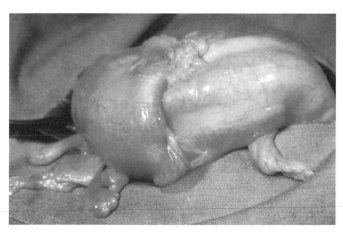

Figure 13.23 Colonic intussusception.

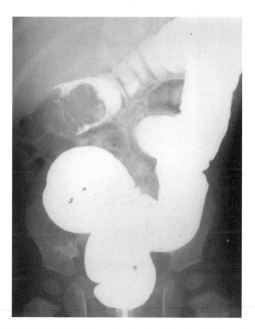

Figure 13.24 Barium enema demonstrating the 'claw sign' in large bowel intussusception.

wall, fat-dense material within the lumen (the intussusceptum) and a 'target' mass, the target comprising an end-on view of the intussusceptum surrounded by the intussusceptions.

Treatment

In children the majority of cases are successfully managed by low-pressure barium enema reduction. This is associated with a 13% recurrence rate. Of those coming to surgery approximately half require resection while in the remainder manual reduction alone is sufficient (Skipper *et al.* 1990).

In adults the conventional treatment is surgical. This is particularly relevant in cases of chronic intussusception where there is a high likelihood of an underlying malignant 'lead point'. After manual reduction, the tumour should be adequately resected and in the absence of necrotic bowel, primary anastomosis performed. Where the patient is not fit for surgery, or the 'lead point' is known to be benign and it would be preferable to avoid surgery, it may be possible to reduce the intussusception endoscopically and remove the polyp via the colonoscope (Kitamura *et al.* 1990).

Colonic pseudo-obstruction

As the name suggests this disorder presents clinically and radiologically as a case of large bowel obstruction in the absence of a mechanical cause. It may present as a single acute episode, recurrent acute episodes or as a chronic disorder.

Over 80% of cases have been associated with some presumed aetiological factor (Dorudi *et al.* 1992). Commonly associated factors appear to be obstetric intervention, pelvic or orthopaedic surgery, underlying medical illness and electrolyte disturbances. In one study more than half the patients were on narcotic medication and over 40% on phenothiazines (Jetmore *et al.* 1992). In the same study, hypocalcaemia was present in 63%, hyponatraemia in 38%, and hypokalaemia in 29%.

No one common pathogenetic mechanism has been identified to link all the aetiological factors. However, it is believed that an imbalance between sympathetic and parasympathetic stimulation to the bowel, with excess sympathetic drive, inhibits colonic activity thus facilitating dilatation (Spira *et al.* 1976; Addison 1983).

Clinical features

The features are those of large bowel obstruction. The patient presents with abdominal distension and although there is often some abdominal discomfort, the pain is generally not severe. Constipation may not be absolute as liquids and flatus can continue to be passed (Dudley and Paterson-Brown 1986). Nausea and vomiting occur later.

On examination there is marked abdominal distension. When abdominal tenderness can be localized to the right iliac fossa, this suggests caecal ischaemia with impending perforation. Bowel sounds may vary in character but are rarely absent (Dorudi *et al.* 1992).

Investigation

Pseudo-obstruction must be distinguished from obstruction due to a mechanical cause. The clinical setting may suggest the possibility of pseudo-obstruction. Plain abdominal X-ray often points to the diagnosis with colonic distension proximal to an area of obstruction, the cut-off often being at the splenic flexure or rectosigmoid junction

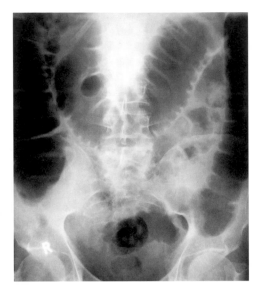

Figure 13.25 Pseudo-obstruction. The whole of the colon is distended. Air is seen in the rectum. There is no evidence of mucosal oedema. Part of the distal ileum is visualized and is of normal calibre.

with no distal distension. Air in the rectum may be identifiable on the plain X-ray film in pseudo-obstruction. Haustral and mucosal patterns are maintained and there is relatively little fluid in the distended bowel (Villar and Norton 1979; Anuras and Shirazi 1984) (Figure 13.25). Where the caecal diameter is greater than 12 cm, there is increased risk of perforation. If perforation has occurred, free air may be seen under the diaphragm.

To exclude a mechanical obstruction confidently, a contrast enema, or colonoscopy should be performed. Contrast enema is probably preferable and water soluble media are safer than barium in case there is an unsuspected perforation.

Emergency colonoscopy can be performed after the use of saline enemas to improve visibility (Strodel *et al.* 1983). One advantage of colonoscopy is the ability to visualize ischaemic mucosa suggesting the need for surgery rather than trying conservative measures. However, the procedure is hazardous and difficult making contrast enema the preferred diagnostic tool.

Management

Conservative

Provided the caecal diameter is less than 12 cm and there is no evidence of perforation, the initial management is conservative with intravenous fluids to correct any electrolyte imbalance and nasogastric aspiration when vomiting is present. Any drugs which might be contributing to the condition should be stopped and treatment of any underlying systemic illness maximized. The prokinetic motility agent cisapride should be commenced (Camilleri *et al.* 1989; MacColl *et al.* 1990). Daily abdominal X-rays should be performed to assess caecal diameter. The majority of cases settle without further intervention 90% resolving within 4 days (23 of 24 patients in one study) (Sloyer *et al.* 1988).

Caecal perforation is associated with a high mortality rate of up to 50%. It should be remembered that the condition develops in patients whose general condition prior to the abdominal scenario was often far from ideal and hence the prognosis following such a catastrophe is poor.

Failure to respond to conservative measures, evidence of deterioration or an increase in caecal diameter are indications for decompression.

Colonoscopy

Colonoscopic decompression is a difficult procedure requiring an expert endoscopist. A minimum of air insufflation should be used. It is sufficient to reach the hepatic flexure without proceeding into the ascending colon or caecum. A long fenestrated intestinal tube can be fed into the bowel and left *in situ* to prevent recurrence (Burke and Shellito 1987). In a review of 169 patients from nine series, colonoscopic decompression was successful in 84% with a 25% recurrence rate. Definitive treatment was achieved in 85% and there was a 2% mortality (Gosche *et al.* 1989).

Surgery

When there are signs of impending perforation or the caecal diameter is greater than 12 cm despite other therapy, surgery is indicated. Placement of a Foley catheter into the caecum to form a caecostomy is the treatment of choice for prevention of perforation. This is usually performed through a small grid iron incision in the right iliac fossa, although it has also been achieved laparoscopically (Soreide *et al.* 1977; Duh and Way 1993).

When caecal ischaemia or perforation is felt to be present, a laparotomy should be performed. The surgery performed will depend upon the viability of the caecum, options varying from a tube caecostomy to resection with or without immediate anastomosis (Dorudi *et al.* 1992).

Irritable bowel syndrome

The irritable bowel syndrome (IBS) is a common clinical disorder the symptoms of which vary in severity from being mildly irritating to incapacitating. Because of the overlap of symptoms spanning the whole gastrointestinal tract, some authors have suggested the term 'irritable gut' as more appropriate (Moriarty 1992). While acknowledging the relationship between the irritable oesophagus, non-ulcer dyspepsia, and IBS, this chapter concentrates on those symptoms presumed to arise from the colon, although it is accepted that some of them may originate in the small intestine. In 1978, Manning *et al.* listed symptoms which when taken together allowed a positive diagnosis of IBS to be made (Manning *et al.* 1978; Thompson 1984, 1986; Longstreth and Wolde-Tsadik 1993) (Table 13.7). Using these criteria it has been possible to compare IBS studies performed in different countries and by different investigators. The more symptoms required for the diagnosis, the greater the specificity. Recently,

Table 13.7 Symptomatic definition of irritable bowel syndrome

Recurrent or continuous presence of the following symptoms for at least 6 months:
Abdominal pain relieved by defecation
Abdominal pain associated with more frequent defecation
Abdominal pain associated with looser stools
Sensation of incomplete evacuation after defecation
Passage of mucus per rectum
Abdominal distension

the presence of persistent or recurrent abdominal pain associated with three of the Manning criteria has been suggested as diagnostic of IBS (Thompson 1984).

Epidemiology

The prevalence of IBS throughout the world is approximately 11–20% depending on the number of symptoms required to make the diagnosis (Thompson 1986; Talley *et al.* 1991; Jones and Lydeard 1992; Longstreth and Wolde-Tsadik 1993). Based on community surveys it has been reported that among non-patient populations the prevalence of IBS-type symptoms is about 15–20% but less than 4% of the community have three or more of the Manning criteria (Longstreth and Wolde-Tsadik 1993). The majority of patients with such symptoms do not consult a doctor and presentation appears to be influenced by psychosocial factors rather than just the severity of symptoms (Welch *et al.* 1985; Smith *et al.* 1990). Compared with non-presenters, patients presenting with IBS do have significantly more serious symptoms (Heaton *et al.* 1991). However, in addition to this they are more anxious about a possible sinister outcome for their symptoms (Kettell *et al.* 1992). They are also more psychologically disturbed (Whitehead *et al.* 1988; Drossman *et al.* 1988).

Pathophysiology

Although in the past the pathophysiology of IBS has been defined as abnormal perception of normal motility or normal perception of abnormal motility, it is now recognized that IBS is a multifactorial illness. The initial two premises need not be mutually exclusive, and other factors may play a part.

Abnormal motility

The normal colon is a relatively active organ with periods of activity alternating with periods of quiescence. There is wide variation in the degree of activity, i.e. the frequency and the amplitude of the contractions, from one individual to another and even considerable day to day variation in the same subject.

Evidence for a motility disorder of the colon or small bowel in IBS has recently been extensively reviewed (McKee and Quigley 1993a,b; Abell and Werkman 1996). Early studies in the colon suggested an increased prevalence of low-frequency, slow wave activity at three cycles per minute (Snape *et al.* 1976; Taylor *et al.* 1978). However, this rhythm did not improve in remission (Taylor *et al.* 1978), could not be reproduced by others (Katschinski *et al.* 1990), and was just as common among psychoneurotic subjects with no gastrointestinal symptoms (Latimer 1983). Initial reports of high-amplitude sigmoid contractions associated with symptoms in the subgroup of patients with pain as their predominant symptom also have not been reproduced (Chaudhary and Truelove 1961; Katschinski *et al.* 1990). Postprandial colonic and jejunal motility does appear to be significantly increased in IBS patients (Narducci *et al.* 1986; Evans *et al.* 1996). The colonic motility response to stress is also increased (Welgan *et al.* 1988). By contrast, in the small bowel, the result of stress is to abolish the migratory motor complex or induce periods of abnormal irregular contraction (Kumar and Wingate 1985). Also noted in the small bowel of IBS patients is the presence of discreet clustered contractions and a shorter period between successive migratory motor complexes in IBS patients with diarrhoea (Kellow and Phillips 1987; Kellow *et al.* 1990). It would appear that there are specific motor abnormalities in the large and small bowel in patients with IBS. However, this is not the case for every patient with the disease and even among those in whom it occurs, its presence may represent an epiphenomenon rather than a cause.

Abnormal sensation

Patients with IBS do appear to have increased visceral perception. When a balloon is inflated in the rectum, patients with IBS have a lower threshold for pain than do controls (Whitehead *et al.* 1990; Prior *et al.* 1990). This altered perception is associated with increased motor activity in the rectum (Prior *et al.* 1990). Prolonged small bowel monitoring demonstrated a similar alteration of perception to physiological events: 61% of prolonged propagated contractions were associated with pain in IBS patients but the equivalent figure for normal subjects was 17% (Kellow and Phillips 1987; Kellow *et al.* 1991). One explanation for these findings would be that in IBS visceral mechanoreceptors have been set at lower thresholds (Levitt *et al.* 1996).

The association with a variety of other non-gastrointestinal symptoms such as dyspareunia, back pain, urinary urgency, and nocturia points towards a generalized alteration in visceral sensation (Whorwell *et al.* 1986; Jamieson and Steege 1996). There is, however, no evidence for any alteration in somatic sensation (Whitehead 1989).

Psychological factors

More than 70% of IBS patients attending hospital will exhibit psychological features or have a psychiatric diagnosis (Whitehead 1989; Gwee *et al.* 1996). They suffer more often from depression, fatigue, and insomnia and tend to be more preoccupied with their somatic symptoms, and more sensitive to them when compared with the general population (Sinha *et al.* 1996).

Childhood experience

Two links have been made between adult IBS and childhood. First, the observation that 'little belly achers grow up to be big belly achers' may apply in IBS and may relate to learned illness behaviour (Apley and Hale 1973). Significantly higher numbers of IBS patients were treated with toys and sweets when they were ill as children compared with the normal population (Whitehead *et al.* 1982; Lowman *et al.* 1987). This learned illness behaviour and encouragement of the sick role may facilitate an exaggerated response to bowel symptoms as adults. Secondly, several reports have documented significant levels of childhood sexual and physical abuse of 20% or more of patients presenting with IBS symptoms (Drossman *et al.* 1990*a*; Felitti 1991; Longstreth and Wolde-Tsadik 1993; Walker *et al.* 1993).

Luminal factors

It has been suggested that IBS patients may display an abnormal response to food and normal luminal contents (McKee and Quigley 1993*b*). In areas of the world where lactase deficiency is common its exclusion has been recommended before making a firm diagnosis of IBS (Fernandez-Banares *et al.* 1993). Malabsorption of other sugars such as fructose and sorbitol has also been demonstrated in patients labelled as IBS (Rumessen and Gudmand-Hoyer 1988; Fernandez-Banares *et al.* 1993). One UK study has documented improvement in 91 of 189 IBS patients by dietary restriction. Various foods such as dairy products, cereals, citrus fruits, tea, coffee, alcohol, additives, and preservatives were excluded. Half of the patients who benefited from dietary restrictions identified two to five foods which upset them (range 1–14) (Nanda *et al.* 1989).

Clinical features and investigation

The classical features of IBS are listed in Table 13.7. Other researchers have attempted to refine these by introducing 46-symptom questionnaires (Talley *et al.* 1989) or scores incorporating examination and investigation as well as history (Kruis *et al.* 1984). In practice, such devices are cumbersome to use and add little to clinical judgement.

Clinical features in favour of the diagnosis of IBS and against such a diagnosis are listed in Tables 13.8 and 13.9, respectively. The diagnosis of IBS should be made on the positive basis of the above symptoms. However, it is reasonable to also exclude other presumed causes. By the time a patient presents to a hospital clinic, he/she will already have been managed by the general practitioner who felt the need for further referral. Such patients tend to be worried about a more sinister diagnosis and are in need of reassurance (Kettell *et al.* 1992).

It is becoming increasingly difficult to satisfy both patient and doctor with a diagnosis based upon history alone. There is an increased tendency towards performing colonoscopy/barium enema and sigmoidoscopy before confirming the label IBS. In addition to this, depending upon the circumstances, it may be appropriate to perform a full blood count, erythrocyte sedimentation rate, thyroid function tests, antigliadin estimation, a lactose hydrogen breath test, 2 week lactose-free diet and stools for organisms and parasites. Therefore, whatever tests a clinician feels he/she needs before giving appropriate reassurance to the patient should be performed at the outset. This is preferable to the 'just one more test' requested at each clinic visit, suggesting to the patient that the doctor is unsure of the cause.

Table 13.8 Features in favour of a diagnosis of irritable bowel syndrome

Pain never awakens from sleep
Pain/frequent defecation limited to a particular time of day (especially the morning)
Small stools
Symptoms for many years
Symptoms disproportionate to signs
Bizarre/unusual description of symptoms
Additional symptoms referable to other gut organs
Additional symptoms referable to outside the gastrointestinal tract
Non-specific childhood abdominal complaints/childhood abuse
Psychiatric illness
On examination:
    Good general health
    Tense/anxious
    Tender palpable sigmoid colon
    Pain on air insufflation at sigmoidoscopy

Table 13.9 Features against a diagnosis of irritable bowel syndrome (IBS)

Non-IBS bowel symptoms—rectal bleeding, steatorrhoea
Recent change in bowel habit
Weight loss (not attributable to depression)
Systemically unwell/fever
Abdominal mass other than sigmoid colon

Table 13.10 Management strategies in the treatment of irritable bowel syndrome

First line	Reassurance and explanation
	Dietary fibre
Second line (symptom specific)	Constipation: bulk laxatives, cisapride
	Diarrhoea: stool chart, loperamide
	Pain: antispasmodics, antidepressants
Third line	Behaviour therapy
	Psychotherapy
Fourth line	Containment

Management (Table 13.10)

The two tenets in the treatment of IBS are a commitment to treat the whole patient and a good doctor/patient relationship. Achieving these does require the investment of time and energy at the outset. It involves convincing the patient that they are believed and not regarded as malingerers. It requires the exploration of patient worries–beliefs–expectations with an attempt to allay fears and meet realistic expectations. It relies upon a confident diagnosis after performing the necessary investigations at the outset. First-line treatment begins with reassurance and explanation. Having performed the appropriate investigations, it is possible to reassure the patient that there is no serious illness causing the symptoms and that he/she has a benign condition. It is possible to proceed to explain simply the nature of the disorder, some physicians concentrating on the oversensitive perception within the patient's bowel. An outline of the natural history of the condition with its remissions and exacerbations is important, avoiding the patient presenting every time symptoms recur.

All patients should be tried on a high-fibre diet which should help both constipation and diarrhoea (Kumar *et al.* 1987; Prior and Whorwell 1987). One side-effect can be to exacerbate bloating and flatulence but this tends to improve with time. Other dietary manipulations may be tried when there is any history of symptoms relating to a specific food or evidence of sugar malabsorption on investigation. For patients with a predominance of wind and/or bloating, avoidance of gas-forming agents such as legumes is beneficial (Levitt *et al.* 1987; Friedman 1991).

Management focuses upon the predominant symptom and attempts to alleviate it pharmacologically. However, it must be borne in mind that no appropriately conducted trial has demonstrated the benefit of any drug in the treatment of IBS (Klein 1988).

Constipation—predominance

Reassessment and maximising of the patient's intake of dietary fibre is still the preferable option. Dietary intake may be supplemented by bulking agents such as ispaghula or psyllium seed preparations. Studies of the motility agent cisapride suggest that it may be beneficial in treating constipation (Muller-Lissner 1987; Van Outryve *et al.* 1991).

Diarrhoea—predominance

Before treating this symptom, it is useful to document its severity by a 2-week stool chart, asking the patient to record both the frequency and consistency. When pharmacological treatment is required, loperimide is the drug of choice as it does not cross the blood/brain barrier. It leads to symptomatic improvement in both urgency and diarrhoea (Cann *et al.* 1984).

Pain—predominance

Anticholinergics, mebeverine and peppermint oil which act to relax the smooth muscle have all been used as 'antispasmodics'. As critical analysis of their use suggests no proven benefit, any trial of therapy should be confined to limited periods of exacerbated symptoms. Such an approach is often justified, bearing in mind the 40–70% placebo response rate in IBS patients (Thompson 1993).

Antidepressant agents, possibly acting by a reduced visceral perception, have a role when pain persists despite the above management. The newer 5-hydroxytryptamine-3 inhibitors appear theoretically to be the most appropriate preparations (Farthing 1991). A possible third-line management, where available and appropriate, involves behaviour or psychotherapy treatment. Behaviour therapy is most applicable to patients who recognize an association between their symptoms and stress. Treatment aims to reduce anxiety and stress levels, providing the patient with ways of dealing with them either through relaxation (Schwarz *et al.* 1990) or hypnosis (Harvey *et al.* 1989).

Psychotherapy is a labour-intensive technique which involves discussion with the patient about their symptoms and attempting to develop a personal coping strategy. By itself (Svedlund *et al.* 1983) and in combination with behavioural approaches (Schwarz *et al.* 1990; Guthrie *et al.* 1991), it is effective in reducing patient symptoms. There is a small subset of patients who despite all these options will continue to complain of severe pain, unresponsive to any intervention. These patients will remain convinced of a sinister underlying cause and have attended many physicians and surgeons for the cure. The object of therapy for such patients must be directed towards acceptance. First, the doctor must accept the diagnosis and resist requests from the patient for repeat investigation. Secondly, the patient must be guided towards acceptance of the diagnosis and its influence on his/her life. The initial step is to agree with the patient a realistic aim, i.e. improved quality of life as opposed to complete cure. Next the doctor must concentrate on how the patient is coping with his/her symptoms rather than the symptoms themselves. Thus the symptoms cease to be the focus of the consultation. Thirdly, regular scheduled visits with the same physician obviate the need to have symptoms to see the doctor. Finally, by discussing all the options the patient can be given responsibility for personal management.

Prognosis

No one has ever died from IBS. However, for some people the symptoms may be sufficiently distressing to make life not worth living. Studies of a long-term outcome of patients diagnosed with IBS vary in their estimates of symptom-free patients over time. Early studies suggested that only one-third of IBS patients experienced freedom from symptoms while more recent studies indicate that one-half to more than two-thirds are symptom-free after 5 years (Chaudhary and Truelove 1962; Otte *et al.* 1986; Harvey *et al.* 1987). Part of the explanation given to the patient when the diagnosis is made must be to inform them of the possible persistence of symptoms whether continuous or episodic. Equally, it must be explained that they will come to no harm because of the disease.

References

Abell TL, Werkman RF. Gastrointestinal motility disorders. *Am. Fam. Physician* 1996; 53: 895–902.

Addison NV. Pseudo-obstruction of the large bowel. *J. R. Soc. Med.* 1983; 76: 252–5.

Agha FP. Intussusception in adults. *Am. J. Radiol.* 1986; 146: 527–31.

Allen-Mersh TG, Henry MM, Nicholls RJ. Natural history of anterior mucosal prolapse. *Br. J. Surg.* 1987; 74: 679–82.

Anuras S, Shirazi SS. Colonic pseudoobstruction. *Am. J. Gastroenterol.* 1984; 79: 525–32.

Apley J, Hale B. Children with recurrent abdominal pain: how do they grow up? *Br. Med. J.* 1973; iii: 7–9.

Arnaud A, Sarles JC, Sielezneff I, *et al.* Sphincter repair without overlapping for fecal incontinence. *Dis. Colon Rectum* 1991; 34: 744–7.

Arnold RP, Rogers D, Cook DA. Medical problems of adults who were sexually abused in childhood. *Br. Med. J.* 1990; 300: 705–8.

Ashraf W, Park F, Lof J, Quigley EM. An examination of the reliability of reported stool frequency in the diagnosis of idiopathic constipation. *Am. J. Gastroenterol..* 1996; 91: 26–32.

Bar-Ziv J, Solomon A. Computed tomography in adult intussusception. *Gastrointest. Radiol.* 1991; 16: 264–6.

Barnes PR, Lennard-Jones JE. Function of the striated anal sphincter during straining in control subjects and constipated patients with a radiologically normal rectum or idiopathic megacolon. *Int. J. Colorectal Dis.* 1988; 3: 207–9.

Barnes PR, Hawley PR, Preston DM, *et al.* Experience of posterior division of the puborectalis muscle in the management of chronic constipation. *Br. J. Surg.* 1985; 72: 475–7.

Barnes PR, Lennard-Jones JE, Hawley PR, *et al.* Hirschsprung's disease and idiopathic megacolon in adults and adolescents. *Gut* 1986; 27: 534–41.

Barrett JA, Brocklehurst JC, Kiff ES, *et al.* Anal function in geriatric patients with faecal incontinence. *Gut* 1989; 30: 1244–51.

Bartolo DC, Jarratt JA, Read NW. The use of conventional electromyography to assess external sphincter neuropathy in man. *J. Neurol. Neurosurg. Psychiatry* 1983; 46: 1115–8.

Bartolo DC, Roe AM, Locke-Edmunds JC, *et al.* Flap-valve theory of anorectal continence. *Br. J. Surg.* 1986; 73: 1012–4.

Bassotti G, Gaburri M, Imbimbo BP, *et al.* Colonic mass movements in idiopathic chronic constipation. *Gut* 1988; 29: 1173–9.

Binnie NR, Papachrysostomou M, Clare N, *et al.* Solitary rectal ulcer: the place of biofeedback and surgery in the treatment of the syndrome. *World J. Surg.* 1992; 16: 836–40.

Blanchard EB, Schwarz SP, Neff DF, *et al.* Prediction of outcome from the self-regulatory treatment of irritable bowel syndrome. *Behav. Res. Ther.* 1988; 26: 187–90.

Bogomoletz WV. Solitary rectal ulcer syndrome. Mucosal prolapse syndrome. *Pathol. Annu.* 1992; 27 Pt 1: 75–86.

Broden B, Snellman B. Procidentia of the rectum studied with cineradiography. A contribution to the discussion of causative mechanism. *Dis. Colon Rectum* 1968; 11: 330–47.

Brook A. Bowel distress and emotional conflict. *J. R. Soc. Med.* 1991; 84: 39–42.

Burke G, Shellito PC. Treatment of recurrent colonic pseudo-obstruction by endoscopic placement of a fenestrated overtube. Report of a case. *Dis. Colon Rectum* 1987; 30: 615–9.

Camilleri M, Malagelada JR, Abell TL, *et al.* Effect of six weeks of treatment with cisapride in gastroparesis and intestinal pseudoobstruction. *Gastroenterology* 1989; 96: 704–12.

Cann PA, Read NW, Holdsworth CD, *et al.* Role of loperamide and placebo in management of irritable bowel syndrome (IBS). *Dig. Dis. Sci.* 1984; 29: 239–47.

Chaudhary NA, Truelove SC. Human colonic motility: a comparative study of normal subjects, patients with ulcerative colitis, and patients with the irritable colon syndrome. I. Resting patterns. *Gastroenterology* 1961; 40: 1–17.

Chaudhary NA, Truelove SC. The irritable colon syndrome: a study of the clinical features, predisposing causes, and prognosis in 130 cases. *Q. J. Med.* 1962; 123: 307–22.

Christiansen J. Advances in the surgical management of anal incontinence. *Baillières Clin. Gastroenterol.* 1992; 6: 43–57.

Christiansen J, Sparso B. Treatment of anal incontinence by an implantable prosthetic anal sphincter. *Ann. Surg.* 1992; 215: 383–6.

Christiansen J, Sorensen M, Rasmussen OO. Gracilis muscle transposition for faecal incontinence. *Br. J. Surg.* 1990; 77: 1039–40.

Costalat G, Garrigues JM, Alquier Y, *et al.* Solitary rectal ulcer syndrome: clinical features, clinical course and treatment. *Ann. Chir.* 1990; 44: 807–16.

Cotler AM, Cohn I. Intussusception in adults. *Am. J. Surg.* 1961; 101: 114–20.

Cruveiheir J. Ulcère chronique du rectum. *Anatomie Pathologique du Corps Humain.* (1829–1842), Vol. 2, Livre 25. Paris: Baillière, 1842: 4

Cuesta MA, Meijer S, Derksen EJ, *et al.* Anal sphincter imaging in fecal incontinence using endosonography. *Dis. Colon Rectum* 1992; 35: 59–63.

Deen KI, Oya M, Ortiz J, *et al.* Randomized trial comparing three forms of pelvic floor repair for neuropathic faecal incontinence. *Br. J. Surg.* 1993; 80: 794–8.

Deen KI, Grant E, Billingham C, *et al.* Abdominal resection rectopexy with pelvic floor repair versus perineal rectosigmoidectomy and pelvic floor repair for full-thickness rectal prolapse. *Br. J. Surg.* 1994; 81: 302–4.

Delorme R. Sur le traitement des prolapsus du rectum totaux pour l'excision de la muquese rectable au rectocolique. *Bull. Membres Soc. Chir. Paris* 1900; 26: 498–9.

Devroede G. Constipation. In: Sleisenger MH, Fordtran JS, eds. *Gastrointestinal disease: pathophysiology/diagnosis/management*, 5th edn. Philadelphia: WB Saunders, 1993: 837–87.

Devroede G, Soffie M. Colonic absorption in idiopathic constipation. *Gastroenterology* 1973; 64: 552–61.

Dietzen CD, Pemberton JH. Perineal approaches for the treatment of complete rectal prolapse. *Neth. J. Surg.* 1989; 41: 140–4.

Dorudi S, Berry AR, Kettlewell MG. Acute colonic pseudo-obstruction. *Br. J. Surg.* 1992; 79: 99–103.

Drossman DA, McKee DC, Sandler RS, *et al.* Psychosocial factors in the irritable bowel syndrome. A multivariate study of patients and nonpatients with irritable bowel syndrome. *Gastroenterology* 1988; 95: 701–8.

Drossman DA, Thompson WG, Talley NJ, *et al.* Identification of subgroups of functional gastrointestinal disorders. *Gastroenterol. Int.* 1990a; 3: 159–72.

Drossman DA, Leserman J, Nachman G, *et al.* Sexual and physical abuse in women with functional or organic gastrointestinal disorders. *Ann. Intern. Med.* 1990b; 113: 828–33.

du Boulay CE, Fairbrother J, Isaacson PG. Mucosal prolapse syndrome—a unifying concept for solitary ulcer syndrome and related disorders. *J. Clin. Pathol.* 1983; 36: 1264–8.

Dudley HA, Paterson-Brown S. Pseudo-obstruction. *Br. Med. J.* 1986; 292: 1157–8.

Duh QY, Way LW. Diagnostic laparoscopy and laparoscopic cecostomy for colonic pseudo-obstruction. *Dis. Colon Rectum* 1993; 36: 65–70.

Duhamel B. Retrorectal and transanal pull-through procedure for the treatment of Hirschprung's disease. *Dis. Colon Rectum* 1964; 7: 455–8.

Duthie GS, Bartolo DC. Anismus: the cause of constipation? Results of investigation and treatment. *World J. Surg.* 1992; 16: 831–5.

Duthie GS, Bartolo DCC, Miller R. Estimation of the incidence of anismus by laboratory tests. *Br. J. Surg.* 1991; 78: A747.

Duthie HL, Bennett RC. The relation of sensation in the anal canal to the functional sphincter length: a possible factor in anal incontinence. *Gut* 1963; 4: 179–82.

Ederle A, Bulighin G, Orlandi PG, *et al.* Endoscopic application of human fibrin sealant in the treatment of solitary rectal ulcer syndrome. *Endoscopy* 1992; 24: 736–7.

Elebute EA, Adesola AO. Intussusception in Western Nigeria. *Br. J. Surg.* 1964; 51: 440–4.

Epstein SE, Ascari WQ, Ablow RC, *et al.* Colitis cystica profunda. *Am. J. Clin. Pathol.* 1966; 45: 186–201.

Evans PR, Bennett EJ, Bak YT, Tennant CC, Kellow JE. Jejunal sensorimotor dysfunction in irritable bowel syndrome: clinical and psychosocial features. *Gastroenterology* 1996; 110: 393–404.

Farthing MJ. 5-Hydroxytryptamine and 5-hydroxytryptamine-3 receptor antagonists. *Scand. J. Gastroenterol.* 1991; 188 (Suppl.): 92–100.

Fasth S, Hedlund H, Svaninger G, *et al.* Functional results after subtotal colectomy and caecorectal anastomosis. *Acta Chir. Scand.* 1983; 149: 623–7.

Felitti VJ. Long-term medical consequences of incest, rape, and molestation. *South Med. J.* 1991; 84: 328–31.

Felix EL, Cohen MH, Bernstein AD, *et al.* Adult intussusception; case report of recurrent intussusception and review of the literature. *Am. J. Surg.* 1976; 131: 758–61.

Felt-Bersma RJ, Klinkenberg-Knol EC, Meuwissen SG. Anorectal function investigations in incontinent and continent patients. Differences and discriminatory value. *Dis. Colon Rectum* 1990; 33: 479–85.

Fernandez-Banares F, Esteve-Pardo M, de Leon R, *et al.* Sugar malabsorption in functional bowel disease: clinical implications. *Am. J. Gastroenterol.* 1993; 88: 2044–50.

Fleshman JW, Peters WR, Shemesh EI, *et al.* Anal sphincter reconstruction: anterior overlapping muscle repair. *Dis. Colon Rectum* 1991; 34: 739–43.

Fleshman JW, Fry RD, Kodner IJ. The surgical management of constipation. *Baillières Clin. Gastroenterol.* 1992; 6: 145–62.

Frenckner B, Euler CV. Influence of pudendal block on the function of the anal sphincters. *Gut* 1975; 16: 482–9.

Friedman G. Diet and the irritable bowel syndrome. *Gastroenterol. Clin. North Am.* 1991; 20: 313–24.

Frykman HM, Goldberg SM. The surgical treatment of rectal procidentia. *Surg. Gynecol. Obstet.* 1969; 129: 1225–30.

Gordon RS, O'Dell KB, Namon AJ, *et al.* Intussusception in the adult—a rare disease. *J. Emerg. Med.* 1991; 9: 337–42.

Gosche JR, Sharpe JN, Larson GM. Colonoscopic decompression for pseudo-obstruction of the colon. *Am. Surg.* 1989; 55: 111–5.

Gottlieb SH, Schuster MM. Dermatoglyphic (fingerprint) evidence for a congenital syndrome of early onset constipation and abdominal pain. *Gastroenterology* 1986; 91: 428–32.

Guthrie E, Creed F, Dawson D, *et al.* A controlled trial of psychological treatment for the irritable bowel syndrome. *Gastroenterology* 1991; 100: 450–7.

Gwee KA, Graham JC, McKendrick MW, Collins SM, Marshall JS, Walters SJ, Read NW. Psychometric scores and persistence of irritable bowel after infectious diarrhoea. *Lancet* 1996; 347: 150–3.

Hallan RI, Williams NS, Melling J, *et al.* Treatment of anismus in intractable constipation with botulinum A toxin. *Lancet* 1988; ii: 714–7.

Harari D, Gurwitz JH, Avorn J, Bohn R, Minaker KL. Bowel habit in relation to age and gender. Findings from the National Health Interview Survey and clinical implications. *Arch. Intern. Med.* 1996; 156: 315–20.

Harvey RF, Mauad EC, Brown AM. Prognosis in the irritable bowel syndrome: a 5-year prospective study. *Lancet* 1987; i: 963–5.

Harvey RF, Hinton RA, Gunary RM, *et al.* Individual and group hypnotherapy in treatment of refractory irritable bowel syndrome. *Lancet* 1989; i: 424–5.

Heaton KW, Ghosh S, Braddon FE. How bad are the symptoms and bowel dysfunction of patients with the irritable bowel syndrome? A prospective, controlled study with emphasis on stool form. *Gut* 1991; 32: 73–9.

Heine JA, Wong WD, Goldberg SM. Surgical treatment for constipation. *Surg. Gynecol. Obstet.* 1993; 176: 403–10.

Hernandez G, Troncoso G, Palencia C, *et al.* Double-blind dose–response study of cisapride in the treatment of chronic functional constipation. *Adv. Therapy* 1988; 5: 121–7.

Hight DW, Hertzler JH, Philippart AI, Benson CD. Linear cauterisation for the treatment of rectal prolapse in infants and children. *Surg. Gynecol. Obstet.* 1982; 154: 400–2.

Hinton JM, Lennard-Jones JE, Young AC. A new method for studying gut transit times using radioopaque markers. *Gut* 1969; 10: 842–7.

Hodgson WJ. The placebo effect. Is it important in diverticular disease? *Am. J. Gastroenterol.* 1977; 67: 157–62.

Holmstrom B, Broden G, Dolk A. Results of the Ripstein operation in the treatment of rectal prolapse and internal rectal procidentia. *Dis. Colon Rectum* 1986; 29: 845–8.

Hosie KB, Kmiot WA, Keighley MR. Constipation: another indication for restorative proctocolectomy. *Br. J. Surg.* 1990; 77: 801–2.

Ihre T, Seligson U. Intussusception of the rectum–internal procidentia: treatment and results in 90 patients. *Dis. Colon Rectum* 1975; 18: 391–6.

Jacobs LK, Lim YJ, Orkin BA. The best operation for rectal prolapse. *Surg. Clin. North Am.* 1997; 77: 49–70.

Jamieson DJ, Steege JF. The prevalence of dysmenorrhea, dyspareunia, pelvic pain, and irritable bowel syndrome in primary care practices. *Obstet. Gynecol.* 1996; 87: 55–8.

Jetmore AB, Timmcke AE, Gathright JB Jr, *et al.* Ogilvie's syndrome: colonoscopic decompression and analysis of predisposing factors. *Dis. Colon Rectum* 1992; 35: 1135–42.

Jones PN, Lubowski DZ, Swash M, *et al.* Is paradoxical contraction of puborectalis muscle of functional importance? *Dis. Colon Rectum* 1987a; 30: 667–70.

Jones PN, Lubowski DZ, Swash M, *et al.* Relation between perineal descent and pudendal nerve damage in idiopathic faecal incontinence. *Int. J. Colorectal Dis.* 1987b; 2: 93–5.

Jones R, Lydeard S. Irritable bowel syndrome in the general population. *Br. Med. J.* 1992; 304: 87–90.

Jorge JMN, Wexner SD, Ger GC, *et al.* Cinedefecography and electromyography in the diagnosis of non-relaxing puborectalis syndrome. *Dis. Colon Rectum* 1993; 36: 668–76.

Kamm MA, Stabile G. Management of idiopathic megarectum and megacolon. *Br. J. Surg.* 1991; 78: 899–900.

Kamm MA, Hawley PR, Lennard-Jones JE. Outcome of colectomy for severe idiopathic constipation. *Gut* 1988a; 29: 969–73.

Kamm MA, Hawley PR, Lennard-Jones JE. Lateral division of the puborectalis muscle in the management of severe constipation. *Br. J. Surg.* 1988b; 75: 661–3.

Karasick S, Ehrlich SM. Is constipation a disorder of defecation or impaired motility?: distinction based on defecography and colonic transit studies. *Am. J. Roentgenol.* 1996; 166: 63–6.

Katschinski M, Lederer P, Ellermann A, *et al.* Myoelectric and manometric patterns of human rectosigmoid colon in irritable bowel syndrome and diverticulosis. *Scand. J. Gastroenterol.* 1990; 25: 761–8.

Kawimbe BM, Papachrysostomou M, Binnie NR, *et al.* Outlet obstruction constipation (anismus) managed by biofeedback. *Gut* 1991; 32: 1175–9.

Keighley MR, Fielding JW, Alexander-Williams J. Results of Marlex mesh abdominal rectopexy for rectal prolapse in 100 consecutive patients. *Br. J. Surg.* 1983; 70: 229–32.

Kekk JO, Staniusas RJ, Coller JA, *et al.* Biofeedback training in useful in faecal incontinence but disappointing in constipation. *Dis. Colon Rectum* 1994; 37: 1271–6.

Kellow JE, Phillips SF. Altered small bowel motility in irritable bowel syndrome is correlated with symptoms. *Gastroenterology* 1987; 92: 1885–93.

Kellow JE, Gill RC, Wingate DL. Prolonged ambulant recordings of small bowel motility demonstrate abnormalities in the irritable bowel syndrome. *Gastroenterology* 1990; 98: 1208–18.

Kellow JE, Eckersley CM, Jones MP. Enhanced perception of physiological intestinal motility in the irritable bowel syndrome. *Gastroenterology* 1991; 101: 1621–7.

Kennedy DK, Hughes ES, Masterton JP. The natural history of benign ulcer of the rectum. *Surg. Gynecol. Obstet.* 1977; 144: 718–20.

Kettell J, Jones R, Lydeard S. Reasons for consultation in irritable bowel syndrome: symptoms and patient characteristics. *Br. J. Gen. Pract.* 1992; 42: 459–61.

Kiff ES, Barnes PR, Swash M. Evidence of pudendal neuropathy in patients with perineal descent and chronic straining at stool. *Gut* 1984; 25: 1279–82.

Kitamura K, Kitagawa S, Mori M, *et al.* Endoscopic correction of intussusception and removal of a colonic lipoma. *Gastrointest. Endosc.* 1990; 36: 509–11.

Klein KB. Controlled treatment trials in the irritable bowel syndrome: a critique. *Gastroenterology* 1988; 95: 232–41.

Konsten J, Baeten CG, Spaans F, *et al.* Follow-up of anal dynamic gracilo-plasty for fecal continence. *World J. Surg.* 1993; 17: 404–8.

Krishnamurthy S, Schuffler MD, Rohrmann CA, *et al.* Severe idiopathic constipation is associated with a distinctive abnormality of the colonic myenteric plexus. *Gastroenterology* 1985; 88: 26–34.

Kruis W, Thieme C, Weinzierl M, *et al.* A diagnostic score for the irritable bowel syndrome. Its value in the exclusion of organic disease. *Gastroenterology* 1984; 87: 1–7.

Kuijpers HC. Treatment of complete rectal prolapse: to narrow, to wrap, to suspend, to fix, to encircle, to plicate or to resect? *World J. Surg.* 1992; 16: 826–30.

Kuijpers HC, Strijk SP. Diagnosis of disturbances of continence and defecation. *Dis. Colon Rectum* 1984; 27: 658–62.

Kuijpers HC, Bleijenberg G. The spastic pelvic floor syndrome. A cause of constipation. *Dis. Colon Rectum* 1985; 28: 669–72.

Kuijpers HC, Bleijenberg G, de Morree H. The spastic pelvic floor syndrome. Large bowel outlet obstruction caused by pelvic floor dysfunction: a radiological study. *Int. J. Colorect. Dis.* 1986; 1: 44–8.

Kumar A, Kumar N, Vij JC, *et al.* Optimum dosage of ispaghula husk in patients with irritable bowel syndrome: correlation of symptom relief with whole gut transit time and stool weight. *Gut* 1987; 28: 150–5.

Kumar D, Wingate DL. The irritable bowel syndrome: a paroxysmal motor disorder. *Lancet* 1985; ii: 973–7.

Kupfer CA, Goligher JC. One hundred consecutive cases of complete pro-lapse of the rectum treated by operation. *Br. J. Surg.* 1970; 57: 482–7.

Lam TC, Lubowski DZ, King DW. Solitary rectal ulcer syndrome. *Baillières Clin. Gastroenterol.* 1992; 6: 129–43.

Lane RH. Clinical application of anorectal physiology. *Proc. R. Soc. Med.* 1975; 68: 28–30.

Lane RH, Todd IP. Idiopathic megacolon: a review of 42 cases. *Br. J. Surg.* 1977; 64: 307–10.

Lane WA. The results of the operative treatment of chronic constipation. *Br. Med. J.* 1908; i: 126–30.

Lasagna L, Mosteller F, von Felsinger JM, *et al.* A study of the placebo response. *Am. J. Med.* 1951; 16: 770–9.

Latimer PR. Colonic psychophysiology. Implications for functional bowel disorders. In: Holzl R, Whitehead WE, eds. *Psychophysiology of the gastrointestinal tract. Experimental and clinical applications.* New York: Plenum Press, 1983: 263–88.

Laurberg S, Swash M, Henry MM. Delayed external sphincter repair for obstetric tear. *Br. J. Surg.* 1988; 75: 786–8.

Lestar B, Penninckx F, Kerremans R. The composition of anal basal pressure. An *in vivo* and *in vitro* study in man. *Int. J. Colorectal Dis.* 1989; 4: 118–22.

Lestar B, Penninckx F, Kerremans R. Biofeedback defaecation training for anismus. *Int. J. Colorectal Dis.* 1991; 6: 202–7.

Levitt MD, Hirsh P, Fetzer CA, *et al.* H2 excretion after ingestion of complex carbohydrates. *Gastroenterology* 1987; 92: 383–9.

Levitt MD, Furne J, Olsson S . The relation of passage of gas an abdominal bloating to colonic gas production. *Ann. Intern. Med.* 1996; 124: 422–4.

Lincoln J, Crowe R, Kamm MA, *et al.* Serotonin and 5-hydroxyindoleacetic acid are increased in the sigmoid colon in severe idiopathic constipation. *Gastroenterology* 1990; 98: 1219–25.

Loening-Baucke V. Biofeedback training in children with functional constipation. A critical review. *Dig. Dis. Sci.*. 1996; 41: 65–71.

Longstreth GF, Wolde-Tsadik G. Irritable bowel-type symptoms in HMO examinees. Prevalence, demographics, and clinical correlates. *Dig. Dis. Sci.* 1993; 38: 1581–9.

Lorigan JG, DuBrow RA. The computed tomographic appearances and clin-ical significance of intussusception in adults with malignant neoplasms. *Br. J. Radiol.* 1990; 63: 257–62.

Lowman BC, Drossman DA, Cramer EM, *et al.* Recollection of childhood events in adults with irritable bowel syndrome. *J. Clin. Gastroenterol.* 1987; 9: 324–30.

Lubowski DZ, Nicholls RJ. Faecal incontinence associated with reduced pelvic sensation. *Br. J. Surg.* 1988; 75: 1086–8.

MacColl C, MacCannell KL, Baylis B, *et al.* Treatment of acute colonic

pseudoobstruction (Ogilvie's syndrome) with cisapride. *Gastroenterology* 1990; 98: 773–6.

MacIntyre IM, Balfour TW. Results of the Lord non-operative treatment for haemorrhoids. *Lancet* 1972; i: 1094–5.

Mackle EJ, Parks TG. The pathogenesis and pathophysioloy of rectal pro-lapse and solitary rectal ulcer syndrome. *Clin. Gastroenterol.* 1986; 15: 985–1002.

Mackle EJ, Mills JOM, Parks TG. The investigation of anorectal dysfunc-tion in the solitary rectal ulcer syndrome. *Int. J. Colorectal Dis.* 1990; 5: 21–4.

MacLeod JH. Management of anal incontinence by biofeedback. *Gastroenterology* 1987; 93: 291–4.

Madigan MR. Solitary ulcer of the rectum. *Proc. R. Soc. Med.* 1964; 57: 403–5.

Madigan MR, Morson BC. Solitary ulcer of the rectum. *Gut* 1969; 10: 871–81.

Madoff RD, Williams JG, Caushaj PF. Fecal incontinence. *N. Engl. J. Med.* 1992; 326: 1002–7.

Mann CV, Hoffman C. Complete rectal prolapse: the anatomical and func-tional results of treatment by an extended abdominal rectopexy. *Br. J. Surg.* 1988; 75: 34–7.

Manning AP, Thompson WG, Heaton KW, *et al.* Towards positive diag-nosis of the irritable bowel. *Br. Med. J.* 1978; 2: 653–4.

Martin CJ, Parks TG, Biggart JD. Solitary rectal ulcer syndrome in Northern Ireland. 1971–1980. *Br. J. Surg.* 1981; 68: 744–7.

McCue JL, Thomson JP. Clinical and functional results of abdominal rectopexy for complete rectal prolapse. *Br. J. Surg.* 1991; 78: 921–3.

McKee DP, Quigley EM. Intestinal motility in irritable bowel syn-drome: is IBS a motility disorder? Part 1. Definition of IBS and colonic motility. *Dig. Dis. Sci.* 1993a; 38: 1761–72.

McKee DP, Quigley EM. Intestinal motility in irritable bowel syn-drome: is IBS a motility disorder? Part 2. Motility of the small bowel, esophagus, stomach, and gall-bladder. *Dig. Dis. Sci.* 1993b; 38: 1773–82.

Miller R, Bartolo DC, Cervero F, *et al.* Anorectal temperature sensation: a comparison of normal and incontinent patients. *Br. J. Surg.* 1987; 74: 511–5.

Miller R, Bartolo DC, Cervero F, *et al.* Anorectal sampling: a comparison of normal and incontinent patients. *Br. J. Surg.* 1988; 75: 44–7.

Miller R, Orrom WJ, Cornes H, *et al.* Anterior sphincter plication and levatorplasty in the treatment of faecal incontinence. *Br. J. Surg.* 1989; 76: 1058–60.

Milner P, Crowe R, Kamm MA, *et al.* Vasoactive intestinal polypeptide levels in sigmoid colon in idiopathic constipation and diverticular disease. *Gastroenterology* 1990; 99: 666–75.

Monson JR, Jones NA, Vowden P, *et al.* Delorme's operation: the first choice in complete rectal prolapse? *Ann. R. Coll. Surg. Engl.* 1986; 68: 143–6.

Moriarty KJ. ABC of colorectal diseases. The irritable bowel syndrome. *Br. Med. J.* 1992; 304: 1166–9.

Muller-Lissner SA. Treatment of chronic constipation with cisapride and placebo. *Gut* 1987; 28: 1033–8.

Nanda R, James R, Smith H, *et al.* Food intolerance and the irritable bowel syndrome. *Gut* 1989; 30: 1099–104.

Narducci F, Bassotti G, Granata MT, *et al.* Colonic motility and gastric emptying in patients with irritable bowel syndrome. Effect of pretreat-ment with octylonium bromide. *Dig. Dis. Sci.* 1986; 31: 241–6.

Nicholls RJ, Simson JNL. Anteroposterior rectopexy in the treatment of solitary rectal ulcer syndrome without overt rectal prolapse. *Br. J. Surg.* 1986; 73: 222–4.

Orrom WJ, Miller R, Cornes H, *et al.* Comparison of anterior sphinctero-plasty and postanal repair in the treatment of idiopathic fecal incontinence. *Dis. Colon Rectum* 1991; 34: 305–10.

Otte JJ, Larsen L, Andersen JR. Irritable bowel syndrome and symptomatic diverticular disease—different diseases? *Am. J. Gastroenterol.* 1986; 81: 529–31.

Parks AG. Anorectal incontinence. *Proc. R. Soc. Med.* 1975; 68: 681–90.

Parks AG, Porter NH, Hardcastle J. The syndrome of the descending perineum. *Proc. R. Soc. Med.* 1966; 59: 477–82.

Parks TG. The usefulness of tests of anorectal function. *World J. Surg.* 1992; 16: 804–10.

Pearl RK, Prasad ML, Nelson RL, *et al.* Bilateral gluteus maximus transposition for anal incontinence. *Dis. Colon Rectum* 1991; 34: 478–81.

Pemberton JH. Further improvements in the surgical treatment of severe chronic constipation. *Gastroenterology* 1992; 102: 2172–4.

Pemberton JH, Rath DM, Ilstrup DM. Evaluation and surgical treatment of severe chronic constipation. *Ann. Surg.* 1991; 214: 403–11.

Penfold JC, Hawley PR. Experiences of Ivalon-sponge implant for complete rectal prolapse at St. Mark's Hospital, 1960–70. *Br. J. Surg.* 1972; 59: 846–8.

Perry RE, Blatchford GJ, Christensen MA, *et al.* Manometric diagnosis of anal sphincter injuries. *Am. J. Surg.* 1990; 159: 112–6.

Pinho M, Yoshioka K, Keighley MR. Long term results of anorectal myectomy for chronic constipation. *Br. J. Surg.* 1989; 76: 1163–4.

Pinho M, Yoshioka K, Keighley MR. Long-term results of anorectal myectomy for chronic constipation. *Dis. Colon Rectum* 1990; 33: 795–7.

Preston DM, Lennard-Jones JE, Thomas BM. Towards a radiologic definition of idiopathic megacolon. *Gastrointest. Radiol.* 1985; 10: 167–9.

Prior A, Whorwell PJ. Double blind study of ispaghula in irritable bowel syndrome. *Gut* 1987; 28: 1510–3.

Prior A, Maxton DG, Whorwell PJ. Anorectal manometry in irritable bowel syndrome: differences between diarrhoea and constipation predominant subjects. *Gut* 1990; 31: 458–62.

Rainey JB, Donaldson DR, Thomson JP. Postanal repair: which patients derive most benefit? *J. R. Coll. Surg. Edinburgh* 1990; 35: 101–5.

Rao SS, Read NW, Davison PA, *et al.* Anorectal sensitivity and responses to rectal distension in patients with ulcerative colitis. *Gastroenterology* 1987; 93: 1270–5.

Read MG, Read NW, Haynes WG, *et al.* A prospective study of the effect of haemorrhoidectomy on sphincter function and faecal continence. *Br. J. Surg.* 1982; 69: 396–8.

Rogers J. Testing for and the role of anal and rectal sensation. *Baillières Clin. Gastroenterol.* 1992; 6: 179–91.

Romero Y, Evans JM, Fleming KC, Phillips SF. Constipation and fecal incontinence in the elderly population. *Mayo Clin. Proc.* 1996; 71: 81–92.

Rumessen JJ, Gudmand-Hoyer E. Functional bowel disease: malabsorption and abdominal distress after ingestion of fructose, sorbitol, and fructose–sorbitol mixtures. *Gastroenterology* 1988; 95: 694–700.

Rutter KR. Electromyographic changes in certain pelvic floor abnormalities. *Proc. R. Soc. Med.* 1974; 67: 53–6.

Rutter KR, Riddell RH. The solitary ulcer syndrome of the rectum. *Clin. Gastroenterol.* 1975; 4: 505–30.

Sainio AP, Halme LE, Husa AI. Anal encirclement with polypropylene mesh for rectal prolapse and incontinence. *Dis. Colon Rectum* 1991; 34: 905–8.

Schmidt RA, Kogan BA, Tanagho EA. Neuroprostheses in the management of incontinence in myelomeningocele patients. *J. Urol.* 1990; 143: 779–82.

Schouten WR, ten Kate FJ, de Graaf EJ, *et al.* Visceral neuropathy in slow transit constipation: an immunohistochemical investigation with monoclonal antibodies against neurofilament. *Dis. Colon Rectum* 1993; 36: 1112–7.

Schrock TR. Examination of anorectum and diseases of anorectum. In: Sleisenger MH, Fordtran JS, eds. *Gastrointestinal disease: pathophysiology/diagnosis/management*, 5th edn. Philadelphia: WB Saunders, 1993: 1494–516.

Schuster MM, Hookman P, Hendrix PR, *et al.* Simultaneous manometric recording to internal and external anal sphincter reflexes. *Bull. Johns' Hopkins Hosp.* 1965; 116: 79–88.

Schwarz SP, Taylor AE, Scharff L, *et al.* Behaviorally treated irritable bowel syndrome patients: a four-year follow-up. *Behav. Res. Ther.* 1990; 28: 331–5.

Schweiger M. Method for determining individual contributions of voluntary and involuntary anal sphincters to resting tone. *Dis. Colon Rectum* 1979; 22: 415–6.

Shafik A. New concept of the anatomy of the anal sphincter mechanism and the physiology of defecation. II. Anatomy of the levator ani muscle with special reference to puborectalis. *Invest. Urol.* 1975; 13: 175–82.

Sinha L, Liston R, Testa T, Moriarty KJ. Anxiety and irritable bowel syndrome. *Lancet* 1996; 347: 617–8.

Siproudhis L, Ropert A, Gosselin A, *et al.* Constipation after rectopexy for rectal prolapse: Where is the obstruction? *Dig. Dis. Sci.* 1993; 38: 1801–8.

Skipper RP, Boeckman CR, Klein RL. Childhood intussusception. *Surg. Gynecol. Obstet.* 1990; 171: 151–3.

Sloyer AF, Panella VS, Demas BE, *et al.* Ogilvie's syndrome. Successful management without colonoscopy. *Dig. Dis. Sci.* 1988; 33: 1391–6.

Smith RC, Greenbaum DS, Vancouver JB, *et al.* Psychosocial factors are associated with health care seeking rather than diagnosis in irritable bowel syndrome. *Gastroenterology* 1990; 98: 293–301.

Snape WJ Jr, Carlson GM, Cohen S. Colonic myoelectric activity in the irritable bowel syndrome. *Gastroenterology* 1976; 70: 326–30.

Snooks SJ, Setchell M, Swash M, *et al.* Injury to innervation of pelvic floor sphincter musculature in childbirth. *Lancet* 1984; ii: 546–50.

Snooks SJ, Henry MM, Swash M. Faecal incontinence due to external anal sphincter division in childbirth is associated with damage to the innervation of the pelvic floor musculature: a double pathology. *Br. J. Obstet. Gynaecol.* 1985a; 92: 824–8.

Snooks SJ, Nicholls RJ, Henry MM, *et al.* Electrophysiological and manometric assessment of the pelvic floor in the solitary rectal ulcer syndrome. *Br. J. Surg.* 1985b; 72: 131–3.

Sonnenberg A, Koch TR. Epidemiology of constipation in the United States. *Dis. Colon Rectum* 1989; 32: 1–8.

Soreide O, Bjerkeset T, Fossdal JE. Pseudo-obstruction of the colon (Ogilve's syndrome), a genuine clinical conditions? Review of the literature (1948–1975) and report of five cases. *Dis. Colon Rectum* 1977; 20: 487–91.

Spira 1A, Rodrigues R, Wolff WI. Pseudo-obstruction of the colon. *Am. J. Gastroenterol.* 1976; 65: 397–408.

Stabile G, Kamm MA, Hawley PR, *et al.* Colectomy for idiopathic megarectum and megacolon. *Gut* 1991; 32: 1538–40.

Stabile G, Kamm MA. Surgery for idiopathic megarectum and megacolon. *Int. J. Colorectal Dis.* 1991; 6: 171–4.

Stabile G, Kamm MA, Hawley PR, *et al.* Results of stoma formation for idiopathic megarectum and megacolon. *Int. J. Colorectal Dis.* 1992a; 7: 82–4.

Stabile G, Kamm MA, Phillips RK, *et al.* Partial colectomy and coloanal anastomosis for idiopathic megarectum and megacolon. *Dis. Colon Rectum* 1992b; 35: 158–62.

Stricker JW, Schoetz DJ Jr, Coller JA, *et al.* Surgical correction of anal incontinence. *Dis. Colon Rectum* 1988; 31: 533–40.

Strodel WE, Nostrant TT, Eckhauser FE, *et al.* Therapeutic and diagnostic colonoscopy in nonobstructive colonic dilatation. *Ann. Surg.* 1983; 197: 416–21.

Stubenbord WT, Thorbjarnarson B. Intussusception in adults. *Ann. Surg.* 1970; 172: 306–10.

Sun WM, Read NW, Donnelly TC. Impaired internal anal sphincter in a subgroup of patients with idiopathic fecal incontinence. *Gastroenterology* 1989; 97: 130–5.

Sun WM, Read NW, Miner PB, *et al.* The role of transient internal sphincter relaxation in faecal incontinence? *Int. J. Colorectal Dis.* 1990; 5: 31–6.

Svedlund J, Sjodin I, Ottosson JO, *et al.* Controlled study of psychotherapy in irritable bowel syndrome. *Lancet* 1983; ii: 589–92.

Swinton NW, Palmer TE. The management of rectal prolapse and procidentia. *Am. J. Surg.* 1960; 99: 144–51.

Talley NJ, Phillips SF, Melton J 3d, *et al.* A patient questionnaire to identify bowel disease. *Ann. Intern. Med.* 1989; 111: 671–4.

Talley NJ, Zinsmeister AR, Van Dyke C, *et al.* Epidemiology of colonic symptoms and the irritable bowel syndrome. *Gastroenterology* 1991; 101: 927–34.

Talley NJ, Weaver AL, Zinsmeister AR, *et al.* Functional constipation and outlet delay: a population-based study. *Gastroenterology* 1993; 105: 781–90.

Talley NJ, Fleming KC, Evans JM, O'Keefe EA, Weaver AL, Zinsmeister AR, Melton LJ 3rd. Constipation in an elderly community: a study of prevalence and potential risk factors. *Am. J. Gastroenterol.* 1996; 91: 19–25.

Taylor I, Darby C, Hammond P. Comparison of rectosigmoid myoelectrical activity in the irritable colon syndrome during relapses and remissions. *Gut* 1978; 19: 923–9.

Tedesco FJ, DiPiro JT. Laxative use in constipation. American College of Gastroenterology's Committee on FDA-related matters. *Am. J. Gastroenterol.* 1985; 80: 303–9.

Thirlby RC. Further improvements in the surgical treatment of severe chronic constipation. *Gastroenterology* 1992; 102: 2172–4.

Thompson WG. Gastrointestinal symptoms in the irritable bowel compared with peptic ulcer and inflammatory bowel disease. *Gut* 1984; 25: 1089–92.

Thompson WG. Irritable bowel syndrome: prevalence, prognosis and consequences. *Can. Med. Assoc. J.* 1986; 134: 111–3.

Thompson WG. Irritable bowel syndrome: pathogenesis and management. *Lancet* 1993; 341: 1569–72.

Tjandra JJ, Fazio VW, Church JM, *et al.* Clinical conundrum of solitary rectal ulcer. *Dis. Colon Rectum* 1992; 35: 227–34.

Tjandra JJ, Fazio VW, Church JM, *et al.* Ripstein procedure is an effective treatment for rectal prolapse without constipation. *Dis. Colon Rectum* 1993; 36: 501–7.

Todd IP. Constipation: results of surgical treatment. *Br. J. Surg.* 1985; 72 (Suppl.): S12–3.

Turnbull GK, Lennard-Jones JE, Bartram CI. Failure of rectal expulsion as a cause of constipation: why fibre and laxatives sometimes fail. *Lancet* 1986; i: 767–9.

Van Outryve M, Milo R, Toussaint J, et al. 'Prokinetic' treatment of constipation-predominant irritable bowel syndrome: a placebo-controlled study of cisapride. *J. Clin. Gastroenterol.* 1991; 13: 49–57.

Vasilevsky CA, Nemer FD, Balcos EG, *et al.* Is subtotal colectomy a viable option in the management of chronic constipation? *Dis. Colon Rectum* 1988; 31: 679–81.

Verduron A, Devroede G, Bouchoucha M, *et al.* Megarectum. *Dig. Dis. Sci.* 1988; 33: 1164–74.

Villar HV, Norton LW. Massive cecal dilation: pseudoobstruction versus cecal volvulus? *Am. J. Surg.* 1979; 137: 170–4.

Wald A, Tunuguntla AK. Anorectal sensorimotor dysfunction in fecal incontinence and diabetes mellitus. Modification with biofeedback therapy. *N. Engl. J. Med.* 1984; 310: 1282–7.

Walker EA, Katon WJ, Roy-Byrne PP, *et al.* Histories of sexual victimization in patients with irritable bowel syndrome or inflammatory bowel disease. *Am. J. Psychiatry* 1993; 150: 1502–6.

Wallace WC, Madden WM. Experience with partial resection of the puborectalis muscle. *Dis. Colon Rectum* 1969; 12: 196–200.

Wassef R, Rothenberger DA, Goldberg SM. Rectal prolapse. *Curr. Probl. Surg.* 1986; 23: 402–51.

Welch GW, Hillman LC, Pomare EW. Psychoneurotic symptomatology in the irritable bowel syndrome: a study of reporters and non-reporters. *Br. Med. J.* 1985; 291: 1382–4.

Welgan P, Meshkinpour H, Beeler M. Effect of anger on colon motor and myoelectric activity in irritable bowel syndrome. *Gastroenterology* 1988; 94: 1150–6.

Wexner SD, Marchetti F, Jagelman DG. The role of sphincteroplasty for fecal incontinence reevaluated: a prospective physiologic and functional review. *Dis. Colon Rectum* 1991; 34: 22–30.

Wexner SD, Cheape JD, Jorge JM, *et al.* Prospective assessment of biofeedback for the treatment of paradoxical puborectalis contraction. *Dis. Colon Rectum* 1992; 35: 145–50.

Whitehead WE. Effects of psychological factors on gastrointestinal function. In: Snape WJJ, ed. *Pathogenesis of functional bowel disease.* New York: Plenum, 1989: 37.

Whitehead WE, Winget C, Fedoravicius AS, *et al.* Learned illness behavior in patients with irritable bowel syndrome and peptic ulcer. *Dig. Dis. Sci.* 1982; 27: 202–8.

Whitehead WE, Bosmajian L, Zonderman AB, *et al.* Symptoms of psychologic distress associated with irritable bowel syndrome. Comparison of community and medical clinic samples. *Gastroenterology* 1988; 95: 709–14.

Whitehead WE, Drinkwater D, Cheskin LJ, *et al.* Constipation in the elderly living at home. Definition, prevalence, and relationship to lifestyle and health status. *J. Am. Geriatr. Soc.* 1989; 37: 423–9.

Whitehead WE, Holtkotter B, Enck P, *et al.* Tolerance for rectosigmoid distension in irritable bowel syndrome. *Gastroenterology* 1990; 98: 1187–92.

Whitehouse FR, Kernohan JW. Myenteric plexus in congenital megacolon. *Arch. Intern. Med.* 1948; 82: 75–111.

Whorwell PJ, Lupton EW, Erduran D, *et al.* Bladder smooth muscle dysfunction in patients with irritable bowel syndrome. *Gut* 1986; 27: 1014–7.

Williams NS, Patel J, George BD, *et al.* Development of an electrically stimulated neoanal sphincter. *Lancet* 1991; 338: 1166–9.

Williams NS, Hallan RI, Koeze TH, *et al.* Anorectal reconstruction. *Br. J. Surg.* 1992; 79: 733–4.

Womack NR, Williams NS, Holmfield JH, *et al.* Pressure and prolapse—the cause of solitary rectal ulceration. *Gut* 1987; 28: 1228–33.

Womack NR, Morrison JF, Williams NS. Prospective study of the effects of postanal repair in neurogenic faecal incontinence. *Br. J. Surg.* 1988; 75: 48–52.

Yoshioka K, Keighley MR. Clinical results of colectomy for severe constipation. *Br. J. Surg.* 1989; 76: 600–4.

Zargar SA, Khuroo MS, Mahajan R. Sucralfate retention enemas in solitary rectal ulcer. *Dis. Colon Rectum* 1991; 34: 455–7.

14 The appendix

Congenital abnormalities

The embryological link between the development of the caecum and appendix explains the association between congenital abnormalities in both sites.

Duplication of the appendix is usually associated with duplication of the caecum, about 80 cases having been reported (Biermann *et al.* 1993). Most commonly one appendix is hypertropic and the second rudimentary (Kabanchuk *et al.* 1990; Mitchell and Nicholls 1990). Alternatively, two well formed, entirely normal appendices, or even three appendices, may occur. If the caecum is normal, the appendix may be double-barrelled, contained within a single muscle coat.

Congenital absence or atresia of the appendix is reported in about 1 in 100 000 appendices (Rolff *et al.* 1992). This may represent an overestimate, some cases attributed to agenesis in fact representing an overlooked intramural appendix confined to the caecal wall. Therefore, if no appendix is apparent, a careful examination of the entire right colon and the ileocaecal area should be performed. True absence of the appendix may be associated with ileal atresia. Alternatively, the appendix may be rudimentary.

Diverticula

Diverticula may be congenital or acquired.

Congenital diverticula of the appendix, characterized by the involvement of all coats of the appendiceal wall and the absence of inflammation, are exceptionally rare (Figure 14.1). Acquired diverticula occur in less than 1% of appendicectomy specimens. Nearly all diverticula represent an acquired mucosal herniation through a defect in the muscle wall. They are essentially 'blow-outs' from raised intraluminal pressure normally caused by a combination of luminal narrowing and muscle hypertrophy. They may also arise in conjunction with appendiceal carcinoids. Diverticula are often multiple and are usually situated along the mesenteric and antimesenteric aspects of the distal third of the appendix. Although frequently asymptomatic, inflammation in the diverticulum presents as a distinct clinical entity that mimics acute appendicitis. Such cases present earlier and with a higher rate of perforation than normal appendicitis (Sharp *et al.* 1990). On account of this significant risk of complication, it is suggested that the incidental finding of an appendiceal diverticulum at laparotomy justifies appendicectomy. Diverticula occur more frequently in patients with cystic fibrosis, being reported in 14% of those with this condition.

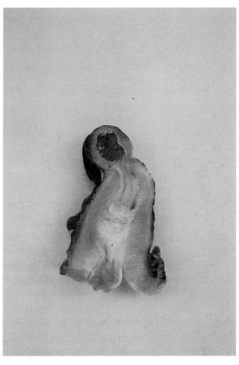

Figure 14.1 Diverticulum of the appendix. Note the involvement of all coats of the appendix wall.

Inflammatory conditions

Acute non-specific appendicitis

Incidence

The importance of acute inflammation of the appendix as a cause of sepsis in the right iliac fossa has been recognized for over 100 years. Acute appendicitis was rare before the twentieth century, its incidence peaking in the 1950, before currently declining to half of this level. This fall in incidence may be partly attributable to changes in hospital coding statistics.

Appendicectomy is still the commonest emergency operation performed in Western Europe, North America, and Australasia but is rare in rural Africa and India. In a study of over 47 000 appendicectomies, operation for histologically proven acute appendicitis was more common in males than females and peaked in the 10–19-year age groups (Primatesta and Goldacre 1994). Both emergency appendicectomy without appendicitis and incidental appendicectomy were more common in women than men (female to male ratio 2:1 and 3:1, respectively) (Primatesta and Goldacre 1994). Wide variations occur in the reported incidence of appendicitis, the severity of inflammation also varying geographically. Acute transmural inflammation is seen in about 25% of African, as opposed to 60% of European appendices removed surgically. Race is a further factor; the incidence of appendicitis in white Americans is 15/100 000 per year, which is 1.5 times greater than that of non-whites. In a study of 100 000 appendicectomies in California, appendicitis was more common in Caucasians and Hispanics than in Negroes and Asians (Luckmann and Davies 1991).

Some studies have found appendicitis to be 10% more common in the summer months (Addiss *et al.* 1990; Luckmann and Davies 1991). Appendicitis is seen more frequently in the second and third decades of life. Females have a slightly greater risk of developing appendicitis than males (relative risk 1.1–1.7 depending on age). The life-time risk of acute inflammation of the appendix in males is 7%, that in females 9%. However, females have a significantly greater life-time risk of having the appendix removed than males (23% versus 12%, respectively) (Addiss *et al.* 1990).

Aetiology and pathogenesis

The aetiology of appendicitis is multifactorial (Table 14.1). Patients with a positive family history are estimated to have 10 times the risk of developing appendicitis compared with those without a family history. However, the major aetiological factor for appendicitis appears to be obstruction of the lumen. Within an obstructed appendix, the pressure of secretions may reach 90 mmHg. The resul-

tant ischaemic damage to the mucosa allows the entry of an increasing number and variety of faecal organisms, initiating the inflammatory process (Baron *et al.* 1992). Bacteriological studies confirm a bacterial transmigration of resident colorectal flora across the wall of inflamed appendices (Baron *et al.* 1992). *Bacteroides* species and *Streptococcus melleri* occur in 60–100% and 50%, respectively, of acute, as opposed to 25% of normal appendices, suggesting that bacterial transmigration occurs with inflammation (Bennion *et al.* 1990; Thadepalli *et al.* 1991). On average, 10 varieties of organism can be grown from acutely inflamed appendices, *Bacteroides fragilis* and *Escherichia coli* occurring in almost all instances (Bennion *et al.* 1990; Hopkins *et al.* 1993). *Peptostreptococcus* are grown in 80% and *Pseudomonas* species in 40% of cases (Bennion *et al.* 1990).

Obstruction of the appendiceal lumen is most frequently caused by a faecolith (Figure 14.2). This represents inspissated faecal material which has formed about a foreign body nidus, growing slowly by the deposition of successive laminae, with occasional calcification. Although such calculi are six times less common than faecoliths, they are associated with a higher incidence of appendiceal perforation (45% versus 20%) (Nitecki *et al.* 1990). When a faecolith co-exists with appendicitis, the inflammation is almost always distal to the obstruction, suggesting the obstruction has contributed to the inflammation. A low roughage diet predisposes to faecolith formation by producing motions that are difficult to propel along the bowel. The geographical variation in both incidence and severity has also been attributed to the lack of fibre in the Western diet.

Other causes of obstruction thought to contribute to appendicitis include constriction of the appendix by peritoneal bands or fibrous adhesions, bezoars and tumours of the appendix or caecum. Carcinoma of the caecum is an uncommon cause of appendicitis, even in elderly patients. In only 2% of patients over the age of 65 years is appendicitis due to caecal carcinoma (Timmermans *et al.* 1992). Lymphoid hyperplasia following viral or bacterial infections

Table 14.1 Causes of appendicitis	
Category	**Cause**
Non-specific obstruction of appendiceal lumen	Faecoliths
	Lymphoid hyperplasia
	Carcinoma of appendix or caecum
	Bezoars
	Peritoneal bands
	Neuronal hyperplasia
Non-obstructed appendicitis Specific	
Bacterial	Tuberculosis
	Actinomycosis
	Schistosomiasis
	Yersinia
Viral	Influenza
	Adenoviruses
	Enteroviruses
	Measles virus
	Mumps
	Cytomegalovirus/HIV
Parasites	*Enterobius*
	Strongyloides
	Amoebiasis
	Ascaris
	Endolumax
	Giardia
	Trichuruasis
	Taeniasis
Inflammatory bowel disease	Ulcerative colitis
	Crohn's disease

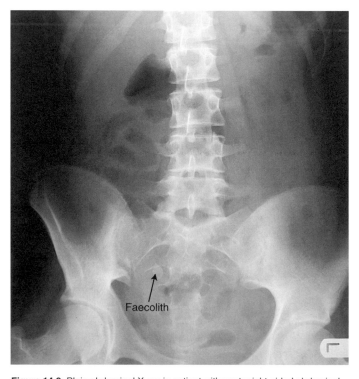

Figure 14.2 Plain abdominal X-ray in patient with acute right-sided abdominal pain showing a faecolith in the appendix and small bowel gas.

may account for the high incidence of appendicitis in childhood. In Africa, lymphoid hyperplasia is noted in 25% of surgically removed acute appendices (Babekir and Devi 1990). In contrast, the inspissated secretions of patients with cystic fibrosis appear to be protective, as the incidence of acute appendicitis in this group is only 2% (Coughlin *et al.* 1990).

The aetiology of so-called 'non-obstructive' appendicitis is controversial. It may represent a functional and intermittent obstruction from the semilunar valve at the base of the appendix or muscular spasm of the appendix itself. The firm motions created by a low roughage diet result in exaggerated muscle activity and a predisposition to muscle spasm. The early epigastric colic of acute appendicitis may be the result of such spasm, rather than inflammation (Gorenstin *et al.* 1996). Neural mechanisms may participate in the adaptation to a low roughage diet. This may be associated with 'neurogenic appendicopathy', which is claimed to account for most cases of fibrous obliteration of the lumen. This condition is characterized by proliferation of nerve fibres, hyperplasia of endocrine cells, and connective tissue infiltration by eosinophils. Neurogenic appendicopathy is claimed to occur in up to 30% of all appendicectomy specimens and up to 80% of macroscopically 'normal' appendicectomies. Subepithelial neuroendocrine cells are identified in 85% of specimens. Half of cases show cells positive for serotonin, one in 10 have somatostatin-positive cells, while cells containing 5-hydroxytryptophan, substance P, bombastin, enteroglucagon, and VIP are occasionally found in the mucosa of both normal appendices and neurogenic appendicopathy. It is postulated that serotonin acts as a neurotransmitter causing the spastic contractions of appendicular colic. Appendicular carcinoids may originate in the frequently multicentric foci of small endocrine cell groups that are localized within the proliferative nerve fibres in the subepithelial stroma.

Acute specific appendicitis

Occasionally, a primary infective cause of appendicitis is attributed to bacteria, viruses, or parasites.

Bacteria implicated in the aetiology of appendicitis include tuberculosis, actinomycosis, schistosomiasis, and yersiniosis.

Tuberculosis

Tuberculous appendicitis is rare in the UK, but represents 2% of appendices removed in India (Nair *et al.* 1993). It is most commonly associated with ileocaecal tuberculosis, although secondary spread from pulmonary infection or apparent primary appendiceal tuberculosis have been recorded. The clinical appearances vary from normal to a thickened, chronically inflamed appendix adherent to adjacent structures. Pathologically tubercle bacilli can be demonstrated in the characteristic caseating granulomata of the appendiceal wall and mesenteric lymph nodes.

Actinomycosis

Actinomyces israelia is a commensal of the mouth which may be seen in, or grown from, 0.05% of appendicectomy specimens (Zagorski *et al.* 1992). However, the presence of *A.israelia* in the lumen of even acutely inflamed appendices does not necessarily imply pathogenicity. Appendicitis can only be attributed to *Actinomyces* if the characteristic branching filaments are present within the inflamed tissues. Appendiceal actinomycosis typically presents as chronic, rather than acute, inflammation. Complications include sinus or fistula formation, either enteric or cutaneous, and liver abscesses from septic embolization along the portal vein.

Schistosomiasis

In areas where it is endemic, schistosomiasis may account for 6% of all removed appendices (Babekir and Divi 1990). The histological features of appendiceal schistosomiasis reflect those of the rest of the colon, namely mucosal ulceration, a prominent eosinophilic reaction in response to the deposition of eggs in the submucosa and a chronic granulomatous inflammation (Adebamowo *et al.* 1991). The resultant fibrosis leads to chronic inflammation with spotty, linear, or amorphous calcification being detected radiologically in 45% of cases.

Yersinia

The appendix may be involved in intestinal yersiniosis, although changes are much more common and more conspicuous in the terminal ileum and mesenteric nodes (Franzin *et al.* 1991; Kanazawa *et al.* 1991). The histological changes in the affected appendix are variable sometimes being indistinguishable from acute non-specific appendicitis. On other occasions the characteristic histological features of yersiniosis are seen in the ileum with granulomata often containing micro-abscesses and lymphoid hyperplasia. The diagnosis is best confirmed by serology.

Acute appendicitis may complicate the course of specific intestinal infections, such as typhoid and paratyphoid fever, bacillary dysentery, and salmonella food poisoning. Salmonella infection accounts for up to 0.05% of cases of acute appendicitis (Zagorski *et al.* 1992). The changes in the appendix in such cases reflect those found in other parts of the intestine. Other bacteria have also been implicated. *Campylobacter jejuni* may produce abdominal pain mimicking appendicitis but has also been recovered from infected appendices. *Campylobacter laridis* and sarcophaga larvae may also be detected in acute appendicitis. Spirochetes (*Brachyspira aalborgi*) are detected in 0.7% of pathologically inflamed, as well as 12% of clinically inflamed, appendices.

Viruses

The clinical features of viral appendicitis are usually ill-defined, although lymphoid hyperplasia may produce appendicitis by luminal narrowing or initiating intussusception. Measles infection is the easiest to recognize histologically by characteristic Warthin–Finkeldey multinucleated giant cells situated in the margins of briskly reactive lymphoid follicles. Adenovirus infection may also produce lymphoid hyperplasia, with focal destruction of the surface epithelium. Cytomegalovirus and Kaposi's sarcoma appendicitis associated with AIDS have been reported, the risk of perforation of the appendix being high (Chetty *et al.* 1993; Neumayer *et al.* 1993) (Figure 14.3a and b). A minority of patients with acute appendicitis do show serological evidence of recent infection with mumps or influenza B viruses. In children influenza viruses, enteroviruses, adenoviruses, and paramyxoviruses may be found in up to two-thirds of cases of appendicitis, influenza virus type C being the most commonly identified. In 80% of such cases *Escherichia coli*, *Pseudomonas aerugonosa*, and *Klebsiella* are also found, suggesting a possible interaction between bacteria and viruses in the aetiology of appendicitis. Consequently, it has been proposed that primary viral infection initiates mucosal barrier damage sufficiently to allow secondary invasion by faecal organisms.

Parasites

Several parasites have been identified in appendicectomy specimens. The reported incidence of infestation of the appendix by oxyuriasis (*Enterobius*) vermicularis, also known as threadworm or pinworm, is

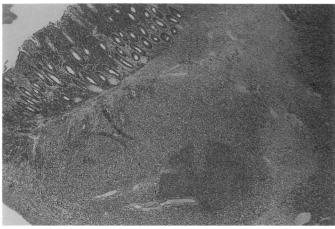

(a)

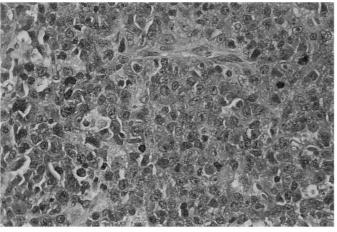

(b)

Figure 14.3 Section from the base of an intestinal ulcer in a patient with AIDS. Cytomegalovirus inclusion bodies are identified (arrowed). (a) H + EX50; (b) H + E × 250.

usually about 5% (Babekir and Devi 1990; Wiebe 1991). It is commonest in the 6–10 year and 21–25 year age groups, being identified in 15% of appendices removed during childhood (Cerva *et al.* 1991; Wiebe 1991) (Figure 14.4). Although male pinworms are more common, there is an association between the release of ova from female pinworms and appendiceal inflammation. Their presence can evoke a marked eosinophilic response resulting in a granulomatous reaction. However, pinworm infestation of the appendix appears to be asymptomatic and only rarely contributes to the development of acute appendicitis. Other infestations, such as *Strongyloides stercoralis* can also give rise to eosinophilic appendicitis. Appendiceal involvement may also occur in amoebic dysentery, although there are reports of amoebiasis apparently localized to the appendix (Malik *et al.* 1994; Siddiqui *et al.* 1994). Several other parasites may be found in appendicectomy specimens, particularly in developing countries. These include *Ascaris lumbricoides* (0.5% of appendicectomy specimens), tophozoites of *Dientamosla fragilis* (5%), *Endolumax nana* (2%), entamobea (1%), cysts of *Giardia intestinalis* (2%), trichuriasis (0.05%), and taeniasis (0.05%) (Cerva *et al.* 1991).

Pathological appearances

The earliest macroscopic abnormality of acute appendicitis is swelling with patchy inflammation of the serosal surface and thin mucopus in the lumen. Swelling and hyperaemia then increase, especially distal to any obstruction, the peritoneal surface becoming dulled by the deposition of fibrin or purulent exudate. Eventually gangrene supervenes, part or all of the organ becoming friable and haemorrhagic, showing greenish-brown patches of necrosis. The lumen is then grossly distended with thick mucopus. The combination of a wall weakened by gangrene and a raised intraluminal pressure from the accumulation of infected exudate in an obstructed lumen, may lead to perforation and peritonitis. Occasionally, the clinical and pathological features are poorly correlated, gangrenous appendicitis occurring within a few hours of the onset of symptoms.

Histologically, acute appendicitis is characterized by oedema and congestion of the appendiceal wall, a transmural infiltration of neutrophil polymorphs often forming small intramural abscesses, ulceration of the mucosa, and a local fibrinopurulent exudate (Figure

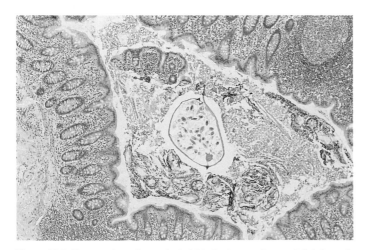

Figure 14.4 Pinworm (oxyuris vermicularis) in the lumen of an acutely inflamed appendix. H&E×100.

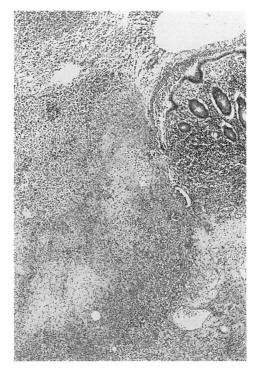

Figure 14.5 Acute appendicitis showing intense active transmural inflammation. The mucosa is ulcerated and there is pus in the lumen. H&E×100.

14.5). Thrombosis may be seen, particularly in the veins and may be associated with necrosis of the wall and perforation. Fibrosis results in the appendix becoming a thickened fibrous cord, with partial or complete obliteration of the lumen.

It is suggested that all surgically removed appendices should be examined pathologically, as unsuspected abnormalities, which may require further treatment are found in up to 5% of cases. Diagnostic difficulty arises, when, in the presence of clinical appendicitis, pathology reveals only mild inflammation confined to the mucosa. This could represent early appendicitis or merely a variation of normal (Wang et al. 1996). Immunoperoxidase staining with fibronectin may then be helpful in distinguishing normal from truly inflamed appendices. It is suggested that five pathological categories be employed; no inflammation, early inflammation, acute inflammation, peri-appendicitis, and other diagnoses (granulomata) (Herd et al. 1992).

Up to 35% of appendices removed electively from asymptomatic patients undergoing unrelated surgery show collections of neutrophil polymorphs in the lumen, focal ulceration of the surface epithelium with pus cells in the adjacent lamina propria and even a few crypt abscesses. Of 117 incidentally removed appendices during gynaecological procedures, abnormalities were detected in 83% and in 17% the findings altered clinical management. Incidentally removed appendices during jejunoileal bypass or urological surgery show about one-third to have some pathological abnormality. In neither study did incidental appendicectomy increase the morbidity or mortality of the procedure, the complication rate of removing non-inflamed appendices being 3%. Therefore, in cases where the pathological changes are slight, other causes for acute abdominal pain should be excluded before the changes are attributed to appendicitis.

Clinical presentation

The classical symptoms and signs of appendicitis are well known, the proportion of children presenting with abdominal pain being 98%, fever 80%, vomiting 80%, and altered bowel habit 20%, respectively (Silen and Tracy 1993; Jeddy et al. 1994). Over 5% of patients will have had similar symptoms on a previous occassion suggesting recurrent appendicitis (Barber et al. 1997). Atypical presentations, with symptoms such as bladder irritation, occasionally occur. However, 15–20% of patients with a typical presentation will have a pathologically normal appendix (Gibney et al. 1992). As age increases, classical presentation becomes less common and delay in diagnosis increases (Braveman et al. 1994). Classical symptoms occur in only 20% of the over 60s, with only half of cases being diagnosed as possible appendicitis on presentation. Seventy per cent of elderly patients present with perforation and complications occur in up to 40% of cases (Shoji and Becker 1994). Consequently, a high index of suspicion is required for the correct diagnosis of appendicitis in elderly patients (Ovrebo et al. 1993).

The position of the appendix has important clinical implications, as it localizes the site of parietal pain during inflammation. Traditional teaching states that the base of the appendix lies opposite the junction of the lateral and middle thirds of a line drawn between the anterior superior iliac spine and the umbilicus (McBurney's point). However, barium studies suggest that in 70% of cases, the base of the appendix is situated at a position lower and more medial than McBurney's point (Karim et al. 1990). The appendix is most often located behind the caecum or with its distal end in the pelvis. Retrocaecal appendices become more common with age, but are less frequent in Negros. About 60% of appendices are retrocaecal. The other positions in which appendices occur are pelvic (30%), subcaecal (3%), pre-ileal (1%), and post-ileal (1%).

Despite most appendices being retrocaecal, appendices in this position are less likely to become inflamed (Shen et al. 1991). Only about 25% of surgically removed acutely inflamed appendices in both Caucasians and Africans are situated retrocaecally, compared with about 40% of pelvic appendices (Ceres et al. 1990). Reports vary as to whether appendices which are 'hidden' from clinical assessment have a greater risk of perforation. Although Guidry and Poole (1994) found that 'hidden' appendices are more likely to present with gangrenous than simple appendicitis (69% versus 5%), others have noted no difference in the incidence of perforation between retrocaecal and other positions (14% versus 18%) (Shen et al. 1991; Hale et al. 1997).

Diagnosis

Accurate diagnosis of acute appendicitis is difficult and controversy exists between balancing the risk of perforation with that of removing normal appendices. The clinical assessment of appendicitis is notoriously inaccurate, the incidence of pathologically normal appendices removed surgically varying from 14% to 36%, most studies world-wide reporting a normal appendicectomy rate of about 20% (Babekir and Devi 1990; Ricci et al. 1991; Sivit et al. 1992). Clinical judgement of appendicitis has an accuracy of about 75%, with a sensitivity of 50–63%, and specificity of 82–95% (Gibney et al. 1992). The false positive rate of clinical assessment is 25%, being 16% for males and 38% for females (Royes et al. 1991). The predictive value of a clinical diagnosis of appendicitis is 90%, the negative predictive value being 30–60% (Grunewald and Keating 1993; Lindsey 1994). However, clinical accuracy in women varies from 55% to 70%, being poorest in those 20–40 years old or halfway through their menstrual cycle (Ricci et al. 1991; Gibney et al. 1992; Webster et al. 1993). In children the clinical accuracy for correctly diagnosing acute appendicitis is 80% and is not improved by biochemical tests (Ovrebo et al. 1993). If the appendix is macroscopically normal, 15–20% of children will have other diseases (small bowel/mesenteric 10%, gynaecological 5%) (Sivit et al. 1992).

The most accurate clinical feature is migration of the pain to the right iliac fossa, which is associated with an odds ratio of 5.1 (John et al. 1993; Eskelinen et al. 1994). Nausea and bowel irregularity are less reliable, while appendicitis is unlikely if symptoms have been present for more than 48 h (John et al. 1993). In children, vomiting occurring before the pain makes the diagnosis unlikely. Useful findings are rigidity (odds ratio 5.0), rebound (odds ratio 3.3), and guarding (odds ratio 3.1) (John et al. 1993; Eskelinen et al. 1994). The presence and pitch of bowel sounds are of little diagnostic value (John et al. 1993). Similarly, tenderness on rectal examination and pyrexia do not improve diagnostic accuracy, particularly if rebound is present (Jeddy et al. 1994).

The reported sensitivity, specificity, and negative predictive value of an elevated white cell count are all about 85%, but is not predictive of perforation. Examining the proportion of neutrophils improves the sensitivity at the expense of specificity (John et al. 1993).

C-reactive protein is elevated in 95% of cases of acute appendicitis compared with 15% of normal appendices (Mazlam and Hodgson 1994). If the C-reactive protein level in blood drawn 12 h after the onset of symptoms is less than 2.5 mg/dl, it is claimed that acute appendicitis can be excluded (Albu et al. 1994). The combination of alterations in white cell count, differential white cell count and C-reactive protein can reduce the negative laparotomy rate from 24% to 16%, sensitivity and positive predictive value being up to 100%, the predicitive value of a negative test being 37%. Peritoneal aspiration cytology is claimed to be useful in diagnosing acute appendicitis and consequently reducing the negative appendicectomy rate. The sensitivity is 91% and specificity 94% corresponding to a positive predictive value of 95% and negative predictive value of 94% (Caldwell and Watson 1994).

In an attempt to improve the accuracy of diagnosis, scoring systems, and probability nomograms have been developed (Owen *et al.* 1992; Eskelinen *et al.* 1994). Although these reduce the negative laparotomy rate, their main benefit is to aid junior doctors in Accident and Emergency departments decide on the necessity for admission, the clinical experience of the surgeon still being important in determining the need for operation. Overall, appendicitis is unlikely if symptoms and signs are equivocal, pain starts in the right iliac fossa, white cell count is less than 10 000/ml or in females during the first 14 days of the menstrual period (Christian and Christian 1992). Operation should be performed early in those over 50 years as atypical or asymptomatic presentations are common. However, if too strict constraints are applied on operation, morbidity rises from 5% to 20% (Milamed and Hedley-Whyte 1994). The assessment of the surgeon in theatre as to the presence of acute inflammation in a given appendix is also variable. The false positive rate, with the surgeon feeling the appendix is inflamed but with normal pathological findings, is 5%, while the reverse situation occurs in 10%.

Radiology can aid in the diagnosis of appendicitis and reduce the negative laparotomy rate. The presence of gas in the appendix occurs in 3% of cases of acute appendicitis, but makes subsequent ultrasonic diagnosis difficult. A gas-filled appendix is thought to be diagnostic of appendicitis if the appendix is caudad to the caecum in the right lower quadrant. However, this finding lacks specificity. The presence of a gas-filled appendix with an meniscus due to a faecolith is, however, specific of appendicitis. A barium enema may also aid diagnosis and reduce the negative laparotomy rate in doubtful cases (Figure 14.6). The reported sensitivity is 83% specificity 86%, accuracy 92%, positive predictive value 88%, and negative predictive value 95% (Sarfati *et al.* 1993). Complete appendiceal filling on either single or double contrast barium enemas excludes a

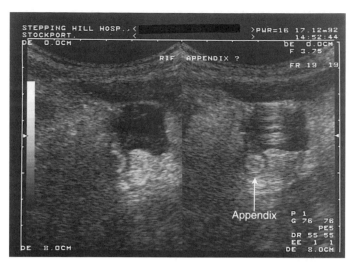

Figure 14.7 Ultrasound scan in patient with RIF pain showing the typical 'polo mint' appearance of the appendix (arrowed). Note also the adjacent free fluid.

diagnosis of appendicitis. Barium enema may show appendiceal filling defects (83% of cases), partial appendiceal filling (44%), non-visualization of the appendix (42%) and appendicular distension (100%). Caution is required in cases of appendiceal abscesses producing extrinsic compression of the caecum, as this may mimic caecal carcinoma. Some feel that barium enemas should be reserved for cases in which the diagnosis is in doubt, others that it should be performed in every case over the age of 50 years when caecal carcinoma may be detected in up to 8% of cases (Bleker and Wereldsma 1989).

Ultrasound scan can correctly diagnose appendicitis in 90% of all cases (Ceres *et al.* 1990; Sivit *et al.* 1992; Jeffrey *et al.* 1994; Reisener *et al.* 1994). Appearances in acute appendicitis may be either a fluid–filled slightly distended structure or a collapsed single tubular structure with slight circumferential wall thickening (Figure 14.7). Increased blood flow in the appendiceal wall detected by colour Doppler suggests appendicitis, but absence of flow cannot definitively distinguish a normal from an abnormal appendix (Quillin and Siegel 1994; Patriquin *et al.* 1996).

Computerized tomography (CT) scanning may also be useful, particularly if faecoliths are present (Sarfati *et al.* 1993; Wong *et al.* 1993; Moser *et al.* 1994; Rao *et al.* 1997). It is also beneficial in diagnosing appendiceal abscesses, especially in elderly patients in whom the presentation is often atypical (Smith *et al.* 1996; Duran *et al.* 1997). However, a caecum filled with faeces can confuse the diagnosis. CT is often more accurate than ultrasound in the diagnosis of acute appendicitis (Balthazar *et al.* 1994; Friedland and Siegel 1997; Lane *et al.* 1997).

Complications

The overall complication rate of simple and gangrenous appendicitis is 5% and 10%, respectively (Keller *et al.* 1996; Hale *et al.* 1997). Perforation results in diffuse peritonitis and an overall complication rate of up to 30% from the widespread bacteraemia and abscess formation (Hopkins *et al.* 1993) (Figure 14.8). With the use of thorough peritoneal lavage and pre-operative antibiotics, wound infection rates of 5% can be expected, even in gangrenous appendicitis (Serour *et al.* 1996). Consequently, absorbable subcuticular sutures for skin closure may be used in almost all cases (Serour *et al.* 1996; Brasel *et al.* 1997). Using such measures there is little need for drains, which in themselves are believed to increase the risk of in-

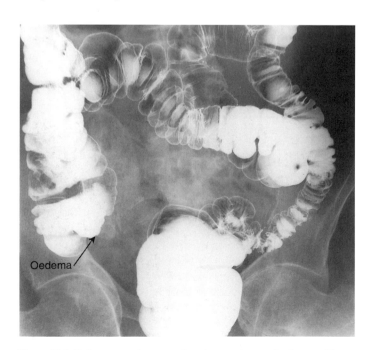

Figure 14.6 Barium enema in a case of a retrocaecal appendix abscess. There is absence of filling of the appendix and mucosal oedema indenting the caecum from behind (arrowed).

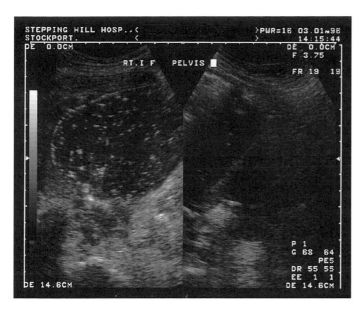

Figure 14.8 Ultrasound scan in a case of appendix abscess. Note the 'snow shower' appearance in a localized collection.

fection. One in 10 adults and one in seven children will be admitted with gangrenous appendicitis (Berends *et al.* 1994; Guidry and Poole 1994). Slow perforation or perforation of a retrocaecal appendix results in containment of the pus by the fibrinous exudate that binds the appendix to adjacent structures, creating an appendix abscess. These may be drained percutaneously or transrectally (Pereira *et al.* 1996). Very occasionally, such an abscess may rupture back into the caecum or fistulate into the adjacent small or large bowel, bladder or abdominal wall.

Infected thrombosis of the veins is usually confined to the small vessels of the appendix. Involvement of larger vessels allows septic emboli to travel to the liver, creating multiple liver abscesses (Mahieu *et al.* 1993) (Figure 14.9). Such suppurative phlebitis has become much rarer since the introduction of antibiotics.

Late complications include fibrous adhesions predisposing to subsequent intestinal obstruction. Proximal obliteration of the lumen by post-inflammatory scarring can result in distension by sterile mucus, forming a mucocele. This may become infected to create an

empyema or rupture, spilling mucus into the peritoneal cavity (pseudo-myxoma peritonei). The mortality of appendicitis has declined steadily over the last 50 years, mainly due to the use of antibiotics. About 60% of deaths occur in those over 70 years (Milamed and Hedley-Whyte 1994), as presentation is less typical and consequently late diagnosis and silent perforation are more common, in this age group. Mortality in those over 60 years is 0.7% but rises to 2% in cases where perforation or abscesses are present.

Treatment

To minimize complications acute appendicitis is best treated as early as possible by appendicectomy. In the diagnosis of right iliac fossa pain of uncertain origin it is suggested that laparoscopy provides diagnostic and therapeutic advantages over conventional surgery (Valla *et al.* 1991; Nowzaradan *et al.* 1993; Jadallah *et al.* 1994; Reissman *et al.* 1994). Laparoscopy gives excellent exposure of the entire abdomen including the appendix regardless of its position while allowing definitive treatment of most of the surgical conditions encountered (Nowzaradan *et al.* 1993; Champault *et al.* 1997) (Figure 14.10). The technique allows an accurate diagnosis of acute appendicitis with a 97% correlation between the clinical assessment on laparoscopy and microscopic evidence of inflammation (Valla *et al.* 1991). Laparoscopy alters the diagnosis in 20% and the management in 15% of patients (Scott and Rosin 1993). On laparoscopy up to 40% of patients with possible appendicitis do not require appendicectomy (Jadallah *et al.* 1994). In a study of right iliac fossa pain in females, appendicitis was diagnosed by laparoscopy in 55% of cases, pelvic inflammatory disease in 22%, and torted fimbral cyst in 3% (Scott and Rosin 1993). Many of these conditions may also be successfully treated laparoscopically (Apelgren *et al.* 1996). Several reports suggest that incidental appendicectomy should be performed in patients undergoing diagnostic laparoscopy for lower abdominal pain (Welch *et al.* 1991; Luthi *et al.* 1993; Jadallah *et al.* 1994). In a study comparing routine and selective removal of appendices identified at laparoscopy, only 13% of the routinely removed appendices did not show some degree of pathological abnormality (Jadallah *et al.* 1994).

Several studies have compared conventional and laparoscopic appendicectomy (Buckley *et al.* 1994; Frazee *et al.* 1994; Hansen *et al.* 1996; McCahill *et al.* 1996). None of these were controlled. In series consisting of over 100 laparoscopic cases operating times are similar between the two techniques (mean duration of open appendicec-

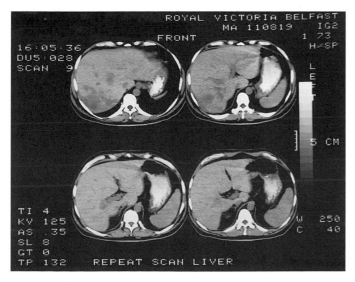

Figure 14.9 CT scan showing multiple liver abscesses.

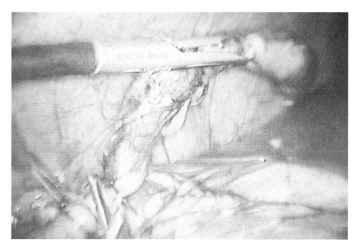

Figure 14.10 Laparoscopic appendicectomy—acutely inflamed appendix about to be divided.

tomy 45 min, laparoscopic appendicectomy 50 min) (Pier *et al.* 1991; Saye *et al.* 1991). With experience, all grades of appendiceal inflammation, including abscesses, can be treated laparoscopically, conversion to open surgery being necessary in 5–10% of cases (Kim *et al.* 1993; Schiffino *et al.* 1993; Buckley *et al.* 1994; Hebebrand *et al.* 1994; Frazee and Bohannon 1996). Minor intra-operative complications occur in about 4% of laparoscopic appendicectomies (Valla *et al.* 1991; Hansen *et al.* 1996). The procedure may be safely performed in children, provided paediatric instruments are used (Valla *et al.* 1991; Misena *et al.* 1993; el Ghoneimi *et al.* 1994)

The postoperative complications following laparoscopic and conventional appendicectomy are similar, although minor complications, particularly wound infections, may be less with the laparoscopic approach (Buckley *et al.* 1994; Williams *et al.* 1994; Panton *et al.* 1996). Removal of the appendix through the trocar or in an entrapment sac protects the wound and may explain the lower incidence of wound infection with the laparoscopic approach. Following laparoscopic appendicectomy about 2% of patients will require a subsequent laparotomy or repeat laparoscopic procedure (Valla *et al.* 1991). Recurrent appendicitis has been reported when a long appendiceal stump was not recognized and resected during laparoscopic appendicectomy (Devereaux *et al.* 1994). Complications following laparoscopic appendicectomy may be reduced by ensuring safe insertion of the Veress needle, employing electrocautery to separate the appendix from the mesoappendix and using an organ retrieval sac for removal of the appendix (McAnena and Wilson 1993; Nowzaradan and Barnes 1993).

Several studies suggest that postoperative pain requirements and pain scores are less with the laparoscopic procedure (Buckley *et al.* 1994; Williams *et al.* 1994). Mean hospital stay is also slightly less following laparoscopic appendicectomy (4.5 days compared to 6 days for the open procedure) (Schiffino *et al.* 1993; Williams *et al.* 1994). Return to full activity occurs at a mean of 14 days after laparoscopic, compared with 25 days following open appendectomy (Saye *et al.* 1991; Vallina *et al.* 1993; Frazee *et al.* 1994).

An intra-abdominal abscess develops in about 2% of patients following appendicectomy (Mosdell *et al.* 1994; Surana and Puri 1994; Pacelli *et al.* 1996). It can normally be detected by ultrasound scan 1–2 weeks after operation (Gorenstein *et al.* 1994) (Figure 14.11).

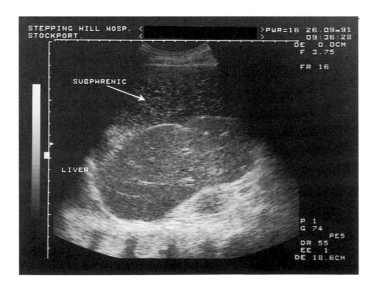

Figure 14.11 Ultrasound scan showing a right subphrenic collection in a case of perforated appendicitis.

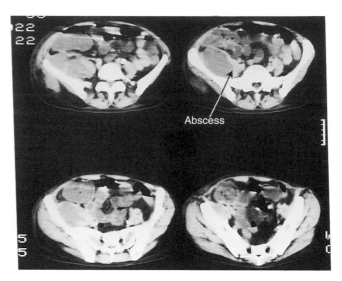

Figure 14.12 CT scan of a right iliac fossa abscess.

Conservative management consists of intravenous antibiotics effective against both aerobes and anaerobes and serial ultrasound scans. Eighty per cent of patients show gradual shrinkage and collapse of the abscess in response to such measures (Gorenstein *et al.* 1994). Those demonstrating enlargement of the collection on serial ultrasound scans frequently respond to percutaneous drainage under ultrasonic or CT control (Gorenstein *et al.* 1994; Moser *et al.* 1994; Pereira *et al.* 1996) so that few patients require further surgical intervention (Figure 14.12).

Appendicitis in pregnancy

Appendicitis is the commonest non-obstetric surgical condition complicating pregnancy. The signs and symptoms are often classical so that overall diagnostic accuracy (75%) is little less than in non-pregnant females (Halvorsen *et al.* 1994). However, diagnosis may be difficult as the clinical presentation resembles several other surgical and medical entities common to pregnancy, while physiological abdominal pain is frequent in the pregnant female. In addition, physical examination of the abdomen is hampered by the pregnant state. The reluctance to use X-rays should be reconsidered in the presence of severely ill or unstable patients (Epstein 1994). Whenever the diagnosis is uncertain, liberal use of surgical and obstetric consultants is warranted. The development of sepsis is associated with uterine contractions and fetal death (Halvorsen *et al.* 1994). Appropriate antibiotics should therefore be used as the consequences of sepsis are severe (Halvorsen *et al.* 1994). After the first trimester the risk of sepsis with its associated fetal mortality outweighs the adverse effects of an anaesthetic. Consequently, to minimize maternal and especially fetal mortality, prompt clinical diagnosis and surgical intervention are necessary (Epstein 1994; Halvorsen 1994). Pregnancy should therefore not divert surgeons from performing appendicectomy promptly once the diagnosis is suspected, while simultaneous Caesarean section should only be performed on obstetric indications (Halvorsen *et al.* 1994).

Chronic non-specific appendicitis

The existence of chronic appendicitis is contentious, some believing it merely represents arrested inflammation rather than a distinct clinical entity. This is supported by the frequently poor correlation between a clinical diagnosis of chronic appendicitis and the pathological findings. In contrast, that spontaneous resolution of acute appendicitis may occur is suggested by the incidence of pathological changes in incidentally removed appendices (Seidman *et al.* 1991; Mattei *et al.* 1994). The incidence of recurrent appendicitis, distinct from acute appendicitis, is claimed to be up to 10% of those with recurrent right iliac fossa pain (Hawes and Whalen 1994). Histological comparison between appendices of those clinically felt to have chronic appendicitis is remarkably similar to specimens removed incidentally from asymptomatic patients. Among those who accept the entity of chronic appendicitis, the incidence of this condition varies from 0.9% to 5% of all appendices removed. This is related to differences in the pathological criteria used for diagnosis. For instance, fibrosis alone cannot be used as an indicator of chronic appendicitis as the amount of appendiceal fibrous tissue increases with age (Andreou *et al.* 1990). Rather, to make a diagnosis of chronic appendicitis, there should be evidence of acute-on-chronic inflammation such as lymphocyte or plasma cell infiltration or the presence of granulation tissue. Unless such histological proof is obtained, it is prudent to seek another cause, rather than attribute recurrent abdominal pain to chronic appendicitis.

Other varieties of appendicitis

Inflammatory bowel disease

The appendix may be involved in both ulcerative colitis and Crohn's disease (Dudley and Dean 1993). Half of both adults and children with ulcerative colitis will have involvement of the right colon and appendix (Zagorski *et al.* 1992). The degree of appendiceal inflammation is similar to that in the caecum in three-quarters of such cases, acute ulcerative appendicitis occurring in one-quarter (Zagorski *et al.* 1992). Similarly, up to 50% of children with Crohn's disease will have ileocolic involvement, the degree of inflammation in the appendix and ileum being similar in two-thirds of cases (Zagorski *et al.* 1992). The pathological features of such cases are identical to Crohn's disease elsewhere in the gastrointestinal tract, with transmural focal lymphoid aggregates, fissuring, ulceration, granulomatous inflammation, and fibrosis.

Granulomatous appendicitis can be the first manifestation of Crohn's disease. Crohn's disease confined solely to the appendix represents approximately 6% of all surgically operated Crohn's disease (Masuo *et al.* 1994). Two-thirds of these cases present as acute appendicitis and one-sixth as appendiceal abscesses. The risk of Crohn's disease developing in the remainder of the bowel is minimal. Therefore, Crohn's disease limited to the appendix may represent either a less aggressive form of the disease or chronic granulomatous appendicitis of unknown aetiology that is a different clinical entity unrelated to Crohn's disease.

Miscellaneous conditions

Intussusception

Intussusception of the appendix is rare, most cases occurring in childhood (Jevon *et al.* 1992). Primary causes of intussusception are a fetal cone-shaped caecum, a thin meso-appendix, and increased, irregular peristalsis. It is more commonly secondary to intraluminal foreign bodies, faecoliths, worms, lymphoid hyperplasia, endometriosis, adenomatous polyps, or adenocarcinoma of the caecum (Jevon *et al.* 1992). Several varieties are described including intus-

susception of the tip into the more proximal appendix, intussusception of the proximal appendix into the caecum, either of which may lead to complete inversion of the appendix and finally intussusception of the proximal into the distal appendix. Clinically, it may present as a transient phenomenon in otherwise asymptomatic patients or as a rock hard caecal mass at laparotomy. Barium enema shows a characteristic coiled spring appearance in the caecum with non-filling of the appendix, while colonoscopy typically reveals a submucosal swelling.

Endometriosis

Involvement of the appendix occurs in 1% of patients with pelvic endometriosis and up to 0.8% of routine appendicectomy specimens. Whether endometriosis can cause acute appendicitis is disputed; luminal obstruction caused by intussusception or haemorrhage into an endometrial focus being suggested as possible factors (Ardies *et al.* 1990). Pre-operative diagnosis is difficult, almost half of cases presenting with symptoms mimicking chronic or cyclical appendicitis. Most cases therefore arise as an incidental finding at laparotomy or as 'appendicitis' (Gonzalez *et al.* 1992). Although ultrasound or CT scanning may aid diagnosis, laboratory tests are of no benefit, the diagnosis usually being made on histological grounds (Normand and Rioux 1992).

Pathologically, in appendiceal endometriosis there are soft, haemorrhagic, pale fibrotic deposits in any layer of the appendix, most commonly the subserosa and outer muscle coat, associated with marked localized muscular thickening. The characteristic finding is of endometrial glands and stroma, often associated with recent or old haemorrhage and fibrosis. Stromal decidualization may occur during pregnancy (Suster and Moran 1990). Appendicectomy is curative (Gonzalez *et al.* 1992).

Vasculitis

Vasculitis can be detected in 0.3% of appendiceal specimens. Seventy-five per cent of these cases will subsequently develop systemic vasculitis, (most commonly polyarteritis nodosum) in the following 10 years. A focal necrotizing arteritis of the appendix has been described as an incidental finding, usually in young women, unrelated to appendicitis or any systemic disease.

Other conditions which can rarely be found in the appendix are dermoid cysts, malacoplakia and appendicular cystic pneumatosis in young children. Torsion of the appendix is also rare, predisposing to acute appendicitis if the appendix is unusually long or has a lax mesentery.

Mucocele of the appendix

Mucoceles are reported in 0.1% of appendicectomies and are more common in females (Loizon *et al.* 1989; Landen *et al.* 1992). The pathogenesis is unknown. Formerly, the term was applied to all mucin-secreting conditions of the appendix, but it is now suggested that it be restricted to three histological types; mucosal hyperplasia (frequently associated with colonic adenocarcinoma); incidental cystadenoma and mucinous cystadenocarcinoma (Younes *et al.* 1995). About 90% of mucinous cystadenomas and 80% of cystadenocarcinomas presented with mucoceles. Mucoceles due to hyperplasia normally measure less than 1 cm. Histology reveals a flattened epithelium, loose connective tissue containing mucin-laden macrophages and giant cells or occasionally a metaplastic appearance (Higa *et al.* 1973). Mucoceles produced by cystadenomas or cystadenocarcinomas are larger and lined by neoplastic epithelium (Higa *et al.* 1973).

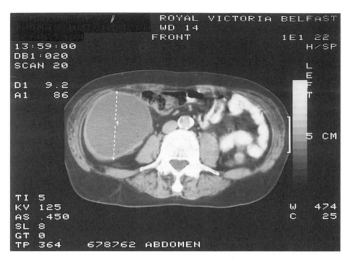

Figure 14.13 CT scan of a patient with appendiceal mucocele and pseudomyxoma peritonei.

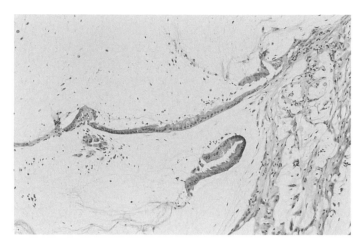

Figure 14.14 Pseudomyxoma peritonei from a mucocele of the appendix. H&E×40.

Clinical signs are non-specific or absent, the abnormality being detected incidentally at laparotomy (Loizon *et al.* 1989; Landen *et al.* 1992). Straight abdominal X-ray may show a calcified, gas-filled appendix (Boyez *et al.* 1985), while ultrasound is often the most useful investigation (Loizon *et al.* 1989). On CT scanning a mucocele appears as a fluid-filled, variable shaped, thin-walled structure containing low-density contents without peri-appendiceal inflammation (Balthazar *et al.* 1988) (Figure 14.13). Mucinous carcinoma appears as a single or multiloculated irregular shaped cystic lesion with solid elements and possible infiltration of the caecum or terminal ileum. Nuclear magnetic resonance imaging is also beneficial, distinguishing between appendiceal mucocele and ovarian carcinoma (Jaluvka *et al.* 1989). Benign mucoceles are satisfactorily treated by appendicectomy, although malignant cases have a bad prognosis because of the risk of pseudo-myxoma peritonei (Loizon *et al.* 1989).

Pseudo-myxoma peritonei

This is the presence of mucinous material, either locally or generally, within the peritoneal cavity. It is caused by rupture of a mucous-filled viscus, usually the appendix, gall-bladder, or a mucinous ovarian cyst into the peritoneal cavity. The appendix accounts for over half of all cases and may be associated with a better survival than pseudo-myxoma arising from other sites (Gough *et al.* 1994; Prayson *et al.* 1994; Hsieh *et al.* 1995). Synchronous involvement of both the appendix and ovary commonly occurs (Young *et al.* 1991; Prayson *et al.* 1994). Rupture of a hyperplastic type mucocele or a cystadenoma of the appendix usually results in the mucus being contained within the right iliac fossa (Figure 14.13). Cystadenocarcinomas which have penetrated the wall may give rise to peritoneal seedlings that produce large volumes of mucus, resulting in generalized pseudo-myxoma peritonei (Higa *et al.* 1973). Rupture of a cystadenocarcinoma also produces generalized pseudo-myxoma peritoneii. Cytological examination of samples of mucus appears to be of limited value in predicting whether an individual case is benign or malignant (Wolff and Ahmed 1976). Pseudo-myxoma peritonei can be distinguished from invasive adenocarcinoma by the presence of inflammation and abscess formation within the wall with an absent desmoplastic reaction (Gibbs 1973). Pre-operative diagnosis can be made by a combination of careful physical examination

and ultrasonography or CT. Echogenic ascites and diffuse low attenuation intra-abdominal masses with scalloping on the surface of liver detected by ultrasound or CT are found in most patients (Nelson *et al.* 1992; Hsieh *et al.* 1995).

Pseudo-myxoma generalized throughout the peritoneal cavity fails to regress after appendicectomy alone but long-term survival can be increased by aggressive excision of all apparent tumour (Smith *et al.* 1992) (Figure 14.14). This significantly improves survival and decreases recurrence rates compared with appendicectomy alone, especially in Dukes' stages B2 and C (Lenroit and Hugier 1989).

Prognosis

The 3-year survival for mild residual disease is 92%, that for moderate disease 48% while that for gross residual tumour is 20%. Recurrence may develop in up to half of patients, necessitating further surgery (Wertheim *et al.* 1994). It has been recommended that adjuvant chemotherapy be restricted to cases where recurrence has developed (Smith *et al.* 1992; Gough *et al.* 1994; Wertheim *et al.* 1994). However, 3-year survival from cytoreductive surgery combined with intra-operative chemotherapy can be 90% (Jacquet *et al.* 1996). A rising carcino-embryonic antigen (CEA) level is suggestive of recurrence (Hsieh *et al.* 1995; Sugarbaker and Jablonski 1995).

Tumours of the appendix

Benign tumours

Benign tumours occur in 0.2% of appendices and comprise two main groups: polyps and adenomas (Higa *et al.* 1973). Appendiceal polyps are similar to those in the rest of the colon and may therefore be metaplastic, hamartomatous, Peutz–Jeghers', or juvenile hamartomatous in type (Kitchen 1953; Shnitka and Sheraniuk 1957). Polyps are distinguished from adenomas solely by the absence histologically of nuclear atypia (Qizilbash 1974) (Figure 14.15). Excessive production of mucus by adenomas causes a large sausage-shaped cystic mass (cystadenoma), mucus invasion of the appendix wall indicating the presence of a mucocele. If a cystadenoma or mucocele ruptures, the mucus is usually contained within the right iliac fossa (localised pseudo-myxoma peritonei) (Higa *et al.* 1973).

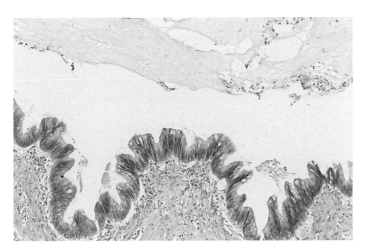

Figure 14.15 Adenoma of the appendix showing dysplastic changes. Note the presence of mucus signifying formation of a mucocele. H&E×40.

Benign lesions of the appendix are usually asymptomatic, being detected incidentally on pathological examination. Cystadenomas and mucoceles have been reported to present as acute appendicitis, a palpable mass, torsion, intussusception, ureteral obstruction, and haematuria (Langsam *et al.* 1984; Sadahiro *et al.* 1991; Landen *et al.* 1992). The combination of an uncomfortable mass in the right lower quadrant and a filling defect in the caecum with non-visualization of the appendix is highly suggestive of cystadenoma or mucocele. Localized pseudo-myxoma peritonei may also present as a right-sided mass (Landen *et al.* 1992). Radiological features suggesting cystadenoma or mucocele are dystrophic calcification with upward and medial displacement of the caecum (Risher *et al.* 1991). CT scan reveals a fluid-filled, variable shaped, thin-walled structure containing low-density contents without peri-appendiceal inflammation (Yoshida *et al.* 1990; Isaacs and Warshauer 1992). Such features may also be detected by ultrasound and magnetic resonance imaging (Macek *et al.* 1992).

On pathological examination, adenomas of the appendix tend to be diffuse and villous, unlike their colorectal counterparts (Wolff and Ahmed 1976). Mucoceles are of three histological types: mucosal hyperplasia; incidental cystadenoma; and mucinous cystade-

nocarcinoma (Higa *et al.* 1973). 'Obstructive' mucoceles caused by mucosal hyperplasia are histologically similar to large bowel hyperplastic or metaplastic polyps and usually measure less than 1 cm. In contrast, mucoceles caused by cystadenomas or cystadenocarcinomas are larger, measuring up to 6 cm (Higa *et al.* 1973).

Benign lesions are cured by appendicectomy, provided the resection limit at the base of the appendix is tumour-free (Higa *et al.* 1973). Adenomas of the appendix therefore have a similar prognosis to those elsewhere in the large bowel. Localized pseudo-myxoma peritonei usually resolves after appendicectomy and excision of local mucin deposits. Cases of appendiceal adenoma or cystadenoma should undergo investigation of the remainder of the colon because of the strong association with synchronous or metachronous colorectal adenomas or carcinoma (Wolff and Ahmed 1976).

Malignant tumours

Primary malignant tumours of the appendix consist of carcinoid tumours and adenocarcinoma (Table 14.2). Involvement of the appendix by secondary tumours is rare.

Carcinoid (endocrine cell) tumours

Incidence and aetiology

The commonest tumour of the appendix is carcinoid, occurring in up to 0.5% of appendicectomy specimens and accounting for 80% of all appendiceal growths (Jetmore *et al.* 1992; Marshall and Bodnarchuk 1993). Carcinoid of the appendix accounts for 15% of all carcinoid tumours and is derived from subepithelial neuroendocrine cells (Shaw 1991; Goddard and Lonsdale 1992). Appendiceal carcinoids occur at all ages (Parkes *et al.* 1993). However, most appendiceal carcinoids occur in adults. The mean age at presentation of classical appendiceal carcinoids is 32 years, that of the mucinous variety being older (58 years) (Anderson *et al.* 1991; Roggo *et al.* 1993). At all ages, carcinoids are more common in women, the female to male ratio being about 4:1 (Moertel *et al.* 1990).

Clinical presentation

The presentation of appendiceal carcinoid is indistinguishable from acute appendicitis in over half of patients (Dhillon *et al.* 1992). Occasionally chronic, recurrent right lower quadrant pain indicates intermittent partial obstruction by the tumour. However, when a

Table 14.2 Comparison of carcinoid and adenocarcinoma of the appendix

	Carcinoid tumour	Adenocarcinoma
Incidence	0.5% of all appendicectomies 80% of all appendiceal growths	0.1% of all appendicectomies Arises in pre-existing adenomas
Presentation	Often incidental finding 'Acute appendicitis' Carcinoid syndrome (metastatic)	'Acute appendicitis' in 70% Abdominal mass
Diagnosis	CT scan MIBG scintigraphy	CT scan Serial CEA assessment
Treatment	Right hemicolectomy required if: tumour larger than 2 cm located at base of appendix invasion (serosa, lymphatics) mucin production high mitotic rate	Right hemicolectomy in all cases except possibly carcinoma *in situ* (5-year survival 60% compared with 20% for appendicectomy alone)
Prognosis	5-year survival 90%	Depends on Duke's stage

carcinoid is found in an acutely inflamed appendix, it is the obstructing factor in only 25% of cases. Most cases not associated with appendicitis represent an incidental finding in appendices removed during laparotomy for other conditions (Nwiloh *et al.* 1990). Symptoms of the carcinoid syndrome are rare and indicate liver metastases. Increased urinary excretion of 5-hydroxyindoleacetic acid (5-HIAA), together with urinary and platelet serotonin concentrations, are useful in monitoring disease progression (Kema *et al.* 1992). CT scanning is helpful in diagnosing an appendiceal tumour and detecting metastases, although confusion occurs in the presence of infection, as the appearances then mimic an appendix abscess (Warshauer *et al.* 1991). Recently, somatostatin analogue or radio-isotope (MIBG) scintigraphy has proved valuable, both pre- and intra-operatively, in detecting metastatic carcinoid tumours (King *et al.* 1993; Kvols *et al.* 1993). The technique is complementary to CT scanning, especially in patients with disseminated pathology, equivocal lesions on CT, or a negative CT and strong clinical or biochemical evidence of a neuroendocrine tumour (King *et al.* 1993). For the detection of liver metastases, CT portography and positron emission tomography are over 90% sensitive while carcinoid heart disease should be investigated initially by echocardiography, supplemented by MR and CT scanning if necessary (Eriksson *et al.* 1993; Pellika *et al.* 1993).

Pathology

Eighty per cent of appendiceal carcinoids measure less than 1 cm in diameter, the proportion measuring 1–2 cm and greater than 2 cm being 14% and 6%, respectively (Roggo *et al.* 1993). About 75% occur at the tip, 15% in the middle, and 10% at the base of the appendix. Two main histological patterns are recognized, one morphologically identical to classical (mid-gut) carcinoids, the other to rectal (hindgut) carcinoids (Shaw and Pringle 1992). Tumours having the macroscopic appearance and infiltrative pattern of a carcinoid tumour, yet the aggressive behaviour of an adenocarcinoma are variously called mucinous carcinoid, goblet cell carcinoid, adenocarcinoid or crypt cell carcinoid (Isaacson 1981, Park *et al.* 1990) (Figure 14.16).

Carcinoid tumours in children tend to be more aggressive than those in adults. Whereas in adults the proportion of cases with tumour confined to the submucosa, serosa or meso-appendiceal fat is 70%, 20%, and 10%, respectively (Roggo *et al.* 1993), the corresponding figures for children are 30%, 40%, and 30% (Parkes *et al.* 1993). Despite this comparatively frequent involvement of the serosa and fat, metastatic spread is rare in classical carcinoids and these tumours are rarely fatal (Lyss 1988). In contrast, metastases, particu-

larly to the ovary, occur in up to 30% of mucinous carcinoids and these tumours may prove fatal from widespread intra-abdominal dissemination (Bak and Asschenfeldt 1988; Seidman *et al.* 1991). Only tumour size has been consistently shown to be related to metastatic potential, tumours over 2 cm being associated with a poor prognosis (Bowman and Rosenthal 1983; Agranovich *et al.* 1991; Goolsby *et al.* 1992; Gouzi *et al.* 1993). However, smaller tumours may occasionally metastasize. The prognosis of classical carcinoids is good, 5-year survival being in the range of 90–100% (Dhillon *et al.* 1992). However, the outlook for mucinous carcinoids is poorer, being intermediate between that of classical carcinoid and well differentiated adenocarcinoma (Berardi and Chen 1989; King *et al.* 1993).

Treatment

The treatment of appendiceal carcinoid is controversial, especially as incidental discovery of the lesion by the pathologist may result in a second, unexpected operation (Rouanet *et al.* 1992). It is accepted that simple appendicectomy is satisfactory treatment for the vast majority of appendiceal carcinoids. Several large series have suggested that indications for further operative treatment (right hemicolectomy) are: (i) lesions larger than 2 cm; (ii) location at the base of the appendix; (iii) invasion of the serosa, lymphatics, or meso-appendix; (iv) mucin production; and (v) cellular pleomorphism with a high mitotic rate (Gouzi *et al.* 1993; Roggo *et al.* 1993). More contentious indications for right hemicolectomy include tumours measuring between 1 and 2 cm, small mucinous carcinoids and tumours in children, as these tend to be more aggressive than those seen in adults (Roggo *et al.* 1993). As mucinous carcinoids metastasize to the ovary in up to 30% of cases, oophorectomy has been recommended for this tumour.

In the presence of liver metastases and carcinoid syndrome, octreotide, a somatostatin analogue, produces symptomatic improvement in 85%, with reduction in urinary 5HIAA in 60%, of patients (Arnold *et al.* 1993; Buchanan 1993). Half of patients experience stabilization of their disease and only 15% progress (Janson and Oberg 1993). However, the initially favourable response is often not maintained and in the presence of far advanced disease, tumour progression occurs in 50% of cases (Arnold *et al.* 1993). Alpha-interferon relieves symptoms in 80% of those with carcinoid syndrome, 60% of patients obtaining a partial response, and 80% stable disease (Bajetta *et al.* 1993; Di Bartolomeo *et al.* 1993). The addition of alpha-interferon should therefore be considered for patients that progress or do not respond to octreotide (Janson and Oberg 1993). Alternatively, the carcinoid syndrome may be treated by hepatic artery occlusion, objective regression occurring in 60% of patients (Moertle *et al.* 1994). Combining this with chemotherapy using 5-fluorouracil and streptozotocin produces an 80% response (Janson *et al.* 1993). However, their effectiveness is often limited, median duration of regression being 4 months for hepatic artery occlusion alone and 18 months when chemotherapy is added (Stokes *et al.* 1993). Finally, in selected patients, liver transplant should be considered (Schweizer *et al.* 1993).

Adenocarcinoma

Incidence and aetiology

Adenocarcinoma of the appendix is found in 0.1% of appendicectomies, corresponding to an estimated incidence of 0.2/100 000 per annum (Nielsen *et al.* 1991). Most, if not all, adenocarcinomas arise in pre-existing adenomas. Two principal growth patterns are seen—cystadenocarcinoma (or mucinous adenocarcinoma), almost invariably arising from a precursor cystadenoma, and, less commonly, a

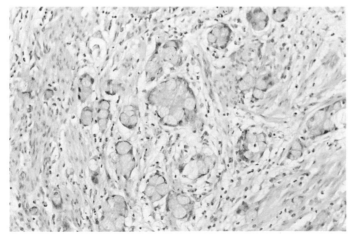

Figure 14.16 Mucinous carcinoid, consisting predominantly of goblet cells, infiltrating the wall of the appendix. H&E×250.

colorectal type tumour, developing from tubular or tubulovillous adenomas (Nitecki *et al.* 1994). The mean age at presentation is about 50 years, males being more commonly affected than females (Gattuso *et al.* 1990).

Clinical presentation

Almost 70% of appendiceal adenocarcinomas present with signs suggestive of acute appendicitis (Lenriot and Huguier 1989) and even at operation, the correct diagnosis is made in less than half of these (Nitecki *et al.* 1994). Most of the remaining cases present as an abdominal mass which may be confused with Crohn's disease, an intussusception, hydronephrosis, or bladder carcinoma (Gilhome *et al.* 1984; Chen and Spaulding 1991). Radiological investigations, such as ultrasound, CT scan, or barium enema, may help in making these distinctions (Janson *et al.* 1992). Rupture of a cystadenocarcinoma sheds malignant mucin-producing cells throughout the peritoneal cavity, producing generalized pseudo-myxoma peritonei. Almost half of those with cystadenocarcinomas will develop pseudo-myxoma peritonei (Nitecki *et al.* 1994). Patients with this condition present with abdominal distension suggestive of ascites, but without shifting dullness (Jougon and Amar 1991). Some cases may mimic a splenic or hepatic mass, or present with uterine prolapse or external fistulation (Snyder and Vandivort 1992). Cytological examination of aspirated mucus and DNA flow cytometry are unhelpful in predicting whether an individual case is benign or malignant (Nielsen *et al.* 1993). However, CT scanning accurately assesses the extent of peritoneal involvement (Nelson *et al.* 1992). Serial CEA measurements are useful in determining the subsequent course of both adenocarcinoma and pseudo-myxoma (Rutledge and Alexander 1992).

Pathology

Adenocarcinoma is identified histologically by the invasion of the appendix wall by neoplastic tissue. Cystadenocarcinomas show abundant extracellular mucin production and tend to be well differentiated while colonic type adenocarcinomas are lacking in mucin and are poorly differentiated (Higa *et al.* 1973). Lymph node metastases are noted in 25% of cases at presentation, being more common in adenocarcinomas than cystadenocarcinomas. Cystadenocarcinomas are generally less virulent than adenocarcinomas, despite their ability to produce pseudo-myxoma peritonei (Young *et al.* 1991). Adenocarcinoma has a malignant potential between that of appendiceal carcinoid and colonic carcinoma, with a predilection to metastasize to the ovary (Rutledge and Alexander 1992). Metastases will subsequently develop in 20% of patients (Noritake *et al.* 1990). Prognosis is determined by Dukes' stage and the degree of differentiation (Andersson *et al.* 1976). Overall 5-year survival is 55%, varying with stage (A, 100%; B, 67%; C, 50%; and D, 6%) and grade (I, 68%, and III, 7%) (Nitecki *et al.* 1994).

Treatment

Tumour invasion is the most important factor determining treatment of appendiceal adenocarcinoma. Right hemicolectomy is the treatment of choice for all lesions with invasion beyond the mucosa, irrespective of histological type or degree of differentiation (Lyss 1988). In the presence of tumour invasion, the 5-year survival for right hemicolectomy is 60%, compared with 20% for appendicectomy alone (Nitecki *et al.* 1994). For lesions confined to the mucosa (*in situ* carcinoma), some suggest there is no survival advantage in performing right hemicolectomy over appendicectomy alone, while others recommend right hemicolectomy for all appendiceal adenocarcinomas (Evans *et al.* 1990). The consensus opinion is that cases truly confined to the mucosa may be treated by appendicectomy alone at the surgeon's discretion. If there is any suggestion that the tumour may have spread beyond the mucosa, right hemicolectomy is indicated (Evans *et al.* 1990; Gattuso *et al.* 1990). Surveillance for synchronous or metachronous tumours is warranted as almost 20% of patients will have, or develop, a second primary malignancy in the gastrointestinal tract (Nitecki *et al.* 1994).

Generalized pseudo-myxoma peritonei is best treated by aggressive surgical debulking of all apparent mucinous tissue (Smith *et al.* 1992). This approach significantly improves survival and decreases recurrence compared with appendicectomy alone (Sugarbaker 1991; Jahne *et al.* 1993). The benefit of aggressive surgery is seen from the 3-year survival for mild, moderate, and gross residual disease being 92%, 48%, and 20%, respectively (Sugarbaker 1991). Although some recommend adjuvant chemotherapy be restricted to cases of proven recurrent pseudo-myxoma 3-year survival of over 90% from combined cytoreductive surgery and intra-operative chemotherapy has been reported (Smith *et al.* 1992). Widespread peritoneal carcinomatosis from adenocarcinoma and cystadenocarcinoma, is an ominous finding. Despite cytoreductive surgery combined with intraperitoneal chemotherapy, 3-year survival is only about 35% (Sugarbaker and Jablonski 1995).

Secondary tumours and non-epithelial lesions

Although it is taught that primary caecal carcinoma may involve the appendix and cause appendicitis in elderly patients, this situation is rare (Armstrong *et al.* 1989). In only 2% of patients over the age of 65 years presenting with appendicitis is a caecal carcinoma found. These tumours behave as, and have a similar prognosis to, other caecal tumours. They are therefore best treated by right hemicolectomy (Rutledge and Alexander 1992). Metastatic tumours infiltrating the appendix may occur in ovarian tumours, being reported in up to 7% of stage I or II and over 50% of stage III or IV ovarian carcinomas (Sonnendecker *et al.* 1989). The appendix may rarely be involved by metastases from other sites, particularly the breast, stomach, and bronchus (Maddox 1990; Carpenter 1991). Secondary tumours are suggested by the bulk of the lesion being extramural, as opposed to intramural, and the absence histologically of adenomatous changes in the mucosa adjacent to the malignant cells. Appendicectomy may limit localized disease but prognosis is determined by the extent of metastatic spread of the primary tumour.

A number of primary appendiceal tumours of non-epithelial origin have been reported, but are exceedingly rare. These include malignant lymphomas (Rao and Aydinalp 1991), Burkitt's lymphoma (Sin *et al.* 1980), smooth muscle tumours (Tarasidis *et al.* 1991), granular cell tumours (Johnston and Helwig 1981), ganglioneuromas (Zarabi and LaBach 1982), and AIDS-associated Kaposi's sarcoma (Zebrowska and Walsh 1991). As the appendix is usually involved by only a small focus of the lesion, appendicectomy often controls local disease. Prognosis is therefore determined by the systemic component of the disease.

References

Addiss DG, Shaffer N, Fowler BS, Tauxe RV. The epidemiology of appendicitis and appendectomy in the United States. *Am. J. Epidemiol.* 1990; 132: 910–25.

Adebamowo CA, Akang EE, Ladipo JK, Ajao OG. Schistosomiasis of the appendix. *Br. J. Surg.* 1991; 78: 1219–21.

Agranovich AL, Anderson GH, Manji M, Acker BD, Macdonald WC, Threlfall WJ. Carcinoid tumour of the gastrointestinal tract: prognostic factors and disease outcome. *J. Surg. Oncol.* 1991; 47: 45–52.

Albu E, Miller BM, Choi Y, Lakhanpal S, Murthy RN, Gerst PH. Diagnostic value of C reactive protein in acute appendicitis. *Dis. Colon Rectum* 1994; 37: 49–51.

Anderson NH, Somerville JE, Johnston CF, Hayes DM, Buchanan KD, Sloan JM. Appendiceal goblet cell carcinoids: a clinicopathological and immunohistochemical study. *Histopathology* 1991; 18: 61–5.

Andersson A, Bergdahl L, Boquist L. Primary carcinoma of the appendix. *Ann. Surg.* 1976; 183: 53–7.

Andreou P, Blain S, Du Boulay CE. A histopathological study of the appendix at autopsy and after surgical resection. *Histopathology* 1990; 17: 427–31.

Apelgren KN, Cowan BD, Metcalf AM, Scott-Conner CE. Laparoscopic appendectomy and the management of gynecologic pathologic conditions found at laparoscopy for presumed appendicitis. *Surg. Clin. North Am.* 1996; 76: 469–82.

Ardies P, Vanwambeke K, Hanssens M, Knockaert D, Penninckx F, Lauwereyns J, Ponette E. Endometriosis of the cecum and appendix: two case reports. *Gastrointest. Radiol.* 1990; 15: 263–4.

Armstrong CP, Ahsan Z, Hinchley G, Prothero DL, Brodribb AJ. Appendicectomy and carcinoma of the caecum. *Br. J. Surg.* 1989; 76: 1049–53.

Arnold R, Neuhaus C, Benning R, Schwerk WB, Trautmann ME, Joseph K, Bruns C. Somatostatin analog sandostatin and inhibition of tumor growth in patients with metastatic endocrine gastroenteropancreatic tumors. *World J. Surg.* 1993; 17: 511–9.

Babekir AR, Devi N. Analysis of the pathology of 405 appendices. *East Afr. Med. J.* 1990; 67: 599–602.

Bajetta E, Zilembo N, Di Bartolomeo M, Di Leo A, Pilotti S, Bochicchio AM. Treatment of metastatic carcinoids and other neuroendocrine tumors with recombinant interferon alpha 2a. A study by the Italian Trials in Medical Oncology Group. *Cancer* 1993; 72: 3099–105.

Bak M, Asschenfeldt P. Adenocarcinoid of the vermiform appendix. A clinicopathologic study of 20 cases. *Dis. Colon Rectum* 1988; 31:605–12.

Balthazar EJ, Megibow AJ, Gordon RB, Whelan CA, Hulnick D. Computed tomography of the abnormal appendix. *J. Comput. Assist. Tomography* 1988; 12: 595–601.

Balthazar EJ, Birnbaum BA, Yee J, Megibow AJ, Roshkow J, Gray C. Acute appendicitis: CT and US correlation in 100 patients. *Radiology* 1994; 190: 31–5.

Barber MD, McLaren J, Rainey JB. Recurrent appendicitis. *Br. J. of Surg.* 1997; 84: 110–2.

Baron EJ, Curren M, Henderson G, Jousimies Somer H, Lee K, Lechowitz K, *et al. Bilophila wadsworthia* isolates from clinical specimens. *J. Clin. Microbiol.* 1992; 30: 1882–4.

Bennion RS, Thompson JE, Baron EJ, Finegold SM. Gangrenous and perforated appendicitis with peritonitis: treatment and bacteriology. *Clin. Ther.* 1990; 12: 31–44.

Berardi RS, Chen H. Goblet cell carcinoid of the appendix. *Int. J. Surg.* 1989; 74: 109–10.

Berends FJ, Vermeulen MI, Leguit P. Perforation rate and diagnostic accuracy in acute appendicitis. *Ned. Tijdschr. Geneeskd.* 1994; 138: 350–4.

Biermann R, Borsky D, Gogora M. Double appendicitis—a rare pathologic entity. *Chirurgie* 1993; 64: 1059–61.

Bowman GA, Rosenthal D. Carcinoid tumors of the appendix. *Am. J. Surg.* 1983; 146: 700–3.

Boyez M, Suzanne A, de St. Maur PP, Valette M. Infected calcified mucocele of the appendix with histologic features of mucinous cystadenoma. *Gastrointest. Radiol.* 1985; 10: 297–8.

Brasel KJ, Borgstrom DC, Weigelt JA. Cost-utility analysis of contaminated appendectomy wounds. *J. Am. Coll. Surg.* 1997; 184: 23–30.

Braveman P, Schaaf VM, Egerter S, Bennett T, Schecter W. Insurance related differences in the risk of ruptured appendix. *N. Engl. J. Med.* 1994; 331: 444–9.

Buchanan KD. Effects of sandostatin on neuroendocrine tumours of the gastrointestinal system. Recent results. *Cancer Res.* 1993; 129: 45–55.

Buckley RC, Hall TJ, Muakkassa FF, Anglin B, Rhodes RS, Scott Conner CE. Laparoscopic appendectomy: Is it worth it? *Am. Surg.* 1994; 60: 30–4.

Caldwell MT, Watson RG. Peritoneal aspiration cytology as a diagnostic aid in acute appendicitis. *Br. J. Surg.* 1994; 81: 276–8.

Carpenter BW. Lymphoma of the appendix. *Gastrointest. Radiol.* 1991; 16: 256–8.

Ceres L, Alonso I, Lopez P, Parra G, Echeverry J. Ultrasound study of acute appendicitis in children with emphasis upon the diagnosis of retrocecal appendicitis. *Pediatr. Radiol.* 1990; 20: 258–61.

Cerva L, Schrottenbaum M, Kliment V. Intestinal parasites: a study of human appendices. *Folia Parasitol. Praha* 1991; 38: 5–9.

Champault C, Taffinder N, Ziol M, Rizk N, Catheline J. Recognition of a pathological appendix during laparoscopy: a prospective study of 81 cases. *Br. J. Surg.* 1997; 84: 671–2.

Chen KT, Spaulding RW. Appendiceal carcinoma masquerading as primary bladder carcinoma. *J. Urol.* 1991; 145: 821–2.

Chetty R, Slavin JL, Miller RA. Kaposi's sarcoma presenting as acute appendicitis in an HIV 1 positive patient. *Histopathology* 1993; 23: 590–1.

Christian F, Christian GP. A simple scoring system to reduce the negative appendicectomy rate.

Coughlin JP, Gauderer MW, Stern RC, Doershuk CF, Izant RJ Jr, Zollinger RM Jr. The spectrum of appendiceal disease in cystic fibrosis. *J. Pediatr. Surg.* 1990; 25: 835–9.

Devereaux DA, McDermott JP, Caushaj PF. Recurrent appendicitis following laparoscopic appendectomy. Report of a case. *Dis. Colon Rectum* 1994; 37: 719–20.

Dhillon AP, Williams RA, Rode J. Age, site and distribution of subepithelial neurosecretory cells in the appendix. *Pathology* 1992; 24: 56–9.

Di Bartolomeo M, Bajetta E, Zilembo N, de Braud F, Di Leo A, Verusio C, D'Aprile M. Treatment of carcinoid syndrome with recombinant interferon alpha 2a. *Acta Oncol.* 1993; 32: 235–8.

Dudley TH Jr, Dean PJ. Idiopathic granulomatous appendicitis, or Crohn's disease of the appendix revisited. *Hum. Pathol.* 1993; 24: 595–601.

Duran JC, Beidle TR, Perret R, Higgins J, Pfister R, Letourneau JG. CT Imaging of acute right lower quadrant disease. *Am. J. Roentgenol.* 1997; 168: 411–6.

el Ghoneimi A, Valla JS, Limonne B, Valla V, Montupet P, Chavrier Y, Grinda A. Laparoscopic appendectomy in children: report of 1379 cases. *J. Pediatr. Surg.* 1994; 29: 786–9.

Epstein FB. Acute abdominal pain in pregnancy. *Emerg. Med. Clin. North Am.* 1994; 12: 151–65.

Eriksson B, Bergstrom M, Lilja A, Ahlstrom H, Langstrom B, Oberg K. Positron emission tomography in neuroendocrine gastrointestinal tumors. *Acta Oncol.* 1993; 32: 189–96.

Eskelinen M, Ikonen J, Lipponen P. Acute appendicitis in patients over the age of 65 years comparison of clinical and computer based decision making. *Int. J. Biomed. Comput.* 1994; 36: 239–49.

Evans DA, Hamid BN, Hoare EM. Primary adenocarcinoma of the appendix. *J. R. Coll. Surg. Edinburgh* 1990; 35: 33–5.

Franzin L, Morosini M, Do D, Borsa M, Scramuzza F. Isolation of *Yersinia* from appendices of patients with acute appendicitis. *Contrib. Microbiol. Immunol.* 1991; 12: 282–5.

Frazee RC, Roberts JW, Symmonds RE, Snyder SK, Hendricks JC, Smith RW, *et al.* A prospective randomized trial comparing open versus laparoscopic appendectomy. *Ann. Surg.* 1994; 219: 725–8.

Frazee RC, Bohannon WT. Laparoscopic appendectomy for complicated appendicitis. *Arch. Surg.* 1996; 131: 509–11.

Friedland JA, Siegel MJ. CT Appearance of acute appendicitis in childhood. *Am. J. Roentgenol.* 1997; 168: 439–42.

Gattuso P, Reddy V, Kathuria S, Abraham KP. Primary adenocarcinoma of the appendix: a review. *Mil. Med.* 1990; 155: 343–5.

Gibbs NM. Mucinous cystadenoma and cystadenocarcinoma of the vermiform appendix with particular reference to pseudomyxoma peritonei. *J. Clin. Pathol.* 1973; 26: 413–16.

Gibney EJ, Ajayi N, Leader M, Bouchier-Hayes D. Emergency appendicectomy: a one year audit. *Ir. J. Med. Sci.* 1992 161: 101–4.

Gilhome RW, Johnston DH, Clark J, Kyle J. Primary adenocarcinoma of the vermiform appendix: report of a series of 10 cases and review of the literature. *Br. J. Surg.* 1984; 71: 553–5.

Goddard MJ, Lonsdale RN. The histogenesis of appendiceal carcinoid tumours. *Histopathology* 1992; 20: 345–9.

Gonzalez Conde R, Aguinaga Manzanos MV, Casas Pinillos S, Cobos Mateos JM, Gonzalez Sanchez JA, Miguel Velasco JE, *et al.* Appendicular endometriosis. Clinicopathologic study of 12 cases. *Rev. Esp. Enferm. Dig.* 1992; 81: 251–5.

Goolsby CL, Punyarit P, Mehl PJ, Rao MS. Flow cytometric DNA analysis of carcinoid tumors of the ileum and appendix. *Hum. Pathol.* 1992; 23: 1340–3.

Gorenstein A, Gewurtz G, Serour F, Somekh E. Postappendectomy intra abdominal abscess: a therapeutic approach. *Arch. Dis. Child.* 1994; 70: 400–2.

Gorenstin A, Serour F, Katz R. Usviatsov I. Appendiceal colic in children: a true clinical entity? *J. Am. Coll. Surg.* 1996; 182: 246–50.

Gough DB, Donohue JH, Schutt AJ, Gonchoroff N, Goellner JR, Wilson TO, *et al.* Pseudomyxoma peritonei. Long term patient survival with an aggressive regional approach. *Ann. Surg.* 1994; 219: 112–9.

Gouzi JL, Laigneau P, Delalande JP, Flamant Y, Bloom E, Oberlin P, Fingerhut A. Indications for right hemicolectomy in carcinoid tumors of the appendix. The French Associations for Surgical Research. *Surg. Gynecol. Obstet.* 1993; 176: 543–7.

Grunewald B, Keating J. Should the 'normal' appendix be removed at operation for appendicitis? *J. R. Coll. Surg. Edinburgh* 1993; 38: 158–60.

Guidry SP, Poole GV. The anatomy of appendicitis. *Am. Surg.* 1994; 60: 68–71.

Hale D, Molloy M, Pearl R, Schutt D, Jaques D. Appendectomy: A contemporary appraisal. *Ann. Surg.* 1997; 225: 252 61.

Halvorsen AC, Brandt B, Andreasen JJ. Appendicitis in pregnancy. Complications and treatment. *Ugeskr. Laeger* 1994; 156: 1308–10.

Hansen JB, Smithers BM, Schache D, Wall DR, Miller BJ, Menzies BL. Laparoscopic versus open appendectomy: prospective randomized trial. *World J. Surg.* 1996; 20: 17–20.

Hawes AS, Whalen GF. Recurrent and chronic appendicitis: the other inflammatory conditions of the appendix. *Am. Surg.* 1994; 60: 217–9.

Hebebrand D, Troidl H, Spangenberger W, Neugebauer E, Schwalm T, Gunther MW. Laparoscopic or classical appendectomy? A prospective randomized study. *Chirurgie* 1994; 65: 112–20.

Herd ME, Cross PA, Dutt S. Histological audit of acute appendicitis. *J. Clin. Pathol.* 1992; 45: 456–8.

Higa E, Rosai J, Pizzimbono CA, Wise L. Mucosal hyperplasia, mucinous cystadenoma and mucinous cystadenocarcinoma of the appendix. *Cancer* 1973; 32: 1525–41.

Hopkins JA, Lee JC, Wilson SE. Susceptibility of intra abdominal isolates at operation: a predictor of postoperative infection. *Am. Surg.* 1993; 59: 791–6.

Hsieh SY, Chiu CT, Sheen IS, Lin DY, Wu CS. A clinical study on pseudomyxoma peritonei. *J. Gastroenterol. Hepatol.* 1995; 10: 86–91.

Isaacs KL, Warshauer DM. Mucocele of the appendix: computed tomographic, endoscopic, and pathologic correlation. *Am. J. Gastroenterol.* 1992; 87: 787–9.

Isaacson P. Crypt cell carcinoma of the appendix (so called adenocarcinoid tumor). *Am. J. Surg. Pathol.* 1981; 5: 213–18.

Jacquet P, Stephens AD, Averbach AM, Chang D, Ettinghausen SE, Dalton RR, Steves MA, Sugarbaker PH. Analysis of morbidity and mortality in 60 patients with peritoneal carcinomatosis treated by cytoreductive surgery and heated intraoperative intraperitoneal chemotherapy. *Cancer* 1996; 77: 2622–9.

Jadallah FA, Abdul Ghani AA, Tibblin S. Diagnostic laparoscopy reduces unnecessary appendicectomy in fertile women. *Eur. J. Surg.* 1994; 160: 41–5.

Jahne J, Lang H, Meyer HJ, Pichlmayr R. Possibilities and limits of surgical therapy of pseudomyxoma peritonei Langenbecks. *Arch. Chir.* 1993; 378: 292–4.

Jaluvka V, Albig M, Hamm B. Magnetic resonance tomography in the differential diagnosis of ovarian tumor and mucocele of the appendix. *Dtsch. Med. Wochenschr.* 1989; 114: 1245–7.

Janson ET, Oberg K. Long term management of the carcinoid syndrome. Treatment with octreotide alone and in combination with alpha interferon. *Acta Oncol.* 1993; 32: 225–9.

Janson ET, Ronnblom L, Ahlstrom H, Grander D, Alm G, Einhorn S, Oberg K. Treatment with alpha interferon versus alpha interferon in combination with streptozocin and doxorubicin in patients with malignant carcinoid tumors: a randomized trial. *Ann. Oncol.* 1992; 3: 635–8.

Jeddy TA, Vowles RH, Southam JA. 'Cough sign': a reliable test in the diagnosis of intra abdominal inflammation. *Br. J. Surg.* 1994; 81: 279.

Jeffrey RB, Jain KA, Nghiem HV. Sonographic diagnosis of acute appendicitis: interpretive pitfalls. *Am. J. Roentgenol.* 1994; 162: 55–9.

Jetmore AB, Ray JE, Gathright JB Jr, McMullen KM, Hicks TC, Timmcke AE. Rectal carcinoids: the most frequent carcinoid tumor. *Dis. Colon Rectum* 1992; 35: 717–25.

Jevon GP, Daya D, Qizilbash AH. Intussusception of the appendix. A report of four cases and review of the literature. *Arch. Pathol. Lab. Med.* 1992; 116: 960–4.

John H, Neff U, Kelemen M. Appendicitis diagnosis today: clinical and ultrasonic deductions. *World J. Surg.* 1993; 17: 243–9.

Johnston J, Helwig EB. Granular cell tumors of the gastrointestinal tract and perianal region. *Dig. Dis. Sci.* 1981; 26: 207–16.

Jougon J, Amar A. Inflammatory pseudotumor of the appendix. Apropos of a case. Review of the literature. *J. Chir.* 1991; 128: 86–8.

Kabanchuk IN, Grechanyi AP, Skorik VT, Dudchenko AG. Two vermiform appendices in one patient. *Klin. Khir.* 1990; 4: 63.

Kanazawa Y, Shimokoshi M, Hasegawa K, Tanabe T, Izumi S, Kageyama M, Ikemura K. Isolation of *Yersinia* from the resected appendix. *Contrib. Microbiol. Immunol.* 1991; 12: 255–9.

Karim OM, Boothroyd AE, Wyllie JH. McBurney's point—fact or fiction? *Ann. R. Coll. Surg. Engl.* 1990; 72: 304–8.

Keller MS, McBride WJ, Vane DW. Management of complicated appendicitis. A rational approach based on clinical course. *Arch. Surg.* 1996; 131: 261–4.

Kema IP, de Vries EG, Schellings AM, Postmus PE, Muskiet FA. Improved diagnosis of carcinoid tumors by measurement of platelet serotonin. *Clin. Chem.* 1992; 38: 534–40.

Kim KU, Kim JK, Won JH, Hong DS, Park HS. Acute appendicitis in patients with acute leukemia. *Korean J. Intern. Med.* 1993; 8: 40–5.

King CM, Reznek RH, Bomanji J, Ur E, Britton KE, Grossman AB, Besser GM. Imaging neuroendocrine tumours with radiolabelled somatostatin analogues and X ray computed tomography: a comparative study. *Clin. Radiol.* 1993; 48: 386–91.

Kitchen AP. Polyps of the intestinal tract. *Br. Med. J.* 1953; 1: 658–9.

Kvols LK, Brown ML, O'Connor MK, Hung JC, Hayostek RJ, Reubi JC, Lamberts SW. Evaluation of a radiolabeled somatostatin analog (I 123 octreotide) in the detection and localization of carcinoid and islet cell tumors. *Radiology* 1993; 187: 129–33.

Landen S, Bertrand C, Maddern GJ, Herman D, Pourbaix A, de Neve A, Schmitz A. Appendiceal mucoceles and pseudomyxoma peritonei. *Surg. Gynecol. Obstet.* 1992; 175: 401–4.

Lane MJ, Katz DS, Ross BA, Clautice-Engle TL, Mindelzun RE, Jeffrey RB Jr. Unenhanced helical CT for suspected acute appendicitis. *Am. J. Roentgenol.* 1997; 168: 405–9.

Langsam LB, Raj PK, Galang CF. Intussusception of the appendix. *Dis. Colon Rectum* 1984; 27: 387–92.

Lenriot JP, Huguier M. Adenocarcinoma of the appendix. A multicenter study from AURC. *Ann. Chir.* 1989; 43: 744–51.

Lindsey D. Missed appendicitis. *Am. J. Emerg. Med.* 1994; 12: 500.

Loizon P, Filali K, Lapeyrie H, Chapuis H. Appendiceal mucoceles. Apropos of 2 cases. *J. Chir.* 1989; 126: 703–5.

Luckmann R, Davis P. The epidemiology of acute appendicitis in California: racial, gender, and seasonal variation. *Epidemiology* 1991; 2: 323–30.

Luthi F, Dusmet M, Merlini M. Pain syndrome in the right iliac fossa and laparoscopy: routine appendectomy or not? *Helv. Chir. Acta* 1993; 60: 39–42.

Lyss AP. Appendiceal malignancies. *Semin. Oncol.* 1988; 15: 129–37.

Macek D, Jafri SZ, Madrazo BL. Ultrasound case of the day. Mucocele of the appendix. *Radiographics* 1992; 12: 1247–9.

Maddox PR. Acute appendicitis secondary to metastatic carcinoma of the breast. *Br. J. Clin. Pract.* 1990; 44: 376–8.

Mahieu X, Boverie J, Lemaire JM, Jacquet N. Pyogenic liver abscess. Diagnostic and therapeutic approach: a case report. *Acta Chir. Belg.* 1993; 93: 220–3.

Malik AK, Hanum N, Yip CH. Acute isolated amoebic appendicitis. *Histopathology* 1994; 24: 87–8.

Marshall JB, Bodnarchuk G. Carcinoid tumors of the gut. Our experience over three decades and review of the literature. *J. Clin. Gastroenterol.* 1993; 16: 123–9.

Masuo K, Yasui A, Nishida Y, Kumagai K. A case of Crohn's disease limited to the appendix, showing a portentous ultrasonographic finding. *J. Gastroenterol.* 1994; 29: 76–9.

Mattei P, Sola JE, Yeo CJ. Chronic and recurrent appendicitis are uncommon entities often misdiagnosed. *J. Am. Coll. Surg.* 1994; 178: 385–9.

Mazlam MZ, Hodgson HJ. Why measure C reactive protein? *Gut* 1994; 35: 5–7.

McAnena OJ, Willson PD. Laparoscopic appendicectomy: diagnosis and resection of acute and perforated appendices. *Baillières Clin. Gastroenterol.* 1993; 7: 851–66.

McCahill LE, Pellegrini CA, Wiggins T, Helton WS. A clinical outcome and cost analysis of laparoscopic versus open appendectomy. *Am. J. Surg.* 1996; 171: 533–7.

Milamed DR, Hedley-Whyte J. Contributions of the surgical sciences to a reduction of the mortality rate in the United States for the period 1968 to 1988. *Ann. Surg.* 1994; 219: 94–102.

Misena L, Ollero Fresno JC, Rodriguez Troncoso V, Sanz Villa N, Rollan Villamarin V. Laparoscopy in pediatric surgery. *Cir Pediatr.* 1993; 6: 178–81.

Mitchell IC, Nicholls JC. Duplication of the vermiform appendix. Report of a case: review of the classification and medicolegal aspects. *Med. Sci. Law* 1990; 30: 124–6.

Moertel CG, Johnson CM, McKusick MA, Martin JK Jr, Nagorney DM, Kvols LK. The management of patients with advanced carcinoid tumors and islet cell carcinomas. *Ann. Intern. Med.* 1994; 120: 302–9.

Moertel CG, Weiland LH, Telander RL. Carcinoid tumor of the appendix in the first two decades of life. *J. Pediatr. Surg.* 1990; 25: 1073–5.

Mosdell DM, Morris DM, Fry DE. Peritoneal cultures and antibiotic therapy in pediatric perforated appendicitis. *Am. J. Surg.* 1994; 167: 313–6.

Moser JJ, Barras JP, Baer HU. Diagnostic surprises in apparently inflammatory masses of the right iliac fossa. *Helv. Chir. Acta* 1994; 60: 653–6.

Nair A, Patel R, Monypenny IJ. Tuberculous peritonitis presenting as coloenteric fistula. *Br. J. Clin. Pract.* 1993; 47: 214–5.

Nelson RC, Chezmar JL, Hoel MJ, Buck DR, Sugarbaker PH. Peritoneal carcinomatosis: preoperative CT with intraperitoneal contrast material. *Radiology* 1992; 182: 133–8.

Neumayer LA, Makar R, Ampel NM, Zukoski CF. Cytomegalovirus appendicitis in a patient with human immunodeficiency virus infection. Case report and review of the literature. *Arch. Surg.* 1993; 128: 467–8.

Nielsen GP, Isaksson HJ, Finnbogason H, Gunnlaugsson GH. Adenocarcinoma of the vermiform appendix. A population study. *APMIS* 1991; 99: 653–6.

Nielsen GP, Jonasson JG, Agnarsson BA, Isaksson HJ. Flow cytometric DNA analysis of adenocarcinomas of the vermiform appendix. Brief report. *APMIS* 1993; 101: 811–4.

Nitecki SS, Karmeli R, Sarr MG. Appendiceal calculi and fecaliths as indications for appendectomy. *Surg. Gynecol. Obstet.* 1990; 171: 185–8.

Nitecki SS, Wolff BG, Schlinkert R, Sarr MG. The natural history of surgically treated primary adenocarcinoma of the appendix. *Ann. Surg.* 1994; 219: 51–7.

Noritake N, Ito Y, Yamakita N, Azuma S, Shimokawa K, Miura K. A case of primary mucinous cystadenocarcinoma of the appendix with elevated serum carcinoembryonic antigen. *Jpn. J. Med.* 1990; 29: 642–6.

Normand JP, Rioux M. Ultrasonographic appearance of appendiceal endometrioma. *Can. Assoc. Radiol. J.* 1992; 43: 141–4.

Nowzaradan Y, Barnes JP Jr. Current techniques in laparoscopic appendectomy. *Surg. Laparosc. Endosc.* 1993; 3: 470–6.

Nowzaradan Y, Barnes JP Jr, Westmoreland J, Hojabri M. Laparoscopic appendectomy: treatment of choice for suspected appendicitis. *Surg. Laparosc. Endosc.* 1993; 3: 411–6.

Nwiloh JO, Pillarisetty S, Moscovic EA, Freeman HP. Carcinoid tumors. *J. Surg. Oncol.* 1990; 45: 261–4.

Ovrebo KK, Eckerbom RM, Haram S, Rokke O. Acute abdomen among children and adolescents. A retrospective study of 470 children and adolescents with acute abdominal pain. *Tidsskr. Nor. Laegeforen* 1993; 113: 3244–7.

Pacelli F, Doglietto GB, Alfieri S, Piccioni E, Sgadari A, Gui D, Crucitti F. Prognosis in intra-abdominal infections. Multivariate analysis on 604 patients. *Arch. Surg.* 1996; 131: 641–5.

Panton ON, Samson C, Segal J, Panton R. A four-year expeience with laparoscopy in the management of appendicitis. *Am. J. Surg.* 1996; 171: 538–41.

Park K, Blessing K, Kerr K, Chetty U, Gilmour H. Goblet cell carcinoid of the appendix. *Gut* 1990; 31: 322–4.

Parkes SE, Muir KR, al Sheyyab M, Cameron AH, Pincott JR, Raafat F, Mann JR. Carcinoid tumours of the appendix in children 1957–1986: incidence, treatment and outcome. *Br. J. Surg.* 1993; 80: 502–4.

Patriquin HB, Garcier JM, Lafortune M, Yazbeck S, Russo P, Jequier S, Quimet A, Filiatrault D. Appendicitis in children and young adults: Doppler sonographic-pathologic correlation. *Am. J. Roentgenol.* 1996; 166: 629–33.

Pellikka PA, Tajik AJ, Khandheria BK, Seward JB, Callahan JA, Pitot HC, Kvols LK. Carcinoid heart disease. Clinical and echocardiographic spectrum in 74 patients. *Circulation* 1993; 87: 1188–96.

Pereira JK, Chait PG, Miller SF. Deep pelvic abscesses in children: transrectal drainage under radiologic guidance. *Radiology* 1996; 198: 393–6.

Pier A, Gotz F, Bacher C. Laparoscopic appendectomy in 625 cases: from innovation to routine. *Surg. Laparosc. Endosc.* 1991; 1: 8–13.

Prayson RA, Hart WR, Petras RE. Pseudomyxoma peritonei. A clinicopathologic study of 19 cases with emphasis on site of origin and nature of associated ovarian tumors. *Am. J. Surg. Pathol.* 1994; 18: 591–603.

Primatesta P, Goldacre MJ. Appendicectomy for acute appendicitis and for other conditions: an epidemiological study. *Int. J. Epidemiol.* 1994; 23: 155–60.

Qizilbash AH. Hyperplastic (metaplastic) polyps of the appendix. *Arch. Pathol.* 1974; 97: 385–9.

Quillin SP, Siegel MJ. Appendicitis: efficacy of color Doppler sonography. *Radiology* 1994; 191: 557–60.

Rao SK, Aydinalp N. Appendiceal lymphoma: a case report. *J. Clin. Gastroenterol.* 1993; 13: 588–90.

Rao PM, Wittenberg J, McDowell RK, Rhea JT, Novelline RA. Appendicitis: use of arrowhead sign for diagnosis at CT. *Radiology.* 1997; 202: 363–6.

Reisener KP, Tittel A, Truong SN, Schumpelick V. Value of sonography in routine diagnosis of acute appendicitis. A retrospective analysis. *Leber Magen Darm.* 1994; 24: 16; 19–22.

Reissman P, Durst AL, Rivkind A, Szold A, Ben Chetrit E. Elective laparoscopic appendectomy in patients with familial Mediterranean fever. *World J. Surg.* 1994; 18: 139–41.

Ricci MA, Trevisani MF, Beck WC. Acute appendicitis. A 5-year review. *Am. Surg.* 1991; 57: 301–5.

Risher WH, Ray JE, Hicks TC. Calcified mucocele of the appendix presenting as ureteral obstruction. *J. La State Med. Soc.* 1991; 143: 29–31.

Roggo A, Wood WC, Ottinger LW. Carcinoid tumors of the appendix. *Ann. Surg.* 1993; 217: 385–90.

Rolff M, Jepsen LV, Hoffmann J. The 'absent' appendix. *Arch. Surg.* 1992; 127: 992.

Rouanet P, Saingra B, Quenet F, Regnier JJ, Simony Lafontaine J, Pujol H. Appendiceal carcinoid tumor of systematic detection. When to propose right hemi colectomy and how to monitor?

Thoughts apropos of a case and review of the literature. *Ann. Chir.* 1992; 46: 919–22.

Royes CA, DuQuesnay DR, Coard K, Fletcher PR. Appendicectomy at the University Hospital of the West Indies (1984–1988). A retrospective review. *West Indian Med. J.* 1991; 40: 159–62.

Rutledge RH, Alexander JW. Primary appendiceal malignancies: rare but important. *Surgery* 1992; 111: 244–250.

Sadahiro S, Ohmura T, Yamada Y, Saito T, Akatsuka S. A case of cecocolic intussusception with complete invagination and intussusception of the appendix with villous adenoma. *Dis. Colon Rectum* 1991; 34: 85–8.

Sarfati MR, Hunter GC, Witzke DB, Bebb GG, Smythe SH, Boyan S, Rappaport WD. Impact of adjunctive testing on the diagnosis and clinical course of patients with acute appendicitis. *Am. J. Surg.* 1993; 166: 660–4.

Saye WB, Rives DA, Cochran EB. Laparoscopic appendectomy: three years' experience. *Surg. Laparosc. Endosc.* 1991; 1: 109–15.

Schiffino L, Mouro J, Karayel M, Levard H, Berthelot G, Dubois F. Laparoscopic appendectomy. A study of 154 consecutive cases. *Int. Surg.* 1993; 78: 280–3.

Schweizer RT, Alsina AE, Rosson R, Bartus SA. Liver transplantation for metastatic neuroendocrine tumors. *Transplant Proc.* 1993; 25: 1973.

Scott HJ, Rosin RD. The influence of diagnostic and therapeutic laparoscopy on patients presenting with an acute abdomen. *J. R. Soc. Med.* 1993; 86: 699–701.

Seidman JD, Andersen DK, Ulrich S, Hoy GR, Chun B. Recurrent abdominal pain due to chronic appendiceal disease. *South Med. J.* 1991; 84: 913–6.

Serour F, Efrati Y, Klin B, Barr J, Gorenstein A, Vinograd I. Subcuticular skin closure as a standard approach to emergency appendectomy in children: prospective clinical trial. *World J. Surg.* 1996; 20: 38–42.

Sharp JF, Nicholson ML, Fossard DP. Diverticulosis of the appendix. *Scott. Med. J.* 1990; 35: 50–1.

Shaw PA. The topographical and age distributions of neuroendocrine cells in the normal human appendix. *J. Pathol.* 1991; 164: 235–9.

Shaw PA, Pringle JH. The demonstration of a subset of carcinoid tumours of the appendix by in situ hybridization using synthetic probes to proglucagon mRNA. *J. Pathol.* 1992; 167: 375–80.

Shen GK, Wong R, Daller J, Melcer S, Tsen A, Awtrey S, Rappaport W. Does the retrocecal position of the vermiform appendix alter the clinical course of acute appendicitis? A prospective analysis. *Arch. Surg.* 1991; 126: 569–70.

Shnitka TK, Sherbaniuk RW. Polyps of the appendix. *Gastroenterology* 1957; 32: 462–5.

Shoji BT, Becker JM. Colorectal disease in the elderly patient. *Surg. Clin. North Am.* 1994; 74: 293–316.

Siddiqui MN, Ahmed R, Shaikh H, Ahmed M. Primary amoebic appendicitis. *Trop. Doctor* 1994; 24: 43–4.

Silen ML, Tracy TF Jr. The right lower quadrant 'revisited'. *Pediatr. Clin. North Am.* 1993; 40: 1201–11.

Sin IC, Ling ET, Prentice RSA. Burkitt's lymphoma of the appendix. Report of two cases *Hum. Pathol.* 1980; 11: 465–70.

Sivit CJ, Newman KD, Boenning DA, Nussbaum Blask AR, Bulas DI, Bond SJ, et al. Appendicitis: usefulness of US in diagnosis in a pediatric population. *Radiology* 1992; 185: 549–52.

Smith JW, Kemeny N, Caldwell C, Banner P, Sigurdson E, Huvos A. Pseudomyxoma peritonei of appendiceal origin. The Memorial Sloan Kettering Cancer Center experience. *Cancer* 1992; 70:396–401.

Smith RC, Verga M, McCarthy S, Rosenfield AT. Diagnosis of acute flank pain: value of unenhanced helical CT. *Am. J. Roentgenol.* 1996; 166: 97–101.

Snyder TE, Vandivort MR. Mucinous cystadenocarcinoma of the appendix with pseudomyxoma peritonei presenting as total uterine prolapse. A case report. *J. Reprod. Med.* 1992; 37: 103–6.

Sonnendecker EW, Margolius KA, Sonnendecker HE. Involvement of the appendix in ovarian epithelial cancer an update. *S. Afr. Med. J* 1989; 76: 667–8.

Stokes KR, Stuart K, Clouse ME. Hepatic arterial chemoembolization for metastatic endocrine tumors. *J. Vasc. Interv. Radiol.* 1993; 4: 341–5.

Sugarbaker PH. Cytoreductive surgery and intra peritoneal chemotherapy with peritoneal spread of cytoadenocarcinoma. *Eur. J. Surg.* 1991; 561: 75–82.

Sugarbaker PH, Jablonski KA. Prognostic features of 51 colorectal and 130 appendiceal cancer patients with peritoneal carcinomatosis treated by cytoreductive surgery and intraperitoneal chemotherapy. *Ann. Surg.* 1995; 221: 124–32.

Surana R, Puri P. Primary wound closure after perforated appendicitis in children. *Br. J. Surg.* 1994; 81: 440–41.

Suster S, Moran CA. Deciduosis of the appendix. *Am. J. Gastroenterol.* 1990; 85: 841–5.

Tarasidis G, Brown BC, Skandalakis LJ, Mackay G, Lauer RC, Gray SW, Skandalakis JE. Smooth muscle tumors of the appendix and colon: a collective review of the world literature. *J. Med. Assoc. Ga.* 1991; 80: 667–83.

Thadepalli H, Mandal AK, Chuah SK, Lou MA. Bacteriology of the appendix and the ileum in health and in appendicitis. *Am. Surg.* 1991; 57: 317–22.

Timmermans LG, Vielle G, Dewulf E. Simulation of appendicitis by tumor like lesion of cecum. *Acta Chir. Belg.* 1992; 92: 191–5.

Valla JS, Limonne B, Valla V, Montupet P, Daoud N, Grinda A, Chavrier Y. Laparoscopic appendectomy in children: report of 465 cases. *Surg. Laparosc. Endosc.* 1991; 1: 166–72.

Vallina VL, Velasco JM, McCulloch CS. Laparoscopic versus conventional appendectomy *Ann. Surg.* 1993; 218: 685–92.

Wang Y, Reen DJ, Puri P. Is a histologically normal appendix following emergency appendicectomy always normal? *Lancet* 1996; 347: 1076–9.

Warshauer DM, Criado E, Woosley JT, Grimmer DL. Infarcted appendiceal carcinoid. CT appearance mimicking appendiceal abscess. *Clin. Imaging* 1991; 15: 182–4.

Webster DP, Schneider CN, Cheche S, Daar AA, Miller G. Differentiating acute appendicitis from pelvic inflammatory disease in women of child-bearing age. *Am. J. Emerg. Med.* 1993; 11: 569–72.

Welch NT, Hinder RA, Fitzgibbons RJ Jr. Laparoscopic incidental appendectomy *Surg. Laparosc. Endosc.* 1991; 1: 116–8.

Wertheim I, Fleischhacker D, McLachlin CM, Rice LW, Berkowitz RS, Goff BA. Pseudomyxoma peritonei: a review of 23 cases. *Obstet. Gynecol.* 1994; 84: 17–21.

Wiebe BM. Appendicitis and *Enterobius vermicularis. Scand. J. Gastroenterol.* 1991; 26: 336–8.

Williams DA, Robinson ME, Geisser ME. Pain beliefs: assessment and utility. *Pain* 1994; 59: 71–8.

Wolff M, Ahmed N. Epithelial neoplasms of the vermiform appendix (parts I and II). *Cancer* 1976; 37: 2493–511.

Wong CH, Trinh TM, Robbins AN, Rowen SJ, Cohen AJ. Diagnosis of appendicitis: imaging findings in patients with atypical clinical features. *Am. J. Roentgenol.* 1993; 161: 1199–203.

Yoshida Y, Kamegawa T, Sugio K, Haraguchi Y, Kitagawa S. Mucocele of the appendix accurately diagnosed using computer tomography. *Clin. Imaging* 1990; 14: 61–3.

Younes M, Katikaneni PR, Lechago J. Association between mucosal hyperplasia of the appendix and adenocarcinoma of the colon. *Histopathology* 1995; 26: 33–7.

Young RH, Gilks CB, Scully RE. Mucinous tumors of the appendix associated with mucinous tumors of the ovary and pseudomyxoma peritonei. A clinicopathological analysis of 22 cases supporting an origin in the appendix. *Am. J. Surg. Pathol.* 1991; 15: 415–29.

Zagorski K, Prokopowicz D, Panasiuk A. Appendicitis and its atypical causes. *Wiad Lek.* 1992; 45: 486–9.

Zarabi M, LaBach JP. Ganglioneuroma causing acute appendicitis. *Hum. Pathol.* 1982; 13: 1143–6.

Zebrowska G, Walsh NM. Human immunodeficiency virus related Kaposi's sarcoma of the appendix and acute appendicitis. Report of a case and review of the literature. *Arch. Pathol. Lab. Med.* 1991; 115: 1157–60.

15 Vascular conditions and lower intestinal bleeding

Vascular conditions affecting the colon include ischaemic colitis and angiodysplasia.

Ischaemic colitis

Incidence

The incidence of ischaemic colitis in the general population is unknown. Existing studies are hospital based and are therefore skewed towards the most severely affected patients. Even hospital studies tend to underestimate the condition as many patients are classified as having infectious colitis or inflammatory bowel disease and transient cases are often missed if investigation is not instituted promptly. Ischaemic colitis accounts for about two-thirds of all patients admitted with intestinal ischaemia (Brandt and Boley 1992). It is suggested that in 50–75% of patients diagnosed as having inflammatory bowel disease beginning after age 50 years, symptoms are actually due to colonic ischaemia. Although young patients are occasionally affected, more than 90% of patients are over 60 years of age (Brandt and Boley 1992; Matsumoto *et al.* 1994). The sex distribution is equal.

Aetiology

The normal blood flow to the colon is the lowest of any part of the intestine and is affected by functional activity such as straining at stool (Levine and Jacobson 1995). This potentially precarious intestinal blood flow can be further affected by changes in the mesenteric vessels or by reduced flow in the systemic circulation (Table 15.1). The preponderance of older patients implies that age-related changes in the vessels are important. In younger patients, constipation may be an important causative factor (Matsumoto *et al.* 1994). Atherosclerosis of the major vessels is rarely the critical event as angiographic studies often reveal these vessels to be patent in the presence of clear evidence of ischaemic colitis (Andriulli *et al.* 1990). Colonic ischaemia is being increasingly recognized in young patients. Causes in this group are vasculitis (especially systemic lupus erythematosus), drug reactions (oestrogens, danazol, vasopressin, gold, psychotropic drugs), sickle cell disease, coagulopathies, and cocaine abuse (Brandt and Boley 1992; Burke *et al.* 1995). Ischaemic colitis is also recognized in competitive long distance runners. Gastrointestinal symptoms occur in up to 30% of marathon runners and a fall in splanchnic blood supply is noted in 80% of these (Michel *et al.* 1994).

Associated colonic diseases (carcinoma, diverticulitis, volvulus, faecal impaction) are found in up to 20% of those with ischaemic colitis (Brandt and Boley 1992). This association is greater than in

Table 15.1 Causes of ischaemic colitis

Category	Causes
Hypotension	Cardiac failure or dysrhythmias
	Shock: allergic, cardiogenic septic, hypovolaemic
Inferior mesenteric artery	Thrombosis
	Embolus
Vasculitis	Systemic lupus erythematosus
	Polyarteritis nodosa
	Rheumatoid arteritis and vasculitis
	Thrombo-angitis obliterans
	Takayasu's arteritis
Iatrogenic/surgical	Aortic aneurysm/aorto-iliac repair
	Lumbar aortography
	Inferior mesenteric artery ligation
Haematological	Sickle-cell disease
	Protein C and S deficiency
	Antithrombin III deficiency
	Exchange transfusions
Drugs	Cocaine
	Oestrogens
	Danazol
	Vasopressin
	Gold
	Psychotropic drugs
Miscellaneous	Long distance running
	Parasitic infections
	Volvulus

the age-matched population. In one study 2% of colorectal carcinomas were proven to have concomitant proximal ischaemic colitis (Seow-Choen *et al.* 1993). In patients with borderline blood flow partial obstruction by these lesions may precipitate ischaemia by causing a fall in flow during straining (Levine and Jacobson 1995). Colonic ischaemia occurs after 2% of elective and up to 60% of emergency operations for aortic aneurysm repair (Mackay *et al.* 1994; Longo *et al.* 1996). Although clinically apparent in 1% of cases, the condition is responsible for 10% of deaths following aortic replacement. Ligation of the inferior mesenteric artery and hypotension are recognized as causative factors.

The colon has a poor blood supply particularly on the left side around the splenic flexure (see Chapter 1, Figure 1.5) At this point the marginal artery linking the left branch of the middle colic artery with the ascending branch of the left colic artery is absent in 7% and tenuous in one-third of individuals. Ischaemic colitis is therefore most common at the splenic flexure and descending colon. Other areas affected include the caecum and rectum (Mackay *et al.*

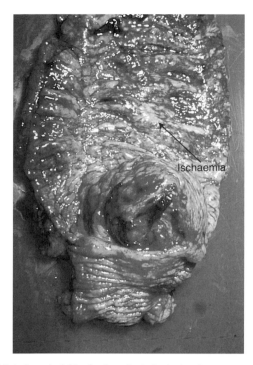

Figure 15.1 Ischaemic right colon in patient who had undergone an aortic aneurysm repair. Note that the caecum in particular is ischaemic (arrowed), as this is the site of a potential weak point in the arterial supply (see Chapter 1, Figure 1.4).

1994), while combined small and large bowel ischaemia is not uncommon (Figure 15.1). In 55% of cases part or all of the splenic flexure and descending colon are affected, in 20% the sigmoid colon, in 10% the ascending colon and in 5% the rectum (Brandt and Boley 1992).

Pathology

The colonic reaction to ischaemia consists of three phases: (i) *acute*, with haemorrhage and necrosis; (ii) *reparative* with granulation tissue and fibrosis; and (iii) *residual* with stricturing. The morphological changes are dependent on the duration and severity of ischaemia.

Macroscopic appearance

In the acute phase the colon is dilated and congested with red, oedematous mucosa. The lumen is filled with altered blood. The wall is thin and friable with an inflammatory peritoneal reaction. Mucosal ulceration varies from slight to extensive when pseudopolyp formation and perforation may occur. Full thickness necrosis, resulting in gangrene, may be patchy. In the resolution phase the bowel wall is thickened, contracted, and indurated. The darkened appearance fades as revascularization and eventually fibrosis develops. Tubular or fusiform strictures tend to occur at the splenic flexure and in some there may be sacculation of the gut wall. Fibrosis is obvious and may extend into the pericolic tissues. Mucosal ulceration is patchy and the submucosa is characteristically widened and filled with granulation tissue. The appearances can mimic segmental Crohn's disease.

Microscopic appearance

Acute changes consist of patchy mucosal and submucosal haemorrhage with oedema and partial mucosal necrosis. The mucosa is raised accounting for the characteristic radiographic 'thumb-print' appearance. Sloughing of the overlying mucosa evacuates the clot and creates an ulcer. Epithelial tubules are covered with fibrin while fibrin thrombi in mucosal and submucosal capillaries are characteristic. The inflammatory cell infiltrate depends on the severity of the ischaemia and colonies of bacteria are often identified in the mucosa. The result is a transient segmental ulcerating colitis. The muscularis is relatively resistant to hypoxia but in severe cases full thickness damage occurs. The microscopic appearances are characteristic and readily distinguished from other causes of bowel inflammation. Crypt abscesses and pseudopolyps are well recognized in this condition and do not indicate ulcerative colitis.

In the reparative phase the mucosa regenerates over the submucosa which is widened and oedematous and contains exuberant granulation and fibrous tissue. This, together with the residual islands of hyperplastic mucosa, may mimic Crohn's disease or chronic ulcerative colitis. When present, iron-laden macrophages are characteristic and confirm the diagnosis. In ischaemic strictures, ulcerated areas show full-thickness mucosal loss, the surface being replaced by granulation tissue (Figure 15.2). The submucosa is widened and filled with a characteristic granulomatous reaction with a marked proliferation of fibroblasts.

Clinical presentation and diagnosis

Colonic ischaemia is more common in elderly female patients with coexisting medical conditions (Reinus and Brandt 1991). It normally presents with the acute onset of crampy, mild left-sided abdominal pain. An urge to defecate often accompanies the pain. Within 24 h there is the passage of small amounts of bright red or maroon blood mixed with the motion. The presence of severe bleeding is so unusual as to question the diagnosis. Physical examination usually reveals only mild to moderate abdominal tenderness over the affected segment. Abdominal distension may be present in the absence of any other findings. Consequently, the correct diagnosis is made initially in 30% of cases (Andriulli *et al.* 1990). Ischaemic colitis associated with obstructing colorectal carcinoma may present dramatically with gangrene or colonic perforation (Halligan *et al.* 1994). Repeated clinical examination is necessary to assess the course of the disease. Increasing abdominal tenderness, guarding, rebound, pyrexia, and paralytic ileus indicate colonic infarction and the need for surgery. Strictures may develop over weeks or months

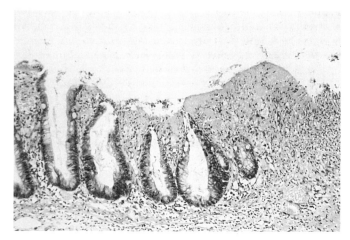

Figure 15.2 Ischaemic colitis. Section taken from the edge of an ischaemic ulcer showing partly ischaemic and ulcerated mucosa. H&E×100.

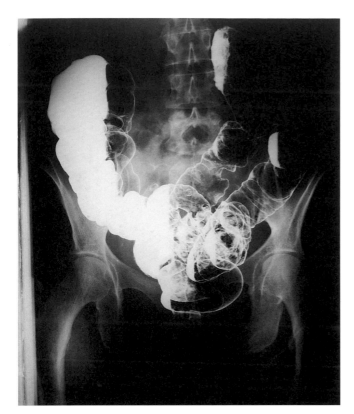

Figure 15.3 Barium enema showing ischaemic colitis at the splenic flexure. Note also the dilatation and pseudo-obstruction of the proximal colon.

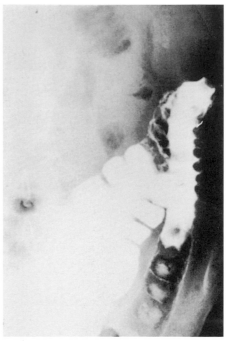

Figure 15.4 Barium enema showing classical 'thumb-printing' or 'saw-tooth pattern' of ischaemic colitis.

and may be clinically silent or produce progressive bowel obstruction. Laboratory tests are of limited benefit, the white cell count being normal in up to one-third of cases. Mesenteric angiography is also of little benefit as it is usually normal even early in the disease. However, in patients undergoing aortic aneurysm repair Doppler flow and intraluminal pH levels can predict ischaemic injury of the colon (Bjorck and Hedberg 1994; Teefey *et al.* 1996).

Diagnostic studies should be performed early as the characteristic thumb-printing disappears within days as the submucosal haemorrhages are either resorbed or evacuated. Plain radiographs may reveal an ileus with thickened intestinal wall and loss of haustration. Spasticity in the affected segment may result in pseudo-obstruction when the normal colon proximal to the site of ischaemia undergoes dilatation (Robson *et al.* 1992) (Figure 15.3). Thumb-printing may be apparent on plain radiographs. The appearances may become more apparent if air is gently inflated into the rectum. In patients without peritonitis, a gentle barium enema should be performed on unprepared bowel within 48 h if the diagnosis is to be made. Water-soluble enemas can be safely used to prepare the bowel prior to barium enema (Hiltunen *et al.* 1991) (Figure 15.4).

Colonoscopy is theoretically more sensitive in diagnosing mucosal abnormalities than barium enema and allows for histological diagnosis (Chatrenet *et al.* 1993). However, caution is required as colonoscopy could theoretically worsen the ischaemia (Wheeldon and Grundman 1990; Johnson 1993). Distension of the colonic lumen to greater than 30 mmHg, which commonly occurs during colonoscopy but not barium enema, diminishes colonic blood flow and progressively decreases the arteriovenous oxygen difference (Brandt and Boley 1992). This may be reduced by insufflating carbon dioxide and if performed carefully, colonoscopy is a safe investigation. On colonoscopy the segmental distribution of haemorrhagic nodules

(thumb-printing) is strongly suggestive, but not conclusive, of the diagnosis unless mucosal gangrene is present. Endoscopic biopsies are often non-specific, but mucosal infarction is pathognomonic. Persistence of supposed thumb-printing implies a different diagnosis such as carcinoma, lymphoma, amyloidosis, or inflammatory bowel disease (Tsai *et al.* 1989). By 1 week the appearances have either resolved or have been replaced by a segmental ulcerative colitis pattern that requires to be distinguished from inflammatory bowel disease.

Treatment

Patients are initially treated conservatively with intravenous fluids. Vasoconstrictive drugs, such as digitalis, should be discontinued. Experimental evidence suggests that broad-spectrum antibiotics reduce the length and severity of bowel damage, but not the risk of perforation (Brandt and Boley 1992). Patients who settle spontaneously require no further treatment. However, they should be followed until resolution occurs as strictures may develop in asymptomatic patients. In those medically unfit for surgery, parenteral nutrition and antibiotic therapy may be considered. Oral steroids are of no advantage and may be dangerous.

In patients requiring surgery, bowel preparation should be avoided as it may precipitate perforation or toxic dilation. The operative specimen should be opened as apparently normal serosal appearances can hide severe underlying mucosal damage (Figure 15.5). Formerly, both ends of bowel were exteriorized for fear of further necrosis. However, some now consider that if the mucosal edges of the resected specimen are viable, primary anastomosis is safe (Brandt and Boley 1992). Colostomy is indicated when long segments of the colon appear externally normal but have infarcted mucosa on sectioning or when the rectum is involved, but not frankly gangrenous. A mucous fistula may be fashioned using diseased bowel as this may heal sufficiently to allow re-anastomosis. However, there is usually insufficient colon to bring to the surface

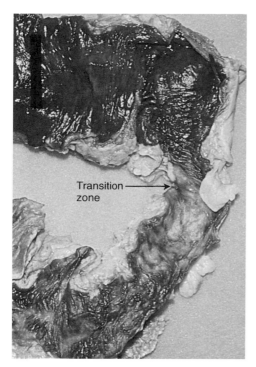

Figure 15.5 Resected specimen in a case of ischaemic colitis showing sharp demarcation between the infarcted and ischaemic segments (arrowed).

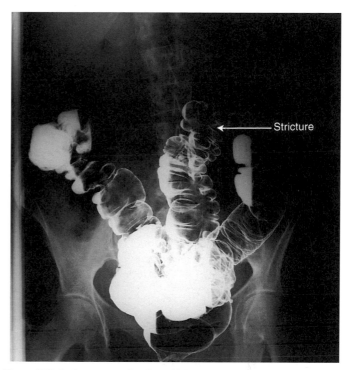

Figure 15.7 Barium enema of patient with healed ischaemic colitis showing pseudo-sacculation and mild stricture formation.

so that a Hartmann's procedure is often indicated. Emergency proctocolectomy is rarely necessary as the rectum is normally viable (Figure 15.6).

The outcome of patients with ischaemic colitis is variable and cannot be predicted at the onset of the disease (Robert *et al.* 1993). Patients who present in shock have a 90% mortality, while those with symptoms persisting beyond 14 days normally develop perforation or a protein-losing enteropathy (Brandt and Boley 1992). In one-third of cases, symptoms resolve spontaneously within 48 h and investigations, which reveal only reversible colonic haemorrhage and oedema, return to normal within 2 weeks. One-fifth of cases go on to severe segmental ulcerating colitis, which may take up to 6 months to heal completely. In almost one-half of cases, the

damage is too severe to heal and irreversible damage occurs. Two-thirds of these cases run a protracted course with either chronic segmental colitis or stricture formation (Figure 15.7). Emergency surgery is required in the remainder.

Angiodysplasia

Incidence and aetiology

Angiodysplasia represents an arteriovenous malformation of uncertain aetiology. Most lesions are acquired and probably result from a degenerative process associated with ageing (Sharma and Gorbien 1995). Factors which may be responsible include intermittent venous obstruction, increased intraluminal pressure, intermittent abnormal arterial flow, and local vascular degeneration (Cappel 1992; Lewis 1993). Mean age at presentation is 65 years and sex incidence is equal (Santos *et al.* 1988; Sharma and Gorbien 1995). Although most patients are elderly, the age range is wide and the abnormalities have been noted in children (Freud *et al.* 1993; de la Torre Mondragon 1995).

The incidence of angiodysplasia among strictly asymptomatic individuals has never been determined, although the prevalence is estimated at 0.8% (Foutch *et al.* 1995). The condition may affect the stomach, small bowel, or colon. In 15% of patients there is simultaneous involvement of the large and small bowel (Cappell 1992; Weinstock *et al.* 1995). Angiodysplasia is responsible for 1–8% of cases of upper gastrointestinal bleeding. Small bowel angiodysplasia accounts for 30–40% of cases of gastrointestinal bleeding of obscure origin and represents the single most common cause for haemorrhage in this subset of patients. Depending on the method of investigation 2–40% of lower intestinal bleeds are attributed to

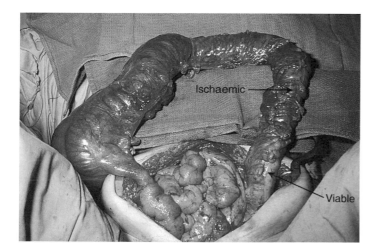

Figure 15.6 Patient with severe ischaemic colitis affecting a large portion of the colon. Note, however, that the mid-descending and sigmoid colons remain viable (arrow).

angiodysplasia, although figures of 2–5% are probably more accurate (Danesh *et al.* 1987; Foutch 1993). The majority of colonic lesions are small (<10 mm) and occur in the right colon (caecum 45%, ascending colon 20%), although any part of the large bowel may be affected (transverse colon 5%, descending colon 5%, sigmoid colon 15%, rectum 10%) (Foutch 1993; Ibach *et al.* 1995).

Pathological diagnosis

Macroscopic appearances of resected specimens are often normal. Postoperative injection with radio-opaque dyes or a silicone rubber compound enables the pathologist to identify the lesions grossly for proper sampling. Alternatively, prolonged intraluminal formalin fixation allows dissection of the mucosa from the muscle wall (Thelmo *et al.* 1992). Histological sections taken from abnormal areas show angiodysplastic lesions characterized by ectatic, engorged submucosal veins, and some dilated venules and capillaries in the mucosal lamina propria (Aldabagh *et al.* 1986).

Clinical presentation

Angiodysplasia may present with overt or occult intestinal haemorrhage. Prior admissions for gastrointestinal bleeding or iron deficiency anaemia are common (Cappell and Gupta 1992; Kepczyk and Kadakia 1995; Gordon *et al.* 1996).

Angiodysplasia has been purported to occur with higher frequency in patients with aortic stenosis (Heyde's syndrome), von Willebrand's disease, cirrhosis, renal failure, and pulmonary disease (Foutch 1993, Natowitz *et al.* 1993). Some report that aortic stenosis is found in up to 25% of patients with gastrointestinal angiodysplasia, others that its incidence is only 2% (Oneglia *et al.* 1993; Gupta *et al.* 1995). It may be that the stenotic aortic valve leads to an acquired, reversible form of von Willebrand's disease (Warkentin *et al.* 1992). In alcoholic cirrhotic patients with colonic vascular ectasias, the prevalence of oesophageal varices is 90% and rectal varices 65% (Naveau *et al.* 1991, 1995). Patients with oesophageal varices have 15 times the risk of colonic vascular ectasias (portal hypertensive colopathy) compared with those without varices (Naveau *et al.* 1991).

Diagnosis

Angiodysplasia may be diagnosed by angiography or colonoscopy. Barium enema is of little benefit (Jaramillo and Slezak 1992). Angiographic features include a vascular tuft, contrast pooling on the anti-mesenteric border of the caecum or ascending colon, a dilated intramural vein and early filling of a draining vein (Figure 15.8). However, these appearances may occasionally be seen in serious pathology such as carcinoma (Belli and Hemingway 1991).

Relative to selective visceral angiography, the diagnostic yield of colonoscopy is 70% (Salem *et al.* 1985). However, colonoscopy is more useful in diagnosing concomitant disease and is potentially therapeutic. Colonoscopy identifies concomitant lesions in between one-third and one-half of cases (diverticula 25%, adenomas 15%, carcinomas in 8%) (Foutch 1993). These associated conditions that may also cause intestinal bleeding are common so that angiodysplasia should only be confidently diagnosed as the source of blood loss if seen to be actively bleeding (Steger *et al.* 1987; Gupta *et al.* 1995). The endoscopic appearances are variable. Most of the vascular dilatations are smaller than 5 mm (66%), flat, and may have a regular or irregular border. Lesions may be single (60%) or multiple. Trans-endoscopic Doppler ultrasonography is claimed to be 90% accurate in confirming or refuting the diagnosis of angiodysplasia

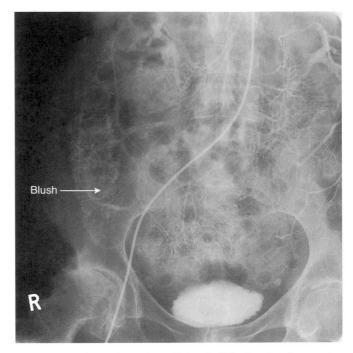

Figure 15.8 Arteriogram in a patient with intestinal bleeding. Note the vascular blush and early filling of the draining veins.

(Jaspersen *et al.* 1994). Due to the approximately 20% correlation between upper and lower non-hereditary gastrointestinal angiodysplasia, the upper and lower tract should be examined by endoscopy prior to elective local resection for bleeding from gastrointestinal angiodysplasia (Cappell 1992). The natural history of angiodysplasia in asymptomatic individuals is benign, significant bleeding within 3 years being very unlikely (Foutch *et al.* 1995).

As co-existent pathology which may also cause bleeding is common, the treatment of angiodysplasia is considered in the section on lower intestinal bleeding.

Lower intestinal bleeding

Incidence and aetiology

Lower intestinal bleeding refers to intraluminal bleeding which arises distal to the ligament of Treitz (Miller *et al.* 1994). Both small and large bowel conditions may be responsible although in up to 20% of cases of presumed lower intestinal bleeding a source proximal to the ligament of Treitz is found (Table 15.2) (Figures 15.9 and 15.10). A large intestinal cause is found in one-quarter of all gastrointestinal bleeding and accounts for 2% of all hospital admissions (Manfredini *et al.* 1994; Ibach *et al.* 1995).

In Western countries, four conditions (haemorrhoids, diverticulosis, neoplasm, and arteriovenous malformation) account for the majority of lower intestinal bleeds (Miller *et al.* 1994; Reinus and Brandt 1994; Helfand *et al.* 1997). Less frequent causes of lower intestinal bleeding include ischaemic colitis, radiation-induced injury, solitary rectal ulcer syndrome (see page 155), endometriosis (see page 200), diversion colitis (see page 194), splanchnic artery aneurysms and gastrointestinal bleeding in runners (Miller *et al.* 1994; Bono 1996). In developing countries infectious colitis accounts

Table 15.2 Causes of lower gastrointestinal bleeding

Small bowel	Large bowel	Incidence (large bowel causes)
Aorto-enteric fistula	Haemorrhoids	50%
Jejunal diverticula	Diverticular disease	20–30%
Ulcers	Arteriovenous malformation	?
Tumours	Tumours	10–15%
Radiation enteritis	Inflammatory bowel disease	5%
Arteriovenous malformation	Radiation enteritis	<1%
Meckel's diverticulum	Focal ulcers	1–5%
Crohn's disease	Infectious colitis	?
Intussusception	Ischaemic colitis	5%
	Idiopathic	5–10%

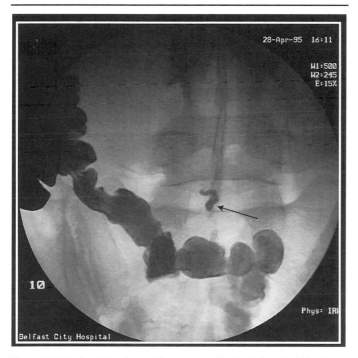

Figure 15.9 Barium follow through in a patient with chronic intestinal bleeding showing a Meckel's diverticulum (arrowed).

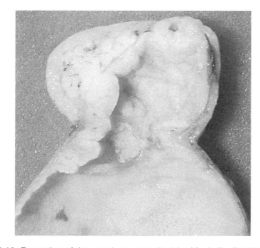

Figure 15.10 Resection of the specimen revealed the Meckel's diverticulum contained gastric mucosa.

for 2–8% and intestinal tuberculosis 2% of cases of intestinal bleeding (Goenka *et al.* 1993).

About half of all cases of lower intestinal bleeding are attributed to haemorrhoids, although up to one-quarter of these may have other coexisting colonic pathology (see Chapter 18). In Western countries diverticular disease accounts for up to 25% of cases of overt and 2–10% of occult intestinal bleeding, being the commonest cause of massive colonic bleeding in the elderly (Makela *et al.* 1993). Benign or malignant neoplasms can be expected in 10–15% of those presenting with rectal bleeding, while ulcerative colitis accounts for about 5% of cases (Makela *et al.* 1993; Norrelund and Norrelund 1996).

Erosion of an abnormally large submucosal muscular artery, usually in the ascending colon, is claimed to cause massive lower intestinal bleeding. The pathological findings in this condition are identical to Dieulafoy's disease of the stomach (Richards *et al.* 1988). The Klippel–Trenaunay syndrome (multiple cutaneous and visceral haemangiomas, severe varicose veins, and prominent limb hypertrophy) can also be associated with significant lower gastrointestinal bleeding from diffuse cavernous haemangiomas of the colon (Myers 1993).

Colonic ulcers may account for up to 5% of cases of rectal bleeding and are often associated with a history of previous non-steroidal anti-inflammatory drug ingestion. In one study, patients with lower intestinal haemorrhage or perforation were more than twice as likely to be consumers of anti-inflammatory drugs than those without these complications (Langman *et al.* 1985). Although ulcers may affect the entire large intestine and the rectum may be affected by ulcers, the caecum (60%), ascending colon (15%), and sigmoid colon (10%) are normally involved by one to four ulcers measuring from a few millimetres up to 3 cm in diameter (Bayerdorffer *et al.* 1987). The sex distribution is equal and although the age range is wide, most patients present in the fifth decade. Embolism to the splanchnic vessels may also cause intestinal bleeding from severe mucosal ulceration. Massive intestinal bleeding has been attributed to atheromicroembolism after cardiac catheterization and to cholesterol crystal embolization (Romano *et al.* 1988).

About 1% of intestinal bleeds are attributed to previous radiotherapy. One-third of radiation-induced intestinal bleeding arises from the large bowel, bleeding usually appearing 2 years after completion of radiotherapy (Zighelboim *et al.* 1993). About 1% of renal transplant recipients experience lower intestinal haemorrhage secondary to colitis from opportunistic infections (40%); pseudomembranous, ischaemic, or uraemic colitis (40%); and idiopathic ulcers of the colon (20%) (Stylianos *et al.* 1988). Mortality in these patients is high (70%) unless withdrawal of immunosuppression and early operative intervention is performed. Rupture of splanchnic artery aneurysms are rare causes of intestinal bleeding (Hong *et al.* 1992). Atherosclerosis is the most common cause of the aneurysm (32%), followed by trauma (22%) and inflammatory lesions (10%) (Psathakis *et al.* 1992). The average age is 40 years but with a wide range (10–85 years). The male to female ratio is 2:1. In 65–80% of cases rupture of the aneurysm is the first clinical manifestation, being associated with a mortality of about 35% (Psathakis *et al.* 1992).

Clinical presentation and diagnosis

A thorough history and examination is required in all cases (Anonymous 1997). Initial diagnostic procedures include rectal examination and proctosigmoidoscopy, nasogastric tube aspiration to

Table 15.3 Comparison of the diagnostic methods of investigating colonic bleeding

Barium enema	Helpful in occult/minimal bleeding
	Abnormality identified may not be source of bleeding
	False positive rate up to 20%
	False negative rate up to 45%
Colonoscopy	Effective in occult and massive haemorrhage
	Diagnosis: correct in 70%; incorrect in 10%; not possible in 20%
	Overall sensitivity 95%
	Therapeutic in many instances
Angiography	Bleeding must be over 1 ml/min
	Identifies site in 75% of cases overall
	Overall sensitivity 75%
	Limits surgical resection in up to 90% of cases
	Complication rate 10%
Radio-isotope scan	Bleeding must be over 0.1 ml/min
	Overall sensitivity 70%
	If scan positive within 2 h, accuracy 85%
	If scan negative, 70% will stop bleeding spontaneously

exclude upper intestinal causes and haematological studies (full blood and platelet count, coagulation screen, biochemical studies). In contrast to upper intestinal bleeding a markedly elevated plasma urea to creatinine ratio is not seen in lower intestinal bleeding. A ratio above 90 is associated with odds for upper gastrointestinal compared with lower intestinal bleeding of 15:1 (Olsen and Andreassen 1991). Patients over the age of 40 years with known haemorrhoids or diverticular disease require investigation of the entire colon as other causes of intestinal bleeding frequently coexist. Definitive investigations include endoscopy, barium enema, angiography, and radio-isotope scanning (Table 15.3).

Endoscopy

Many consider colonoscopy the investigation of choice in the diagnosis of colorectal bleeding, urgent colonoscopy more often being diagnostic than urgent visceral angiography (Bono 1996; Metcalf *et al.* 1996). In addition, colonoscopy may be therapeutic, allowing haemostasis to be achieved in up to 20% of cases (Jensen and Machicado 1988). Complete colonoscopy to the caecum is possible in about 90% of cases, even in acute rapid bleeding (Church 1991). A correct diagnosis is possible in two-thirds of patients, the diagnosis being incorrect in 10% with no bleeding site being identified in about 20% (Goenka *et al.* 1993). The sensitivity of colonoscopy in all cases of rectal bleeding is 95% which is superior to angiography (75%) and scintigraphy (70%). Emergency colonoscopy is also valuable in cases of massive intestinal bleeding, accounting for 5% of all colonoscopies (Giorgio *et al.* 1990). The procedure may be performed without preparation relying on the cathartic effect of blood to clear the colon. However, an oral purge is more effective in cleansing the colon of stool, clots, and blood, the bleeding point being identified in two-thirds of cases even after massive bleeding (Caos *et al.* 1986). Patients with occult bleeding should undergo both upper and lower intestinal endoscopy. This detects the source in half of cases, although the diagnostic yield is significantly higher with gastroscopy than with colonoscopy (45% gastroscopy, 25% colonoscopy) (Zuckerman and Benitez 1992).

Intra-operative endoscopy is an useful adjunct to pre-operative endoscopy, allowing appropriate excisional surgery rather than blind colonic resection (Berry *et al.* 1988; Whelan *et al.* 1989; Lopez *et al.* 1996). Using this technique, intra-operative endoscopy is successful in 90% of cases and provides information that alters the planned operation in one-third of cases. In patients who continue to lose blood despite extensive normal investigations video panendoscopy, employing a segmental advance and look technique, allows visualization and transillumination of the entire gut and identifies mucosal disease in up to 90% of cases (Flickinger *et al.* 1989). Using this technique to guide surgical resection, bleeding can be totally controlled in three-quarters of patients during a mean follow-up period of 2 years.

Barium enema

Single contrast barium enema is generally inaccurate in the assessment of lower intestinal bleeding. Double contrast barium enema is helpful in patients with occult bleeding as these patients have either ceased to bleed or are bleeding at a rate which is below the threshold of sensitivity of diagnostic methods that depend on real-time loss of an intestinal marker (angiography or radio-isotope scanning). However, most clinicians favour colonoscopy to barium enema as it identifies the source of bleeding and allows biopsy of any suspicious area that might be identified radiologically (Noyer and Simon 1991). Identification of diverticular disease on barium enema does not indicate that this is the source of bleeding, so that the false positive rate of barium enema can be as high as 20% and false negative rate 45% (Church 1991). In one study comparing double contrast barium enema against colonoscopy, the sensitivity of barium was 89% and specificity 97% (Jaramillo and Slezak 1992). The sensitivity of barium enema for carcinoma, polyps, and inflammatory bowel disease was 100%, 98%, and 73% respectively. The authors concluded that barium enema is very effective at diagnosing carcinoma and polyps greater than 1 cm, the most frequent causes of bleeding, but less effective in diagnosing rarer causes of lower intestinal bleeding. A non-diagnostic barium enema therefore requires a colonoscopy while a non-diagnostic colonoscopy suggests a small bowel cause for the bleeding.

In a randomized trial comparing colonoscopy with the combination of flexible sigmoidoscopy and double contrast barium enema, colonoscopy detected more polyps under 1 cm and arteriovenous malformations but fewer cases of diverticulosis (Rex *et al.* 1990). There was no significant difference in the detection of cancers or polyps greater than 1 cm. Flexible sigmoidoscopy and double contrast barium enema may therefore be a more cost-effective strategy for the detection of colonic neoplasms in those presenting with rectal bleeding under the age of 55 years. In those over this age, initial colonoscopy is the more cost-effective method of investigation (Rex *et al.* 1990).

Angiography

For angiography to be positive, the bleeding rate requires to be at least 1 mL per minute so that the technique is most helpful in patients with profuse intestinal haemorrhage (Buchman and Bulkley 1987; Freud *et al.* 1993). Selective visceral angiography reveals the anatomical source of bleeding in 75% of patients, allowing the surgical resection to be limited in 90% of these (Imdahl *et al.* 1991). The diagnostic yield of emergency visceral angiography is 15% (Jensen and Machicado 1988). Complications (thrombosis of the femoral artery and pseudoaneurysm formation) occur in up to 10% of cases (Sharma *et al.* 1992).

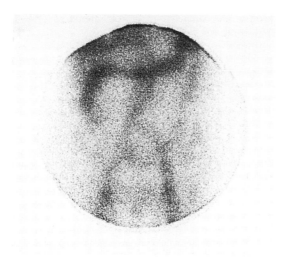

Figure 15.11 Indium-labelled red cell scan in a patient with intestinal bleeding. Blood is seen in the ascending, transverse, and descending colon, suggesting angiodysplasia of the right colon.

Radio-isotope scanning

Nuclear scintigraphy has the theoretical advantages of being non-invasive, not interfering with diagnostic or therapeutic manoeuvres and displaying accumulated as opposed to momentary blood loss (Figure 15.11). Interpretation may be confused by blood and isotope being carried upstream so that in some cases it is only possible to distinguish the source as being from the small or large bowel. Technetium-99m is rapidly accumulated into the reticuloendothelial system and is therefore primarily indicated for rapid blood loss. *In vivo* labelling of red blood cells is technically simple but resolution is poor due to non-specific labelling of other tissues. *In vitro* labelling of autologous red blood cells is more complex to prepare but provides good specificity. With such techniques technetium-labelled red-cell scanning can identify the bleeding site provided the blood loss is in excess of 0.1 ml/min (Ryan *et al.* 1992).

About 60% of radio-isotope scans performed for intestinal bleeding will be positive (Nicholson *et al.* 1989; Dusold *et al.* 1994). In patients requiring emergency surgery scintigraphy locates the bleeding site pre-operatively in about 70% of cases and may therefore limit the extent of colectomy required (Bearn *et al.* 1992) (Figure 15.11). In lower intestinal bleeding, the sensitivity of the technique is 97%, specificity 85%, with positive and negative predictive values of 95% and 92%, respectively (Nicholson *et al.* 1989). Scans which are positive within the first 2 h are 85% accurate in correctly identifying the site of the bleeding (Dusold *et al.* 1994). In patients with early negative scans, later imaging at 3–24 h may provide objective evidence of the presence of continued intermittent haemorrhage (Jacobson and Cerqueira 1992). Bleeding settles spontaneously in 70% of patients with an entirely negative scan, the risk of rebleeding over the following 2 years being 25% (Orecchia *et al.* 1985). In some cases ultrasound or CT scanning identifies segmental wall thickening and typical target lesions (Ranschaert *et al.* 1994; Ettore *et al.* 1997).

Treatment

Acute lower gastrointestinal bleeding stops spontaneously in about three-quarters of patients so that an initial conservative approach is indicated (Reinus and Brandt 1994). About 15% of patients will require transfusion of more than four units of blood and up to two-thirds may undergo some form of intervention to control bleeding

(40% therapeutic endoscopy, 25% surgery, 1% therapeutic angiography) (Jensen and Machicado 1988). Uncontrolled case studies have reported reduction or cessation of bleeding in subjects managed with conjugated oestrogens (Spath-Schwalbe *et al.* 1993), although the results from two prospective randomized controlled trials are conflicting (Foutch 1993). Octreotide may be useful in bleeding from angiodysplasia (Rossini *et al.* 1993).

Colonoscopy is a useful therapeutic tool in lower intestinal bleeding. Bleeding polyps are effectively managed by polypectomy. Residual bleeding from the polypectomy site is often related to aspirin therapy and may be treated by endoscopic band ligation (Slivka *et al.* 1994). Many consider endoscopic therapy to be the treatment of choice for managing colonic angiodysplasia (Gupta *et al.* 1995). A single treatment with injection or coagulation therapy (Bipolar probe, heater probe, or argon laser) is claimed to be successful in 85% of patients, three-quarters having no further bleeding 3–7 years following treatment (Cottone *et al.* 1991; Lau *et al.* 1992). Those who do rebleed often respond to further endoscopic treatment so that only 5% will come to surgery because of persistent bleeding (Imdahl *et al.* 1991). In one study, Doppler ultrasound revealed that injection therapy sclerosed 90% of angiodysplastic lesions within 2 weeks, rebleeding responding to repeat injections (Jaspersen *et al.* 1994). Similarly, injection or laser therapy appears to be an effective (80% control of bleeding) and safe (5% complication rate) therapeutic option in diverticular disease or radiation enteritis, provided the bleeding site has been identified (Kim and Marcon *et al.* 1993; Zighelboim *et al.* 1993).

Therapeutic angiographic techniques include infusing intra-arterial vasopressin, the effects of which tend to be short-lived, and embolization with polyvinyl alcohol particles, which is claimed to achieve immediate haemostasis in up to 90% of cases (Guy *et al.* 1992) (Figure 15.8). However, there is a risk of infarction while up to one-third of patients will rebleed within 1 month.

Indications for surgery include profuse haemorrhage, failure of endoscopic or angiographic therapy and patients with large circumferential cavernous angiomas, such as the Klippel–Trenaunay syndrome (Myers 1993). About 25% of patients will eventually require surgery, with 10% needing an emergency operation for rapid blood loss (Manunta *et al.* 1989; Pricolo and Shellito 1994). Those with angiodysplasia and aortic stenosis are best treated initially by aortic valve replacement as this often cures the bleeding (Alam and Lewis 1991).

If the bleeding site is known, segmental resection is associated with a lower operative mortality and morbidity when compared with total abdominal colectomy (Manunta *et al.* 1989). However, blind segmental resection is associated with a rebleeding rate of 10%. Some authors suggest aggressive pre-operative evaluation can identify the bleeding site in up to 60% of cases, allowing segmental resection to be performed (Manunta *et al.* 1989), others that investigation can unnecessarily delay surgical therapy in the actively haemorrhaging patient (Baker and Senagore 1994). In a study of patients undergoing surgery for massive lower intestinal bleeding, the rebleeding rate at 1 year for subtotal colectomy was 0%, segmental resection with positive angiography 14% and segmental resection with negative angiography 42% (Parkes *et al.* 1993). Morbidity (83%) and mortality (57%) were also highest for those undergoing segmental resection in patients with negative angiography. The authors concluded that segmental resection should be performed when the bleeding site has been identified angiographically, with total abdominal colectomy being reserved for massive bleeding with negative angiography.

If the bleeding site is unknown but there are clues suggesting it to be right-sided, a right hemicolectomy is preferred (Milewski and Schofield 1989; Reinus and Brandt 1994). In older patients, in whom both angiodysplasia and diverticulosis may coexist the extent of resection is unaltered by the presence of diverticulosis so that left-sided resection should only be used when there is proof of left-sided bleeding. If there are no clues to the source of bleeding, 'equivocal' indications of a left-sided source, or the presence of bilateral disease, total abdominal colectomy is indicated (Milewski and Schofield 1989; Reinus and Brandt 1994; Billingham 1977).

The overall mortality of those requiring surgery is about 25%, ranging from 10% in those undergoing urgent surgery to almost 100% in severely hypotensive patients who require colectomy and exteriorization of the bowel (Buchman and Bulkley 1987; Bender *et al.* 1991). In those undergoing elective or urgent surgery morbidity and mortality following total abdominal colectomy and segmental resection are similar (10%) (Baker and Senagore 1994). Mortality is related to age and the amount of blood transfused, being unaffected by type of anastomosis and delay before operation (Bender *et al.* 1991). Once more than 10 units of blood have been transfused, the mortality following total abdominal colectomy rises dramatically (Bender *et al.* 1991). Life table analysis reveals similar rebleeding rates (5–10%) among medically and endoscopically treated patients, with coagulopathy being the only factor that predicts rebleeding (Richter *et al.* 1989). Surgically treated patients have half the rebleeding of the non-operative groups. The overall mortality of lower intestinal bleeding is 5%, increasing to 15% in those with severe bleeding (Makela *et al.* 1993). Although mortality increases with age, elderly patients with lower intestinal bleeding do well, even when surgery is required (Reinus and Brandt 1991). An individual's age, by itself, should therefore not preclude aggressive medical or surgical care.

References

Alam M, Lewis JW Jr. Cessation of gastrointestinal bleeding from angiodysplasia after surgery for idiopathic hypertrophic subaortic stenosis. *Am. Heart J.* 1991; 121: 608–10.

Aldabagh SM, Trujillo YP, Taxy JB. Utility of specimen angiography in angiodysplasia of the colon. *Gastroenterology* 1986; 91: 725–9.

Andriulli A, Pera A, Gindro T, Astegiano M, Verme G. Intestinal ischemia: nosographic framework and risk factors. *Minerva Med.* 1990; 81: 55–60.

Anonymous. Case records of the Massachusetts General Hospital. Weekly clinicopathological exercises. Case 7-1997. A 14-year-old girl with recurrent painless rectal bleeding. *New Eng. J. Med.* 1997; 336: 641–8.

Baker R, Senagore A. Abdominal colectomy offers safe management for massive lower GI bleed. *Am. Surg.* 1994; 60: 578–81.

Bayerdorffer E, Sommer A, Weingart J, Ottenjann R. Gastrointestinal bleeding in solitary colonic ulcers. *Deutsch. Med. Wochenschr.* 1987; 112: 53–6.

Bearn P, Persad R, Wilson N, Flanagan J, Williams T. 99mTechnetium labelled red blood cell scintigraphy as an alternative to angiography in the investigation of gastrointestinal bleeding: clinical experience in a district general hospital. *Ann. R. Coll. Surg. Engl.* 1992; 74: 192–9.

Belli AM, Hemingway AP. Malignant 'angiodysplasia'. *Clin. Radiol.* 1991; 44: 31–3.

Bender JS, Wiencek RG, Bouwman DL. Morbidity and mortality following total abdominal colectomy for massive lower gastrointestinal bleeding. *Am. Surg.* 1991; 57: 536–40.

Berry AR, Campbell WB, Kettlewell MG. Management of major colonic haemorrhage. *Br. J. Surg.* 1988; 75: 637–40.

Billingham RP. The cannadrum of lower gastrointestinal bleeding. *Surg. Clin. North Am.* 1997; 77: 241–52.

Bjorck M, Hedberg B. Early detection of major complications after abdominal aortic surgery: predictive value of sigmoid colon and gastric intramucosal pH monitoring. *Br. J. Surg.* 1994 ; 81: 25–30.

Bono MJ. Lower gastrointestinal tract bleeding. *Emer. Med. Clin. North Am.* 1996; 14: 547–56.

Brandt LJ, Boley SJ. Colonic ischemia. *Surg. Clin. North Am.* 1992; 72: 203–29.

Buchman TG, Bulkley GB. Current management of patients with lower gastrointestinal bleeding. *Surg. Clin. North Am.* 1987; 67: 651–64.

Burke AP, Sobin LH, Virmani R. Localized vasculitis of the gastrointestinal tract. *Am. J. Surg. Pathol.* 1995; 19: 338–49.

Caos A, Benner KG, Manier J, McCarthy DM, Blessing LD, Gogel HK. Colonoscopy after Golytely preparation in acute rectal bleeding. *J. Clin. Gastroenterol.* 1986; 8: 46–9.

Cappell MS. Spatial clustering of simultaneous nonhereditary gastrointestinal angiodysplasia. Small but significant correlation between nonhereditary colonic and upper gastrointestinal angiodysplasia. *Dig. Dis. Sci.* 1992; 37: 1072–7.

Cappell MS, Gupta A. Changing epidemiology of gastrointestinal angiodysplasia with increasing recognition of clinically milder cases: angiodysplasia tend to produce mild chronic gastrointestinal bleeding in a study of 47 consecutive patients admitted from 1980–1989. *Am. J. Gastroenterol.* 1992; 87: 201–6.

Chatrenet P, Friocourt P, Ramain JP, Cherrier M, Maillard JB. Colonoscopy in the elderly: a study of 200 cases. *Eur. J. Med.* 1993; 2: 411–3.

Church JM. Analysis of the colonoscopic findings in patients with rectal bleeding according to the pattern of their presenting symptoms. *Dis. Colon Rectum* 1991; 34: 391–5.

Cottone C, Disclafani G, Genova G, Modica G, Pardo S, Romeo G, *et al.* Use of BICAP in a case of colon angiodysplasia. *Surg. Endosc.* 1991; 5: 99–100.

Danesh BJ Spiliadis C Williams CB Zambartas CM. Angiodysplasia—an uncommon cause of colonic bleeding: colonoscopic evaluation of 1050 patients with rectal bleeding and anaemia. *Int. J. Colorect. Dis.* 1987; 2: 218–22.

de la Torre Mondragon L, Vargas Gomez MA, Mora Tiscarreno MA, Ramirez Mayans J. Angiodysplasia of the colon in children. *J. Pediatr. Surg.* 1995; 30: 72–5.

Dusold R, Burke K, Carpentier W, Dyck WP. The accuracy of technetium 99m labeled red cell scintigraphy in localizing gastrointestinal bleeding. *Am. J. Gastroenterol.* 1994; 89: 345–8.

Ettore GC, Francisco G, Garribba AP *et al.* Helical CT angiography in gastrointestinal bleeding of obscure origin. *Am. J. Roentgenol.* 1997; 168:727–31.

Flickinger EG, Stanforth AC, Sinar DR, MacDonald KG, Lannin DR, Gibson JH. Intraoperative video panendoscopy for diagnosing sites of chronic intestinal bleeding. *Am. J. Surg.* 1989; 157: 137–44.

Foutch PG. Angiodysplasia of the gastrointestinal tract. *Am. J. Gastroenterol.* 1993; 88: 807–18.

Foutch PG, Rex DK, Lieberman DA. Prevalence and natural history of colonic angiodysplasia among healthy asymptomatic people. *Am. J. Gastroenterol.* 1995; 90: 564–7.

Freud E, Kidron D, Gornish M, Barak R, Golinski D, Zer M. The value of precise preoperative localization of colonic arteriovenous malformation in childhood. *Am. J. Gastroenterol.* 1993; 88: 443–6.

Giorgio P, Lorusso D, Di Matteo G, Chicco G. The role of emergency colonoscopy in colorectal hemorrhage. *Minerva Dietol. Gastroenterol.* 1990; 36: 19–22.

Goenka MK, Kochhar R, Mehta SK. Spectrum of lower gastrointestinal hemorrhage: an endoscopic study of 166 patients. *Indian J. Gastroenterol.* 1993; 12: 129–31.

Gordon S, Bensen S, Smith R. Long-term follow-up of older patients with iron deficiency anemia after a negative GI evaluation. *Am. J. Gastroenterol.* 1996; 91: 885–9.

Gupta N, Longo WE, Vernava AM 3rd. Angiodysplasia of the lower gastrointestinal tract: an entity readily diagnosed by colonoscopy and primarily managed nonoperatively. *Dis. Colon Rectum* **1995; 38: 979–82.**

Guy GE, Shetty PC, Sharma RP, Burke MW, Burke TH. Acute lower gastrointestinal hemorrhage: treatment by superselective embolization with polyvinyl alcohol particles. *Am. J. Roentgenol.* 1992; 159: 521–6.

Halligan MS, Saunders BP, Thomas BM, Phillips RK. Ischaemic colitis in association with sigmoid carcinoma: a report of two cases. *Clin. Radiol.* 1994; 49: 183–4.

Helfand M, Marton KI, Zimmer-Gembeck MJ, Sox HC Jr. History of visible rectal bleeding in a primary care population Initial assessment and 10-year follow-up. *JAMA* **1997; 277: 44–8.**

Hiltunen KM, Kolehmainen H, Vuorinen T, Matikainen M. Early water soluble contrast enema in the diagnosis of acute colonic diverticulitis. *Int. J. Colorectal Dis.* 1991; 6: 190–2.

Hong GS, Wong CY, Nambiar R. Massive lower gastrointestinal haemorrhage from a splenic artery pseudoaneurysm. *Br. J. Surg.* 1992; 79: 174.

Ibach MB, Grier JF, Goldman DE, LaFontaine S, Gholson CF. Diagnostic considerations in evaluation of patients presenting with melena and non-diagnostic esophagogastroduodenoscopy. *Dig. Dis. Sci.* 1995; 40: 1459–62.

Imdahl A, Salm R, Ruckauer K, Farthmann EH. Diagnosis and management of lower gastrointestinal hemorrhage. Retrospective analysis of 233 cases. *Langenbecks Arch. Chir.* 1991; 376: 152–7.

Jacobson AF, Cerqueira MD. Prognostic significance of late imaging results in technetium 99m labeled red blood cell gastrointestinal bleeding studies with early negative images. *J. Nuclear Med.* 1992; 33: 202–7.

Jaramillo E, Slezak P. Comparison between double contrast barium enema and colonoscopy to investigate lower gastrointestinal bleeding. *Gastrointest. Radiol.* 1992; 17: 81–3.

Jaspersen D, Korner T, Schorr W, Hammar CH. Diagnosis and treatment control of bleeding colorectal angiodysplasias by endoscopic Doppler sonography: a preliminary study. *Gastrointest. Endosc.* 1994; 40: 40–4.

Jensen DM, Machicado GA. Diagnosis and treatment of severe hematochezia. The role of urgent colonoscopy after purge. *Gastroenterology* 1988; 95: 1569–74.

Johnson H Jr Management of major complications encountered with flexible colonoscopy. *J. Natl Med. Assoc.* 1993; 85: 916–20.

Kepczyk T, Kadakia SC. Prospective evaluation of gastrointestinal tract in patients with iron deficiency anemia. *Dig. Dis. Sci.* 1995; 40: 1283–9.

Kim YI, Marcon NE. Injection therapy for colonic diverticular bleeding. A case study. *J. Clin. Gastroenterol.* 1993; 17: 46–8.

Langman MJ, Morgan L, Worrall A. Use of anti inflammatory drugs by patients admitted with small or large bowel perforations and haemorrhage. *Br. Med. J.* 1985; 290: 347–9.

Lau WY, Chu KW, Yuen WK, Poon GP, Li AK. Bleeding angiodysplasia of the gastrointestinal tract. *Aust. N.Z. J. Surg.* 1992; 62: 344–9.

Levine JS, Jacobson ED. Intestinal ischemic disorders. *Dig Dis. Sci.* **1995; 13: 3–24.**

Lewis B. Obscure gastrointestinal bleeding. *Mt. Sinai J. Med.* 1993; 60: 200–8.

Longo WE, Lee TC, Barnett MG, Vernava AM, Wade TP, Peterson GJ, *et al.* Ischemic colitis complicating abdominal aortic aneurysm surgery in the U.S. veteran. *J. Surg. Res.* 1996; 60: 351–4.

Lopez MJ, Cooley JS, Petros JG, Sullivan JG, Cave DR. Complete intraoperative small-bowel endoscopy in the evaluation of occult gastrointestinal bleeding using the sonde enteroscope. *Arch. Surg.* 1996; 131: 272–7.

Mackay C, Murphy P, Rosenberg IL, Tait NP. Case report: rectal infarction after abdominal aortic surgery. *Br. J. Radiol.* 1994; 67: 497–8.

Makela JT, Kiviniemi H, Laitinen S, Kairaluoma MI. Diagnosis and treatment of acute lower gastrointestinal bleeding. *Scand. J. Gastroenterol.* 1993; 28: 1062–6.

Manfredini R, Gallerani M, Salmi R, Calo G, Pasin M, Bigoni M, Fersini C. Circadian variation in the time of onset of acute gastrointestinal bleeding. *J. Emerg. Med.* 1994; 12: 5–9.

Manunta A, Camilleri G, Di Saverio G, Bergamaschi R, Giani L. Acute colonic hemorrhage. Importance of a preoperative localization of the origin of bleeding in patients requiring emergency surgery. *Minerva Chir.* 1989; 44: 1261–6.

Matsumoto T, Iida M, Kimura Y, Nanbu T, Fujishima M. Clinical features in young adult patients with ischaemic colitis. *J. Gastroenterol. Hepatol.* 1994; 9: 572–5.

Metcalf JV, Smith J, Jones R, Record CO. Incidence and causes of rectal bleeding in general practice as detected by colonoscopy. *Br. J. Gen. Pract.* 1996; 46: 161–4.

Michel H, Larrey D, Blanc P. Hepato digestive disorders in athletic practice. *Presse Med.* 1994; 23: 479–84.

Milewski PJ, Schofield PF. Massive colonic haemorrhage the case for right hemicolectomy. *Ann. R. Coll. Surg. Engl.* **1989; 71: 253–9.**

Miller LS, Barbarevech C, Friedman LS. Less frequent causes of lower gastrointestinal bleeding. *Gastroenterol. Clin. North Am.* **1994; 23: 21–52.**

Myers BM. Treatment of colonic bleeding in Klippel Trenaunay syndrome with combined partial colectomy and endoscopic laser. *Dig. Dis. Sci.* 1993; 38: 1351–3.

Natowitz L, Defraigne JO, Limet R. Association of aortic stenosis and gastrointestinal bleeding (Heyde's syndrome). Report of two cases. *Acta Chir. Belg.* 1993; 93: 31–3.

Naveau S, Bedossa P, Poynard T, Mory B, Chaput JC. Portal hypertensive colopathy. A new entity. *Dig. Dis. Sci.* 1991; 36: 1774–81.

Naveau S, Leger Ravet MB, Houdayer C, Bedossa P, Lemaigre G, Chaput JC. Nonhereditary colonic angiodysplasias: histomorphometric approach to their pathogenesis. *Dig. Dis. Sci.* 1995; 40: 839–42.

Nicholson ML, Neoptolemos JP, Sharp JF, Watkin EM, Fossard DP. Localization of lower gastrointestinal bleeding using *in vivo* technetium 99m labelled red blood cell scintigraphy. *Br. J. Surg.* 1989; 76: 358–61.

Norrelund N, Norrelund H. Colorectal cancer and polyps in patients aged 40 years and over who consult a GP with rectal bleeding. *Family Practice* 1996; 13: 160–5.

Noyer C, Simon D. Air contrast barium enema versus colonoscopy: the debate continues. *Am. J. Gastroenterol.* 1991; 86: 1274–5.

Olsen LH, Andreassen KH. Stools containing altered blood plasma urea: creatinine ratio as a simple test for the source of bleeding. *Br. J. Surg.* 1991; 78: 71–3.

Oneglia C, Sabatini T, Rusconi C, Gardini A, Paterlini A, Buffoli F, Graffeo M. Prevalence of aortic valve stenosis in patients affected by gastrointestinal angiodysplasia. *Eur. J. Med.* 1993; 2: 75–8.

Orecchia PM, Hensley EK, McDonald PT, Lull RJ. Localization of lower gastrointestinal hemorrhage. Experience with red blood cells labeled *in vitro* with technetium Tc 99m. *Arch. Surg.* 1985; 120: 621–4.

Parkes BM, Obeid FN, Sorensen VJ, Horst HM, Fath JJ. The management of massive lower gastrointestinal bleeding. *Am. Surg.* **1993; 59: 676–8.**

Pricolo VE, Shellito PC. Surgery for radiation injury to the large intestine. Variables influencing outcome. *Dis. Colon Rectum* 1994; 37: 675–84.

Psathakis D, Muller G, Noah M, Diebold J, Bruch HP. Present management of hepatic artery aneurysms. Symptomatic left hepatic artery aneurysm, right hepatic artery aneurysm with erosion into the gallbladder and simultaneous colocholecystic fistula a report of two unusual cases and the current state of etiology, diagnosis, histology and treatment. *J. Vasc. Dis.* 1992; 21: 210–5.

Ranschaert E, Verhille R, Marchal G, Rigauts H, Ponette E. Sonographic diagnosis of ischemic colitis. *J. Belg. Radiol.* 1994; 77: 166–8.

Reinus JF, Brandt LJ. Lower intestinal bleeding in the elderly. *Clin. Geriatric Med.* **1991; 7: 301–19.**

Reinus JF, Brandt LJ. Vascular ectasias and diverticulosis. Common causes of lower intestinal bleeding. *Gastroenterol. Clin. North Am.* **1994; 23: 1–20.**

Rex DK, Weddle RA, Lehman GA, Pound DC, O'Connor KW, Hawes RH, *et al.* Flexible sigmoidoscopy plus air contrast barium enema versus colonoscopy for suspected lower gastrointestinal bleeding. *Gastroenterology* 1990; 98: 855–61.

Richards WO, Grove Mahoney D, Williams LF. Hemorrhage from a Dieulafoy type ulcer of the colon: a new cause of lower gastrointestinal bleeding. *Am. Surg.* 1988; 54: 121–4.

Richter JM, Christensen MR, Colditz GA, Nishioka NS. Angiodysplasia. Natural history and efficacy of therapeutic interventions. *Dig. Dis. Sci.* 1989; 34: 1542–6.

Robert JH, Mentha G, Rohner A. Ischaemic colitis: two distinct patterns of severity. *Gut* 1993; 34: 4–6.

Robson NK, Khan SM, Rawlinson J, Dewbury KC. Ischaemic colitis: clinical, radiological and pathological correlation in three cases. *Clin. Radiol.* 1992; 46: 337–9.

Romano TJ, Graham SM, Chuong J, Ballantyne GH, Modlin IM, Sussman J, West AB. Bleeding colonic ulcers secondary to atheromatous microemboli after left heart catheterization. *J. Clin. Gastroenterol.* 1988; 10: 693–8.

Rossini FP, Arrigoni A, Pennazio M. Octreotide in the treatment of bleeding due to angiodysplasia of the small intestine. *Am. J. Gastroenterol.* 1993; 88: 1424–7.

Ryan P, Styles CB, Chmiel R. Identification of the site of severe colon bleeding by technetium labeled red cell scan. *Dis. Colon Rectum* 1992; 35: 219–22.

Salem RR, Wood CB, Rees HC *et al.* A comparison of colonoscopy and selective visceral angiography in the diagnosis of colonic angiodysplasia. *Ann. R. Coll. Surg. Engl.* 1985; 67: 225–6.

Santos JC Jr, Aprilli F, Guimaraes AS, Rocha JJ. Angiodysplasia of the colon: endoscopic diagnosis and treatment. *Br. J. Surg.* 1988; 75: 256–8.

Seow Choen F, Chua TL, Goh HS. Ischaemic colitis and colorectal cancer: some problems and pitfalls. *Int. J. Colorectal Dis.* 1993; 8: 210–2.

Sharma R, Gorbien MJ. Angiodysplasia and lower gastrointestinal tract bleeding in elderly patients. *Arch. Intern. Med.* 1995; 155: 807–12.

Sharma VS, Valji K, Bookstein JJ. Gastrointestinal hemorrhage in AIDS: arteriographic diagnosis and transcatheter treatment. *Radiology* 1992; 185: 447–51.

Slivka A, Parsons WG, Carr Locke DL. Endoscopic band ligation for treatment of post polypectomy hemorrhage. *Gastrointest. Endosc.* 1994; 40: 230–2.

Spath-Schwalbe E, Preclik G, Heimpel H. Successful treatment of recurrent lower gastrointestinal hemorrhage in intestinal angiodysplasia with an estrogen progesterone combination. *Z. Gastroenterol.* 1993; 31: 447–9.

Steger AC, Galland RB, Hemingway A, Wood CB, Spencer J. Gastrointestinal haemorrhage from a second source in patients with colonic angiodysplasia. *Br. J. Surg.* 1987; 74: 726–7.

Stylianos S, Forde KA, Benvenisty AI, Hardy MA. Lower gastrointestinal hemorrhage in renal transplant recipients. *Arch. Surg.* 1988; 123: 739–44.

Teefey SA, Roarke MC, Brink JA, Middleton WD, Balfe DM, Thyssen EP, Hildebolt CF. Bowel wall thickening: differentiation of inflammation from ischemia with color Doppler and duplex US. *Radiology* 1996; 198: 547–51.

Thelmo WL, Vetrano JA, Wibowo A, DiMaio TM, Cruz Vetrano WP, Kim DS. Angiodysplasia of colon revisited: pathologic demonstration without the use of intravascular injection technique. *Hum. Pathol.* 1992; 23: 37–40.

Tsai HH, Howden CW, Thomson TJ. Probable Crohn's colitis mimicking ischaemic colitis in a young adult. *Scott. Med. J.* 1989; 34: 406–7.

Warkentin TE, Moore JC, Morgan DG. Aortic stenosis and bleeding gastrointestinal angiodysplasia: is acquired von Willebrand's disease the link? *Lancet* 1992; 340: 35–7.

Weinstock LB, Larson RS, Stahl DJ, Fleshman JW. Diffuse microscopic angiodysplasia a previously unreported variant of angiodysplasia. Report of a case. *Dis. Colon Rectum* 1995; 38: 428–32.

Wheeldon NM, Grundman MJ. Ischaemic colitis as a complication of colonoscopy. *Br. Med. J.* 1990; 301: 1080–1.

Whelan RL, Buls JG, Goldberg SM, Rothenberger DA. Intra operative endoscopy. University of Minnesota experience. *Am. Surg.* 1989; 55: 281–6.

Zighelboim J, Viggiano TR, Ahlquist DA, Gostout CJ, Wang KK, Larson MV. Endoscopic laser coagulation of radiation induced mucosal vascular lesions in the upper gastrointestinal tract and proximal colon. *Am. J. Gastroenterol.* 1993; 88: 1224–7.

Zuckerman G, Benitez J. A prospective study of bidirectional endoscopy (colonoscopy and upper endoscopy) in the evaluation of patients with occult gastrointestinal bleeding. *Am. J. Gastroenterol.* 1992; 87: 62–6.

16 Other forms of colitis

Radiation colitis

Incidence and aetiology

Radiation proctitis and colitis are a major side-effect of pelvic radiotherapy. The vast majority of patients have received radiation for gynaecological or genitourinary malignancy, with up to 90% of cases arising after treatment of cervical carcinoma (Dawson *et al.* 1987; Monserat *et al.* 1989). Consequently, there is a strong female predominance with a median age at presentation of 55 years (Dawson *et al.* 1987). In one study of radiotherapy for prostatic carcinoma, multivariate analysis identified previous bowel disease or surgery, anterior rectal dose, and average rectal dose as the factors most closely related with high risk of proctitis (Smit *et al.* 1990). The anterior rectal dose was the most important indicator. The actuarial 2-year incidence of moderate or severe proctitis was 20% for anterior rectal doses less than 75 Gy, compared with 60% in doses greater than this (Smit *et al.* 1990).

Pathological appearances

The macroscopic appearances in acute radiation proctitis are loss of the vascular pattern, while in the chronic condition, the bowel shows a fusiform stenosis with serosal fibrosis and adhesions. The earliest histological changes in acute proctitis include nuclear pyknosis, flattening of the cells, loss of nuclear polarity, enlargement of nuclei, reduced mitotic activity, and mucin depletion (Figure 16.1). The surface epithelium is lost and the lamina propria and crypt

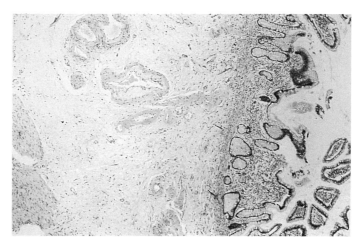

Figure 16.2 Post-irradiation effect in the small intestine. Note the hyalinized thickening of small blood vessel walls in the submucosa and occasional bizarre fibroblasts. H&E×40.

epithelium are infiltrated by eosinophils. In chronic proctitis the most characteristic changes are seen within connective tissue and include oedema, fibrosis, telangiectasia, and fibroblasts with bizarre nuclei. The mucosa is atrophic and may show distorted crypt architecture and cellular atypia. The prominent vascular lesions include swelling of endothelial cells, thrombosis and arteriosclerotic changes (Figure 16.2). Smooth muscle hypertrophy and myenteric plexus damage are also apparent (Varma *et al.* 1986). It is not certain whether these changes represent a primary effect of the radiation or secondary ischaemic damage. A rare complication is proctitis cystica profunda. The fully developed lesion consists of a focal expansion of the submucosa by dilated cystic spaces lined by a single layer of benign epithelial cells (Geisinger *et al.* 1990).

Clinical presentation

Rectal bleeding is the most frequent symptom, occurring in three-quarters of cases (Monserat *et al.* 1989). Radiation colitis accounts for 1% of lower intestinal bleeding (Rhee *et al.* 1991). Bleeding occurs from mucosal friability and neovascular telangiectasias. One-quarter of patients experience alteration in bowel habit (Monserat *et al.* 1989). Symptoms include urgency, frequency, and occasionally faecal incontinence. Other symptoms include passage of mucus, tenesmus, abdominal distension, and colicky abdominal pain. The presentation may mimic ulcerative colitis (Itzkowitz *et al.* 1986). Complications occur in 75% of patients who receive additional postoperative radiation. Most symptoms develop about 1 year after radiotherapy, but the range is wide (1 month to 40 years) (Monserat *et al.* 1989; Fischer *et al.* 1990). Dysfunction of the internal anal

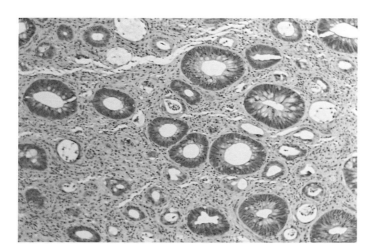

Figure 16.1 Irradiation colitis in a patient following radiotherapy for cervical carcinoma. H&E×100.

sphincter contributes to the anorectal symptoms. Anal manometry reveals that the maximum resting anal canal pressure and the physiological sphincter length are significantly lower than in controls (Varma *et al.* 1986). External sphincter squeeze pressure is not affected. Proctograms reveal a significant reduction in the rectal volumes at sensory threshold, constant sensation and maximal tolerance, and in rectal compliance (Varma *et al.* 1985).

Diagnosis consists of a combination of history, endoscopic appearances, and histology. On sigmoidoscopy, the rectal mucosa in acute radiation proctitis appears oedematous with a loss of vascular pattern. In chronic disease, the mucous membrane is granular and haemorrhagic, with loss of mucosal folds. Magnetic resonance (MR) scanning can prove beneficial (Sovik *et al.* 1993).

The renewal of interest in high-dose contact irradiation in the treatment of early rectal carcinoma and epidermoid tumours of the anus has focused attention on the long-term complications of intense local irradiation. In a study of late radiation-induced proctitis stricturing developed in 50% and fistula formation in 30% (Fischer *et al.* 1990) (Figures 16.3 and 16.4). Progression of lesions to the small bowel or urinary tract occurred in almost two-thirds. Surgery was required in 50% with strictures and in 90% of fistulas. Conservative management was successful in one-half of all patients. Overall radiation induced mortality was 25%. Factors significantly influencing mortality were coexisting injuries of the small bowel or urinary tract. Age, stage of primary malignant disease, and previous laparotomy did not influence outcome. After a median observation period of 11 years, 60% of patients were alive, of whom half had a fair outcome; 35% continued to have slight or moderate symptoms and 15% had disabling symptoms. One-quarter of patients had died from unrelated causes and 15% from recurrent cancer. The authors concluded that because radiation-induced proctitis is likely to

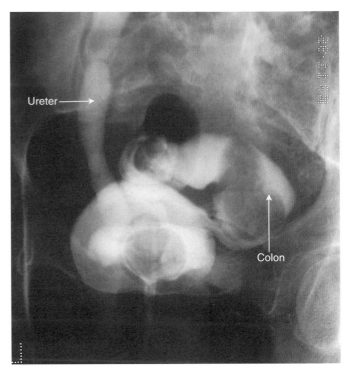

Figure 16.4 Nephrogram in a patient who had received irradiation for a bladder tumour. Note the colovesical fistula into the sigmoid colon and the hydronephrosis.

progress, it cannot be characterized as a harmless manifestation of late radiation injuries (Fischer *et al.* 1990).

Patients receiving abdominal or pelvic radiotherapy are at increased risk of developing colorectal carcinoma or other malignancies such as lymphoma (Sibly *et al.* 1985). This is related to the cytological atypia which is apparent histologically. In colonic adenocarcinoma a change occurs in colonic mucus from normal sulphomucin to sialomucin. In radiation-damaged colon, sialomucin and dysplasia appear significantly more often than in controls and may be a marker of malignant transformation (Dawson *et al.* 1987). In acute proctitis, despite the bizarre histological epithelial cell appearances, flow cytometry reveals the cells to be DNA diploid (Pearson *et al.* 1992). However, biopsies from long-standing cases may contain aneuploid DNA profiles, indicating those patients are at increased risk of malignancy in the irradiated tissues (Pearson *et al.* 1992).

Treatment

Many patients with mild symptoms can be treated medically, although the results are variable (Buchi 1991). Surgical correction may be considered only after recurrent cancer has been excluded and an assessment of rectal function and continence performed. New management approaches include abdominopelvic partitioning, radioprotective medications, formalin installation, and vascularized colonic grafts (Saclarides 1997). 5-ASA enemas do not appear to be effective in the treatment of radiation proctitis (Baum *et al.* 1989). However, a 4-week course of 3.0 g oral sulphasalazine plus 20 mg twice daily rectal prednisolone enemas produces significant clinical and endoscopic improvement (Kochhar *et al.* 1991). In patients with ulcerating lesions sucralfate enemas administered twice daily for 3 weeks is claimed to produce clinical and sigmoidoscopic improvements in 80% of patients (Kochhar *et al.* 1990, 1991). Sodium pentosanpolysulphate also produces a complete response in 80%, a

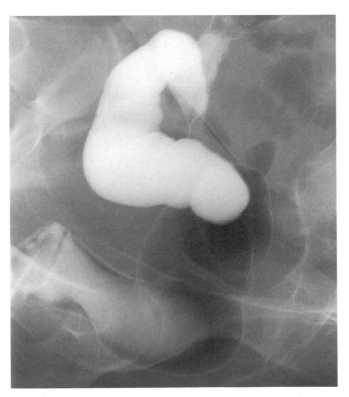

Figure 16.3 Stricturing of the colon following radiotherapy.

partial response in 10%, with 10% failing to respond to therapy (Grigsby *et al.* 1990). Treatment with endoluminal formalin is claimed to stop bleeding permanently in 85% of patients (Lucarotti *et al.* 1991; Seow-Choen *et al.* 1993). It is possible that long-term sequelae of radiotherapy may be prevented by daily hydrocortisone enemas for 3–6 weeks starting in the third week of irradiation (Szepesi *et al.* 1990). The non-steroidal anti-inflammatory agent piroxicam may also be useful in significantly decreasing the incidence of colonic neoplasia (Northway *et al.* 1990).

Significant uncontrollable gastrointestinal bleeding due to radiation colitis has previously required colectomy, proctectomy, arterial ligation, or embolization. Recently, endoscopic laser therapy for haemorrhagic proctitis has proved effective in controlling this problem without recourse to surgery. Laser therapy is effective in obliterating telangiectasias and may be performed as an out-patient procedure (Taylor *et al.* 1993). However, two to three treatments, separated by 6 months are needed and 75% of patients require maintenance therapy for recurrent bleeding from telangiectasias that develop after initial therapy (Taylor *et al.* 1993). Hyperbaric oxygenation therapy is suggested as an alternative to surgical intervention in those with severe haemorrhage (Nakada *et al.* 1993).

About 10% of patients require surgery (Jao *et al.* 1986). The indications for surgery are radiation proctitis with haemorrhage, rectovaginal fistula, rectal stricture, and small bowel obstruction. Symptomatic relief is achieved in 75% of cases but is significantly less (55%) in those with radiation-induced fistulas. Postoperative morbidity is 65% and mortality 10% (Jao *et al.* 1986). Postoperative faecal and internal fistulas of the intestine, bladder, and vagina result from necrosis and perforation secondary to dissection of adhesions, opening of tissue planes, and careless manipulation of the bowel. Morbidity and mortality are not significantly influenced by the site or type of lesion. Morbidity is lower after colostomy alone (45%) than after more aggressive operations (80%), transverse loop colostomy and descending colostomy being safer than sigmoid colostomy (Jao *et al.* 1986). A permanent stoma is necessary in 70% of patients. However, radical resection of the radiation-damaged rectum has been shown to be a safe and reliable treatment for rectovaginal fistulas, rectal strictures, and proctitis unresponsive to medical measures (Lucarotti *et al.* 1991).

In those undergoing anastomoses a variety of procedures are possible. Low anterior resection and coloanal anastomosis may be performed without a reservoir. To avoid urgency and frequency a coloanal J-reservoir with coloanal sleeve anastomosis has been advocated (Lucarotti *et al.* 1991). The selective use of the Parks' coloanal pull-through anastomosis has been advocated for patients suffering from severe radiation injuries of the rectum (Gazet 1985). It is claimed to obviate the need for a difficult dissection of the lower rectum and separation of tissues damaged by radiation and avoids the need for eversion techniques. Continence is good or excellent in three-quarters, although one-third will require dilatation for anastomotic stricture. Long-term follow up suggests that recurrence of haemorrhage, fistulas, perineal pain, or tenesmus is very unlikely (Gazet 1985).

Collagenous colitis

Incidence and aetiology

Collagenous colitis was first described in 1976 by Lindstrom as an unusual cause of persistent, watery diarrhoea (Jarlov *et al.* 1994;

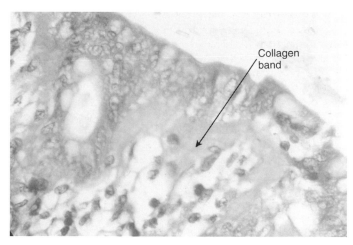

Figure 16.5 Collagenous colitis. Note the marked thickening of the subepithelial collagen band (arrowed) (see colour plates).

Maxson *et al.* 1994). It is characterized by a histologically distinctive band of collagen under the surface epithelium of the colon (Stampfl and Friedman 1991) (Figure 16.5). The clinical situation is associated with two histological varieties, collagenous colitis and lymphocytic (microscopic) colitis (Ettinghausen 1993; Veress *et al.* 1995). Some consider these to be two separate entities. Similarities include age, symptomatology, and non-diagnostic radiographic and endoscopic studies. However, in lymphocytic colitis the male-to-female ratio is equal while collagenous colitis is associated with a female predominance (80%) (Giardiello *et al.* 1989). Other differences include dissimilar histocompatibility phenotypes and a collagen band on biopsies of collagenous but not lymphocytic colitis (van Tilburg *et al.* 1990; Giardiello *et al.* 1992) (Figure 16.6). These findings suggest that lymphocytic and collagenous colitis may be related yet distinct disorders (Lee *et al.* 1992; Veress *et al.* 1995). However, one study found that over a 5-year follow-up that the thickness of the collagen table varied with time, such that when thickening was minimal, morphological features in those originally diagnosed as collagenous colitis were indistinguishable from microscopic colitis (Sylwestrowicz *et al.* 1989). In about one-fifth of patients histological features of both conditions exist (Bogomoletz *et al.* 1991). Collagenous colitis and microscopic colitis are therefore probably

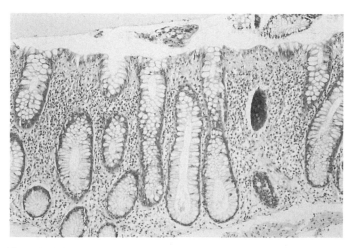

Figure 16.6 Lymphocytic colitis. Note the marked lymphocytic response and absence of the collagen band. H&E×100

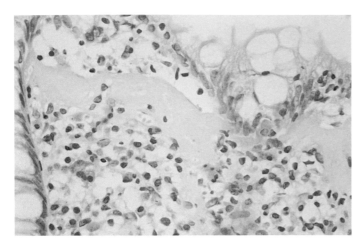

Figure 16.7 Collagenous colitis showing the collagen band and an inflammatory infiltrate. H&E×250.

part of the same spectrum of colonic mucosal response comprising a watery diarrhoea-colitis syndrome (Sylwestrowicz *et al.* 1989).

Since 1976, increasingly more cases have been reported and the condition is now recognized as a distinct clinical entity (Gubbins *et al.* 1991). Most patients are middle-aged (mean age 55 years) but the age range of many series is wide (18–80 years) (Velasco *et al.* 1992; Angos *et al.* 1993; Jarlov *et al.* 1994). The condition is also well recognized as a cause of chronic diarrhoea in children (Gremse *et al.* 1993). The condition is rare, with an estimated prevalence of 1/100 000 population. Thickening of the surface epithelium occurs in up to 5% of all colonic biopsies but few of these patients have symptoms suggestive of collagenous colitis (Gledhill and Cole 1984). However, in patients presenting with persistent diarrhoea and otherwise normal looking colon, histological evidence of collagenous colitis is found in 5% and microscopic colitis in 15% of biopsies (Gineston *et al.* 1989).

The aetiology of collagenous colitis remains obscure (Zins *et al.* 1995; Halaby *et al.* 1996). The thickening of the subepithelial collagen layer may be a response to chronic inflammation or a local abnormality of collagen synthesis (Stampfl and Friedman 1991) (Figure 16.7). The precise mechanism of the diarrhoea in collagenous colitis is also unclear, and it has not been possible to link the diarrhoea directly to the excess collagen deposition. The relationship between collagenous colitis and lymphocytic colitis remains to be defined. An association with non-steroidal anti-inflammatory drugs (NSAIDs) has been implicated (Giardiello *et al.* 1990). Many patients with collagenous colitis have been on NSAIDs, diarrhoea following their use after an average of 5 years (Riddell *et al.* 1992). In some patients, diarrhoea improves after withdrawing NSAIDs and recurs after rechallenging with the drugs (Riddell *et al.* 1992). The pathogenesis of NSAID enteropathy is a multistage process involving specific biochemical and subcellular organelle damage followed by a relatively non-specific tissue reaction (Bjarnason *et al.* 1993).

There appears to be a link with coeliac disease (McCashland *et al.* 1992). In both collagenous colitis and lymphocytic (microscopic) colitis the colorectal mucosa shows surface epithelial damage with intraepithelial lymphocytes that is strikingly similar to the small intestinal findings in coeliac disease (Greenson *et al.* 1990). Coeliac disease may also show subepithelial collagen deposition resembling that seen in collagenous colitis. In addition, there is a very high incidence of coeliac disease among patients with collagenous colitis. Coeliac disease is found in 40% of patients with collagenous colitis

who have a small bowel biopsy (DuBois *et al.* 1989). Despite the morphological similarities to coeliac disease, antireticulin antibodies are not associated with collagenous or lymphocytic colitis (Greenson *et al.* 1990).

Although its aetiology is unknown, the possibility has been raised that autoimmunity may play a part in both lymphocytic and collagenous colitis (Angos *et al.* 1993). Human leucocyte antigen (HLA) typing suggests that lymphocytic colitis is a distinct form of chronic intestinal inflammatory disease associated with HLA class I phenotypes. The HLA patterns noted previously in other gastrointestinal disorders, including ulcerative colitis and Crohn's disease, are not apparent in those with lymphocytic or collagenous colitis (van Tilburg *et al.* 1990; Giardiello *et al.* 1992). Humoral factors in the faeces may also be responsible as faecal stream diversion results in resolution of the histological and clinical features (Jarnerot *et al.* 1995).

Pathological appearances

The colon is grossly normal without any macroscopic evidence of inflammation. Histological examination is therefore necessary for the diagnosis.

In collagenous colitis the characteristic biopsy findings are a combination of increased mucosal inflammation as well as subepithelial collagenous thickening. The normal membrane measures 3–7 μm with about 5% of all colorectal biopsies showing significant thickening greater than 10 μm, without clinically having diarrhoea suggestive of collagenous colitis (Gledhill and Core 1984). Thickening of the subepithelial collagen layer greater than 15 μm with or without mucosal inflammatory changes is suggestive of the condition (Velasco *et al.* 1992). The collagenous thickening has qualitative as well as quantitative differences from normal, which can be highlighted by Masson trichrome stains. Major problems in diagnosing collagenous colitis arise from focusing solely on the subepithelial region without attention to inflammatory changes. The mucosal inflammatory changes include increased lamina propria plasma cells, prominent intraepithelial lymphocytes, and in some cases, numerous eosinophils. Immunostaining of the lymphoid infiltrate reveals an increase in intraepithelial lymphocytes in collagenous colitis due to an influx of CD8-positive cells. There are striking similarities between lymphocytic colitis and collagenous colitis, but subepithelial collagen thickening is seen primarily in collagenous colitis (Lazenby *et al.* 1989). In up to one-fifth of cases the histological features may show a mixed pattern of lymphocytic and collagenous colitis. The most distinctive features of lymphocytic colitis are increased intraepithelial lymphocytes, particularly in the surface epithelium, surface epithelial damage, increased lamina propria chronic inflammation, and minimal crypt distortion or active cryptitis (Lazenby *et al.* 1989). These features are distinctive from other causes of diarrhoea. Inflammatory bowel disease shows prominent crypt distortion and greater active inflammation, in addition to minimal intraepithelial lymphocytes. Acute colitis occasionally demonstrates prominent surface epithelial damage, but is otherwise dissimilar from lymphocytic colitis. The diarrhoea is secondary to anion secretion from prostaglandins synthesized locally in response to mucosal hypoxia (Rask Madsen *et al.* 1983). The collagen table thickening characteristic of the condition appears to play no part in the diarrhoea (Lee *et al.* 1992).

Clinical presentation

Patients with collagenous colitis present with chronic, watery, non-bloody diarrhoea with normal endoscopic findings. Many have previously been diagnosed as having irritable bowel syndrome (Brady and McKee 1993). Diarrhoea may have been present from a few months to 20 years, the average being 5 years (Gubbins et al. 1991; Angos et al. 1993). The number of bowel movements ranges from two to 12 bowel movements a day (mean 5) (Angos et al. 1993). Although, occasionally, diarrhoea is slight or absent, the volume of fluid passed per day may be over a litre (Leigh et al. 1993; Jarlov et al. 1994). There is usually no associated weight loss, anaemia or hypoalbuminaemia, although patients with coeliac disease may have laboratory evidence of small bowel dysfunction and malabsorption. In severe cases steatorrhoea or protein-losing enteropathy may occur (Jarlov et al. 1994).

There is a high prevalence of arthritis (up to 80%) and auto-antibodies (50%) in lymphocytic colitis but no increase in frequency of histocompatibility antigens (DR3, B8) associated with well-defined autoimmune disease (Angos et al. 1993; Kingsmore et al. 1993). About 10% of patients will have monoarticular reactive arthritis and one-fifth have coexisting autoimmune illness (Angos et al. 1993). Collagenous colitis should therefore be considered in the differential diagnosis of diarrhoea occurring in patients with known autoimmune diseases or arthritis. The condition may also occasionally be seen in patients with known inflammatory bowel disease (Chandrate et al. 1987).

A characteristic of the condition is that laboratory, stool, endo-scopic, and radiological investigations are normal (Gubbins et al. 1991; Velasco et al. 1992). In such patients the cost-yield of random colonic biopsies is low. It has therefore been suggested to confine biopsies to patients with relatively severe or debilitating symptoms, with diarrhoea that sounds 'organic' (e.g. nocturnal stools, frequent watery stools, weight loss, elevated sedimentation rate), or in pa-tients who are immunosuppressed (Marshall et al. 1995). However, in one study two of five patients had non-specific mucosal granular-ity and irregularity of the rectosigmoid on double contrast barium enema (Feczko et al. 1991). However, the diagnosis is generally only made histologically. It is suggested that patients with persistent ab-dominal symptoms, particularly diarrhoea, and normal endoscopy should therefore undergo routine biopsy (Velasco et al. 1992). Rectal biopsy alone is a relatively poor method of making the diagnosis as the disease may be focal (Tanaka et al. 1992; Jarlov et al. 1994). Flexible sigmoidoscopy with multiple biopsy specimens from several sites can make the diagnosis in up to 60–90% of cases (Carpenter et al. 1992; Tanaka et al. 1992; Jarlov et al. 1994). Should left-sided biopsy specimens show a normal collagen band but an inflamed mucosa, total colonoscopy with multiple specimens including the caecum may be required to establish the diagnosis (Tanaka et al. 1992). Jejunal biopsy should also be considered because of the asso-ciation with coeliac disease.

Patients with associated coeliac disease often do not respond to a gluten-free diet (DuBois et al. 1989; Jarlov et al. 1994). This lack of response to a gluten-free diet may be more apparent in lymphocytic than collagenous colitis (Sylwestrowicz et al. 1989). Some of these patients may respond to the addition of steroids to dietary manipulation.

Treatment

The outcome of collagenous colitis is variable, with the possibility of spontaneous recovery or, more frequently, of remission (Roblin et al. 1991; Zins et al. 1995). The clinical course is benign; in only one case has the condition been felt to contribute to a patient's death (Widgren et al. 1990; Halaby et al. 1996). Patients with NSAID-induced enteropathy obtain symptomatic relief from stopping the drugs (Bjarnason et al. 1993). Diarrhoea may be controlled sympto-matically with drugs such as loperamide (Pimentel et al. 1995). Although there is no specific treatment, several forms of treatment have been tried. In one study after empirical therapy for 15 months 60% of patients showed histological resolution and symptom relief (Carpenter et al. 1992). Oral sulphasalazine and azulfidine is claimed to produce symptomatic response in almost three-quarters of cases (Velasco et al. 1992; Brady and McKee 1993). Omeprazole is claimed to achieve rapid and total abolition of clinical signs and a significant reduction of the collagen band (Roblin et al. 1991). Several authors have obtained symptomatic improvement with pred-nisolone (Jarlov et al. 1994; Zins et al. 1995). In one prospective study, the clinicopathological effect of prednisolone was associated with a significant decrease in stool frequency (Sloth et al. 1991). However, the effect was transitory, as the diarrhoea recurred when prednisolone treatment was discontinued. The authors recommend that treatment with prednisolone be restricted to periods of acute diarrhoeal episodes (Sloth et al. 1991).

Diversion colitis

Incidence and aetiology

Diversion colitis refers to the inflammatory changes that occur in the defunctioned segment of the large intestine following diversion of the faecal stream (Haque et al. 1993). Colonoscopy studies reveal that 75–90% of defunctioned colons demonstrate inflammation after an average of 30 weeks following diversion (Orsay et al. 1993; Whelan et al. 1994). Up to 75% of children who undergo surgical diversion for chronic pseudo-obstruction or Hirschprung's disease will develop diversion colitis (Ordein et al. 1992). The inflammation arises independently and does not represent a recurrence of the con-dition which necessitated the colostomy, the proximal bowel 'in continuity' being normal in nearly all cases (Whelan et al. 1994). There is evidence that diversion colitis represents a nutritional-deficiency syndrome based upon a local mucosal requirement for short chain fatty acids (Agarwal and Schimmel 1989). Nutrition of colonic epithelial cells is mainly from short chain fatty acids (acetic and n-butyric acids) produced by bacterial fermentation in the colonic lumen. Incomplete starvation of colonic epithelial cells through lack of these compounds in the lumen leads, in the short term, to hypoplasia of the mucosa and, if chronic, to full-blown di-version colitis (Rabasa et al. 1992; Haque et al. 1993). The inflam-mation is compounded by stasis of intestinal contents with bacterial invasion of the mucous membrane (Nobels et al. 1989). In diversion colitis the total bacterial count is normal, but with an altered flora. Strict anaerobes, principally of the genus Eubacterium and Bifidobacterium, are reduced while aerobes (enterobacteria) are in-creased (Neut et al. 1989).

Pathological appearances

Subclinical inflammation is almost inevitable in defunctioned bowel, being independent of the time since the colostomy was fashioned (Roe et al. 1993; Whelan et al. 1994). Biopsies show non-specific acute and chronic inflammation (Ordein et al. 1992). Lymphoid hy-perplasia is a distinctive histological feature of diversion colitis (Drut and Dent 1992; Toolenaar et al. 1993). Other features include non-specific changes with mild to moderate lymphocytic infiltrates in the lamina propria, mild architectural alterations of the crypts, slight decrease in crypt numbers, and apthous ulcers (Komorowski *et al.* 1990; Geragthy and Charles 1994). Apthous ulceration, Paneth cell metaplasia, and crypt abscesses simulating ulcerative colitis are uncommon, being observed almost exclusively in the more severe cases (Ma *et al.* 1990; Haque *et al.* 1993; Roe *et al.* 1993). Granulomata raise the possibility of Crohn's disease. Distinction from ulcerative colitis and Crohn's disease is therefore possible in most cases. The severity of inflammation can increase with the length of time since the bowel has been defunctioned (Ordein *et al.* 1992). Generally, colitis is mild in 50%, moderate in 45%, and severe in 5% of cases. Large ulceration may be seen in severe cases (Lu *et al.* 1995). Submucosal carcinoids have been described in association with diversion colitis (Griffiths *et al.* 1992).

Clinical presentation and diagnosis

An accurate diagnosis is dependent on the clinical history, comparison of histological morphology in both colonic segments, and the response to therapy (Komorowski *et al.* 1990). Clinical symptoms develop in a wide range of those with a defunctioned colon, depending on the length of time the colon has been diverted (Haas *et al.* 1990; Ma *et al.* 1990). Symptoms develop from a few months to many years after stoma formation. Patients may present with a blood-stained mucus discharge, tenesmus, or pain (Ma *et al.* 1990). Children complain of diffuse, poorly localized abdominal pain. Blood in the stools occurs in 20% of children, although the diagnosis may be suspected in up to three-quarters of those who do not pass blood (Ordein *et al.* 1992). Occasionally, haemorrhage can be massive.

Colonoscopy can detect abnormalities in about three-quarters of cases (Whelan *et al.* 1994). Routine biopsy reveals histological inflammation in 10% of those with apparently normal colonoscopy. As abnormalities are so frequent, some advocate regular endoscopy of the bowel distal to a colostomy (Haas *et al.* 1990). Colonoscopic findings include mucous plugs, friable mucosa, petechia, erythema, ulcers, exudate, and nodules, polyps, or carcinoma (Ma *et al.* 1990; Roe *et al.* 1993). Double contrast barium enema can identify lymphoid follicular hyperplasia in 30% of patients (Lechner *et al.* 1990). The condition is associated with progressive involution of the rectal stump. Proctogram studies show an appreciable decrease in rectal volume in all cases, by a mean of 35%. However, there is no change in rectal sensation or compliance. (Roe *et al.* 1993). Strictures can occur (Harig *et al.* 1989).

Treatment

Diversion colitis can be treated medically or surgically (Ferguson and Siegel 1991). Local steroids may be effective (Haas *et al.* 1990). Treatment with 5-aminosalicylic acid enemas also results in both endoscopic and histological resolution (Haas *et al.* 1990). A recent concept is treatment with enemas containing short chain fatty acids (Haque and West 1992; Rabassa *et al.* 1992). One controlled trial found that endoscopic and histological findings of diversion colitis were not improved by irrigation of short chain fatty acids for 14 days but a longer treatment period may be required (Guillemot *et al.* 1991; Harig *et al.* 1989). A characteristic feature is that the inflammation is reversible in all but the most severe cases if bowel continuity is restored (Nobels *et al.* 1989). Stomal closure may be performed in up to 70% of patients and is effectively curative (Whelan *et al.* 1994). After re-anastomosis, barium enema changes return to normal in one-fifth of cases (Lechner *et al.* 1990). Despite

the role of bacteria in causing diversion colitis there is no increased risk of infection following colostomy closure (Orsay *et al.* 1993). Removal of the excluded colon is seldom necessary (Haas *et al.* 1990).

References

Agarwal VP, Schimmel EM. Diversion colitis: a nutritional deficiency syndrome? *Nutr. Rev.* 1989; 47: 257–61.

Angos R, Idoate MA, Zozaya JM, Munoz M, Conchillo F. Collagenous colitis: clinicopathologic study of 6 new cases. *Rev. Esp. Enferm. Dig.* 1993; 83: 161–7.

Baum CA, Biddle WL, Miner PB. Failure of 5 aminosalicylic acid enemas to improve chronic radiation proctitis. *Dig. Dis. Sci.* 1989; 34: 758–60.

Bjarnason I, Hayllar J, MacPherson AJ, Russell AS. Side effects of nonsteroidal anti inflammatory drugs on the small and large intestine in humans. *Gastroenterology* 1993; 104: 1832–47.

Bogomoletz WV, Flejou JF. Newly recognized forms of colitis: collagenous colitis, microscopic (lymphocytic) colitis, and lymphoid follicular proctitis. *Semin. Diagn. Pathol.* 1991; 8: 178–89.

Brady SK, McKee DD. Collagenous colitis: a cause of chronic diarrhea. *Am. Fam. Phys.* 1993; 48: 1081–4.

Buchi K. Radiation proctitis: therapy and prognosis. *JAMA* 1991; 265: 1180–6.

Carpenter HA, Tremaine WJ, Batts KP, Czaja AJ. Sequential histologic evaluations in collagenous colitis. Correlations with disease behavior and sampling strategy. *Dig. Dis. Sci.* 1992; 37: 1903–9.

Chandratre S, Bramble MG, Cooke WM, Jones RA. Simultaneous occurrence of collagenous colitis and Crohn's disease. *Digestion* 1987; 36: 55–60.

Dawson PM, Galland RB, Rees HC. Mucin abnormalities in the radiation damaged colon. *Dig. Surg.* 1987; 4: 19–21.

Drut R, Drut RM. Hyperplasia of lymphoglandular complexes in colon segments in Hirschsprung's disease: a form of diversion colitis. *Pediatr. Pathol.* 1992; 12: 575–81.

DuBois RN, Lazenby AJ, Yardley JH, Hendrix TR, Bayless TM, Giardiello FM. Lymphocytic enterocolitis in patients with 'refractory sprue'. *JAMA* 1989; 262: 935–7.

Ettinghausen SE. Collagenous colitis, eosinophilic colitis, and neutropenic colitis. *Surg. Clin. North Am.* 1993; 73: 993–1016.

Feczko PJ, Mezwa DG. Nonspecific radiographic abnormalities in collagenous colitis. *Gastrointest. Radiol.* 1991; 16: 128–32.

Ferguson CM, Siegel RJ. A prospective evaluation of diversion colitis. *Am. Surg.* 1991; 57: 46–9.

Fischer L, Kimose HH, Spjeldnaes N, Wara P. Late progress of radiation induced proctitis. *Acta Chir. Scand.* 1990; 156: 801–5.

Gazet JC. Parks' coloanal pull through anastomosis for severe, complicated radiation proctitis. *Dis. Colon Rectum* 1985; 28: 110–14.

Geisinger KR, Scobey MW, Northway MG, Cassidy KT, Castell DO. Radiation induced proctitis cystica profunda in the rat. *Dig. Dis. Sci.* 1990; 35: 833–9.

Geraghty JM, Charles AK. Aphthoid ulceration in diversion colitis. *Histopathology* 1994; 24: 395–7.

Giardiello FM, Lazenby AJ, Bayless TM, Levine EJ, Bias WB, Ladenson PW, *et al.* Lymphocytic (microscopic) colitis. Clinicopathologic study of 18 patients and comparison to collagenous colitis. *Dig. Dis. Sci.* 1989; 34: 1730–8.

Giardiello FM, Hansen FC 3d, Lazenby AJ, Hellman DB, Milligan FD, Bayless TM, Yardley JH. Collagenous colitis in the setting up of nonsteroidal anti-inflammatory drugs and antibiotics. *Dig. Dis. Sci.* 1990; 35: 257–60.

Giardiello FM, Lazenby AJ, Yardley JH, Bias WB, Johnson J, Alianiello RG, *et al.* Increased HLA A1 and diminished HLA A3 in lymphocytic colitis compared to controls and patients with collagenous colitis. *Dig. Dis. Sci.* 1992; 37: 496–9.

Gineston JL, Sevestre H, Descombes P, Viot J, Sevenet F, Davion T, *et al.* Biopsies of the endoscopically normal rectum and colon: a necessity. Incidence of collagen colitis and microscopic colitis. *Gastroenterol. Clin. Biol.* 1989; 13: 360–3.

Gledhill A, Cole FM. Significance of basement membrane thickening in the human colon. *Gut* 1984; 25: 1085–8.

Greenson JK, Giardiello FM, Lazenby AJ, Pena SA, Bayless TM, Yardley JH. Antireticulin antibodies in collagenous and lymphocytic (microscopic) colitis. *Mod. Pathol.* 1990; 3: 259–60.

Gremse DA, Boudreaux CW, Manci EA. Collagenous colitis in children. *Gastroenterology* 1993; 104: 906–9.

Griffiths AP, Dixon MF. Microcarcinoids and diversion colitis in a colon defunctioned for 18 years. Report of a case. *Dis. Colon Rectum* 1992; 35: 685–8.

Grigsby PW, Pilepich MV, Parsons CL. Preliminary results of a phase I/II study of sodium pentosanpolysulfate in the treatment of chronic radiation induced proctitis. *Am. J. Clin. Oncol.* 1990; 13: 28–31.

Gubbins GP, Dekovich AA, Ma CK, Batra SK. Collagenous colitis: report of nine cases and review of the literature. *South Med. J.* 1991; 84: 33–7.

Guillemot F, Colombel JF, Neut C, Verplanck N, Lecomte M, Romond C, *et al.* Treatment of diversion colitis by short chain fatty acids. Prospective and double blind study. *Dis Colon Rectum* 1991; 34: 861–4.

Haas PA, Fox TA Jr, Szilagy EJ. Endoscopic examination of the colon and rectum distal to a colostomy. *Am. J. Gastroenterol.* 1990; 85: 850–4.

Haque S, West AB. Diversion colitis 20 years a growing. *J. Clin. Gastroenterol.* 1992; 15: 281–3.

Halaby IA, Rantis PC, Vernana AM III, Longo WE. Collagenous colitis: pathogenesis and management. *Dis. Colon Rectum* 1996; 39: 573–8.

Haque S, Eisen RN, West AB. The morphologic features of diversion colitis: studies of a pediatric population with no other disease of the intestinal mucosa. *Hum. Pathol.* 1993; 24: 211–9.

Harig JM, Soergel KH, Komorowski RA, Wood CM. Treatment of diversion colitis with short chain fatty acid irrigation. *N. Engl. J. Med.* 1989; 320: 23–8.

Itzkowitz SH. Conditions that mimic inflammatory bowel disease. Diagnostic clues and potential pitfalls. *Postgrad. Med.* 1986; 80: 219–31.

Jao SW, Beart RW Jr, Gunderson LL. Surgical treatment of radiation injuries of the colon and rectum. *Am. J. Surg.* 1986; 151: 272–7.

Jarlov AE, Gjorup IE, Thomsen OO. Collagenous colitis. *Ugeskr. Laeger.* 1994; 156: 194–6.

Jarnerot G, Tysk C, Bohr J, Eriksson S. Collagenous colitis and fecal stream diversion. *Gastroenterology* 1995; 109: 449–55.

Kingsmore SF, Kingsmore DB, Hall BD, Wilson JA, Gottfried MR, Allen NB. Co-occurrence of collagenous colitis with seronegative spondyloarthropathy: report of a case and literature review. *J. Rheumatol.* 1993; 20: 2153–7.

Kochhar R, Mehta SK, Aggarwal R, Dhar A, Patel F. Sucralfate enema in ulcerative rectosigmoid lesions. *Dis Colon Rectum* 1990; 33: 49–51.

Kochhar R, Patel F, Dhar A, Sharma SC, Ayyagari S, Aggarwal R, *et al.* Radiation induced proctosigmoiditis. Prospective, randomized, double blind controlled trial of oral sulfasalazine plus rectal steroids versus rectal sucralfate. *Dig. Dis. Sci.* 1991; 36: 103–7.

Komorowski RA. Histologic spectrum of diversion colitis. *Am. J. Surg. Pathol.* 1990; 14: 548–54.

Lazenby AJ, Yardley JH, Giardiello FM, Jessurun J, Bayless TM. Lymphocytic ('microscopic') colitis: a comparative histopathologic study with particular reference to collagenous colitis. *Hum. Pathol.* 1989; 20: 18–28.

Lechner GL, Frank W, Jantsch H, Pichler W, Hall DA, Waneck R, Wunderlich M. Lymphoid follicular hyperplasia in excluded colonic segments: a radiologic sign of diversion colitis. *Radiology* 1990; 176: 135–6.

Lee E, Schiller LR, Vendrell D, Santa Ana CA, Fordtran JS. Subepithelial collagen table thickness in colon specimens from patients with microscopic colitis and collagenous colitis. *Gastroenterology* 1992; 103: 1790–6.

Leigh C, Elahmady A, Mitros FA, Metcalf A, al Jurf A. Collagenous colitis associated with chronic constipation. *Am. J. Surg. Pathol.* 1993; 17: 81–4.

Lu ES, Lin T, Harms BL, Gaumnitz EA, Singaram C. A severe case of diversion colitis with large ulcerations. *Am. J. Gastroenterol.* 1995; 90: 1508–10.

Lucarotti ME, Mountford RA, Bartolo DC. Surgical management of intestinal radiation injury. *Dis. Colon Rectum* 1991; 34: 865–9.

Ma CK, Gottlieb C, Haas PA. Diversion colitis: a clinicopathologic study of 21 cases. *Hum. Pathol.* 1990; 21: 429–36.

Marshall JB, Singh R, Diaz-Arias AA. Chronic, unexplained diarrhea: are biopsies necessary if colonoscopy is normal? *Am. J. Gastroenterol.* 1995; 90: 372–6.

Maxson CJ, Klein HD, Rubin W. Atypical forms of inflammatory bowel disease. *Med. Clin. North Am.* 1994; 78: 1259–73.

McCashland TM, Donovan JP, Strobach RS, Linder J, Quigley EM. Collagenous enterocolitis: a manifestation of gluten sensitive enteropathy. *J. Clin. Gastroenterol.* 1992; 15: 45–51.

Monserat R, Bronstein M, Fuentes D, Garnica E, Palao R, Isern AM, *et al.* Colitis caused by radiation: 20 years' experience. *GEN* 1989; 43: 46–8.

Nakada T, Kubota Y, Sasagawa I, Suzuki H, Yamaguchi T, Ishigooka M, Kakizaki H. Therapeutic experience of hyperbaric oxygenation in radiation colitis. Report of a case. *Dis. Colon Rectum* 1993; 36: 962–5.

Neut C, Colombel JF, Guillemot F, Cortot A, Gower P, Quandalle P, *et al.* Impaired bacterial flora in human excluded colon. *Gut* 1989; 30: 1094–8.

Nobels F, Colemont L, Van Moer E. A case of diversion rectitis. *Acta Clin. Belg.* 1989; 44: 202–4.

Northway MG, Scobey MW, Cassidy KT, Geisinger KR. Piroxicam decreases postirradiation colonic neoplasia in the rat. *Cancer* 1990; 66: 2300–5.

Ordein JJ, Di Lorenzo C, Flores A, Hyman PE. Diversion colitis in children with severe gastrointestinal motility disorders. *Am. J. Gastroenterol.* 1992; 87: 88–90.

Orsay CP, Kim DO, Pearl RK, Abcarian H. Diversion colitis in patients scheduled for colostomy closure. *Dis. Colon Rectum* 1993; 36: 366–7.

Pearson JM, Kumar S, Butterworth DM, Schofield PF, Haboubi NY. Flow cytometric DNA characteristics of radiation colitis a preliminary study. *Anticancer Res.* 1992; 12: 1647–9.

Pimentel RR, Achkar E, Bedford R. Collagenous colitis. A treatable disease with an elusive diagnosis. *Dig. Dis. Sci.* 1995; 40: 1400–4.

Rabassa AA, Rogers AI. The role of short chain fatty acid metabolism in colonic disorders. *Am. J. Gastroenterol.* 1992; 87: 419–23.

Rask Madsen J, Grove O, Hansen MGJ. Colonic transport of water and electrolytes in a patient with secretory diarrhoea due to collagenous colitis. *Dig. Dis. Sci.* 1983; 28: 1141–6.

Rhee JC, Lee KT. The causes and management of lower GI bleeding: a study based on clinical observations at Hanyang University Hospital. *Gastroenterol. Jpn.* 1991; 26 (Suppl. 3): 101–6.

Riddell RH, Tanaka M, Mazzoleni G. Non steroidal anti inflammatory drugs as a possible cause of collagenous colitis: a case control study. *Gut* 1992; 33: 683–6.

Roblin X, Becot F, Abinader J, Piquemal A, Monnet D, Carre JL. Value of omeprazole in the treatment of collagenous colitis. *Ann. Gastroenterol. Hepatol.* 1991; 27: 177–8.

Roe AM, Warren BF, Brodribb AJ, Brown C. Diversion colitis and involution of the defunctioned anorectum. *Gut* 1993; 34: 382–5.

Saclarides TJ. Radiation injuries of the gastrointestinal tract. *Surg. Clin. North Am.* 1997; 77: 261–8.

Seow-Choen F, Goh HS, Eu KW, Ho YH, Tay SK. A simple and effective treatment for hemorrhagic radiation proctitis using formalin. *Dis. Colon Rectum* 1993; 36: 135–8.

Sibly TF, Keane RM, Lever JV, Southwood WFW. Rectal lymphoma in radiation injured bowel. *Br. J. Surg.* 1985; 72: 879–80.

Sloth H, Bisgaard C, Grove A. Collagenous colitis: a prospective trial of prednisolone in six patients. *J. Intern. Med.* 1991; 229: 443–6.

Smit WG, Helle PA, van Putten WL, Wijnmaalen AJ, Seldenrath JJ, van der Werf Messing BH. Late radiation damage in prostate cancer patients treated by high dose external radiotherapy in relation to rectal dose. *Int. J. Radiat. Oncol. Biol. Phys.* 1990, 18: 23–9.

Sovik E, Lien HH, Tveit KM. Postirradiation changes in the pelvic wall. Findings on MR. *Acta Radiol.* 1993; 34: 573–6.

Stampfl DA, Friedman LS. Collagenous colitis: pathophysiologic considerations. *Dig. Dis. Sci.* 1991; 36: 705–11.

Sylwestrowicz T, Kelly JK, Hwang WS, Shaffer EA. Collagenous colitis and microscopic colitis: the watery diarrhoea colitis syndrome. *Am. J. Gastroenterol.* 1989; 84: 763–8.

Szepesi S, Jacobi V, Vecsei P, Bottcher HD. Treatment of radiogenic colitis with a rectal foam containing cortisol. Clinical and pharmacologic data. *Strahlenther Onkol.* 1990; 166: 271-4.

Tanaka M, Mazzoleni G, Riddell RH. Distribution of collagenous colitis: utility of flexible sigmoidoscopy. *Gut* 1992; 33: 65–70.

Taylor JG, DiSario JA, Buchi KN. Argon laser therapy for hemorrhagic radiation proctitis: long term results. *Gastrointest. Endosc.* 1993; 39: 641–4.

Toolenaar TA, Freundt I, Huikeshoven FJ, Drogendijk AC, Jeekel H, Chadha Ajwani S. The occurrence of diversion colitis in patients with a sigmoid neovagina. *Hum. Pathol.* 1993; 24: 846–9.

van Tilburg AJ, Lam HG, Seldenrijk CA, Stel HV, Blok P, Dekker W, Meuwissen SG. Familial occurrence of collagenous colitis. A report of two families. *J. Clin. Gastroenterol.* 1990; 12: 279–85.

Varma JS, Smith AN, Busuttil A. Correlation of clinical and manometric abnormalities of rectal function following chronic radiation injury. *Br. J. Surg.* 1985; 72: 875–8.

Varma JS, Smith AN, Busuttil A. Function of the anal sphincters after chronic radiation injury. *Gut* 1986; 27: 528–33.

Velasco M, Poniachik J, Chesta J, Brahm J, Latorre R, Smok G. Microscopic colitis and collagenous colitis. An entity not yet reported in Chile. *Rev. Med. Chil.* 1992; 120: 880–5.

Veress B, Lofberg R, Bergman L, Microscopic colitis syndrome. *Gut* 1995; 36: 880–6.

Whelan RL, Abramson D, Kim DS, Hashmi HF. Diversion colitis. A prospective study. *Surg. Endosc.* 1994; 8: 19–24.

Widgren S, MacGee W. Collagenous colitis with protracted course and fatal evolution. Report of a case. *Pathol. Res. Pract.* 1990; 186: 303–6.

Zins BJ, Sandborn WJ, Tremaine WJ. Collagenous and lymphocytic colitis: subject review and therapeutic alternatives. *Am. J. Gastroenterol.* 1995; 90: 1394–400.

17 Colorectal trauma and miscellaneous conditions

Colorectal trauma

Aetiology

Most cases of trauma occur in those in the second and third decades of life (Morgado *et al.* 1992). Intra-abdominal trauma may be caused by blunt or penetrating injuries. In European countries, blunt trauma accounts for 80% of cases (55% road traffic accidents), while in America and South Africa, penetrating injuries are more common (Nagel *et al.* 1991; Thompson *et al.* 1994). In blunt trauma the overall risk of bowel injury is 10% (Feliciano 1991). Blunt injury may crush the colon against the vertebral column, burst the colon in a seat-belt-type injury or shear it in vertical deceleration injuries (Rutledge *et al.* 1991). Crushing and bursting injuries tend to cause full thickness disruption but shearing forces may only cause submucosal damage. In penetrating injuries, the colon (particularly the transverse and sigmoid) ranks third after the small bowel and stomach to be damaged. Tissue damage from gunshot wounds is related to the kinetic energy of the bullet on impact ($1/2\ MV^2$), high velocity bullets (>600 m/s) causing cavitation 30 times the diameter of the bullet (Georgi *et al.* 1991) (Figures 17.1 and 17.2). Irrespective of cause, multiple injuries are common. In principally blunt trauma, damage to other intra-abdominal organs occurs in 40% of patients, craniocerebral trauma in 25% and thoracic injuries in 10% (Nagel *et al.* 1991). The abdominal organs commonly injured in abdominal gunshot or shrapnel wounds are the colon (50%), small bowel (40%), liver (33%), major vessels

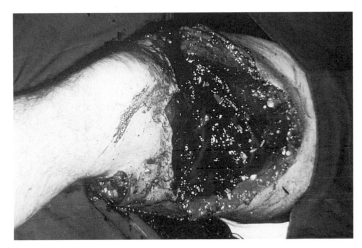

Figure 17.2 High-velocity gunshot wound to the thigh. Note the cavitation effect causes extensive tissue damage far exceeding the diameter of the bullet.

(20%), diaphragm (15%), stomach (15%), spleen (15%), and kidney (15%) with associated extra-abdominal injuries being present in 25% of cases (Georgi *et al.* 1991) (Figure 17.3). Civilian rectal injuries are caused by low-velocity firearms (70%), blunt trauma (20%) and stab wounds, iatrogenic or self-inflicted injuries (10%) (Thompson *et al.* 1994) (Figure 17.4).

Clinical assessment

A careful physical examination is mandatory and should be conducted simultaneously with restoration of oxygenation and intra-

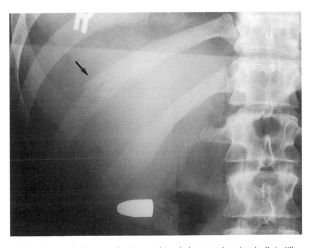

Figure 17.1 Low-velocity gunshot wound to abdomen showing bullet still present in abdominal cavity. Note also rib fracture (arrowed).

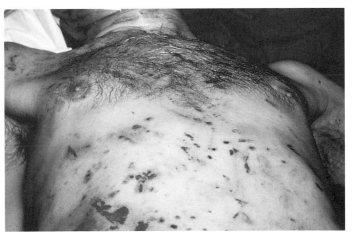

Figure 17.3 Shrapnel wounds from a bomb explosion. Injuries to multiple organs are common in such cases.

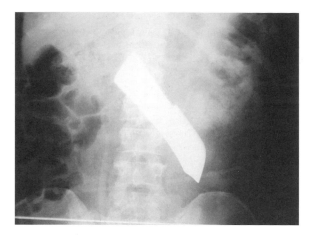

Figure 17.4 Knife wound to the abdomen.

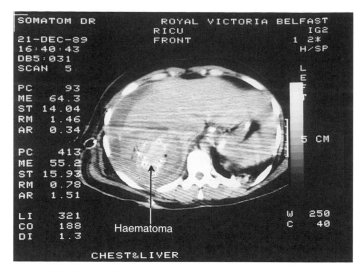

Figure 17.5 CT scan of patient with gunshot wound to the chest and abdomen showing haematoma in the liver. Note the linear scattering artefact caused by fragments of the bullet at the entry wound.

vascular volume. In cases of blunt trauma, features which suggest a possible severe intra-abdominal injury are: (ii) auto–pedestrian impacts; (ii) falls from heights; (iii) ejection or extraction from a vehicle; (iv) hypotension; (v) penetrating injuries which traverse the chest or abdomen; and (vi) beatings (Flint 1994). Digital rectal examination should routinely be performed but if normal does not exclude a rectal injury. If a rectal injury is suspected, sigmoidoscopy is indicated, the presence of intraluminal blood detecting 70% of rectal injuries (Ivatury et al. 1991). In patients with abdominal stab wounds repeated examination by the same surgical team accurately detects significant injuries, being more informative than local wound exploration (Flint 1994). A breech in the peritoneum, even when omentum is protruding, is not an indication for surgery as 40% of these cases will have no significant intra-abdominal injury (Huizinga and Baker 1987). In contrast, over 85% of gunshot wounds in proximity to the peritoneal cavity will have significant intra-abdominal injuries, the negative laparotomy rate being less than 15% (Flint 1994). Surgical emphysema may represent a delayed presentation of colonic trauma (Balachandran and Allen 1991). The most dependable physical signs of intra-abdominal injury are: (i) localized tenderness and guarding; (ii) abdominal distension; and (iii) absent bowel sounds (Flint 1994). On multivariate analysis the principal predictors of serious intra-abdominal injury are major associated injuries to the chest and pelvis, a history of hypotension and a base deficit exceeding −3 mmol/l (Mackersie et al. 1989). Other laboratory tests, such as haematocrit or serum amylase are unhelpful as they are often normal in the presence of significant intra-abdominal injury.

Erect chest X-rays are useful in assessing perforation and associated chest injuries but abdominal radiographs have little benefit other than in locating missiles (Figure 17.1). Diagnostic peritoneal lavage is helpful in assessing intra-abdominal injury, the complication rate (false positive and negative results, catheter misplacement, iatrogenic injury) being 6% (Flint 1994). In an otherwise normal diagnostic peritoneal lavage, elevated lavage amylase levels are highly specific for isolated small bowel or pancreatic, but not colonic injury (McAnena et al. 1991). However, in one study the lavage was positive in only 70% of those with operatively proven penetrating injuries of the colon, the overall false-negative rate being 30% (Obeid et al. 1984). The accuracy of lavage was 73% for gunshot wounds of the colon and 64% for stab wounds (Obeid et al. 1984). Computerized tomography (CT) scanning may be considered in those in whom non-operative treatment is contemplated or in whom peritoneal lavage cannot be performed (Kirton et al. 1997) (Figure

17.5). In unstable patients the associated delay can be dangerous. Children with CT evidence of active haemorrhage have a different spectrum of injuries than that seen in adults (Taylor et al. 1994). Despite the high rate of haemodynamic instability most children with CT findings of active haemorrhage survive (Taylor et al. 1994). CT signs of intestinal injury include pneumoperitoneum, a sentinel clot adjacent to the bowel wall, bowel wall thickening or free fluid with CT characteristics different from clot (Rizzo et al. 1989). These findings are non-specific as only 44% of those with pneumoperitoneum after an injury are proven to have bowel perforation at operation (Bulas et al. 1989). In addition, it is expensive and expert radiological interpretation is required for an accurate diagnosis (Flint 1994). Ultrasound scanning is cheaper but is associated with a false negative rate of 12% (Hoffman et al. 1992). If bowel perforation is suspected, a water soluble enema may be performed (Figure 17.6). Laparoscopy has been successfully used in both blunt and penetrating abdominal trauma avoiding the need for non-therapeutic laparotomy. In one report of diagnostic laparoscopy in 28 patients with abdominal gunshot wounds the accuracy was 100% with

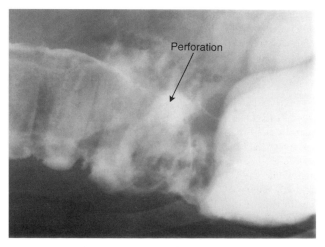

Figure 17.6 Water soluble enema showing a perforated descending colon (arrowed) from a bullet wound. The patient also had a damaged left kidney.

no morbidity in patients with negative laparoscopy (Sosa *et al.* 1993). In patients with penetrating thoracoabdominal injuries, thoracoscopy alters the management in over 40% of cases and obviates laparotomy if the diaphragm has not been penetrated (Jones *et al.* 1991).

A number of indices assessing the severity of abdominal injury are available. The simplest is the Flint Severity Score (Flint *et al.* 1981). Colon injuries are divided into: (i) isolated colon injury, minimal contamination, no shock, minimal delay; (ii) through and through perforation, lacerations, moderate contamination; and (iii) severe tissue loss, devascularization, heavy contamination. The Penetrating Abdominal Trauma Index (PATI) is derived by combining the scores of each injured organ as determined at operation (Huber and Thal 1990; Thompson *et al.* 1996). Each organ is assigned a number based on the severity of injury that is multiplied by a coefficient that represents the likelihood of complications to that organ. It is very effective at predicting intra-abdominal morbidity (Nelkin and Lewis 1989). The major disadvantage, that it does not include injuries to other body regions, may be overcome by using the Injury Severity Score (ISS).

Treatment

Patients who have ceased bleeding or who have lost less than 15% of their circulating volume will respond to rapid infusion of 2 litres of crystalloid. Recurrence of hypotension indicates persistent bleeding and strongly suggests surgery will be required. Aggressive preoperative volume expansion in those with penetrating torso injuries and shock should be avoided as the ensuing recurrent haemorrhage may be rapidly fatal (Kowalenko *et al.* 1992). In patients requiring surgery, antibiotic therapy, particularly those effective against *Bacteroides* species, is indicated (Demetriades *et al.* 1991). A single dose is usually sufficient unless contamination is marked (Thompson *et al.* 1994). Although drains are frequently used in the treatment of trauma patients, there is no evidence to support their use specifically for the colon injury (Huber and Thal 1990). In heavily contaminated wounds, delayed primary closure may be indicated.

Over the last few years several studies have provided evidence that primary repair is safe in colonic injuries, even when multiple penetrations have occurred (Thompson *et al.* 1996). Traditional war-time management of colonic injuries consisted of exteriorizing the colonic wound as a colostomy. Much of the concern now expressed about treating patients with a colostomy is based on the morbidity and extra hospitalization associated with its closure. In one retrospective study no statistically significant difference was found in morbidity between colostomy (27%) and primary repair (20%) (Ridgeway *et al.* 1989). Mean hospital stay for primary repair patients was 10 days and for colostomy patients 25 days (initial and colostomy closure admissions). As patients are generally young, colostomy closure is performed in over 90% of cases (Ridgeway *et al.* 1989). The morbidity of colostomy closure in trauma cases is 10–20%, consisting principally of wound infections and intestinal obstruction (Rehm *et al.* 1993). The mortality of colostomy closure in trauma cases is significantly less than in non-traumatized patients (0.2% versus 1.4%) (Thal and Yeary 1980). Colostomy is therefore still a safe method of treating colon injuries. Colostomy may be performed at the site of injury or by a diverting colostomy (transverse or sigmoid) proximal to a repair (Ridgeway *et al.* 1989). Subsequent closure in experienced hands does not carry a significant complication rate (Rehm *et al.* 1993).

Exteriorization was developed to overcome the complications of colostomy in cases where primary closure was considered unsafe. This technique consists of repairing the colon injury with or without resection and anastomosis and exteriorizing the repaired segment on the abdominal wall. The repaired bowel is returned to the abdomen after 5–10 days, once healing has been demonstrated. If healing fails to occur, the exteriorized segment can be converted to a colostomy. Failure to heal with conversion to stoma occurs in 20–50%, with further morbidity or intestinal obstruction in up to 25% (Huber and Thal 1990). The procedure is effective but hospital stay is longer than with primary anastomosis. The technique is advocated in cases where delay in performing surgery might make primary anastomosis unwise (Thompson *et al.* 1994). However, compared with intraperitoneal primary closure, mortality and hospital stay are both significantly greater, even in the presence of multiple colonic injuries (Thompson *et al.* 1996).

Primary repair of a colon injury may involve simple closure. This is usually selected for injuries ranging from serosal tears to involvement of a small percentage of the wall circumference. Adequate wall debridement may be necessary to provide adequate wall apposition. Resection and anastomosis are appropriate for major wall injury or blood vessel injury that affects the viability of the colon. Primary repair of selected colon injuries is becoming increasingly popular, many series reporting primary repair in about 60% of cases (Huber and Thal 1990; Miller and Schache 1996). Prospective randomized trials reveal that the mortality rate (under 4%) is similar to that of colostomy, but morbidity is significantly lower (Demetriades *et al.* 1992; Thompson *et al.* 1994).

The resurgence of interest in primary repair has followed appreciation that postoperative morbidity and mortality are determined primarily by the initial injury rather than the type of surgery performed (Chappuis *et al.* 1991; Miller and Schache 1996) (Table 17.1). In a study of 1000 colonic injuries, primary repair, including suture repair and resection with anastomosis, was performed in 61%, colostomy in 28%, exteriorized repairs in 8.5%, while the remaining 2.5% had the colonic vessels ligated for exsanguinating haemorrhage (Burch *et al.* 1991). The odds ratios for adverse outcomes (defined as a faecal fistula, abdominal abscess, stomal complication, or death from multisystem failure) for primary repair, colostomy, and exteriorized repair were 1.0, 1.9, and 2.0, respectively (Burch *et al.* 1991). Neither mild pre-operative hypotension nor gross faecal contamination are contraindications to primary repair as, when present, morbidity and mortality are no greater following primary repair than after colostomy (Nelkin and Lewis 1989; Ridgeway *et al.* 1989). However, in the presence of a combination of significant contamination, hypotension, multiple associated injuries, and delay in performing surgery of greater than 6–8 h, colostomy is probably advisable (Thompson *et al.* 1994). Contraindications to primary closure are therefore poor quality tissue to suture, doubtful vascularity, severe pancreaticoduodenal injury, vascular graft or major urinary leak (Huber and Thal 1990; Thompson *et al.* 1994). Primary repair of the left colon is associated with the same morbidity and mortality as the right colon, so that left colon injuries are not a contraindication to primary repair (Huber and Thal 1990). On-table lavage may be used for left colon injuries but does not appear to affect morbidity or mortality (Danne 1991; Thompson *et al.* 1994). There is no evidence to suggest that colonic gunshot wounds should be treated differently from stab injuries, so that it is safe to perform primary anastomosis (Thompson *et al.* 1994). Injury severity indices have a positive predictive value in identifying those who can safely undergo primary repair. Primary anastomosis should be considered in patients with a PATI or ISS of less than 25 or a Flint score of less than 2 unless spillage is large, there is a large transfusion requirement or surgery has been delayed (Nelkin and

Table 17.1 Surgical options in colonic trauma

Colostomy, either at site of injury or proximal to a repair:
Advisable if combination of hypotension, significant contamination, multiple associated injuries or delay in performing surgery
Safe, as no initial anastomosis
90% of colostomies closed
Morbidity of colostomy closure 10–25%
Mortality of colostomy closure lower than in non-traumatized patients, as patients generally young
Total mean hospital stay, including colostomy closure, 25 days

Exteriorization of repaired colonic wound on the abdominal wall:
Suitable if delay in performing primary anastomosis
If healing evident, bowel returned to abdomen after 5–10 days
If failure to heal (20–50%), colostomy can be formed, but at cost of increased morbidity and hospital stay
Hospital stay longer than primary anastomosis

Primary anastomosis, with or without resection of the traumatised segment:
Resection of the traumatized segment
Possible in about 60% of most series
Mortality (4%) similar to overall mortality of colostomy formation and closure
Morbidity similar or less than that of colostomy formation and closure
Outcome of left and right colon injuries similar

Lewis 1989). However, in one prospective trial with the average PATI score of 24 for the colostomy group and 26 for the primary repair group, septic-related complications were 18% in the colostomy and 21% in the primary repair group. There were no suture line failures in the primary repair/anastomosis group (Chappuis *et al.* 1991).

In cases of rectal injury small and isolated rectal or rectosigmoid perforations may be repaired primarily without faecal diversion (Ivatury *et al.* 1991) (Figure 17.7). The value of distal rectal irrigation remains to be proven, but it may be indicated in high-energy injuries of the rectum.(Ivatury *et al.* 1991). In more severe injuries the rectum should be completely defunctioned by a loop or end colostomy (Ivatury *et al.* 1991; Rehm *et al.* 1993; Thompson *et al.* 1994). The overall incidence of pelvic abscess in rectal injury is 5% (Ivatury *et al.* 1991). Some feel that faecal matter should be removed by repeated rectal washouts to prevent continuing sepsis and promote healing in the pararectal tissues. Others report that this procedure has no effect on septic complications (Ivatury *et al.* 1991). There is also debate in civilian injuries as to whether in cases with an intact peritoneum, the rectum should be left alone or extensively mobilized to delineate the injury and drain the pararectal tissues (Thomas *et al.* 1990; Thompson *et al.* 1994). Before colostomy closure the distal limb should be assessed for stricture or fistula formation by contrast studies. Those who have sustained sphincter damage should be assessed by anorectal manometry to determine whether they would be best served by a permanent colostomy or sphincter reconstruction.

Postoperative morbidity and mortality are determined by the pathophysiological events caused by the initial injury including hypotension, faecal contamination and the presence of other injuries (Thompson *et al.* 1994). Overall hospital mortality is about 2% (Morgado *et al.* 1992). Most deaths after 48 h are due to multiple organ failure. The severity of the initial injury is reflected by the mortality of abdominal gunshot wounds being 7–15% compared with 5% for stab wounds (Georgi *et al.* 1991; Thompson *et al.* 1994). Morbidity is also related to the severity of the injury, as reflected by the extent of blood transfusion (Morgado *et al.* 1992). Septic complications occur in 15–30% of patients requiring less than

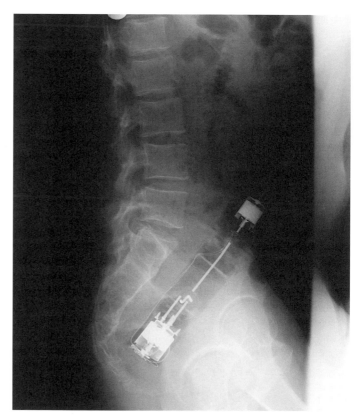

Figure 17.7 A foreign body ('vibrator') inserted in the rectum. Such instruments often cause surprisingly little mucosal damage.

4 units of blood compared with 75% of those receiving a larger transfusion (Nelkin and Lewis 1989). Septic complications following gunshot wounds are principally due to faecal contamination of the psoas muscle following the bullet passing through the large bowel and can be more common if bullet fragments are retained (Poret *et al.* 1991; Demetriades and Charalambides 1993). Prolonged hypotension is a major factor contributing to increased mortality.

Mortality is 5% for pre-operative hypotension, 25% for intra-operative hypotension and 60% if shock occurs both before and during surgery (Burch *et al.* 1991). Morbidity is related to the degree of faecal spillage, being 20% following minor spillage compared with 60% with major contamination (Nelkin and Lewis 1989; Georgi *et al.* 1991). Delay in operation from the time of injury increases the degree of contamination and consequently the complication rate. Morbidity and mortality are also strongly related to the number of associated injuries (Burch *et al.* 1991; Morgado *et al.* 1992). In the presence of two or less associated injuries, the risk of septic complication is 33% compared with 80% if more than two other injuries are present (Georgi *et al.* 1991). Age is generally not considered a major risk factor (Nelkin and Lewis 1989). Removal of an injured spleen does not have an adverse influence on the incidence of serious infective complications in the early postoperative period in patients with injuries to the spleen, the colon, or both (Huizinga and Baker 1993).

Miscellaneous disorders

Pneumatosis coli

Pneumatosis coli is an uncommon disorder characterized by the development of cysts on the bowel wall. The aetiology is unknown. Pneumatosis coli is associated with a large number of conditions. Associated intestinal conditions include inflammatory bowel disease, intestinal obstruction, surgery involving bowel anastomoses, peptic ulcer disease, and pyloric stenosis (Rogy *et al.* 1990). Non-gastrointestinal disorders which have been linked with pneumatosis coli include chronic obstructive airways disease, cystic fibrosis, connective tissue diseases, trichlorethylene exposure, steroid therapy, and previous transplantation (Rogy *et al.* 1990). An associated cause is much more likely to be present in pneumatosis cystoides intestinalis of the small bowel, which represents 85% of all cases, pneumatosis coli generally being idiopathic (Galandiuk and Fazio 1986). The cysts contain high levels of hydrogen, and nitrogen, smaller volumes of nitrous oxide and carbon dioxide and traces of methane, butane, and ethane. By examining the various associated conditions, three hypotheses on the pathogenesis of pneumatosis coli have been developed: mechanical, bacterial invasion, and high hydrogen pressures.

The 'mechanical hypothesis' suggests that gas is forced into the bowel, usually through a breach in the mucosa (Galandiuk and Fazio 1986). This is supported by the association with peptic ulcer disease and is consistent with the increased incidence among patients after bowel surgery or colonoscopy. Gas may be forced submucosally at the site of an anastomosis or by the high pressure generated by an obstructive lesion. Alternatively, alveolar rupture in those with chronic obstructive airways disease would allow air to track retroperitoneally and to enter the bowel wall via the mesentery. However, as the gas within the cysts has a high hydrogen content this hypothesis seems unlikely.

The 'bacterial invasion hypothesis' proposes the penetration through the mucosa of gas-forming bacteria. This is supported by the response to metronidazole and the high concentration of hydrogen in the cysts, which is a product of bacterial, as opposed to mammalian cell, metabolism (Ellis 1980; Jauhonen *et al.* 1987). However, against this there is little evidence of mucosal inflammation in pneumatosis coli (Rogy *et al.* 1990). The most acceptable

hypothesis postulates a high partial pressure of hydrogen in the lumen of the bowel (Forgacs *et al.* 1973; van der Linden and Marsell 1979) and is supported by the high hydrogen content of the cysts (Hughes *et al.* 1966). Hydrogen excretion is also higher in these patients (van der Linden and Marsell 1979; Christl *et al.* 1993). It has also been demonstrated that patients with pneumatosis coli are totally lacking or highly deficient in the hydrogen-metabolizing bacteria of the colon (McKay *et al.* 1985; Christl *et al.* 1993). As such organisms metabolize more than 75% of hydrogen produced in the colon of normal subjects, their deficiency could account for the development of pneumatosis coli.

Pathology

Macroscopic appearance

Pneumatosis coli appears as multiple, sessile, or pedunculated gas-filled cysts on the serosal and mucosal surfaces varying from a few millimetres to several centimetres. Mucosal cysts tend to be situated on the mesenteric border, while serosal cysts give the bowel a crepitant consistency.

Microscopic appearance

All layers of the bowel wall may be involved, although the muscular layer is the least affected (Figure 17.8). Histological examination of the cyst lining reveals prominent foreign body giant cells and macrophages (Ghahremani *et al.* 1974).

Clinical presentation

The importance of the condition is that it may be misdiagnosed or that an underlying cause may be missed. Pneumatosis coli is generally benign. However, fulminant cases do occur; in children associated with necrotizing enterocolitis and in adults in relation to Crohn's disease and pseudomembranous colitis. The benign form of pneumatosis coli usually presents with the symptoms of 'irritable bowel syndrome', such as abdominal distension, the passage of large amounts of gas, frequent stools, tenesmus, and colicky abdominal pain. Stools may be blood-stained. In the fulminant form, severe abdominal pain may occur as a result of necrotizing enterocolitis, resulting in peritonitis. There may be little to find on examination, although a large, dilated loop of intestine or non-tender crepitant masses may be palpable. If the cysts rupture, pneumoperitoneum without evidence of peritonitis may be detectable.

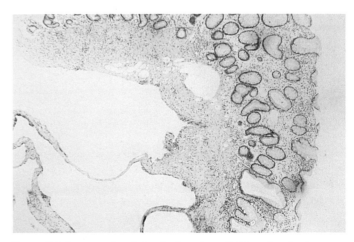

Figure 17.8 Pneumatosis coli. Section from the wall of the colon showing dilated gas filled spaces within the submucosa. The spaces are lined by foreign body type giant cells. H&E×25.

Diagnosis

Plain abdominal X-ray is often diagnostic, revealing clusters of translucent cysts along the edge of the bowel wall. Pneumoperitoneum may be present as an incidental finding and occurs from rupture of a serosal cyst without full thickness perforation of the bowel. The cysts indenting into the lumen may be seen on barium enema as filling defects which may be mistaken for polyps or ulcerative colitis (Figure 17.9). The sigmoid colon is affected in 90% of cases. Generally, the filling defects can be distinguished from solid lesions by their radiolucency. During colonoscopy a multitude of submucosal cysts can be seen projecting into the lumen-like large, sessile polyps. The cysts vary in size from being a few millimetres to several centimetres in diameter and the mucosa overlying them ranges from pale to an haemorrhagic appearance. Ultrasound or CT are claimed to be more sensitive at detecting intramural gas than plain radiographs.

Treatment

The most widely reported form of treatment is with oxygen therapy (Rogy et al. 1990; Grieve and Unsworth 1991). As hydrogen and nitrogen concentrations within the cysts are high, increasing the partial pressure of oxygen in the circulation with concomitant reduction in the pressure of nitrogen, creates a pressure gradient encouraging the absorption of hydrogen and nitrogen from the cysts. Various concentrations of oxygen as well as hyperbaric oxygen have all been used successfully, although permanent cure is rarely obtained (Holt et al. 1978). High oxygen concentration consists of administrating 75% oxygen via a modified head tent to maintain the arterial oxygen saturation above 200 mmHg (Forgacs et al. 1973).

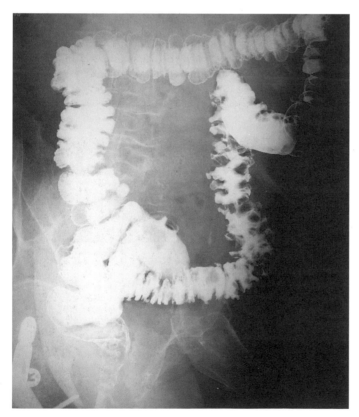

Figure 17.9 Barium enema of pneumatosis coli. The air-filled cysts give appearances that may be confused with polyposis, ulcerative colitis or diverticular disease.

Hyperbaric oxygen at 2.5 atmospheres is effective without risk of pulmonary toxicity and requires only a short course of treatment.

An alternative therapeutic approach has aimed at reducing the production of hydrogen. Treatment of one patient with an elemental diet produced resolution of symptoms and an associated reduction in hydrogen excretion (van der Linden 1979). It was hypothesized that the elemental diet was absorbed entirely in the small bowel, reducing the substrate available to hydrogen-forming colonic bacteria. Improvement has also been noted in response to metronidazole (Jauhonen et al. 1987; Tak et al. 1992) and broad-spectrum antibiotics (Holt et al. 1978). The absence of hydrogen-metabolizing bacteria in patients with pneumatosis coli is an important finding and may offer a means of therapy for the future.

Surgery is reserved for the fulminant form of pneumatosis coli (Woodward et al. 1995). It is important to recognize pneumatosis coli as the cause of free gas in the peritoneum as it can be managed conservatively.

Endometriosis

Endometriosis is the presence of normal endometrial tissue outside the uterus. Typically, it involves the reproductive organs and peritoneum. It is present in 8–18% of young women and up to 30% of those requiring gynaecological surgery (Zwas and Lyon 1991). In a comprehensive review that is still relevant, MacAfee and Greer (1960) found intestinal involvement in 880 (12%) of 7177 cases of endometriosis. The sigmoid colon and rectum were involved in 72% of cases with intestinal involvement, followed by the small intestine, then the caecum and finally the appendix (MacAfee and Greer 1960). Intestinal endometriosis requiring treatment accounts for 5% of all cases of endometriosis, with only 0.7% undergoing intestinal resection (Borsellino et al. 1993).

The most likely explanation for the pathogenesis of endometriosis is that fragments of shed endometrium reflux out of the fallopian tubes during menstruation. The ectopic implants undergo the same cycle of maturation and shedding under hormonal control as does normal endometrium. The increased frequency of diagnosis in recent years relates not only to the introduction of laparoscopy (endometriosis is detected in 20% of all gynaecological laparoscopies) but also to an absolute increase associated with the greater number of menstrual cycles now experienced by women.

Pathology

Macroscopic appearance

The implanted endometrial fragments proliferate on the serosa with some penetration into the bowel wall. However, the invading endometrial tissue rarely breaches the mucosa, explaining why blood loss is a late and uncommon feature. Reactive fibrosis causes adhesions to surrounding structures.

Microscopic appearance

Typical endometrial tissue invading first the serosa and extending more deeply is present (Figure 17.10). The 'endometrioma' contains characteristic chocolate coloured material representing the products of shed endometrial tissue and blood, which cannot escape. Fibrosis and marked smooth muscle hypertrophy identify the response of the bowel wall to the invading endometrial tissue.

Clinical presentation

The average age of women with colonic endometriosis at the time of diagnosis is 40 years, ranging from 24 to 58 years (Graham and Mazier 1988). The majority of cases (95%), have no gastrointestinal

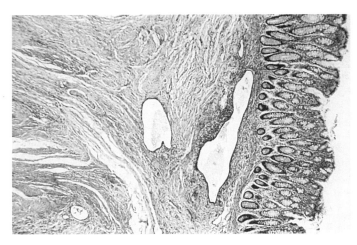

Figure 17.10 Endometriosis of the colon. Endometriosis glands with surrounding stroma present within the submucosa and muscularis propria of the colon. H&E×40.

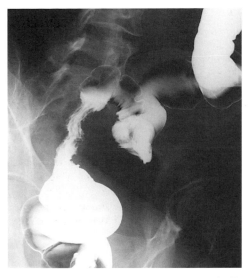

Figure 17.11 Barium enema of a young female who presented with rectal bleeding and partial intestinal obstruction thought to be due to Crohn's disease.

symptoms and the diagnosis of colonic involvement is made incidentally at laparoscopy (Zwas and Lyon 1991). When symptoms do occur the most frequent are intermittent, colicky abdominal pain, deep rectal pain, constipation or diarrhoea, and rectal bleeding (Sharpe 1992; Miller *et al.* 1994). Colin and Russell (1990) reported that diarrhoea occurred in 33% of patients, constipation and tenesmus in 20% and abdominal distension or rectal bleeding in 10%. In only a minority are the symptoms described as cyclical. However, one series reported that in seven of 10 cases of rectal bleeding, the bleeding was associated with the menstrual cycle (Graham and Mazier 1988).

When the appendix is the site of involvement, the majority of cases are asymptomatic (Panganiban and Cornog 1972). If symptoms do occur they have a strong cyclical pattern and it has been suggested that in women presenting with acute appendicitis on the day prior to menstruation the diagnosis of endometrial appendicitis should be considered (Uohara and Kovara 1975).

At least one of the four classical symptoms of endometriosis (infertility, dysmenorrhoea with pelvic pain, dyspareunia, and menstrual problems) is present in two-thirds of patients with colonic involvement (Kistner *et al.* 1977). Caecal involvement may also cause right iliac fossa discomfort and may be complicated by intussusception.

The most important aspects of physical examination are the rectal and vaginal examinations. The most frequent findings are of pelvic tenderness, a mass palpable rectally or vaginally and nodularity in the pouch of Douglas or uterosacral ligaments. These findings may be most obvious just prior to or during menstruation and both tenderness and mass size reduce between menses. The principal complications of intestinal endometriosis are obstruction, bleeding, and intussusception. Perforation with peritonitis can occur in the appendix but not the colorectum. Isolated cases of adenosquamous carcinoma have been reported in long-standing colonic endometriosis. Many conditions may be mimicked by, and require to be distinguished from, intestinal endometriosis, including primary and secondary tumours, Crohn's disease, and radiation enteritis (Croom *et al.* 1984) (Figures 17.11 and 17.12).

Diagnosis

There are no radiological or diagnostic imaging findings specific for endometriosis and unequivocal diagnosis requires microscopic examination.

Endometrial deposits are found on the serosal surface or in the muscle wall of the bowel. The mucosal surface remains intact. Viewed at laparoscopy they are usually much less than 5 cm in diameter and have a greyish hue. They may give the appearance of an annular tumour growing around the bowel wall or invading into the serosa. When multiple lesions are seen they resemble metastatic deposits. The majority of cases are diagnosed as incidental findings at laparoscopy. The diagnosis may be confirmed histologically on biopsy.

Colonoscopic examination is difficult in these patients because of pelvic tenderness and bowel immobility. The findings may often be normal because the mucosa remains intact. In other cases an external compression indenting the bowel wall and causing compression can be noted. A bluish submucosal discoloration may be detected before menstruation or bleeding may occasionally be seen (Graham and Mazier 1988). Histological specimens will usually be normal as

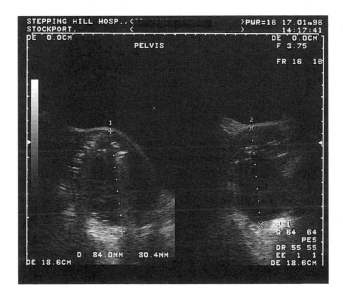

Figure 17.12 Ultrasound scan of the patient in Figure 17.11, showing a large pelvic mass. Laparotomy revealed endometriosis and bilateral tubo-ovarian abscesses which were causing extrinsic compression of the colon.

only the mucosa is biopsied (Graham and Mazier 1988). The most useful role of endoscopy is to confirm normal mucosa when the laparoscopic or radiological findings suggest a carcinoma. This avoids unnecessary or radical surgery. In future endoscopic ultrasound may prove beneficial in diagnosis (Hirata *et al.* 1994).

Barium enema examination will usually reveal an abnormality (61 of 63 patients in one study; Zwas and Lyon 1991). The most common findings are of external compression or of intramural filling defects. Stricturing can also be seen. Ultrasonography and CT can locate the endometrial cysts and thickened loops of bowel confirming the diagnosis if the characteristic chocolate material is aspirated. Because of the non-specific nature of these findings the correct diagnosis is made pre-operatively in less than 50% of cases (Graham and Mazier 1988). Laparotomy generally only increases the pre-operative diagnostic rate by revealing the presence of extra-colonic endometriosis thus raising the possibility of colonic involvement. In cases that have not undergone pre-operative endoscopy it should be performed during laparotomy to exclude colorectal adenocarcinoma (Farinon and Vadora 1980). Frozen section histological examination of a biopsy from a lesion will also confirm the benign nature of the disease.

Treatment

The management of all patients must first be to exclude malignancy. In the majority of cases this will require histological diagnosis, a biopsy specimen being obtained at laparoscopy or occasionally laparotomy.

Asymptomatic deposits which are found incidentally require no treatment. In patients with mild to moderate symptoms the initial management is medical. The principle of conservative treatment is to inhibit the cyclical changes of ectopic endometrium, allowing resorption of the necrotic tissue with resolution. Danazol 400 mg, b.d. and an oestrogen/progesterone combination are both effective treatments (Luciano and Pitkin 1984). While danazol is the more effective, it has significant side-effects and the combined oral contraceptive pill is the drug of initial choice. Treatment with a gonadotrophin-releasing hormone agonist has also been used (Dmowski *et al.* 1989). The results of hormonal therapy may be disappointing, failure being reported in up to 70% of cases (Graham and Mazier 1988). Oestrogen treatment has been implicated in the development of endometrioid carcinoma (Duun *et al.* 1993). The response to treatment may, if necessary, be assessed by serial laparoscopy.

When symptoms are severe, intestinal obstruction is present or medical management has failed, surgery is the treatment of choice. The options for surgery include ablation or excision of the localized deposit at laparoscopy or laparotomy, resection of the affected segment of the bowel or hysterectomy with bilateral salpingo-oophorectomy (Panebianco *et al.* 1994). Laparoscopy has the advantage of not only assessing the extent of disease but allows therapeutic procedures. Superficial disease can be resected laparoscopically with scissors (Nezhat *et al.* 1992; Sharpe and Redwime 1992). Deeper lesions requiring full-thickness resection and closure of the bowel or segmental resection have also been treated by laparoscopically assisted colectomy (Nezhat *et al.* 1992; Garcha *et al.* 1996). The choice of surgical therapy is dependent upon the age of the patient, their desire for further family, the extent of the bowel involvement, and of involvement of other organs. Complete control of symptoms can be obtained by surgical resection (Graham and Mazier 1988). If this fails to control symptoms, postoperative hormonal therapy should be considered (Townell and Vanderwalt 1984).

Melanosis coli

Melanosis coli was first described over 150 years ago. The pigment causing this appearance has been identified as lipofuscin, possibly coming from degeneration of intracytoplasmic organelles (Ghadially and Parry 1966) (Figure 17.13).

The reported incidence of melanosis coli varies between less than 1% and 30% of the population (Wittoesch *et al.* 1958; Clark *et al.* 1985). Such wide variation may reflect regional differences but more likely represents differing methods of diagnosis, macroscopic inspection having a lower yield than histological assessment of the proximal colon at autopsy.

Melanosis coli is due to pigment-laden macrophages within the submucosa (Figure 17.14). A variety of aetiological factors have been suggested including the possibility that slow colonic transit leads to prolonged exposure of the mucosa to damaging agents. This hypothesis would appear to be incorrect (Badiali *et al.* 1985; Clark *et al.* 1985). A more tenable link is that between laxative usage and melanosis coli. It occurs after long-term intake of anthraquinones and has no functional consequences (Muller–Lissner 1993). In one study pigment deposition was found in three-quarters of patients on anthracene laxatives and in none in a control group (Badiali *et al.* 1985). The mean time from starting laxatives to the appearance of melanosis coli is 9 months and it is generally reversible over a 12-month period on stopping the medication.

Melanosis coli is an asymptomatic condition. It can be seen at endoscopy and should alert the physician to the possibility of laxative abuse. The majority of cases are not seen endoscopically and require a biopsy for diagnosis (Badiali *et al.* 1985).

Early reports suggested a possible association with carcinoma of the colon (Ghadially and Parry 1966). However, in patients with known melanosis coli the incidence of carcinoma is very low and it can be considered a benign disorder (Earnest and Hixon 1993; Nusko *et al.* 1993). However, the risk of adenoma development in

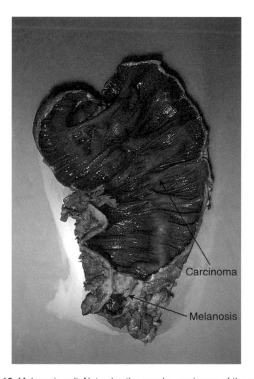

Figure 17.13 Melanosis coli. Note also the annular carcinoma of the rectum (arrowed) (see colour plates).

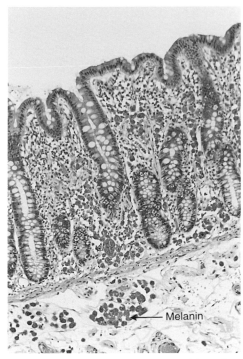

Figure 17.14 Melanosis coli showing the melanin containing cells, principally in the submucosa. H&E×250.

patients with melanosis coli relative to those without the condition is 2.2 (Nusko *et al.* 1993).

Volvulus

Incidence

In Western countries, volvulus accounts for under 5% of all cases of intestinal obstruction and less than 10% of all colonic obstructions (Allen 1990; Bagarani *et al.* 1993; Cabano *et al.* 1993). Half of all cases involve the sigmoid colon, 40% the caecum, with 10% occurring at other sites, principally the transverse colon (Halliday *et al.* 1993; Khoda *et al.* 1993). Occasionally, there may be synchronous involvement of the caecum and sigmoid colon by volvulus (Theure and Cheadle 1991; Moore *et al.* 1992). In developing countries volvulus accounts for up to 20% of acute intestinal obstruction and 10% of all emergency operations (Ofiaeli 1993). The estimated incidence in developing countries is 12 per 100 000 per year (Schagen-van-Leeuwen 1985). Racial and environmental differences are apparent in that the condition, particularly sigmoid volvulus, is more common in American Negroes, African Bantus, and Indians (Degiannis *et al.* 1996). It has been stated that volvulus principally affects older men, but a wide age range is reported, up to 15% of cases occurring in children (Allen 1990; Smith *et al.* 1990; Oncu *et al.* 1991). A male/female ratio of 3:1 is reported for sigmoid volvulus and 1:3 for caecal volvulus, others report an equal sex incidence (Allen 1990; Smith *et al.* 1990; Oncu *et al.* 1991).

Aetiology and pathophysiology

Volvulus is a torsion of the bowel on its mesentery. The two principal areas of the colon with sufficiently long mesentery to allow volvulus are the caecum and sigmoid colon. The main factors required for the occurrence of volvulus are a long, freely mobile segment of colon and its associated mesocolon together with a short

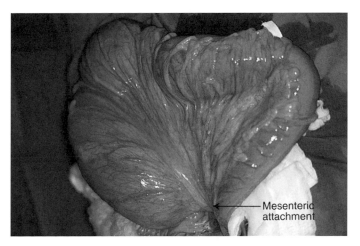

Figure 17.15 Sigmoid volvulus (untwisted) showing the long mesocolon and narrow mesenteric attachment (arrowed).

mesenteric attachment of the proximal and distal mesocolic limbs (Figure 17.15). In the sigmoid colon the mesentery forms a narrow inverted 'V' while in the caecum incomplete peritoneal attachment of the right colon is the major factor allowing the mobile colon to tort. The transverse colon may twist if there is a long transverse mesocolon associated with closely approximated flexures (Halliday 1993; Khoda *et al.* 1993). These peritoneal abnormalities are present in 10–20% of the population so that other factors must be present to precipitate torsion. These include distension of the colon by faeces or gas, such as occurs from chronic constipation or obstruction from a distal carcinoma, adhesions from previous surgery, congenital malrotation, coeliac disease, Chagas' disease, pregnancy, and the puerperium (Jones and Fazio 1989; Koziol and Price 1990; Lord *et al.* 1996). Two-thirds of patients are from psychiatric institutions, are bedridden or use constipating drugs (Theuer and Cheadle 1991), while predisposing factors are present in one-third of children (Smith *et al.* 1990).

If the above factors are present, the colon can intermittently rotate clockwise or anticlockwise through 180° or 360° about its narrow mesenteric attachment. The bowel can also twist along its long axis to a variable degree. In the sigmoid the twist is normally counterclockwise about the axis of the sigmoid mesentery accompanied by an axial torsion about the axis of the bowel (Janzen and

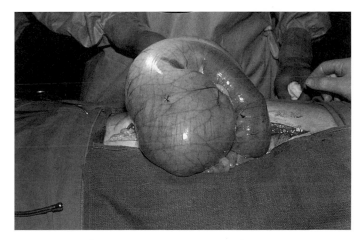

Figure 17.16 Sigmoid volvulus showing counter-clockwise rotation about the axis of the sigmoid mesentery.

Heap 1992) (Figure 17.16). In caecal volvulus the twist is most often clockwise. The result of such rotation is a closed-loop obstruction. Proximal obstruction occurs, the extent of which is dependent on the competence of the ileocaecal valve.

If the torsion is moderate, the bowel remains viable, peristalsis forcing gas and liquid into the involved segment from which they cannot escape, resulting in rapid distension of the bowel. If unrelieved, necrosis, maximal at the site of torsion, occurs, followed by perforation and peritonitis. If the torsion is severe, strangulation occurs, occluding first the veins and then the arteries. Thrombosis of the mesenteric vessels then results, leading to perforation. Repeated torsion causes scarring and thickening of the mesocolon (McCalla *et al.* 1985).

Clinical presentation

Symptoms

The commonest presentation of sigmoid volvulus is recurrent, subacute attacks of abdominal pain and distension, which often resolve spontaneously. A chronic clinical course is seen in psychiatric or elderly patients. The condition is also seen in 2% of patients with a spinal injury, constipation occurring in these patients as a result of immobility and drug treatment (Fenton *et al.* 1993). The chronic presentation occurs as an insidious onset of recurrent episodes of extreme abdominal distension associated with constipation, minimal abdominal pain, and no vomiting. The distension may intermittently settle.

An acute presentation of sigmoid volvulus is preceded by a similar but less severe, previous episode in one-third of patients (Pahlman *et al.* 1989). There is a sudden onset of generalized cramps associated with a steady continuous pain in 90% of patients and tenderness in the left lower quadrant (Porro Novo *et al.* 1989). Complete constipation for both faeces and flatus occurs in most cases, associated with a repeated, unsuccessful desire to defecate. Occasionally a small stool is passed which empties the rectum. Vomiting may occur but is neither frequent nor copious. Acute volvulus of the transverse colon presents in a similar manner to that of sigmoid volvulus, mesenteric ischaemia being a prominent feature (Halliday *et al.* 1993). In children abdominal pain (66%), vomiting (10%), and constipation (10%) occur (McCalla *et al.* 1985; Smith *et al.* 1990).

Caecal volvulus may also have an acute, subacute, or chronic presentation; the acute presentation accounting for 80% of cases. In acute caecal volvulus there is a sudden onset of severe abdominal pain, vomiting, constipation, and abdominal distension. Subacute cases present with a gradual onset of abdominal discomfort or distension, pain, and tenderness. The chronic presentation consists of transient episodes of right lower quadrant pain, tenderness, and intermittent distension.

Signs

Abdominal distension is the principal finding. Tenderness is often minimal, even in the presence of a severely ischaemic bowel. Tachycardia and hypotension suggest ischaemia and are associated with a poor prognosis. In children abdominal findings include distension (70%), tenderness (40%), and a mass (10%) (Smith *et al.* 1990).

Diagnosis

An elevated temperature and white cell count are suggestive of ischaemic bowel, but the diagnosis is essentially made by radiology. Plain radiographs of sigmoid volvulus reveal marked distension of

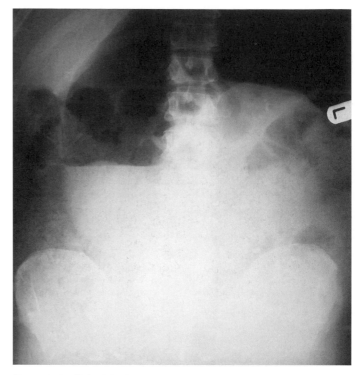

Figure 17.17 Plain abdominal X-ray of sigmoid volvulus (1.5 turns). Note the dilated loop is in the right upper quadrant and the presence of gas in the ascending colon .

the sigmoid colon with air–fluid levels situated in the right side showing an 'omega' sign, together with moderate distension of the remainder of the colon (Figure 17.17). The plain radiograph is diagnostic in 35% and suggestive of volvulus in 60% of cases.

A plain radiograph of caecal volvulus reveals a large air-filled loop of colon occupying the left upper quadrant with its convex surface facing the left lower quadrant (owing to clockwise rotation) (Figure 17.18). The caecal shadow is therefore not in its normal position and there is small bowel obstruction with collapse of the distal colon (Ismail *et al.* 1993). A single air–fluid level is present in caecal volvulus, whereas multiple levels occur in sigmoid volvulus. However, the diagnosis is often missed, diagnostic difficulties occurring particularly in patients with gross small bowel dilatation or peritonitis. In children the classic radiological omega sign of volvulus is present on plain films in only 30% of the cases, barium enema often being of more benefit (diagnostic in 60% of cases) (McCalla *et al.* 1985; Smith *et al.* 1990).

Plain films of volvulus of the transverse colon reveals a 'double closed loop' with air–fluid levels in the twisted transverse and ascending colons due to obstruction at the hepatic flexure and a competent ileocaecal valve. The appearances may be mimicked by a duplication of the proximal colon (Ho and Goh 1992) or a transomental herniation (Siddins and Cade 1990). Radiographic features of a splenic flexure volvulus are: (i) a markedly dilated, air-filled colon with an abrupt termination at the anatomical splenic flexure; (ii) two widely separated air–fluid levels, one in the transverse colon and the other in the caecum; (iii) an empty descending and sigmoid colon; and (iv) a characteristic beak at the anatomical splenic flexure at a barium enema examination (Mindelzun and Stone 1991).

If plain radiographs are not diagnostic, barium studies may be performed, confirming the diagnosis in 70% (Kunin *et al.* 1992). In sigmoid volvulus, there is a characteristic outline of the proximal

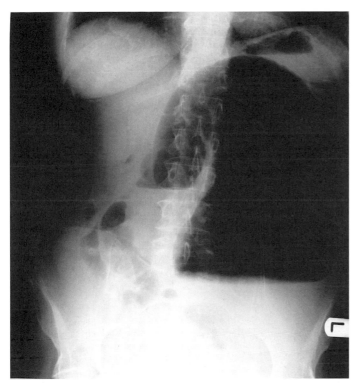

Figure 17.18 Plain abdominal film of caecal volvulus. The dilated colon occupies the left upper quadrant. There is gas in the small bowel but not in the distal colon.

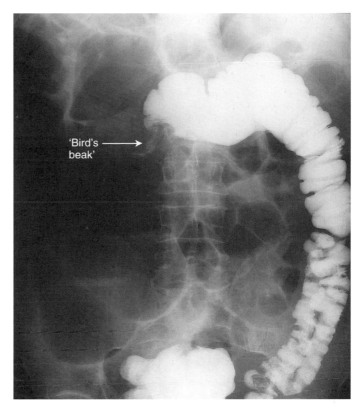

Figure 17.19 Barium enema in caecal volvulus showing the typical 'birds beak' deformity.

part of the rectum which smoothly narrows down to the site of obstruction, giving a 'bird's beak' deformity. Occasionally, barium enema relieves the obstruction in which case a large redundant sigmoid colon fills with barium. Barium enema of caecal volvulus also shows a 'bird's beak' deformity but located at the site of torsion in the right lower quadrant (Figures 17.19 and 17.20). If a CT scan is performed a characteristic 'whirl' sign is apparent in caecal volvulus (Frank *et al.* 1993; Catalano 1996). Barium enema of a transverse colon volvulus reveals a blockage at the splenic flexure or an unusually mobile or malpositioned transverse colon.

Sigmoidoscopy confirms the diagnosis in over half of the cases of sigmoid volvulus by identifying and often relieving the site of obstruction (Sroujieh *et al.* 1992). Spiral folds of twisted mucosa may be seen just proximal to the site of obstruction. Caecal volvulus is easily differentiated from acute gastric dilatation by passage of a nasogastric tube.

Treatment

Current knowledge suggests that primary prevention of colonic volvulus is not possible, so morbidity and mortality can only be reduced by rapid diagnosis and immediate adequate treatment of the acute presentation (Jones and Fazio 1989). Individualization of treatment is appropriate in medically compromised patients or in special circumstances and sound clinical judgement still has an important role in the treatment of volvulus.

Patients presenting with acute sigmoid volvulus should be treated initially by a non-operative attempt to untwist and decompress the affected bowel. This is traditionally performed using a rigid sigmoidoscope but more recently, many authors have employed colonoscopy, if necessary under radiological control (Jones and Fazio 1989; Forde 1992). Colonoscopic decompression can be obtained in

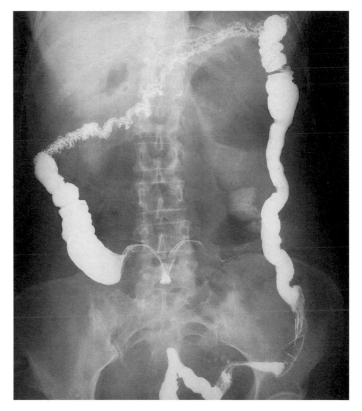

Figure 17.20 Barium enema in a case of reduced caecal volvulus. Note the oedema of the transverse colon and the deformity of the caecum.

80% and reduction of the volvulus in 40% (Strodel and Brothers 1989; Clemente *et al.* 1990). The point of obstruction is usually 15–25 cm from the anus and can be identified by twisting of the rectal mucosa just before the obstruction is reached. If the mucosa is ulcerated or necrotic, the procedure should be abandoned because of the risk of perforation. In the presence of viable mucosa passage of a flatus tube results in rapid decompression from passage of flatus and fluid faeces. The flatus tube should remain *in situ* for 2–3 days as recurrence is common on removal (Wyman 1989). Non-operative treatment of acute sigmoid volvulus is successful in 75% of cases of sigmoid volvulus, although the response in children may not be as good as in adults (Smith *et al.* 1990; Salim 1991; Theur and Cheadle 1991). Salim (1991) claims that percutaneous deflation of acute sigmoid volvulus is a simple, rapid, and safe method enabling successful sigmoidoscopic decompression with avoidance of emergency surgery in many instances.

Non-operative treatment may also be attempted in caecal volvulus using a colonoscope. In contrast to sigmoid volvulus, the success rate is only 30% and occasionally colonoscopy may precipitate a further volvulus (Le Neel 1989; Theur 1991). If decompression fails, a hydrostatic barium enema can reduce the volvulus in half of the cases. Recently, decompressing the colon under fluoroscopic guidance has been described which may be considered in selected, ill patients (Bender *et al.* 1993). Although non-operative measures are usually successful in relieving acute sigmoid volvulus, without further treatment recurrent twisting will occur in 30–90% of patients (Smith *et al.* 1990; Oncu *et al.* 1991). In addition, conservative management after detorsion often results in decompensation of the concurrent illnesses and a significant mortality rate of about 10% (Le Neel 1989).

Mortality of colonic volvulus is significant, being closely related to the viability of the bowel and the age and general condition of the patient. Most authors report an overall mortality of 10–20% (Pahlman *et al.* 1989; Oncu *et al.* 1991; Hiltunen *et al.* 1992). Morbidity is up to 40%, usually due to respiratory problems in an elderly population (Kunin *et al.* 1992). Mortality is least with the first attack (7%), increasing with each subsequent acute episode, being 20% with the second and 40% with the third attack (Cabano *et al.* 1993). In contrast, operative mortality is of the order of 5% for the elective situation but may be up to 40% in emergency cases, particularly if gangrene is present (Le Neel 1989; Buffin *et al.* 1992). Therefore, although repeated non-operative decompression can be successful (Theur 1991), the high risk of recurrence with its associated mortality means that surgery is indicated for most cases (Keller and Aeberhard 1990). This is best performed during the same hospital admission, after the patient has been stabilized and the bowel prepared (Le Neel 1989; Buffin *et al.* 1992). However, patients over 70 years with a first episode of volvulus are at particularly high risk of dying if subjected to surgical intervention. Non-operative detorsion alone should be considered for this subgroup of patients (Peoples *et al.* 1990).

Emergency surgery is indicated for the 25% of cases in whom conservative measures fail and in those with gangrenous mucosa or impending perforation on colonoscopy. It is generally agreed that if the bowel is of dubious viability, resection of the affected segment is required. In such circumstances, both limbs of the bowel should be brought out to the surface as a double-barrelled (Paul-Mickulitz) colostomy if possible, as this facilitates later closure of the stoma. If there is insufficient length to bring out both limbs, the distal limb should be closed and returned to the abdomen as a Hartmann's procedure (Oncu *et al.* 1991).

There is debate as to the procedure which should be performed if the bowel is viable at laparotomy. Some suggest that untwisting of the bowel and fixation of the caecum or sigmoid (caecopexy or mesosigmoidopexy) is successful in many cases (Baker and Wardrop 1992). Mesosigmoidoplasty, which consists of shortening the mesosigmoid by incision along its axis and transverse suture may be used in children as well as adults (Ponticelli *et al.* 1989; Akgun 1996). Salim (1991) advocates colopexy by banding as a simple elective procedure with a low recurrence rate and fewer complications than mesenteropexy and resectional surgery. Recently both caecopexy and mesosigmoidopexy have been successfully performed laparoscopically and this may in future allow treatment in high risk or elderly patients who are poor candidates for conventional bowel surgery (Miller *et al.* 1992; Chiulli *et al.* 1993; Pruett 1993; Shoop and Sackier 1993). However, subsequent recurrence rates for colopexy procedures of over 40% have been reported so that these authors recommend immediate resection of the affected segment. Hiltunen and colleagues (1992) found that detorsion and sigmoidopexy was associated with a 25% incidence of recurrent volvulus. Consequently, many believe that a primary sigmoid resection should be performed and the bowel exteriorized as a stoma (Hartmann's or Paul-Mickulitz) or anastomosed primarily at the lower ends of both limbs. Primary anastomosis has the attraction of avoiding multistage procedures in patients who are often elderly or with multiple diseases and has an acceptable hospital stay (12–18 days) (Johanet *et al.* 1991). If at operation the bowel is not adequately prepared, primary anastomosis may still be performed using on-table lavage (Conti *et al.* 1993) (Figure 17.21). Alternatively, an intracolonic bypass, anchoring a pliable latex tube to the mucosa and submucosa, 3 cm proximal to a site of the anastomosis can be inserted and is later spontaneously evacuated via the rectum (Rosati *et al.* 1992).

Bagarani and colleagues (1993) performed a prospective, randomized trial of the surgical treatment of sigmoid volvulus. Patients with viable bowel underwent either mesosigmoidopexy or resection and primary anastomosis. Those with gangrenous bowel had either a Hartmann's procedure or resection and primary anastomosis. Overall mortality was 13%, being significantly higher in those with gangrene (21%) compared with those with viable bowel (6%). In those with viable bowel, the success rate in patients treated with resection-anastomosis was higher than that of mesosigmoidopexy (90% versus

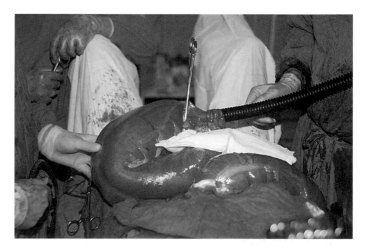

Figure 17.21 On-table lavage in a case of sigmoid volvulus, allowing primary resection and anastomosis.

71%). In the case of gangrenous bowel Hartmann's procedure resulted in a better patient outcome, mortality rates being 12% and 33%, respectively. They concluded that the therapeutic approach to sigmoid volvulus should depend on the presence of gangrenous colon, the treatment of choice being resection with primary anastomosis in patients with viable colon and Hartmann's procedure in patients with gangrenous colon.

Conservative management of caecal volvulus consists of colonoscopic decompression or hydrostatic barium enema. A few cases will resolve spontaneously (Ostergaard and Halvorsen 1990). If conservative measures fail, which is likely in over 70% of cases, or there is evidence of peritonitis, right hemicolectomy is the procedure of choice (Friedman *et al.* 1989). Recurrence following caecopexy is common and caecostomy has little role in the modern management of caecal volvulus in all but the most ill of patients. Ostergaard and Halvorsen (1990) reviewed patients with caecal volvulus treated by untwisting; caecopexy; caecostomy; or resection. After a mean follow up of 12 years, 43%, 38%, 33% and 69%, respectively remained symptom free. They concluded that resection gives the best long-term results with acceptable mortality and morbidity and should be the treatment of choice for caecal volvulus. However, the other procedures may be considered a safer temporizing option in poor risk individuals. Volvulus of the transverse colon is also best treated by resection and primary anastomosis (extended right hemicolectomy), although the anastomosis may be delayed if there is marked dilatation or questionable viability of the small bowel (Halliday *et al.* 1993; Khoda *et al.* 1993).

References

Akgun Y. Mesosigmoplasty as a definitive operation in treatment of acute sigmoid volvulus. *Dis.Colon Rectum* 1996; 39: 579–81.

Allen JC. Sigmoid volvulus in pregnancy. *J. R. Army Med. Corps* 1990; 136: 55–6.

Badiali D, Marcheggiano A, Pallone F, *et al.* Melanosis of the rectum in patients with chronic constipation. *Dis. Colon Rectum* 1985; 28: 241–5.

Bagarani M, Conde AS, Longo R, Italiano A, Terenzi A, Venuto G. Sigmoid volvulus in West Africa: a prospective study on surgical treatments. *Dis. Colon Rectum.* 1993; 36: 186–90.

Baker D, Wardrop P. Mesosigmoplasty as a definitive operation for sigmoid volvulus. *Br. J. Surg.* 1992; 79: 1384.

Balachandran KS, Allan A. Surgical emphysema: a delayed presentation of colonic trauma in multisystem injury. *Injury* 1991; 22: 165–6.

Bender GN, Do Dai DD, Briggs LM. Colonic pseudo obstruction: decompression with a tricomponent coaxial system under fluoroscopic guidance. *Radiology* 1993; 188: 395–8.

Borsellino G, Buonaguidi A, Veneziano S, Borsellino V, Mariscalco G, Minnici G. Endometriosis of the large intestine. A report of 2 clinical cases. *Minerva Ginecol.* 1993; 45: 443–7.

Buffin RP, Dabrowski A, Kaskas M, Helfrich P, Sabbah M. Volvulus of the sigmoid colon. Emergency resection and anastomosis. *J. Chir.* 1992; 129: 254–6.

Bulas DI, Taylor GA, Eichelberger MR. The value of CT in detecting bowel perforation in children after blunt abdominal trauma. *Am. J. Radiol.* 1989; 153: 561–4.

Burch JM, Martin RR, Richardson RJ, Muldowny DS, Mattox KL, Jordan GL Jr. Evolution of the treatment of the injured colon in the 1980s. *Arch. Surg.* 1991; 126: 979–83.

Cabano F, Vezzulli I, Venegoni A, Resta E, De Medici A. Sigmoid volvulus. *Minerva Chir.* 1993; 31: 48: 549–57.

Catalano O. Computed tomographic appearance of sigmoid volvulus. *Abdom. Imaging* 1996; 21: 314–7.

Chappuis CW, Frey DJ, Dietzen CD, Panetta TP, Buechter KJ, Cohn I Jr. Management of penetrating colon injuries. A prospective randomized trial. *Ann. Surg.* 1991; 213: 492–7.

Chiulli RA, Swantkowski TM. Sigmoid volvulus treated with endoscopic sigmoidopexy. *Gastrointest Endosc.* 1993; 39: 194–6.

Christl SU, Gibson GR, Murgatroyd PR, Scheppach W, Cummings JH. Impaired hydrogen metabolism in pneumatosis cystoides intestinalis. *Gastroenterology* 1993; 104: 392–7.

Clark JC, Collan Y, Eide TJ, *et al.* Prevalence of polyps in an autopsy series from areas with varying incidence of large bowel cancer. *Int. J. Cancer* 1985; 36: 179–86.

Clemente Ricote G, Banares Canizares R, Sebastian Domingo JJ, Rabago Torre L, Menchen PL, Senent C, *et al.* Colonoscopic approach in the therapy of sigmoid volvulus. *Rev. Esp. Enferm. Dig.* 1990; 77: 129–32.

Conti F, Gentilli S, Voghera P, Dalbo R, Boltri F. Intra operative irrigation during colonic resection and anastomosis in colonic obstruction. *Minerva Chir.* 1993; 48: 133–6.

Croom RD 3d, Donovan ML, Schwesinger WH. Intestinal endometriosis. *Am. J. Surg.* 1984; 148: 660–7.

Danne PD. Intra operative colonic lavage: safe single stage, left colorectal resections. *Aust. N.Z. J. Surg.* 1991; 61: 59–65.

Degiannis E, Levy RD, Sliwa K, Hale MJ, Saadia R. Volvulus of the sigmoid colon at Baragwanath Hospital. *S. Afr. J. Surg.* 1996; 34: 25–8.

Demetriades D, Charalambides D. Gunshot wounds of the colon: role of retained bullets in sepsis. *Br. J. Surg.* 1993; 80: 772–3.

Demetriades D, Lakhoo M, Pezikis A, Charalambides D, Pantanowitz D, Sofianos C. Short course antibiotic prophylaxis in penetrating abdominal injuries: ceftriaxone versus cefoxitin. *Injury* 1991; 22: 20–4.

Demetriades D, Pantanowitx D, Charambides D. Gunshot wounds of the colon: role of primary repair. *Ann. R. Coll. Surg. Engl.* 1992; 74: 391–4.

Dmowski WP, Radwanska E, Binor Z, Tummon I, Pepping P. Ovarian suppression induced with Buserelin or danazol in the management of endometriosis: a randomized, comparative study. *Fertil. Steril.* 1989; 51: 395–400.

Duun S, Roed Petersen K, Michelsen JW. Endometrioid carcinoma arising from endometriosis of the sigmoid colon during estrogenic treatment. *Acta Obstet. Gynecol. Scand.* 1993; 72: 676–8.

Earnest DL, Hixon LJ. Other diseases of the colon and rectum. In: Sleisenger MII, Fordtran JS, eds. *Gastrointestinal disease: pathophysiology/ diagnosis/ management*, 5th edn. Philadelphia: WB Saunders, 1993: 1537–70.

Ellis BW. Symptomatic treatment of primary pneumatosis coli with metronidazole. *Br. Med. J.* 1980; 280: 763–4.

Farinon AM, Vadora E. Endometriosis of the colon and rectum: an indication for peroperative coloscopy. *Endoscopy* 1980; 12: 136–9.

Feliciano DV. Diagnostic modalities in abdominal trauma. *Surg. Clin. North Am.* 1991; 71: 241–56.

Fenton Lee D, Yeo BW, Jones RF, Engel S. Colonic volvulus in the spinal cord injured patient. *Paraplegia* 1993; 31: 393–7.

Flint LM. Assessment of abdominal trauma. *Curr. Pract. Surg.* 1994; 6: 65–9.

Flint LM, Vitale GC, Richardson JD. The injured colon. *Ann. Surg.* 1981; 193: 619–23.

Forde KA. Therapeutic colonoscopy. *World J. Surg.* 1992; 16: 1048–53.

Forgacs P, Wright PH, Wyatt AP. Treatment of intestinal gas cysts by oxygen breathing. *Lancet* 1973; i: 579–82.

Frank AJ, Goffner LB, Fruauff AA, Losada RA. Cecal volvulus: the CT whirl sign. *Abdom. Imaging* 1993; 18: 288–9.

Friedman JD, Odland MD, Bubrick MP. Experience with colonic volvulus. *Dis. Colon Rectum* 1989; 32: 409–16.

Galandiuk S, Fazio VW. Pneumatosis cystoides intestinalis. A review of the literature. *Dis. Colon Rectum* 1986; 29: 358–63.

Garcha IS, Perloe M, Strawn EY, Mason EM. Laparoscopic resection of sigmoid endometrioma. *Am. Surgeon* 1996; 62: 274–5.

Georgi BA, Massad M, Obeid M. Ballistic trauma to the abdomen: shell fragments versus bullets. *J. Trauma* 1991; 31: 711–5.

Ghadially FN, Parry EW. An electron microscope and histochemical study of melanosis coli. *J. Pathol. Bacteriol.* 1966; 92: 313–7.

Ghahremani GG, Port RB, Beachley MC. Pneumatosis coli in Crohn's disease. *Am. J. Dig. Dis.* 1974; 19: 315–23.

Graham B, Mazier WP. Diagnosis and management of endometriosis of the colon and rectum. *Dis. Colon Rectum* 1988; 31 :952–6.

Grieve DA, Unsworth IP. Pneumatosis cystoides intestinalis: an experience with hyperbaric oxygen treatment. *Aust. N.Z. J. Surg.* 1991; 61: 423–6.

Halliday KE, Bellamy E, Ellis BW. Volvulus of the splenic flexure and spleen. *Eur. J. Surg.* 1993; 159: 383–4.

Hiltunen KM, Syrja H, Matikainen M. Colonic volvulus. Diagnosis and results of treatment in 82 patients. *Eur. J. Surg.* 1992; 158: 607–11.

Hirata N, Kawamoto K, Ueyama T, Iwashita I, Masuda K. Endoscopic ultrasonography in the assessment of colonic wall invasion by adjacent diseases. *Abdom. Imaging* 1994; 19: 21–6.

Ho YH, Goh HS. Duplication of the proximal colon mimicking volvulus: a case report. *Aust. N.Z. J. Surg.* 1992; 62: 983–5 .

Hoffman R, Nerlich M, Muggia Sullman M, Pohlemann T, Wipperman B, Regel G, Tscherne H. Blunt abdominal trauma in cases of multiple trauma evaluated by ultrasonography: a prospective analysis of 291 patients. *J. Trauma* 1992; 32: 452–8.

Holt S, Stewart IC, Heading RC, Macpherson AI. Resolution of primary pneumatosis coli. *J. R. Coll. Surg. Edinburgh* 1978; 23: 297–9.

Huber PJ, Thal ER. Management of colon injuries. *Surg. Clin. North Am.* 1990; 70: 561–73.

Hughes DT, Gordon KC, Swann JC, Bolt GL. Pneumatosis cystoides intestinalis. *Gut* 1966; 7: 553–7.

Huizinga WK, Baker LW. Selective management of abdominal and thoracic stab wounds with established peritoneal penetration: the eviscerated omentum. *Am. J. Surg.* 1987; 153: 564–8.

Huizinga WK, Baker LW. The influence of splenectomy on infective morbidity after colonic and splenic injuries. *Eur. J. Surg.* 1993; 159: 579–84.

Ismail A, Arai Y, Atri M. Residents' corner. Answer to case of the month #20. Cecal volvulus. *Can. Assoc. Radiol. J.* 1993; 44: 315–7.

Ivatury RR, Licata J, Gunduz Y, Rao P, Stahl WM. Management options in penetrating rectal injuries. *Am. Surg.* 1991; 57: 50–5.

Janzen DL, Heap SW. Organo axial volvulus of the sigmoid colon. *Australas. Radiol.* 1992; 36: 332–3.

Jauhonen P, Lehtola J, Karttunen T. Treatment of pneumatosis coli with metronidazole. Endoscopic follow up of one case. *Dis. Colon Rectum* 1987; 30: 800–1.

Johanet H, Costil P, Saliou C, Marmuse JP, Benhamou G, Charleux H. Emergency treatment of sigmoid volvulus. One stage resection with mechanical staplers. *Ann. Chir.* 1991; 45: 38–41.

Jones IT, Fazio VW. Colonic volvulus. Etiology and management. *Dig. Dis.* 1989; 7: 203–9.

Jones JW, Kitahama A, Webb WR, McSwain N. Emergency thoracoscopy: a logical approach to chest trauma management. *J. Trauma* 1991; 31: 280–4.

Keller A, Aeberhard P. Emergency resection and primary anastomosis for sigmoid volvulus in an African population. *Int. J. Colorectal Dis.* 1990; 5: 209–12.

Khoda J, Sebbag G, Lantzberg L. Volvulus of the transverse colon. Apropos of three cases. *Ann. Chir.* 1993; 47: 451–4.

Kirton OC, Wint D, Thrasher B *et al.* Stab wounds to the back and flank in the hemodynamically stable patient: a decision algorithm based on contrast-enhanced computed tomography with colonic opacification. *Am. J. Surg.* 1997; 173: 189–93.

Kistner RW, Siegler AM, Behrman SJ. Suggested classification for endometriosis: relationship to infertility. *Fertil. Steril.* 1977; 28 :1008–10.

Kowalenko T, Stern S, Dronen S, Wang X. Improved outcome with hypotensive resuscitation of uncontrolled hemorrhagic shock in a swine model. *J. Trauma* 1992; 33: 349–53.

Koziol KA, Price LM. Colonic volvulus as a complication of celiac sprue. *J. Clin. Gastroenterol.* 1990; 12: 633–5.

Kunin N, Letoquart JP, La Gamma A, Mambrini A. Volvulus of the colon. Apropos of 37 cases. *J. Chir.* 1992; 129: 531–6.

Le-Neel JC, Farge A, Guiberteau B, Kohen M, Leborgne J. Volvulus of the sigmoid colon. *Ann. Chir.* 1989; 43: 348–51.

Lord SA, Boswell WC, Hungerpiller JC. Sigmoid volvulus in pregnancy. *Am. Surg.* 1996; 62: 380–2.

Luciano AA, Pitkin RM. Endometriosis: approaches to diagnosis and treatment. *Surg. Annu.* 1984; 16: 297–312.

MacAfee CHG, Greer HLH. Intestinal endometriosis: a report of 29 cases and a survey of the literature. *J. Obstet. Gynaecol. Br. Emp.* 1960; 67: 539–55.

Mackersie RC, Tiwary AD, Shackford SR, Hoyt DB. Intraabdominal injury following blunt trauma. *Arch. Surg.* 1989; 124: 809–13.

McAnena OJ, Marx JA, Moore EE. Contributions of peritoneal lavage enzyme determinations to the management of isolated hollow visceral abdominal injuries. *Ann. Emerg. Med.* 1991; 20: 834–7.

McCalla TH, Arensman RM, Falterman KW. Sigmoid volvulus in children. *Am. Surg.* 1985; 514–19.

McKay LF, Eastwood MA, Brydon WG. Methane excretion in man: a study of breath, flatus, and faeces. *Gut* 1985; 26: 69–74.

Miller BJ, Schache DJ. Colorectal injury: where do we stand with repair? *Aust. NZ. J. Surg.* 1996; 66: 348–52.

Miller LS, Barbarevech C, Friedman LS. Less frequent causes of lower gastrointestinal bleeding.*Gastroenterol. Clin. North Am.* 1994; 23: 21–52.

Miller R, Roe AM, Eltringham WK, Espiner HJ. Laparoscopic fixation of sigmoid volvulus. *Br. J. Surg.* 1992; 79: 435.

Mindelzun RE, Stone JM. Volvulus of the splenic flexure: radiographic features. *Radiology* 1991; 181: 221–3.

Moore JH, Cintron JR, Duarte B, Espinosa G, Abcarian H. Synchronous cecal and sigmoid volvulus. Report of a case. *Dis. Colon Rectum* 1992; 35: 803–5.

Morgado PJ, Alfaro R, Morgado PJ Jr, Leon P. Colon trauma clinical staging for surgical decision making. Analysis of 119 cases. *Dis. Colon Rectum* 1992; 35: 986–90.

Muller Lissner SA. Adverse effects of laxatives: fact and fiction. *Pharmacology* 1993; 47 (Suppl. 1): 138–45.

Nagel M, Saeger HD, Massoun H, Buschulte J. Injuries of the small and large intestine in the traumatized abdomen. *Unfallchirurg* 1991; 94: 105–9.

Nelkin N, Lewis F. The influence of injury severity on complications rates after primary closure or colostomy for penetrating colon trauma. *Ann. Surg.* 1989; 209: 439–47.

Nezhat F, Nezhat C, Pennington E, Ambroze W Jr. Laparoscopic segmental resection for infiltrating endometriosis of the rectosigmoid colon: a preliminary report. *Surg. Laparosc. Endosc.* 1992; 2: 212–6.

Nusko G, Schneider B, Muller G, Kusche J, Hahn EG. Retrospective study on laxative use and melanosis coli as risk factors for colorectal neoplasma. *Pharmacology* 1993; 47 (Suppl. 1): 234–41.

Obeid FN, Sorensen V, Vincent G. Inaccuracy of diagnostic peritoneal lavage in penetrating colonic trauma. *Arch. Surg.* 1984; 119: 906–8.

Ofiaeli RO. Volvulus of the sigmoid colon a re appraisal. *Trop. Doct.* 1993; 23: 23–4.

Oncu M, Piskin B, Calik A, Yandi M, Alhan E. Volvulus of the sigmoid colon. *S. Afr. J. Surg.* 1991; 29: 48–9.

Ostergaard E, Halvorsen JF. Volvulus of the caecum. An evaluation of various surgical procedures. *Acta Chir. Scand.* 1990; 156: 629–31.

Pahlman L, Enblad P, Rudberg C, Krog M. Volvulus of the colon. A review of 93 cases and current aspects of treatment. *Acta Chir. Scand.* 1989; 155: 53–6.

Panebianco V, Poli A, Blandino R, Pistritto A, Puzzo L, Grasso A, Petino AG. Low anterior resection of the rectum using mechanical anastomosis in intestinal endometriosis. *Minerva Chir.* 1994; 49: 215–7.

Panganiban W, Cornog JL. Endometriosis of the intestines and vermiform appendix. *Dis. Colon Rectum* 1972; 15: 253–60.

Peoples JB, McCafferty JC, Scher KS. Operative therapy for sigmoid volvulus. Identification of risk factors affecting outcome. *Dis. Colon Rectum* 1990; 33: 643–6.

Ponticelli A, Mastrobuono I, Matarazzo E, Zaccara A, Appetito C, Inserra A, Alessandri A. Mesosigmoidoplasty in the treatment of sigmoid volvulus in children. *S. Afr. J. Surg.* 1989; 27: 105–7.

Poret HA, Fabian TC, Croce MA, Bynoe RP, Kudsk KA. Analysis of septic morbidity following gunshot wounds to the colon: the missile is an adjuvant for abscess. *J. Trauma* 1991; 31: 1088–94.

Porro Novo N, Flores Miranda E, Castells Avello R, Cuan Corrales R. Volvulus of the colon. Presentation of 22 cases. *Rev. Esp. Enferm. Apar. Dig.* 1989; 75: 583–8.

Pruett B. Laparoscopic colectomy for sigmoid volvulus. *J. Miss. State. Med. Assoc.* 1993; 34: 73–5.

Rehm CG, Talucci RC, Ross SE. Colostomy in trauma surgery: friend or foe? *Injury* 1993; 24: 595–6.

Ridgeway CA, Frame SB, Rice JC, Timberlake GA, McSwain NE Jr, Kerstein MD. Primary repair vs. colostomy for the treatment of penetrating colon injuries. *Dis. Colon Rectum* 1989; 32: 1046–9.

Rizzo MJ, Federle MP, Griffiths BG. Bowel and mesenteric injury following blunt trauma: evaluation with CT. *Radiology* 1989; 173: 143–8.

Rogy MA, Mirza DF, Kovats E, Rauhs R. Pneumatosis cystoides intestinalis (PCI). *Int. J. Colorect. Dis.* 1990; 5: 120–4.

Rosati C, Smith L, Deitel M, Burul CJ, Baida M, Borowy ZJ, Bryden P. Primary colorectal anastomosis with the intracolonic bypass tube. *Surgery* 1992; 112: 618–22.

Rutledge R, Thomason M, Oller D, Meredith W, Moylan J, Clancy T, et al. The spectrum of abdominal injuries associated with the use of seat belts. *J. Trauma* 1991; 31: 820 5.

Salim AS. Management of acute volvulus of the sigmoid colon: a new approach by percutaneous deflation and colopexy. *World J. Surg.* 1991; 15: 68–72.

Schagen Van Leeuwen JH. Sigmoid volvulus in a West African population *Dis. Colon Rectum* 1985; 28: 712–16.

Sharpe DR, Redwine DB. Laparoscopic segmental resection of the sigmoid and rectosigmoid colon for endometriosis. *Surg. Laparosc. Endosc.* 1992; 2: 120–4.

Shoop SA, Sackier JM. Laparoscopic cecopexy for cecal volvulus. Case report and a review of the literature. *Surg. Endosc.* 1993; 7: 450–4.

Siddins MT, Cade RJ. Hepatocolonic vagrancy: wandering liver with colonic abnormalities. *Aust. N.Z. J. Surg.* 1990; 60: 400–3.

Smith SD, Golladay ES, Wagner C, Seibert JJ. Sigmoid volvulus in childhood. *South Med. J.* 1990; 83: 778–81.

Sosa JL, Markley M, Sleeman D, Puente I, Carrillo E. Laparoscopy in abdominal gunshot wounds. *Surg. Laparosc. Endosc.* 1993; 3: 417–9.

Sroujieh AS, Farah GR, Jabaiti SK, el Muhtaseb HH, Qudah MS, Abu Khalaf MM. Volvulus of the sigmoid colon in Jordan. *Dis. Colon Rectum* 1992; 35: 64–8.

Strodel WE, Brothers T. Colonoscopic decompression of pseudo obstruction and volvulus. *Surg. Clin. North Am.* 1989; 69: 1327–35.

Tak PP, Van Duinen CM, Bun P, et al. Pneumatosis cystoides intestinalis in intestinal pseudoobstruction. Resolution after therapy with metronidazole. *Dig. Dis. Sci.* 1992; 37: 949–54.

Taylor GA, Kaufman RA, Sivit CJ. Active hemorrhage in children after thoracoabdominal trauma: clinical and CT features. *Am. J. Roentgenol.* 1994; 162: 401–4.

Thal ER, Yeary EC. Morbidity of colostomy closure following colon trauma. *J Trauma* 1980; 20: 287–90.

Theuer C, Cheadle WG. Volvulus of the colon. *Am. Surg.* 1991; 57: 145–50.

Thomas DD, Levison MA, Dykstra B, Bender J. Management of rectal injuries: dogma versus practice. *Am. Surg.* 1990; 56: 507–11.

Thompson SR, Huizinga WK, Baker LW. Bowel trauma. *Curr. Pract. Surg.* 1994; 6: 70–7.

Thompson SR, Baker A, Baker LW. Bowel trauma. *J. R. Coll. Surg. Edinburgh* 1996; 41: 20–4.

Townell NH, Vanderwalt JD. Intestinal endometriosis. *Postgrad. Med. J.* 1984; 60: 514–7.

Uohara JK, Kovara TY. Endometriosis of the appendix. Report of twelve cases and review of the literature. *Am. J. Obstet. Gynecol.* 1975; 121: 423–6.

van der Linden W, Marsell R. Pneumatosis cystoides coli associated with high H_2 excretion. Treatment with an elemental diet. *Scand. J. Gastroenterol.* 1979; 14: 173–4.

Wittoesch JH, Jackman RJ, McDonald JR. Melanosis coli: general review and a study of 887 cases. *Dis. Colon Rectum* 1958; 1: 172–80.

Woodward A, Lai L, Burgess B, Beynon J, Carr ND. A case of pneumatosis coli managed by restorative proctectomy and ileal pouch-anal anastomosis. *Int. J. Colorect. Dis.* 1995; 10: 181–2.

Wyman A, Zeiderman MR. Maintaining decompression of sigmoid volvulus. *Surg. Gynecol. Obstet.* 1989; 169: 265.

Zwas FR, Lyon DT. Endometriosis. An important condition in clinical gastroenterology. *Dig. Dis. Sci.* 1991; 36: 353–64.

18 Benign anal conditions

Anorectal abscesses

An anorectal abscess represents a cavity filled with pus and lined by a pyogenic membrane at any position from the lower rectum to the anal skin. The condition is closely associated with fistula in ano, the pathogenesis of the two conditions being similar.

Incidence

The exact incidence of anorectal abscesses is unknown. Perianal abscesses are the most common site, occurring in 43–70% of cases, followed by ischiorectal abscesses (23–39% of cases) (Winslett *et al.* 1988). The intersphincteric and supralevator spaces are involved in about 20% and 10% of cases, respectively.

Age and sex distribution

Most patients with anal sepsis are aged between 30 and 60 years (Isbister 1995). The male to female predominance is about 2:1. This may be related to less fastidious anal hygiene, greater anal sweating, and rougher clothing in males.

Aetiology

The major factor in formation of anorectal abscesses is extension of infection in the anal glands. In children, congenital dilatation of the ducts or thickening of the dentate line (an anorectal band) are possible causes. In adults, obstruction of the anal glands by foreign material, inflammation, or stenosis is the most likely initiating event. As a result of blockage , the internal opening is identified in only 25% of acute abscesses (Seow-Choen *et al.* 1993). Infection of the anal glands leads to an intersphincteric abscess which can spread to form abscesses at other sites in the anorectum (Figure 18.1). In the few cases (up to 20%) in which an infected anal gland cannot be detected, the abscess may have resulted from infection of an abrasion in the lining of the anal canal. This abrasion is nearly always caused by trauma such as a treatment of haemorrhoids (particularly injection sclerotherapy), infection of a perianal haematoma, or trauma from foreign bodies, anal intercourse, rough clothing, or the passage of hard faeces. Entry of organisms into the abrasion then leads to cellulitis and abscess formation. This is the probable mechanism in homosexuals, a group known to have a significantly higher incidence of anal sepsis and poor healing than heterosexuals (Carr *et al.* 1991).

In about 5% of cases of anorectal sepsis there is an underlying systemic disease, such as diabetes, leukaemia, or tuberculosis (Winslett *et al.* 1988; Myers 1994). One-third of AIDS patients develop anorectal problems. More commonly inflammatory bowel

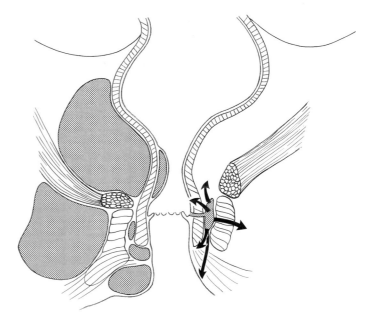

Figure 18.1 Aetiology of anal abscesses. An infected anal gland leads to an inter-sphincteric abscess which can then spread to cause infection at other sites.

disease or hidradenitis is identified. Anorectal abscesses occur in 15% of cases of Crohn's disease, depending on the site of bowel affected. Rarely, anorectal abscesses may be secondary to haematogenous spread from a septic focus elsewhere. Cases of perirectal abscesses nearly always demonstrate underlying pelvic sepsis from appendicitis, diverticulitis, or salpingitis, rather than a primary infection in the anal glands.

Bacteriology

Bacteriological studies show the predominance of 'gut-derived' organisms in anorectal abscesses. In up to 80% of abscesses *Bacteroides*, *Escherichia coli*, or *Streptococcus faecalis* can be identified. The presence of such organisms raises the possibility of an associated fistula (Kufahl and Andreasen 1992). Skin-derived *Staphylococcus aureus* does not suggest an underlying fistula, being cultured in 10% or less of anorectal abscesses associated with fistulas. In contrast, it can be grown in 30% of cases in which no fistula is apparent. Culture from an anorectal abscess is therefore of prognostic value in assessing recurrent sepsis and fistula formation (Kufahl and Andreassen 1992; Seow-Choen *et al.* 1993). Occasionally, tuberculosis or actinomycosis may be identified. The presence of these organisms, or other opportunistic infections, such as cryptococcus, suggests impaired immunity, as may be found in

AIDS or renal failure. Tetanus may also complicate anorectal sepsis, while worm infestation (*Trichuris trichuria* and *Enterobius vermicularis*) has also been implicated.

Pathology

Microscopically, the majority of anorectal abscesses show a pyogenic type of inflammatory reaction. Giant cells are frequently encountered, presumably as a response to the presence of faecal material in the abscess or associated fistulous tracts. When present, giant cells also raise the possibility of Crohn's disease or tuberculosis.

Classification

Anorectal abscesses are classified according to the principal tissue space involved. They may therefore be *intersphincteric, perianal, ischiorectal, submucosal, high intermuscular, supralevator,* or *pelvirectal* (Figure 18.2). Once infection is established it will spread along the path of least resistance. From the intersphincteric space spread can occur inferiorly (perianal abscess) or superiorly, either inside (intramuscular) or outside (supralevator) the bowel wall. Spread through the external sphincter at any level results in an ischiorectal abscess. Spread can also occur in a circumferential direction within any space. In the ischiorectal space pus can cross the deep posterior retro-anal space of Courtney resulting in a 'horseshoe' abscess.

Clinical presentation

Symptoms

Anorectal abscesses are tender and can be exquisitely painful. Spontaneous discharge, either internally or externally, relieves the pain. Persistent discharge suggests an underlying fistula in ano.

Signs

The classical rubor, calor, dolor, and tumour of an abscess cavity are usually present. In a perianal abscess, a red inflamed, tender, and possibly fluctuant swelling is apparent near the anus (Figure 18.3). Rectal examination is normal above the level of the visible

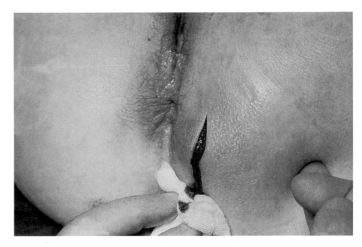

Figure 18.3 Ischiorectal abscess showing the features of acute inflammation.

swelling. Although similar findings may be present in an ischiorectal abscess, the swelling is frequently more diffuse and brawny. It may be bilateral with necrosis of the overlying skin. A small area of black gangrene suggests the possibility of extensive tissue necrosis. Rectal examination reveals tenderness, bulging, and induration in the anal canal in the presence of pyrexia and constitutional upset. High intramuscular or pelvirectal abscesses rarely have any external findings. Both should be palpable on digital rectal examination. Thickening of the anal wall is detectable by endoluminal ultrasound (Solomon *et al.* 1995).

Complications

Anorectal abscesses recur in up to one-third of patients. Following surgery recurrence rates of 6–16% are reported (Doberneck 1987). Frequent recurrence raises the possibility of Crohn's disease or hidradenitis suppurivata. Another frequent complication is that the anorectal abscess bursts through the skin, creating an anal fistula. A fistulous track can be identified in up to 40% of abscesses at the time of presentation. In studies on anorectal sepsis, fistulas occur in 6% of all abscesses (Doberneck 1987) and 8% and 2.5% of perianal and ischiorectal abscesses, respectively (Winslett *et al.* 1988). Cases with supralevator or intersphincteric abscesses are associated with a higher incidence of fistula or with diffuse peritonitis. When confronted with an anorectal abscess it is important to consider possible underlying immunosuppressed states such as diabetes, leukaemia, or AIDS. In these situations an anorectal abscess can run a very aggressive course and frequently be life-threatening (Angel *et al.* 1991). The mortality from perianal sepsis in haematological malignancy can be as high as 50%, but is normally about 20%. Wound healing in both haematological malignancy and those with AIDS is poor.

Treatment

Non-operative treatment of anorectal sepsis is rarely successful as perianal cellulitis almost invariably progresses to suppuration rather than spontaneous resolution. Relying on broad-spectrum antibiotics may therefore only delay surgery and result in more complex lesions. Surgical drainage is therefore nearly always indicated, irrespective of the patient's age (Abercrombie and George 1992). Bacteriological swabs should be taken as the presence of gut-derived organisms suggests the presence of an underlying fistula.

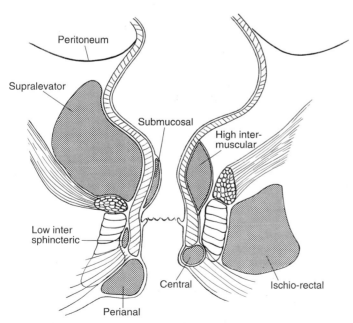

Figure 18.2 The tissue spaces that may be affected by ano-rectal sepsis.

Perianal abscesses may be drained by simply 'de-roofing' them using a cruciate incision. Intersphincteric abscesses can be drained into the anal canal after identifying the internal opening with a probe, or by partial division of the internal sphincter. Ischiorectal abscesses require de-roofing and breaking down of any septa or loculi in the involved ischiorectal space. If there has been supralevator extension into the pelvirectal space, fibres of the levator ani should be separated to allow adequate drainage. The transsphincteric fistula can then be dealt with at a later date.

Most interest has concerned the timing of surgery for an underlying fistula. Retrospective studies have shown that 50–75% of patients with perianal abscesses undergoing simple drainage will not have recurrent sepsis (Vasilevsky and Gordon 1985). The risk that inexperienced surgeons may create an artificial internal opening or sphincter damage in the acute phase has led to the suggestion that an examination under anaesthetic should be performed 1–2 weeks after drainage of the abscess to identify possible internal openings (Vasilevsky and Gordon 1985), although this is generally not done. Others also suggest that anorectal abscesses should be treated initially by simple incision and drainage alone as up to 85% of patients so treated will have no further sepsis within 1 year (Doberneck 1987; Seow-Choen *et al.* 1993). Treating identifiable fistulas at the time of simple drainage further lessens the risk of recurrent sepsis but altered anal function or incontinence in between 10% and 30% of cases with sphincter defects being detectable by endo-anal ultrasound (Seow-Choen *et al.* 1993; Felt-Bersma *et al.* 1995). Consequently, if a fistulous track is identified at the time of abscess drainage, it should only be laid open by a skilled and well trained surgeon. In immunosuppressed patients, both a conservative and an early surgical approach have been advocated (Corfitsen *et al.* 1992). Extensive perineal sepsis with a 'free-floating' anus requires combined antibiotic therapy, repeated vigorous debridement and occasionally a diverting colostomy.

Anal fistula

An anal fistula represents a chronic granulating track connecting an external opening in the perianal skin with an internal opening in the anal canal or rectum. If only one opening is apparent the terms blind fistula or perianal sinus are used. It is rare to have more than a single internal opening but the external opening may be multiple.

Incidence

In studies on anorectal sepsis, fistulas occur in 6% of all abscesses (Doberneck 1987) and in 8% and 2.5% of perianal and ischiorectal abscesses, respectively (Winslett *et al.* 1988). Those with supralevator or intersphincteric abscesses are associated with a higher incidence of fistulas. However, approximately one-third of patients presenting with an anal fistula will have no history of a previous abscess. Most patients with anal fistula are between 30 and 60 years. The average age is 38 years (Vasilevsky and Gordon 1985).

Aetiology

Anal fistulas may be either primary or secondary. Most anal fistulas are primary, the principal aetiological factor being infection of the anal glands leading to an intersphincteric abscess which discharges through the skin producing a fistulous connection between the anorectum and skin (Shouler *et al.* 1986). The intersphincteric

Table 18.1 The causes of anal fistula

Cause	Feature
Primary cause	
Infection of the anal glands	Accounts for 90% of all anal fistulas
Secondary causes	
Crohn's disease	Develops in over 20% of Crohn's patients
Ulcerative colitis	Develops in about 10% of UC patients
Trauma	Surgical, obstetric, radiotherapeutic
Tuberculosis	Accounts for 15% of fistulas in developing countries
Lymphogranuloma venerum	
Actinomycosis	
Anal canal tumour	

abscess acts as a reservoir for repeated infections, the chronic fistulous track being kept open by the presence of columnar epithelium lining the inner portion of the track. Infection of the anal glands is said to occur in up to 90% of fistulas. Consequently, anal fistulas are not identified in anorectal sepsis caused by non-intestinal organisms (Kufahl and Andreasen 1992). The chronicity of fistulas does not appear to be related to either the virulence or numbers of organisms identified. The predominant organisms are *E. coli* (22%), *Enterococcus* species (16%), and *Bacteroides fragilis* (20%).

Approximately 10% of fistulas can be attributed to a specific cause such as Crohn's disease, lymphogranuloma venerum, tuberculosis, or actinomycosis (Fry *et al.* 1992) (Table 18.1). Over 20% of patients with Crohn's disease will develop an anal fistula at some time during their illness (Figure 18.4). Anal fistulas were noted in 112 of 329 cases of Crohn's disease seen at St Mark's Hospital, the incidence of anal fistula with small bowel, large bowel, and rectal Crohn's disease being 10%, 25%, and 35%, respectively (Marks *et al.* 1981). Fistulas also occur in up to 14% of patients with ulcerative colitis, probably due to infection of small anal cracks or fissures.

Uncommon but important causes of anal fistula are colloid carcinoma of the anal canal, prostatic cancer, vulval carcinoma, tuberculosis, actinomycosis, lymphogranuloma venereum and diverticular disease (Josey 1988; Shukla *et al.* 1988). A pelvic abscess which has burst through the levator ani muscle may also produce a fistula.

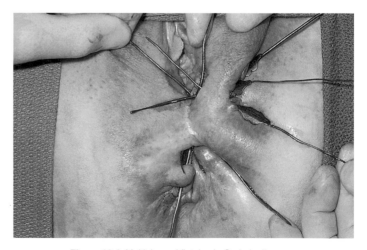

Figure 18.4 Multiple anal fistulas in Crohn's disease.

Fistulas may also be related to trauma including surgical, obstetrical or radiotherapeutic procedures (Nino-Murcia and Friedland 1988). While anal gland infection accounts for 90% of the causes of anal fistulas, the proportion attributed to trauma, ulcerative colitis, Crohn's disease, and tuberculosis is 4%, 1.5%, 1.5%, and 0.2%, respectively. In children, fistulas may arise from infected anal glands, as in adults (Shafer *et al.* 1987), or may be congenital in origin (Pople and Ralphs 1988; Poenaru and Yazbeck 1993). In the latter case, it is thought that invagination of the proctodeum into the hindgut creates an anorectal band which predisposes to infection of the intramuscular anal glands. Persistence of anal fistulas may be related more to non-specific epithelialization of the track than to a chronically infected anal gland (Lunniss *et al.* 1995).

Classification

An anal fistula may spread in a similar manner to abscesses; upward, downward, and around the anal canal, along the various tissue planes and spaces. This results in the fistulous track extending into either a trans-sphincteric, intersphincteric, subcutaneous, or suprasphincteric position. The relative proportion of each of these types of fistula in most general surgical units is about 60%, 30%, 8%, and 2%, respectively (Vasilevsky and Gordon 1985) (Figure 18.5). Approximately 10% and 20% of patients will have horseshoe or high fistulas, respectively (Saino and Husa 1985). In addition, fistulas extending distally to the skin may be grouped as type I, while those with an initial proximal high track have been called type II. Parks and Stitz (1976) classified a high fistula as one in which any part of the fistulous track, not just the internal opening, extends above the puborectalis. This may occur in several situations such as extra-sphincteric fistulas, supra-sphincteric fistulas or when there is supralevator extension from trans-sphincteric or ntrasphincteric tracts. A trans-sphincteric fistula with a high penetration of the sphincter mechanism, most commonly between the puborectalis and the deep part of the external sphincter will also result in a high fistula.

Pathology

Histologically, there is an acute on chronic inflammatory picture, together with prominent giant cells. It is important to distinguish the foreign body reaction seen in these circumstances from that of Crohn's disease or tuberculosis. Infection leads to surrounding fat necrosis, secondary vasculitis, and degeneration in striated muscle with the formation of giant hyperchromatic nuclei. In chronic cases fibrosis may be marked.

Clinical presentation

Symptoms

The typical symptoms of an anal fistula are intermittent discharge and recurrent sepsis.

Signs

Inspection may reveal the external opening as a papilla of granulation tissue, with or without evidence of mucopurulent discharge (Figure 18.6). The external opening is usually single, and if multiple implies a more complex fistula. The position of the opening has important clinical implications. Spread of pus from an infected anal gland is possible in the horizontal as well as the vertical plane. Fistulas with their external openings anterior to a transverse line drawn through the anus usually run down directly to the anal canal, while those posterior to this line run a curved course to reach the anal canal in the mid-line (Goodsall 1900). Whereas this is true for high fistulas, low anal fistulas generally follow a direct path to the anus, irrespective of the position of the opening on the anal circumference. No matter where the actual internal and external openings may occur, the horseshoe track around the circumference of the anus is constant. It follows closely the sling of the puborectalis

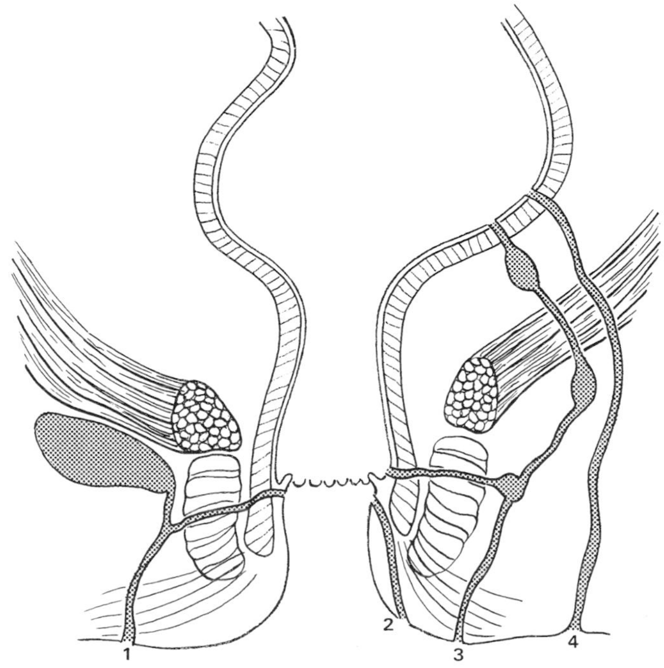

Figure 18.5 Classification of anal fistulas. 1 = Ischiorectal. 2 = Perianal. 3 = Trans-sphincteric (and pelvi-rectal). 4 = Supra-levator.

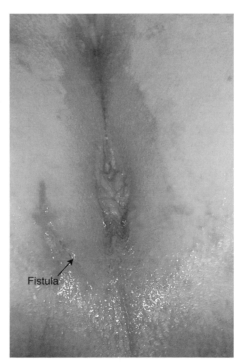

Figure 18.6 Anal fistula with opening at the 7 o'clock position (arrowed).

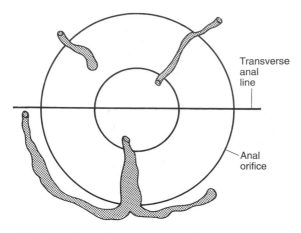

Figure 18.7 Goodsall's rule. Fistulae anterior to a line drawn transversely across the anus tend to run a straight, those posterior a curved, course to the anus.

muscle lying external to the uppermost part of the external sphincter and below or external to the lowermost part of the levator ani (Figure 18.7).

An anterior horseshoe fistula is likely if the anterior opening is greater than 2.5 cm from the anal verge, or if the fistulas are multiple or recurrent (Aluwihare 1987). Despite claims that Goodsall's rule is followed in 97% of cases, others suggest it is only accurate when applied to complete submuscular anal fistulas with posterior external anal openings, when 90% will track to the mid-line (Cirocco and Reilly 1993). The radial course predicted by Goodsall is seen in only half of anterior fistulas. Although the external opening may be multiple, there is always a single internal opening.

Diagnosis

Rectal examination may reveal an area of induration, suggesting the site of the internal opening. Circumferential, intersphincteric, or supralevator spread can also be detected. Proctoscopy and sigmoidoscopy should be performed but are frequently unhelpful. Several methods have been devised to identify the tracks of anal fistulas (Table 18.2). Injection of radio-opaque dye (fistulography) is felt by some to be beneficial, identifying the primary track in all, a secondary track in 60% and the internal opening in 20% of cases (Weisman *et al.* 1992). Others suggest that radiology is of limited value, as rectal examination by a consultant assesses 78% of anal

Table 18.2 Techniques available to diagnose anal fistulas	
Technique	Author
Visualization of internal opening using:	Aluwihare 1987
Hydrogen peroxide	Cheong *et al.* 1993
Fistulography	Weisman *et al.* 1992
Endoanal ultrasound	Law *et al.* 1989,
	Buchmann 1990
	Hussain *et al.* 1996
	Farouk *et al.* 1997
CT/MR and isotope scanning	Hussain *et al.* 1996,
	de Souza *et al.* 1996
Anal manometry	Lewis *et al.* 1994

tracks more accurately than ultrasound (Henrichsen and Christiansen 1986; Choen *et al.* 1991).

Other specific causes of fistulation, such as Crohn's disease, tuberculosis, or lymphogranuloma venerum should be sought. The appearances of an anal fistula may be closely mimicked by hidradenitis suppurivata. However, in this infection of the apocrine glands the tracks are short, multiple, do not track deeply close to the sphincters and the anal verge is not affected. The inguinal and axillary regions may also be involved. A spontaneously discharging fistula on the peri-urethral skin may be caused by a urethral stricture leading to obstruction and subsequent infection in the peri-urethral glands. Although an anal fistula may occasionally occur at this anterior site, induration around the track should be easily palpable. An anal carcinoma may also present as an anal fistula (Nelson *et al.* 1985). In female patients an anterior fistula may be mimicked by a Bartholin gland infection, while a high intersphincteric abscess with pelvic extension may simulate gynaecological disease (Evaldson 1986). Endoanal ultrasound is an accurate method of identifying anal sphincter defects with a sensitivity and specificity of 100% for external anal sphincter; 100% and 95%, respectively, for internal anal sphincter defects (Deen *et al.* 1993; Alexander *et al.* 1994; Tio and Kallimanis 1994). In one study the accuracy of clinical examination in correctly locating anal fistulas was 50%, that of both electromyography and anal manometry 75%, while that of endoanal ultrasound 100% (Sultan *et al.* 1994). Further information can be obtained by injecting hydrogen peroxide into the fistulous tract prior to performing ultrasound (Cheong *et al.* 1993).

Magnetic resonance imaging shows abnormalities not detected by pre-operative digital examination (Lunniss *et al.* 1994; Van Beers *et al.* 1996) (Figure 18.8) The fistulous tracks with their secondary extensions and abscesses are readily seen as low signal on T1-weighted images and high signal areas on alternative (STIR) images (Barker *et al.* 1994; Semelka *et al.* 1997). Visualization of complex fistulous systems with sparse secretion can be improved by using saline as a contrast agent (Myhr *et al.* 1994). Concordance rates between MRI and operative findings are 85% for presence and course of the primary track, 90% for the presence and site of secondary extensions or abscesses, and 97% for the presence of 'horseshoeing' (Barker *et al.* 1994; deSouza *et al.* 1996; Hussain *et al.* 1996).

Complications

An untreated anal fistula may occasionally heal spontaneously if the lining of the granulation tissue is covered by squamous epithelium. This most commonly occurs if a subcutaneous fistula has arisen from an anal fissure, or in the case of a chronic low transphincteric fistula (Garcia-Aguilar *et al.* 1996. Left untreated, the periodic release of pus from the openings prevents the formation of new fistulous tracks, so that fistulas do not become more complicated in nature. Carcinoma may arise in a long-standing fistula, the incidence being estimated at 0.1%. This has been attributed to chronic irritation of the granulation tissue of the track, although a more likely explanation is malignancy occurring in columnar epithelium from congenital duplication of the hindgut. Carcinoma complicating anal fistulas is best treated by abdominoperineal resection.

Treatment

Recently, conservative measures, such as autologous fibrin glue, have been used to occlude complex, recurrent, or cancerous fistulas (Abel *et al.* 1990). In cases of Crohn's or AIDS fistulas, fibrin glue decreases the discharge, but healing is less likely than with other

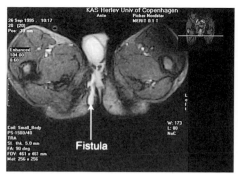 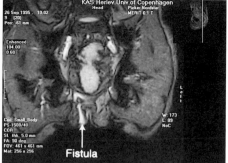

Figure 18.8 T2 weighted sagittal and coronal MR scans of a patient with a high Crohn's anal fistula (arrowed).

causes. The majority of anal fistulas are therefore best treated surgically.

Low intra- or trans-sphincteric fistulas, running below the sphincters, irrespective of age, are successfully treated by laying open of the fistula (Garcia-Aguilar *et al.* 1996). There appears to be little difference between fistulotomy and fistulectomy with primary closure. Time to healing may be slightly quicker with fistulectomy but recurrence rates at 1 year are similar (4%) (Kronborg 1985; Parkash *et al.* 1985). Laying open is the treatment of choice for low fistulas as it is a definitive (2–6% recurrence of anal sepsis) and safe (0.5–4% prolonged impairment of continence) procedure (Piazza and Radhakrishnan 1990; Fucini 1991). Recurrence is most commonly due to a missed track (Vasilevsky and Gordon 1985; Garcia-Aguilar *et al.* 1996). However, persistence in trying to identify the openings results in healing in most cases. Normal continence, leakage of mucus, flatus, or faeces occur in 80%, 10%, 5%, and 5%, respectively. Multiple previous fistula surgery and a gutter-shaped, firm scar are important in determining postoperative incontinence (Sainio and Husa 1985).

For high trans- and supra-sphincteric fistulas, preservation of the puborectalis is important in maintaining continence. In these circumstances, one-stage fistulotomy and occlusion of the internal opening is associated with a 20–30% recurrence rate and between 15% and 40% impairment of continence. In contrast, staged fistulotomy, using a Seton suture is a safe and effective method of treating high or complicated anorectal fistulas (Garcia-Aguilar *et al.* 1996) (Figure 18.9). The indications for Seton suture insertion include prevention of fibrosis around complex fistulas, anterior high transphincteric fistulas in females, anorectal Crohn's disease, massive sepsis with free floating anus, and AIDS (McCourtney and Finlay 1995). Seton fistulotomy with counter drainage is the treatment of choice for horseshoe fistulas associated with abscesses. Recurrent fistulas occur in 18% of cases treated by a Seton, compared with almost one-third of those undergoing simple fistulotomy (Held *et al.* 1986). Setons cure 85% of high fistulas often without causing major incontinence, although up to 60% of cases experience at least some disturbance of sphincter function (Garcia-Olmo *et al.* 1994; Graf *et al.* 1995). Recurrent fistulas occur in 3% of cases following Seton suture insertion, major faecal incontinence requiring a pad occurring in 5% of cases.

Alternative techniques include preservation of the external sphincter and this may be associated with a lower recurrence rate, an intersphincteric approach with total sphincter conservation (Matos *et al.* 1993) or re-routing the extra-sphincteric portion of the fistula (Mann and Clifton 1985).

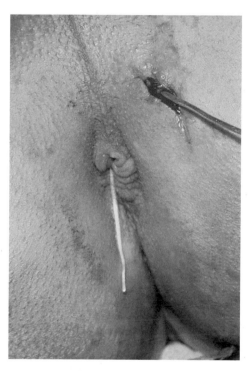

Figure 18.9 Track of high anal fistula outlined prior to insertion of a Seton suture.

A sliding anorectal mucosal flap can be used to close the internal opening after fistula excision and counter-drainage of the fistula track (Fazio 1987; Rutten and Buth 1988; Klotz and Buchmann 1993). Complete healing occurs after an average of 2 months with preservation of sphincter function in almost all cases (Marti and Koscinki 1992). Advancement flaps are particularly useful in anterior fistulas in females, which are associated with a high risk of sphincter disturbance by other techniques, including Setons (Shemesh *et al.* 1988; Pescatori *et al.* 1995). Following mucosal advancement flaps, 80% of patients will be asymptomatic with about 20% experiencing minor soiling or incontinence of flatus (Aguilar *et al.* 1985; Leong and Seow-Choen 1995). For extra-sphincteric fistulas, fistula excision, plastic transfer of mucosa for closure of the internal opening with preservation of sphincter function is advised.

In studies of rectovaginal fistulas that persist after previous treatment, three-quarters of simple fistulas and 40% of complex fistulas healed following further treatment (MacRae *et al.* 1995; Mazier *et al.* 1995). Healing following sphincteroplasty and fistulectomy was

86%, coloanal anastomosis 67%, advancement flap 30%, and gracilis transposition 100%. The authors suggest that advancement flap repair is generally not recommended for persistent complex fistulas or for simple fistulas that have failed a previous advancement flap repair (MacRae *et al.* 1995).

Anal fissure

Anal fissure is a common condition the exact incidence of which is unknown (Isbister and Prasad 1995*a*). Fissures can occur at any age, including infancy, but are most frequently seen in young or middle-aged adults. Although both sexes are equally affected, anterior fissures are more common in women than men, accounting for 10% of all fissures in females, but only 1% of fissures in males. Anal fissure occurs more commonly in Western countries, probably related to the low fibre diet consumed in these regions.

Aetiology

Anal fissures are caused by a mixture of dietary and mechanical factors (Jensen 1987). The passage of hard stool is the principal underlying factor leading to spasm of the internal sphincter (Keck *et al.* 1995). It was formerly thought that the faecal bolus created a linear tear which began at the anal valve and extended towards the anal margin. However, the anal valve is only rarely involved. Weakness in the anal wall posteriorly along with infection and subsequent ulceration in the anal glands, which are more common posteriorly, partly accounts for the tendency of anal fissures to be located at this site. The anal orifice normally forms an anteroposterior slit. With straining, the anorectal angle is modified and the posterior anal canal becomes less well supported than the anterior portion and therefore is maximally subjected to the trauma of the faecal bolus.

Anal blood flow studies have shown that in 85% of the population, the posterior commisure is less well perfused than the rest of the anal canal (Schouten *et al.* 1994). The blood supply is further compromised by contusion of the vessels as they pass vertically through the muscle fibres of the internal sphincter during increased sphincter tone. This accounts for the pain and poor healing of anal fissures. The relatively high frequency of anterior fissures in females can be explained by an additional weak area occurring between the vulva, vagina, and perineal body (Corby *et al.* 1997). Loss of elasticity of the epithelium below the dentate line predisposes to the delayed healing and chronicity of anal fissures. Loss of elasticity may be exacerbated by chronic diarrhoea, the passage of alkaline faeces, or irritant laxative abuse. Surgery which results in a mid-line wound may also account for some fissures if the wound deepens to the level of the internal sphincter. In some cases infection, histoplasmosis (Recondo *et al.* 1991), proctocolitis or Crohn's disease may also give rise to fissures. Traumatic fissures may occur in up to 50% of homosexuals (Carr *et al.* 1991).

Rectal examination is a poor assessment of anal incontinence (Sainio 1985). Most manometric studies suggest that the resting and maximal anal pressure in patients with anal fissures are elevated (McNamara *et al.* 1992; Melange *et al.* 1992; Xynos *et al.* 1993; Farouk *et al.* 1994; Romano *et al.* 1994; Horvath *et al.* 1995).

Pathology

Histologically, an anal fissure shows features of non-specific inflammation. The edges of a chronic fissure are thickened and under-mined with adjacent oedema and a heavy lymphocyte and plasma cell infiltration. Fibrosis is seen throughout the internal sphincter (Brown *et al.* 1989).

Clinical presentation

Symptoms

Acute anal fissures are characterized by severe pain on defecation associated with the passage of a small amount of bright red blood on the motion or paper.

Signs and differential diagnosis

An anal fissure is always situated superficial to the lower third of the internal sphincter. Initially, the floor of the fissure consists of the subcutaneous fibres of the longitudinal muscle. Failure of the fissure to heal leads to erosion of longitudinal muscle revealing the circular fibres of the internal sphincter at the base of the fissure. The presence of even a small fissure results in intense spasm of the internal sphincter, which becomes worse once the internal sphincter fibres are exposed. Fibrosis of the sphincter in the presence of this spasm leads in time to a tightly contracted internal sphincter (Notaras 1988).

The typical fissure is a longitudinal ulcer usually located posteriorly in the mid-line and extending anywhere from the dentate line to the anal verge. These findings may be mimicked by several other anal conditions. In pruritis ani the cracks are multiple, superficial and never extend as far as the dentate line. In ulcerative colitis fissures are multiple, broad, inflamed, and occur some distance away from the mid-line. They occur in 7% of patients with colitis. The ulcers of Crohn's disease are more oedematous, have larger skin tags, and may be painless. The appearances in tuberculosis are similar but there is a tendency for the ulcer to be large and irregular with eroded edges. Either squamous or adenocarcinoma of the anus may present with ulceration. By this stage they are usually extensive and clinically apparent at the anus on digital examination. The primary chancre of syphilis may be very similar to an anal fissure but is often bilateral, covered in a serous discharge and associated with inguinal lymphadenopathy; although commonly painless, pain may be a prominent feature and associated condylomata are frequent. In leukaemia the lesions are indurated and frequently infected. Stenosis of the internal sphincter may occur in chronic laxative abuse due to the lack of the dilating action of faeces.

Complications

At the lower end of the fissure, low-grade infection and lymphatic oedema may result in the formation of a tag-like swelling, a 'sentinel pile'. Even after the fissure has healed fibrosis may result in a permanent skin tag (Petros *et al.* 1993). However, spontaneous healing may occur in 70% of Crohn's fissures (Sweeney *et al.* 1988). At the craniad end of the fissure oedema and fibrosis of the anal valves may result in a hypertrophied anal papilla or anal polyp (Figure 18.10). The lateral edges of the fissure may become fibrotic and indurated in chronic cases, while pruritis ani may result from a persistent discharge or insufficient local hygiene. Infection of the fissure leads to a perianal abscess which may burst into the anal canal. Alternatively it may extend as a short, low fistulous track close to the mid-line posteriorly or open into the perianal skin. Loss of elasticity may be exacerbated by chronic diarrhoea, the passage of alkaline faeces or irritant laxative abuse. Surgery which results in a mid-line wound may also account for some fissures if the wound

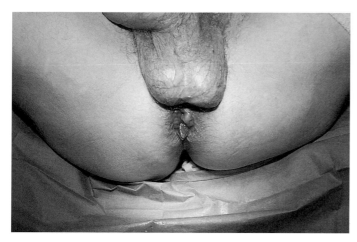

Figure 18.10 Prolapsed anal polyp.

deepens to the level of the internal sphincter. In some cases infection, histoplasmosis (Recondo *et al.* 1991), proctocolitis, or Crohn's disease may also give rise to fissures. Traumatic fissures may occur in up to 50% of homosexuals (Carr *et al.* 1991).

Treatment

Conservative treatments

Non-surgical measures cure up to 40% of patients at 5 years, although one-quarter of these will subsequently develop a recurrence. Frezza *et al.* (1992) found no significant difference in the mean time to healing of acute (45 days versus 40 days) or chronic (40 days versus 30 days) anal fissures in patients treated conservatively or surgically. The use of local ointments is safe and without side-effects, while dietary bulk and laxatives are important in maintaining healing of anal fissures. In a study comparing lignocaine, hydrocortisone, and a combination of Sitz baths and bran, fissure healing was 60%, 82%, and 87%, respectively (Jensen 1986). Glycerine trinitrate ointment may also prove beneficial (Lund *et al.* 1996; Watson *et al.* 1996).

Anal dilatation

Immediate pain relief occurs following 95% of anal dilatations, although minor soiling and incontinence of flatus or faeces occur in 20%, 12%, and 2% of cases, respectively (Romano *et al.* 1994) (Table 18.3). Anal dilatation successfully treats about 55% of anal fissures without risk of wound complications, but about 25% of patients will develop some degree of incontinence (90% of these being

Table 18.3 Comparison of anal dilatation and sphincterotomy for anal fissure

	Anal dilatation	Sphincterotomy
Healing at 1 month	55–95%	95%
Incontinence:	20% (3–39%)	5% (3–15%)
Minor soiling	20%	5%
of flatus	12%	2%
of faeces	2%	1%
Wound problems	0%	2–10%
Recurrent fissure	16% (10–30%)	6% (3–29%)

females) (MacDonald *et al.* 1992; Saad and Omer 1992). In a study comparing conservative therapy, dilatation, and subcutaneous sphincterotomy, it was suggested that dilatation should be performed first, sphincterotomy being reserved for treatment failures (Giebel and Horch 1989). Anal dilatation, precisely performed with a Parks' retractor is successful in curing 95% of fissures.

Sphincterotomy

Internal sphincterotomy heals over 90% of anal fissures, the mean time to healing being about 3 weeks (Saad and Omer 1992; Blessing 1993; Xynos *et al.* 1993) (Table 18.3). In Crohn's disease, nearly 90% of fissures will eventually heal following sphincterotomy (Wolkomir and Luchtefeld 1993). Sphincterotomy produces a global, symmetrical decrease in anal canal resting pressure and a significant increase in manometric asymmetry of the resting anal canal by creating a detectable segmental defect (Williams *et al.* 1995).

Minor complications include pain, pruritus, wound abscess, discharge, delayed healing, bleeding, faecal impaction, minor incontinence, and urgency and occur in 15% of patients (Pernikoff *et al.* 1994). Wound problems, such as bruising or infection occur in under 10% of cases (Pons and Muntada 1989; Saad and Omer 1992). Most series comparing dilatation with sphincterotomy suggest that dilatation is associated with a higher recurrence rate (10–30% versus 3–29%) with greater impairment of continence (7–39% versus 3–15%).

Results with lateral, posterior, or bilateral sphincterotomies are generally similar (Khubchandani and Reed 1989; Saad and Omer 1992). Most reports suggest that lateral sphincterotomy is associated with a shorter healing time, lower recurrence, and less problem with incontinence (Pernikoff *et al.* 1994). Performing a subcutaneous, as opposed to open, sphincterotomy, gives pain relief in 95%, although minor soiling (5%), incontinence of flatus (2%), or faeces (1%) do occur (Pernikoff *et al.* 1994). Closed sphincterotomy is also associated with a shorter hospital stay (mean 1.7 days versus 2.3 days) and similar healing (97% versus 95%) to the open procedure (Kortbeek *et al.* 1992; Pernikoff *et al.* 1994). However, combining fistula excision and sphincterotomy results in about 40% of patients experiencing pain for up to 1 month and a higher incidence of incontinence for both flatus (35%) and faeces (5%) (Saad and Omer 1992). Recurrence of anal fissure following sphincterotomy is reported in 0–7% of cases, compared with 16% after anal dilatation (Simkovic 1989; Pernikoff *et al.* 1994; Farouk *et al.* 1997). Careful patient selection, absence of pre-operative continence problems, and meticulous surgical techniques are necessary to achieve this type of result (Pernikoff *et al.* 1994; Prohm and Bonner 1995). C-anoplasty should be done when strictures are present while excision of the protruding internal sphincter is recommended in patients who present with an excessively elongated, tight anal canal with a partially protruding internal sphincter (Oh *et al.* 1995).

Recently, cryotherapy, lasers, botulin toxin, and topical nitroglycerine have been used to treat anal fissures (Senagore *et al.* 1993; Watson *et al.* 1996). Cryotherapy controls pain in 85% of anal fissures (Krasznay 1990), while the carbon dioxide laser is claimed to have a 2% recurrence rate and fewer complications than other procedures (Babaev *et al.* 1990). Botulin toxin or nitroglycerine act by paralysing or relaxing the sphincters, allowing the fissure to heal (Jost and Schimrigk 1994; Gorfine 1995; Lund and Scholefield 1997). Patients with recurrent fissures and weak anal sphincters may be successfully treated by advancement flaps (Nyam *et al.* 1995).

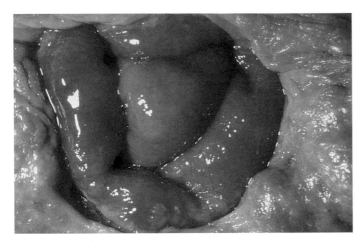

Figure 18.11 Haemorrhoids appearing on straining highlighting the dilatation of the anal cushions.

Haemorrhoids

Haemorrhoids occur in very few species other than humans and have been recognized since antiquity. The definition currently most widely accepted is that haemorrhoids represent an hypertrophy of the normal anal cushions lying in the upper part of the anal canal (Figure 18.11).

Incidence

The exact number of patients affected by haemorrhoids has never been documented, but the prevalence is estimated at 1 in 25 of the population (Cohen 1985). It is estimated that 50–90% of all individuals will complain of haemorrhoids at least once in their lives (Nelson *et al.* 1995). The reported prevalence of haemorrhoids is 86%, being similar in those with or without symptoms. Similarly, 80% of all men and 60% of all women were found to have skin tags representing external haemorrhoids. This makes it the most frequent anal pathology accounting for up to 50% of patients attending a proctology clinic.

Age and sex distribution

Haemorrhoids can occur at any age, including children. The frequency of skin tags increases in women at the beginning of the second, and in men the fourth, decade, respectively. There is a direct proportional relationship with increasing age, at least 50% of patients over 50 years having some degree of haemorrhoids. This may be related to weakening of the anal canal supporting tissue and decrease in the basal anal pressure with age (Hiltunen and Malikamen 1985).

Aetiology

Persistent straining at stool is a major factor leading to haemorrhoids. Although this is commonly due to constipation, tenesmus, persistent diarrhoea, or an enlarged prostate gland may also result in prolonged straining (Akande and Esho 1989). However, constipation *per se* cannot be the sole factor. Haemorrhoids are more common in white people and higher socio-economic groups, while constipation is more frequent in black people and lower socio-economic groups (Johanson and Sonnenberg 1990).

It is recognized that patients with haemorrhoids, especially young males, have a higher basal pressure than controls (Chen *et al.* 1989; Lin 1989; Sun *et al.* 1992). There is controversy whether the maximal squeeze pressure varies significantly from controls (Hiltunen and Matikainen 1985; Sun *et al.* 1992). However, haemorrhoidectomy does result in a reduction in the basal and squeeze pressures to normal levels, suggesting that these changes are more likely to be an effect, rather than the cause, of enlarged anal cushions (Ho *et al.* 1995). Patients with haemorrhoids are also noted to have significantly more ultra-slow wave activity than controls (42% versus 5%), the slow wave activity also returning to normal following haemorrhoidectomy. The abnormally high pressures may be related to increased vascular pressure in the anal cushions or pain, as there is no significant difference in internal sphincter thickness between those with, and those without, haemorrhoids (Sun *et al.* 1992). Patients with haemorrhoids are also more likely to have abnormal perineal descent due to pudendal neuropathy than controls (Heslop 1987; Bruck *et al.* 1988). Although some authors suggest a significant correlation between anal manometry and the degree of haemorrhoids, duration of symptoms and the presence of bleeding (Hiltunen and Matikainen 1985), other reports have not found such an association. It therefore appears that patients with haemorrhoids are not necessarily constipated but exhibit abnormal anal pressure and compliance (Gibbons *et al.* 1988).

Although haemorrhoids are common in those with oesophageal varices, the prevalence of haemorrhoids is not significantly increased in this group relative to controls (Hosking *et al.* 1989). True anorectal varices should be distinguished from haemorrhoids, as bleeding from them can be severe (Weinshel *et al.* 1986; Heaton *et al.* 1993) and their appearances on CT scan, if large, may mimic a rectal carcinoma (Ben-Chetrit and Bal-Ziv 1992).

Patients developing haemorrhoids at an early age may show evidence of a familial tendency to haemorrhoids with possible weakness in the walls of the haemorrhoidal veins. An additional factor may be persistence of the anorectal band, a remnant of the anorectal sinus, which results in elevation of the rectal neck pressure with straining at defecation and the initiation of haemorrhoids.

A deficiency of the sphincter following operations for anal fistulas may result in a haemorrhoid due to loss of the normal support for the venous plexus. Pregnancy is one of the commonest causes for haemorrhoids in women. In this case haemorrhoids can be attributed to the increased vascularity and laxity of the tissues, along with the pelvic venous obstruction caused by the fetus. Postpartum, there is not necessarily a return to complete normality.

There is no evidence to support a causative relationship between rectal carcinoma and haemorrhoids.

Three major theories for the formation of haemorrhoids have been proposed.

1. Haemorrhoids represent abnormal varicosities of the internal (submucous) haemorrhoidal venous plexus, a network of tributaries of the middle and superior haemorrhoidal veins. In portal hypertension or in defecation and straining, these varicosities bulge into the anal lumen (Ganguly *et al.* 1995). Against this theory is that dilatation of the internal venous plexus (the 'corpus cavernosum recti') appears to be a feature of normal anal anatomy and the histological features of haemorrhoidectomy specimens are virtually indistinguishable from those of normal anorectal submucosa.

2. Haemorrhoids are caused by transphincteric reflux of blood associated with an abnormal distension of arteriovenous anastomoses located at the same site as the anal cushions.

3. The theory currently receiving most support is that stretching of the submucosal fibres of the longitudinal muscle allows downward displacement of the anal cushions. Internal haemorrhoids therefore arise from congestion and hypertrophy of the corpus cavernosum recti cushion above the dentate line. Communication with vessels below the dentate line results in the formation of external haemorrhoids. Repeated venous congestion or thrombosis detaches the mucosa from the muscular coat leading to intermittent, and eventually permanent, prolapse of the mucosa and perineal skin. Support for this theory comes from tissue oximetric and thermoconduction studies, which suggest that the bright red rectal bleeding associated with haemorrhoids is related to the middle and inferior haemorrhoidal arteries supplying the cushions, rather than to bleeding from a venous plexus.

Pathology

Histologically, haemorrhoidectomy specimens often resemble normal anorectal mucosa (Kaftan and Haboubi 1995). Occasionally, there is an increase in the venous sinus lumen to wall thickness ratio (Morgado *et al.* 1988) along with increased fibrosis of the internal sphincter. Submucosal neuronal hyperplasia is seen in one-fifth of haemorrhoidectomy specimens. Third-degree haemorrhoids may become sclerotic with painful epidermal metaplasia and dilatation of the surface venules.

Clinical presentation

Symptoms

Haemorrhoids commonly present with anal pain or discomfort, pruritis ani, rectal bleeding, or faecal soiling. The symptoms of haemorrhoids are therefore non-specific and mimic a multitude of other anal conditions. Although patients with haemorrhoids may have mild sensory deficit, continence is usually maintained by other mechanisms.

Signs

Haemorrhoids are consistently seen in the right anterior, right posterior, and left lateral positions, corresponding to the 11, 7, and 3 o'clock positions of the lithotomy position. This is probably due to differences in the number of branches between the right and left superior haemorrhoidal artery, although injection studies have failed to demonstrate this (Figure 18.12). Secondary piles may arise between the primary piles. Haemorrhoids are classified according to the degree of prolapse. Internal haemorrhoids arise in the upper two-thirds of the anal canal, lined by columnar epithelium. External haemorrhoids arise from the lower skin-covered portion of the canal. However, with time haemorrhoids will appear external to the anus. First-degree haemorrhoids are due to bulging of the corpus cavernosum recti into the anal lumen without prolapse. In second-degree haemorrhoids there is prolapse upon straining which spontaneously reduces. The corpus cavernosum recti cannot maintain perfect continence and patients may complain of mucosal discharge. Third-degree haemorrhoids show a permanent prolapse that can be replaced digitally, while fourth-degree haemorrhoids cannot be replaced.

Diagnosis

Proctoscopy is the mainstay of the diagnosis of haemorrhoids with good correlation between observers. In cases of rectal bleeding, sigmoidoscopy is recommended for patients over 40 years because of

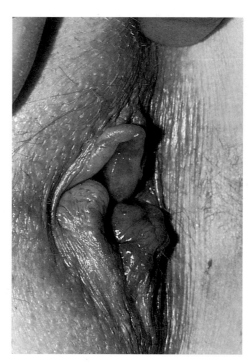

Figure 18.12 Haemorrhoids in the classical 3, 7, and 11 o'clock positions.

the significant risk of colorectal carcinoma. In cases of rectal bleeding thought to be due to haemorrhoids, colonoscopy reveals an unsuspected carcinoma in 1%, angiodysplasia in a further 1%, and benign polyps in 22% (Pines *et al.* 1987).

Complications

Excessive straining may result in thrombosis of an internal haemorrhoid, while haemorrhoidal rupture creates a perianal haematoma (Figure 18.13). The ensuing oedema affects all three cushions, producing a circumferential mucosal prolapse. Chronic perianal venous engorgement or anal haematoma leads to further sclerosis and the development of anal skin tags. Secondary haemorrhage, ulceration and pyelophlebitis with subsequent anal stricture may all then

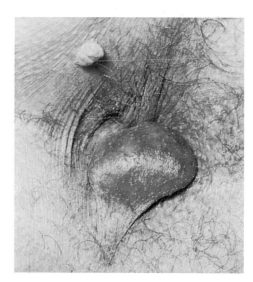

Figure 18.13 Perianal haematoma.

occur. The risk of infection with possible portal pyaemia is particularly present in immunocompromised or haematological patients. Chronic venous congestion results in redundant perianal skin or anal skin tags. Perianal haematomas represent thrombosis within thin-walled vessels of the external venous plexus. This presents as a hard, well defined blue-coloured lump without oedema of the other anal cushions. Other complications of haemorrhoids include prostatic venous congestion caused by milking of the prostate with hard stools and urethral discharge with recurrent *E. coli* bacteruria.

Treatment

Medication

Non-operative treatments remain the mainstay of haemorrhoidal therapy (Dennison *et al.* 1988; Ferguson 1988). A high roughage diet and simple ointments relieve symptoms in 45% of patients with haemorrhoids and remains an important first treatment (Bleday *et al.* 1992). Local ointments will produce a 75–90% improvement in symptoms within 3 weeks (Smith and Moodie 1988). Patients with complications such as thrombosed haemorrhoids can be adequately treated with Sitz baths, ice bags, and ointments. However, medical therapy does not alter anal manometry pressures and improvements are often transient.

Sclerotherapy

The role of sclerotherapy is declining and should be confined to first- or second-degree haemorrhoids (Bruhl 1993) (Table 18.4). Pain occurs in 60% of cases, being severe in 10% (Mann *et al.* 1988). Sclerotherapy initially cures 84% of haemorrhoidal bleeding and 56% of mucosal prolapse (Varma *et al.* 1991). However, its long-term effectiveness in controlling bleeding is doubtful. Although 88% of patients are satisfied with the treatment, control of bleeding at 1 month is only about 40% (Mann *et al.* 1988). In a prospective randomized trial, there was no significant difference in bleeding up to 6 months with bulk laxatives alone compared with bulk laxatives combined with sclerotherapy (Senapati and Nicholls 1988).

Rubber band ligation (RBL) (Table 18.4)

Compared with sclerotherapy, RBL is associated with a significantly better outcome (90% patient satisfaction compared with 70%), particularly for symptoms of bleeding and prolapse (Weinstein *et al.* 1987) (Figure 18.14). Following RBL, 45–90% of patients will become asymptomatic, with up to 85% of patients remaining asymptomatic at 1 year (Bleday *et al.* 1992). Severe pain is experienced by 10% of patients (Choi *et al.* 1985). Over 80% of patients experience pain within the first 24 h following banding (Hardwick and Durdy 1994). Injection of local anaesthetic alleviates the sensa-

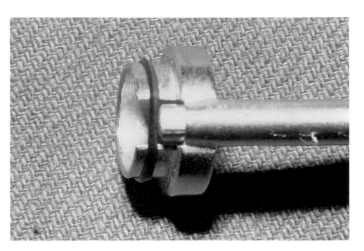

Figure 18.14 Rubber band applicator.

tion of fullness, but severe pain from improper placement of bands too low requires removal. Minor complications such as urinary retention or infection occur in about 5% of patients (Bat *et al.* 1993). About 60% of patients will require more than one treatment and approximately 2% require hospital admission for prolonged bleeding (Bat *et al.* 1993). Severe pelvic sepsis has been reported following RBL (Scarpa *et al.* 1988; Quevedo-Bonilla *et al.* 1988).

Following RBL excellent results are obtained in 75%, a good response in 20% and no improvement in 5% of cases (Cermak *et al.* 1992). Overall patient satisfaction is 80–95% (Bat *et al.* 1993). Combining sclerotherapy with RBL has little additional benefit (Choi *et al.* 1985). However, a high roughage diet is important, recurrent haemorrhoids occurring in up to 85% of patients who remain constipated, compared with 15% of those who are on bran (Jensen *et al.* 1989; Mattana *et al.* 1989). Consequently, haemorrhoidectomy within 2 years is required in 1–6% of cases undergoing RBL (Alemdaroglu and Ulualp 1993). Meta-analysis reveals that rubber band ligation is recommended as the initial mode of therapy for grade 1–3 haemorrhoids (MacRae and McLeod 1995). Although haemorrhoidectomy shows better response rates, it is associated with more complications and pain than rubber band ligation, thus should be reserved for patients who fail to respond to rubber band ligation (MacRae and McLeod 1995).

Coagulation

Infra-red coagulation (IRC) offers good treatment for first- and second-degree haemorrhoids, being safer and associated with less pain than sclerotherapy, rubber band ligation or haemorrhoidectomy (O'Holleran 1990) (Table 18.4; Figure 18.15). At 1 month, 66% of patients undergoing IRC will be asymptomatic, 27% will have some improvement, and 7% no improvement (Sorf *et al.* 1993). However, although significantly more patients are symptom-free than with sclerotherapy at 3 months (80% versus 60%), there is no difference at 1 or 4 years (Walker *et al.* 1990). Combining IRC with conservative measures will relieve symptoms in up to 85% of patients. Following IRC 20% of patients will experience pain, 13% mild discomfort, and 10% minor bleeding (Zinberg *et al.* 1989, Sorf *et al.* 1993).

The use of the direct current probe is claimed to give good results in up to 95% of cases (Zinberg *et al.* 1989). However, the number of treatments, results, and complications are similar to both

Table 18.4 Comparison of techniques to treat reducible haemorrhoids

	Sclerotherapy	Rubber band ligation	Infra-red coagulation
Pain overall	60%	80%	23%
Pain severe	10%	30%	10%
Minor complications	5%	5%	5%
Recurrence rate	60%	15%	33%
Patient satisfaction	70–85%	80–95%	90%

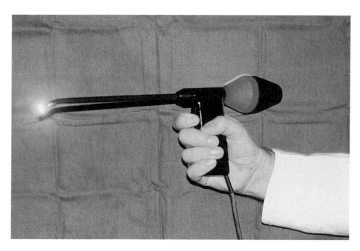

Figure 18.15 Infra-red coagulator for treating haemorrhoids.

sclerotherapy and IRC (Varma *et al.* 1991). As it is slower and frequently more painful, it appears to offer little advantage over these procedures, although it may be of use in third- or fourth-degree haemorrhoids (Zinberg *et al.* 1989; Varma *et al.* 1991). Bipolar diathermy is quicker and better tolerated than the direct current probe, both techniques giving 80% resolution of symptoms (Hinton and Morris 1990). Cryosurgery, using nitrous oxide, is effective and safe in selected patients, although a profuse serous discharge occurs in two-thirds of cases (Rudd 1989; Tanaka 1989). Up to 50% of patients can be treated as day cases, 90% returning to work within 3 weeks. The technique is claimed to be associated with less pain (14% versus 100%), bleeding and anal stenosis than haemorrhoidectomy (Gonzalez *et al.* 1995). However, recurrence at 5 years (5%) is greater than for haemorrhoidectomy. Consequently, cryotherapy now appears to have no advantage over other procedures. The technique may still have a role in controlling life-threatening bleeding from haemorrhoidal varices or managing severe symptoms in elderly, unfit patients. An alternative technique is laser haemorrhoidectomy, which is claimed to produce similar results to haemorrhoidectomy, with a lower incidence of post-procedure pain (Leff 1992; Smith 1992; Chia *et al.* 1995).

Surgical procedures

Anal dilatation or sphincterotomy alone has little place in the treatment of uncomplicated haemorrhoids (Mathai *et al.* 1996). Although the reduction in anal pressures is greater than with haemorrhoidectomy, poor results occur in 25% of patients, particularly in females or the elderly. Anal dilatation alone fails to relieve symptoms in 70% of cases, while one-quarter experience some degree of incontinence (Mortensen *et al.* 1987; MacDonald *et al.* 1992). However, in acutely prolapsed haemorrhoids, lateral sphincterotomy alone results in 80% of patients requiring no further treatment within 2 years (De Roover *et al.* 1989). The remainder will only require rubber band ligation and 90% of patients will be very satisfied with the outcome (De Roover *et al.* 1989). In patients undergoing haemorrhoidectomy, performing a simultaneous sphincterotomy reduces postoperative narcotic requirements from 100% to 20%, urinary retention from 40% to 4%, pain with the first motion from 96% to 6%, and faecal soiling from 58% to 6% (Asfar *et al.* 1988). Postoperative stricture formation is also reduced , with no increase in hospital stay or time to healing (Carditello 1991; Latteri *et al.* 1991; Eu *et al.* 1995). Simple ligation of the vascular pedicle,

without excision of the haemorrhoidal tissue, is claimed to give a 2% recurrence rate, no side-effects, reduced pain, and hospital stay (Maskow and Kirchner 1990). It may be performed with, or without, anal dilatation and is claimed to be a satisfactory alternative to haemorrhoidectomy (Serdev 1990; Rudin and Ragimov 1990).

Haemorrhoidectomy

About 15% of patients will fail to respond to non-surgical techniques and require haemorrhoidectomy (Arthur 1990). Recurrence at 5 years following haemorrhoidectomy is 4% (Dultsev and Rivkin 1989). The procedure is associated with a significant degree of urinary problems and postoperative pain. Following haemorrhoidectomy, up to 15% of male patients will experience urinary retention (Lyngdorf *et al.* 1986). Non-steroidal anti-inflammatory drugs, a caudal injection but not injecting the haemorrhoidectomy wounds with local anaesthetic, reduces postoperative pain following haemorrhoidectomy (Chester *et al.* 1990; Marsh *et al.* 1993; Richman 1993). Postoperative pain may also be reduced by giving faecal softeners pre- or postoperatively (London *et al.* 1987). Performing haemorrhoidectomy with diathermy is quicker than scissor haemorrhoidectomy, and is associated with less bleeding and less oral, but not parenteral, analgesia (Seow-Choen *et al.* 1992; Andrews *et al.* 1993).

Surgical haemorrhoidectomy may be performed by open, closed, submucosal, or radical techniques (Figure 18.16). The standard open Milligan and Morgan haemorrhoidectomy may be complicated by haemorrhage (3%), urinary difficulties (20%), urinary retention (2%), anal stenosis (2–10%) and incontinence of flatus (2%) (Tajana 1989; Johnstone and Isbister 1992). Over half of patients will require narcotic analgesia in the first 24 h, 2% require antibiotics and mean hospital stay is 2.5 days (Robinson *et al.* 1990; Bleday *et al.* 1992). Closing the haemorrhoidectomy wound, rather than leaving it open as in the traditional Milligan and Morgan procedure, results in less severe pain (30% versus 50%), reduced need for dilatation (0% versus 20%), greater primary healing (90% versus 0% within 12 days), and less pruritis and time to a normal bowel movement (Robinson *et al.* 1990; Neto *et al.* 1992). In pregnant females, closed haemorrhoidectomy under local anaesthetic is safe and removes pain with three-quarters of patients requiring no further surgery (Saleeby *et al.* 1991). Patients with circumferential haemorrhoids may be treated by either radical or four pile excision (Seow-Choen and Low 1995). A recent study compared complications of elective haemorrhoidectomy with emergency surgery for acutely

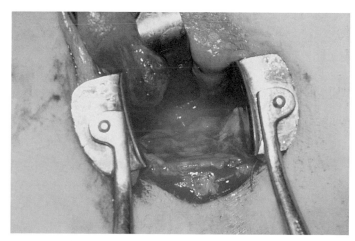

Figure 18.16 Surgical haemorrhoidectomy.

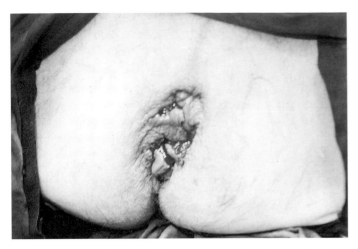

Figure 18.17 Finished haemorrhoidectomy showing skin and mucosal bridges which reduce the incidence of anal stenosis.

prolapsed, thrombosed, or gangrenous haemorrhoids (Eu *et al.* 1994). The incidence of secondary haemorrhage (5%), blood transfusion (2%), reoperation to secure haemostasis (1%), incontinence (5%), portal pyaemia (0%), and recurrent haemorrhoids (6%) were identical in the two groups. However, the incidence of anal stenosis was twice that in those undergoing emergency surgery compared with an elective (3%) procedure (Figure 18.17).

Pilonidal sinus

Pilonidal sinus is a foreign body granuloma related to the presence of hairs in an epidermal invagination. It is normally located between the buttocks but may occur in the interdigital webs, umbilicus, axilla, scalp, perineum, anus, amputation stumps, or penis.

Incidence

Pilonidal sinus is most frequently seen in males between the ages of 20 and 29 years. In children, however, the female to male ratio is 4:1 (Sondenaa *et al.* 1995). It tends to occur in hirsute patients, such as those of Mediterranean origin (Figure 18.18). Approximately

half of patients attending hospital with pilonidal disease present with an abscess.

Aetiology

The aetiology of pilonidal sinus has been attributed to a congenital origin, an acquired origin or a combination of the two (Isbister and Prasad 1995*b*). The congenital theory holds that hormonal changes at puberty are responsible for reactivation of latent embryonal remnants, such as sexual glands, spina bifida scars, or neural crests (Yabe and Furakawa 1995). The acquired theory suggests that hairs are drawn into the epidermal lining of the natal cleft by the constant movement of the buttocks, explaining the prevalence among barbers and drivers. The combined theory is the most satisfactory explanation. This suggests that there is a congenital invagination of the epithelium through which hairs can enter, creating a foreign body reaction (acquired component) with subsequent secondary infection. This explanation satisfies the pathological findings of free hairs within the sinus cavity and the absence of epithelium lining the sinus. Electron microscopy studies confirm that the needle-like projections of the hair help to pierce the skin. The length of the hairs is such as to suggest that the primary source of hair is from the scalp.

Bacteriology

Anaerobic organisms only (*Bacteroides* and anaerobic cocci) are isolated in 77% of pilonidal abscesses, aerobic organisms (*E. coli*, *Proteus*, and *Streptococcus faecalis*) only in 4%, while 17% of cases show mixed anaerobic and aerobic infection (Sondenaa *et al.* 1995).

Clinical presentation

Symptoms

Pilonidal sinus may be asymptomatic or present with a discharge or recurrent abscess. A discharge is noted in two-thirds of cases while swelling and pain occur in 50% and 35% (Sondenaa *et al.* 1995).

Signs

The macroscopic appearance is of one or more primary pits seen in the natal cleft, secondary tracts opening lateral to the cleft. The differential diagnosis is between anal fistula, hidradenitis suppurivata, furuncle, and scratching lesions with an underlying abscess (Figure 18.19).

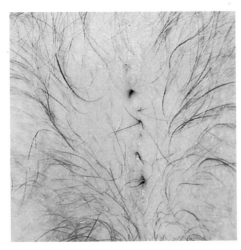

Figure 18.18 Typical hair containing multiple openings of pilonidal sinus.

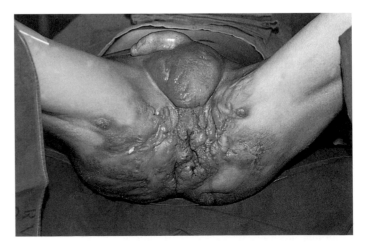

Figure 18.19 Case of extensive hidradenitis suppurivata (see colour plates)

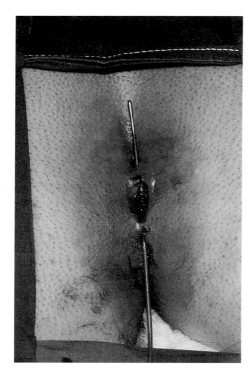

Figure 18.20 Pilonidal sinus presenting as an abscess.

Complications

Abscess formation is the most common complication, while the perianal region may occasionally be involved circumferentially by pilonidal sinuses (Figure 18.20). About 40 cases of carcinoma (squamous cell and spinocellular) arising in pilonidal cysts have been reported (Jeddy *et al.* 1994). Although recurrence or metastases occur in up to 40%, wide local excision can result in a cure in about 90%. Infectious complications, such as anaerobic meningitis or superinfection with tuberculosis have also been noted.

Treatment

Various conservative methods have been tried, with variable success (Armstrong and Barcia 1994; Stephens and Stephens 1995). Phenol injection is reported to give similar results to surgery, the patient staying in hospital 1–2 days and returning to work within 2 weeks (Schneider *et al.* 1994). One injection is usually sufficient, although up to five may be necessary, discomfort being minimal. Seventy per cent of sinuses will heal over a median period of 2 months. Although conservative measures do not address the causative factors of pilonidal sinus, recurrence at 1 year is claimed to be 6%. Surgery aims to correct the congenital epidermal invagination by excision, prevent hairs entering the invagination by shaving, and prevent wound infection (Purkiss 1993).

Simple incision and drainage is the immediate treatment of a pilonidal abscess. It relieves symptoms and allows early return to work in all cases (Fuzun *et al.* 1994). Complete healing occurs in 60% of patients, the cases with multiple or lateral tracts tending to require definitive surgery at a later date. Recurrence occurs in 25% of those with initial healing and the overall cure rate at 18 months is 75%. Excision of the pilonidal pit at the time of surgery for abscess reduces recurrence by up to 40% (Khaira and Brown 1995). Performing primary closure with instillation of antibiotic into the abscess cavity is reputed to give a low recurrence rate (13%), with

rapid return to work (mean 13 days). Alternatively a Bascom's procedure or a V–Y flap may be performed (Khatri *et al.* 1994; Mosquerra and Quayle 1995).

Elective laying open of the sinus tract is associated with a low recurrence rate, but slow healing. The importance of shaping the wound to allow adequate drainage and flexible use of antibiotics has been emphasized. Several procedures have been devised to speed up wound closure and return to work. A randomized trial of Eusol and silastic foam dressings to the open wound found no difference in the time to hospital discharge or full healing (Walker *et al.* 1991). Partially closing the wound, leaving a small opening for drainage allows more rapid healing, although recurrence ranges widely. Primary closure may be performed vertically, horizontally or obliquely. A Z or W-plasty decreases tissue tension and flattens the natal cleft, resulting in a reduction in recurrence of up to 50% (Manterola *et al.* 1991). Creation of a rhomboid flap is associated with seroma in 10% of cases and a hospital stay of 9 days, although recurrences at 1 year are very uncommon.

Recurrence after primary closure is 4–8%. A variation of primary closure has been developed by Bascom (1987) . He argues that radical excision is unwarranted, even in recurrent disease. His procedure is claimed to deal with the cause of pilonidal sinus, by performing primary pit closure, and improve wound healing by avoiding skin pulling away from bone (Bascom 1987). The technique is said to cause little disability, result in primary wound healing, and require minimal postoperative care (Bascom 1987). Initial results are favourable, no recurrences being reported after several years (Obeid 1988).

Comparisons of whether the excised wound should be left open or sutured, suggest that there is benefit from the latter. The mean time to healing following excision and packing, marsupialization of the wound edge and primary wound closure is about 15, 8, and 2 weeks (Kronborg 1985). Excision of the sinus with primary wound closure is reported to result in greater overall healing (98% versus 72%), fewer early complications (27% versus 38%), less infection (13% versus 30%), fewer follow-up visits, less sick leave, greater wound healing, and comparable complications at 1 year (30% versus 25%), than leaving the wound open (Sondenaa *et al.* 1995). Primary subcuticular closure is claimed to give better pain relief without any apparent disadvantages, over interrupted, non-absorbable sutures (Aaser and Gruner 1992). It is therefore claimed that excision and open packing should be abandoned in favour of primary closure, often performed under local anaesthetic.

Anal dermatological conditions

The principal symptom of anal skin conditions is pruritis ani.

Pruritis ani

Pruritis may be classified as primary (idiopathic) or secondary to another disease. It represents an unpleasant itching in the anal region inducing an irresistible urge to scratch. A deep set anus, heavy hair distribution, or sphincter incompetence, results in the leakage of faeces and subsequent mechanical and chemical skin irritation (Stolz *et al.* 1990). There may be a related fall in anal pressure on rectal distension. Although candida is common, there is no difference in the microflora in patients with and without pruritis (Silverman *et al.* 1989). Patients with primary pruritis have a reduced threshold for itching. Stimuli causing no complaints in normal individuals, causes intense itching in these susceptible individuals. Psychological overlay is common, representing feelings of rejection, guilt, sexual eroticism, or stress. Scratching evokes a skin reaction characterized by redness, excoriation, weeping, and possible suppuration (perianal dermatitis). Sensitization leads to papule and vesicle formation (acute perianal eczema). Chronic perianal eczema is the result of lichenification of the skin. Pruritis is one of the commonest symptoms in coloproctology. It is more frequent in the 30–60-year age group, males being four times more commonly affected than females. Although 45–70% of cases of pruritis ani were formerly thought to be idiopathic, a careful examination will find a contributory cause, often skin conditions, in almost all cases. The perianal and perineal areas can be involved in several dermatological conditions, that are not necessarily specific to these regions (Table 18.5).

Dermatitis (eczema)

Dermatitis may occur because of irritant, contact, or infectious factors. Benzocaine, camphor, cocoa butter, lanolin, turpentine, phenol, iodine, neomycin, and antihistamines have all been implicated in causing contact dermatitis. Perianal dermatitis has been related to a contact allergy to clotrimazole and haemorrhoidal preparations (Stolz *et al.* 1990).

The intense itching creates a cycle which leads to chronic inflammatory changes (chronic inflammatory dermatitis). Eventually, the skin becomes thickened (lichenified dermatitis) with prominent skin excoriation and either hyper- or hypopigmentation. Patch-testing, Gram staining, candida cultures, and skin biopsy may be necessary for successful diagnosis. Treatment consists of regular bathing, lotions rather than ointments and avoiding irritants or tight clothing. Topical steroids are suitable only for acute allergic contact dermatitis.

Hidradenitis suppurivata (Figure 18.21)

This is a chronic inflammatory condition characterized by abscesses, fistulas, and scarring. It results from chronic infection of the apocrine glands of the perianal region. It accounts for up to one-third of recurrent perianal abscesses. Symptoms include pain, swelling, purulent discharge, and pruritis present for an average of 6 years. Missed diagnosis on presentation is common, with the proportion of cases diagnosed as having a pilonidal sinus being 28%, anal fistula 37%, or anorectal abscess 16% (Wiltz *et al.* 1990). Twelve per cent of patients have diabetes and a further 12% marked obesity (Wiltz *et al.* 1990). Recurrence after treatment was found in two-thirds of cases. It has been suggested that recurrence might be related to associated *Chlamydia trachomonas* infection. Hidradenitis can initially be treated by oral antibiotics. Abscesses, however, should be drained. No operation is ideal, but wide local excision and healing by secondary intention is best in most instances.

A number of general dermatological conditions may affect the perianal region, including psoriasis, pemphigus vulgaris, Behçet's disease and lichen sclerosus et atrophicus.

Table 18.5 Causes of pruritis ani		
Primary		Itch–scratch cycle
		Poor local hygiene
		Excessive sweating
Secondary		
	Local anal conditions	Anal fistula
		Haemorrhoids
		Rectal prolapse
		Anal fissure
		Anal carcinoma
		Pruritis vulva
Infections		
	Bacterial	Erythrasma
		Syphilis
		Gonorrhoea
	Viral	Anal warts
	Parasitic	Threadworms
		Scabies
		Pediculosis pubis
	Fungal	Candida
		Epidermophyton
		Trichophyton
Dermatological conditions		Dermatitis
		Psoriasis
		Behçet's disease
		Pemphigus vulgaris
		Benign familial pemphigus
		Dyskeratosis follicularis
		Lichen sclerosus et atrophicans
		Acanthosis nigrans
		Hidradenitis suppurivata

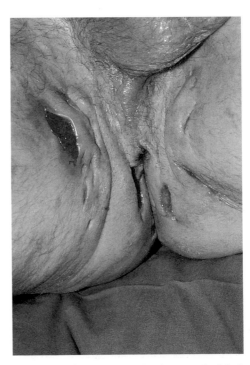

Figure 18.21 Hidradenitis suppurivata showing extensive infected tissue

References

Abel ME, Chiu YS, Russell TR, Volpe PA. Autologous fibrin glue in the treatment of rectovaginal and complex fistulas. *Dis. Colon Rectum* 1990; 36: 447–9.

Abercrombie JF, George BD. Perianal abscess in children. *Ann. R. Coll. Surg. Engl.* 1992; 74: 385–6.

Aguilar PS, Plasencia G, Hardy TG Jr, Hartmann RF, Stewart WR. Mucosal advancement in the treatment of anal fistula. *Dis. Colon Rectum* 1985; 28: 496–8.

Akande B, Esho JO. Relationship between haemorrhoids and prostatism: results of a prospective study. *Eur. Urol.* 1989; 16: 333–4.

al Salem AH, Laing W, Talwalker V. Fistula-in-ano in infancy and childhood. *J. Pediatr. Surg.* 1994; 29: 436–8.

Alemdaroglu K, Ulualp KM. Single session ligation treatment of bleeding hemorrhoids. *Surg. Gynecol. Obst.* 1993; 177: 62–4.

Alexander AA, Miller LS, Liu JB, Feld RI, Goldberg BB. High resolution endoluminal sonography of the anal sphincter complex. *J. Ultrasound Med.* 1994; 13: 281–4.

Aluwihare AP. Evaluation of acute anal sepsis, and anterior horseshoe fistula. *Ann. Acad. Med. Singapore* 1987; 16: 509–10.

Andrews BT, Layer GT, Jackson BT, Nicholls RJ. Randomized trial comparing diathermy hemorrhoidectomy with the scissor dissection Milligan–Morgan operation. *Dis. Colon Rectum* 1993; 36: 580–3.

Angel C, Patrick CC, Lobe T, Rao B, Pui CH. Management of anorectal/perineal infections caused by *Pseudomonas aeruginosa* in children with malignant diseases. *J. Pediatr. Surg.* 1991; 26: 487–9.

Armstrong JH, Barcia PJ. Pilonidal sinus disease. The conservative approach. *Arch. Surg.* 1994; 129: 914–7.

Arthur KE. Hemorrhoids. Medico-surgical treatment. *Revista Med. Panama* 1990; 15: 3–12.

Asfar SK, Juma TH, Ala-Edeen T. Hemorrhoidectomy and sphincterotomy. A prospective study comparing the effectiveness of anal stretch and sphincterotomy in reducing pain after hemorrhoidectomy. *Dis. Colon Rectum* 1988; 31: 181–5.

Babaev OG, Skobelkin OK, Khodzhanepesov K. Treatment of fissure in ano by the method of laser coagulation. *Khirurgiia* 1990; 6: 21–4.

Barker PG, Lunniss PJ, Armstrong P, Reznek RH, Cottam K, Phillips RK. Magnetic resonance imaging of fistula in ano: technique, interpretation and accuracy. *Clin. Radiol.* 1994; 49: 7–13.

Bat L, Melzer E, Koler M, Dreznick Z, Shemesh E. Complications of rubber band ligation of symptomatic internal hemorrhoids. *Dis. Colon Rectum* 1993; 36: 287–90.

Ben-Chetrit E, Bar-Ziv J. Thrombosed hemorrhoid mimicking rectal carcinoma at CT. *Acta Radiol.* 1991; 33: 457–8.

Ben-Chetrit E, Bar-Ziv J. Thrombosed hemorrhoid mimicking rectal carcinoma at CT. *Acta Radiol.* 1992; 33: 457–8.

Bleday R, Pena JP, Rothenberger DA, Goldberg SM, Buls JG. Symptomatic hemorrhoids: current incidence and complications of operative therapy. *Dis. Colon Rectum* 1992; 35: 477–8.

Blessing H. Late results after individualized lateral internal sphincterotomy. *Helv. Chir. Acta* 1993; 59: 603–7.

Brown AC, Sumfest JM, Rozwadowski JV. Histopathology of the internal anal sphincter in chronic anal fissure. *Dis. Colon Rectum* 1989; 32: 680–3.

Bruck CE, Lubowski DZ, King DW. Do patients with haemorrhoids have pelvic floor denervation? *Int. J. Colorectal Dis.* 1988; 3: 210–4.

Bruhl W. Diagnosis and therapy of hemorrhoids. New knowledge in sclerotherapy. *Fortschritte Med.* 1993; 111: 39–42.

Carditello A. Hemorrhoidectomy by Arnous and Parnaud's method: its role in the magnitude of postoperative pain. *Chir. Ital.* 1991; 43: 200–5.

Carr ND, Mercey D, Slack WW. Non-condylomatous, perianal disease in homosexual men. *Br. J. Surg.* 1991; 76: 1064–6.

Cermak J, Hubik J, Toberny M, Gurlich R. Treatment of hemorrhoids with elastic ligature. *Rozhl. Chir.* 1992; 71: 429–32.

Chen WS, Leu SY, Wang FM. The roles of hemorrhoidectomy and lateral internal sphincterotomy in the treatment of hemorrhoids—clinical and manometric study. *Chung Hua i Hsueh Tsa Chih—Chinese Medical* 1989; 43: 255–6.

Cheong DM, Nogueras JJ, Wexner SD, Jagelman DG. Anal endosonography for recurrent anal fistulas: image enhancement with hydrogen peroxide. *Dis. Colon Rectum* 1993; 36: 1158–60.

Chester JF, Stanford BJ, Gazet JC. Analgesic benefit of locally injected bupivacaine after hemorrhoidectomy. *Dis. Colon Rectum* 1990; 33: 487–9.

Chia YW, Darzi A, Speakman CT, Hill AD, Jameson JS, Henry MM. CO_2 laser haemorrhoidectomy—does it alter anorectal function or decrease pain compared to conventional haemorrhoidectomy? *Int. J. Colorectal Dis.* 1995; 10: 22–4.

Choen S, Burnett S, Bartram CI, Nicholls RJ. Comparison between anal endosonography and digital examination in the evaluation of anal fistulae. *Br. J. Surg.* 1991; 78: 445–7.

Choi J, Freeman JB, Touchette J. Long-term follow-up of concomitant band ligation and sclerotherapy for internal hemorrhoids. *Can. J. Surg.* 1985; 28: 523–4.

Cirocco WC, Reilly JC. Challenging the predictive accuracy of Goodsall's rule for anal fistulas. *Dis. Colon Rectum* 1993; 35: 537–42.

Cohen Z. Symposium on outpatient anorectal procedures. Alternatives to surgical hemorrhoidectomy. *Can. J. Surg.* 1985; 28: 230–1.

Corby H, Donnelly VS, O'Herlihy C, O'Connell PR. Anal canal pressures are low in women with postpartum anal fissure. *Br. J. Surg.* 1997; 84: 86–8.

Corfitsen MT, Hansen CP, Christensen TH, Kaae HH. Anorectal abscesses in immunosuppressed patients. *Eur. J. Surg.* 1992; 158: 51–3.

De Roover DM, Hoofwijk AG, van Vroonhoven TJ. Lateral internal sphincterotomy in the treatment of fourth degree haemorrhoids. *Br. J. Surg.* 1989; 76: 1181–3.

de Souza NM, Hall AS, Puni R, Gilderdale DJ, Young IR, Kmiot WA. High resolution magnetic imaging of the anal sphincter using a dedicated endoanal coil. Comparison of magnetic resonance imaging with surgical findings. *Dis. Colon Rectum* 1996; 39: 926–34.

Deen KI, Kumar D, Williams JG, Olliff J, Keighley MR. Anal sphincter defects. Correlation between endoanal ultrasound and surgery. *Ann. Surg.* 1993; 218: 201–5.

Dennison AR, Wherry DC, Morris DL. Hemorrhoids. Nonoperative management. *Surg. Clin. North Am.* 1988; 68: 1401–9.

deSouza NM, Puni R, Gilderdale DJ, Bydder GM. Magnetic resonance imaging of the anal sphincter using an internal coil. *Magnetic Resonance Q.* 1995; 11: 45–56.

Doberneck RC. Perianal suppuration: results of treatment. *Am. Surg.* 1987; 53: 569–72.

Dultsev YV, Rivkin VL. Treatment of haemorrhoids at the Moscow Research Institute of Proctology. *Int. Surg.* 1989; 74: 7–9.

Eu KW, Seow-Choen F, Goh HS. Comparison of emergency and elective haemorrhoidectomy. *Br. J. Surg.* 1994; 81: 308–10.

Eu KW, Teoh TA, Seow-Choen F, Goh HS. Anal stricture following haemorrhoidectomy: early diagnosis and treatment. *Aust. N.Z. J. Surg.* 1995; 65: 101–3.

Evaldson GR. Pararectal abscess with pelvic extension simulating gynecological disease. *Acta Obstet. Gynecol. Scand.* 1986; 65: 803–4.

Farouk R, Duthie GS, MacGregor AB, Bartolo DC. Sustained internal sphincter hypertonia in patients with chronic anal fissure. *Dis. Colon Rectum* 1994; 37: 424–9.

Farouk R, Monson JR, Duthie GS. Technical failure of lateral sphincterotomy for the treatment of chronic anal fissure: a study using endoanal ultrasonography. *Br. J. Surg.* 1997; 84: 84–5.

Fazio VW. Complex anal fistulae. *Gastroenterol. Clin. North Am.* 1987; 16: 93–114.

Felt-Bersma RJ, van Baren R, Koorevaar M, Strijers RL, Cuesta MA. Unsuspected sphincter defects shown by anal endosonography after anorectal surgery. A prospective study. *Dis. Colon Rectum* 1995; 38: 249–53.

Ferguson EF Jr. Alternatives in the treatment of hemorrhoidal disease. *South Med. J.* 1988; 81: 606–10.

Frezza EE, Sandei F, Leoni G, Biral M. Conservative and surgical treatment in acute and chronic anal fissure. A study on 308 patients. *Int. J. Colorectal Dis* 1992; 7: 188–9.

Fry RD, Birnbaum EH, Lacey DL. Actinomyces as a cause of recurrent perianal fistula in the immunocompromised patient. *Surgery* 1992; 111: 591–4.

Fucini C. One stage treatment of anal abscesses and fistulas. A clinical appraisal on the basis of two different classifications. *Int. J. Colorectal Dis.* 1991; 6: 12–6.

Fuzun M, Bakir H, Soylu M; Tansug T, Kaymak E, Harmancioglu O. Which technique for treatment of pilonidal sinus—open or closed? *Dis. Colon Rectum* 1994; 37: 1148–50.

Ganguly S, Sarin SK, Bhatia V, Lahoti D. The prevalence and spectrum of colonic lesions in patients with cirrhotic and noncirrhotic portal hypertension. *Hepatology* 1995; 21: 1226–31.

Garcia-Aguilar J, Belmonte C, Wong WD, Goldberg SM, Madoff RD. Anal fistula surgery. Factors associated with recurrence and incontinence. *Dis. Colon Rectum* 1996; 39: 723–9.

Garcia-Olmo D, Vazquez Aragon P, Lopez Fando J. Multiple setons in the treatment of high perianal fistula. *Br. J. Surg.* 1994; 81: 136–7.

Gibbons CP, Bannister JJ, Read NW. Role of constipation and anal hypertonia in the pathogenesis of haemorrhoids. *Br. J. Surg.* 1988; 75: 656–60.

Giebel GD, Horch R. Treatment of anal fissure: a comparison of three different forms of therapy. *Nippon Geka Hokan—Arch. Jpn. Chir.* 1989; 58: 126–33.

Gonzalez AR, de Oliveira O Jr, Verzaro R, Nogueras J, Wexner SD. Anoplasty for stenosis and other anorectal defects. *Am. Surg.* 1995; 61: 526–9.

Goodsall DH. In: Goodsall DH and Miles WE, eds. *Diseases of the anus and rectum*, Part 1. London: Longmans, 1900.

Gorfine SR. Treatment of benign anal disease with topical nitroglycerin. *Dis. Colon Rectum* 1995; 38: 453–6.

Graf W, Pahlman L, Ejerblad S. Functional results after seton treatment of high transsphincteric anal fistulas. *Eur. J. Surg.* 1995; 161: 289–91.

Hardwick RH, Durdey P. Should rubber band ligation of haemorrhoids be performed at the initial outpatient visit? *Ann. R. Coll. Surg. Engl.* 1994; 76: 185–7.

Heaton ND, Davenport M, Howard ER. Incidence of haemorrhoids and anorectal varices in children with portal hypertension. *Br. J. Surg.* 1993; 80: 616–830.

Held D, Khubchandani I, Sheets J, Stasik J, Rosen L, Riether R. Management of anorectal horseshoe abscess and fistula. *Dis. Colon Rectum* 1986; 29: 793–7.

Henrichsen S, Christiansen J. Incidence of fistula-in-ano complicating anorectal sepsis: a prospective study. *Br. J. Surg.* 1986; 73: 371–2.

Heslop JH. Piles and rectoceles. *Aust. N.Z. J. Surg.* 1987; 57: 935–8.

Hiltunen KM, Matikainen M. Anal manometric findings in symptomatic hemorrhoids. *Dis. Colon Rectum* 1985; 28: 807–9.

Hinton CP, Morris DL. A randomized trial comparing direct current therapy and bipolar diathermy in the outpatient treatment of third-degree hemorrhoids. *Dis. Colon Rectum* 1990; 33: 931–2.

Ho YH, Seow-Choen F, Goh HS. Haemorrhoidectomy and disordered rectal and anal physiology in patients with prolapsed haemorrhoids. *Br. J. Surg.* 1995; 82: 596–8.

Horvath KD, Whelan RL, Golub RW, Ahsan H, Cirocco WC. Effect of catheter diameter on resting pressures in anal fissure patients. *Dis. Colon Rectum* 1995; 38: 728–31.

Hosking SW, Smart HL, Johnson AG, Triger DR. Anorectal varices, haemorrhoids, and portal hypertension. *Lancet* 1989; i: 349–52.

Hussain SM, Stoker J, Schouten WR, Lameris JS. Fistula in ano: endoanal sonography versus endoanal MR imaging in classification. *Radiology* 1996; 200: 475–81.

Isbister WH. Fistula in ano: a surgical audit. *Int. J. Colorectal Dis.* 1995; 10: 94–6.

Isbister WH, Prasad J. Fissure in ano. *Aust. N.Z. J. Surg.* 1995a; 65: 107–8.

Isbister WH, Prasad J. Pilonidal disease. *Aust. N.Z. J. Surg.* 1995b; 65: 561–3.

Jeddy TA, Vowles RH, Southam JA. Squamous cell carcinoma in a chronic pilonidal sinus. *Br. J. Clin. Pract.* 1994; 48: 160–1.

Jensen SL. Treatment of first episodes of acute anal fissure: prospective randomised study of lignocaine ointment versus hydrocortisone ointment or warm sitz baths plus bran. *Br. Med. J. (Clin. Res.)* 1986 3; 292: 1167–9.

Jensen SL. Maintenance therapy with unprocessed bran in the prevention of acute anal fissure recurrence. *J. R. Soc. Med.* 1987; 80: 296–8.

Jensen SL, Harling H, Tange G, Shokouh-Amiri MH, Nielsen OV. Maintenance bran therapy for prevention of symptoms after rubber band ligation of third-degree haemorrhoids. *Acta Chir. Scand.* 1988; 154: 395–8.

Jensen SL, Harling H, Arseth-Hansen P, Tange G. The natural history of symptomatic haemorrhoids. *Int. J. Colorectal Dis.* 1989; 4: 41–2.

Johanson JF, Sonnenberg A. The prevalence of hemorrhoids and chronic constipation. An epidemiologic study. *Gastroenterology* 1990; 98: 380–6.

Johnstone CS, Isbister WH. Inpatient management of piles: a surgical audit. *Aust. N.Z. J. Surg.* 1992; 62: 720–4.

Jones IT, Fazio VW, Jagelman DG. The use of transanal rectal advancement flaps in the management of fistulas involving the anorectum. *Dis. Colon Rectum* 1987; 30: 919–23.

Josey WE. Anovaginal fistula presenting as a vulvar ulcer. A report of two cases in postmenopausal women. *Reprod. Med.* 1988; 33: 857–8.

Jost WH, Schimrigk K. Therapy of anal fissure using botulin toxin. *Dis. Colon Rectum* 1994; 37: 1321–4.

Kaftan SM, Haboubi NY. Histopathological changes in haemorrhoid associated mucosa and submucosa. *Int. J. Colorectal Dis.* 1995; 10: 15–8.

Keck JO, Staniunas RJ, Coller JA, Barrett RC, Oster ME. Computer generated profiles of the anal canal in patients with anal fissure. *Dis. Colon Rectum* 1995; 38: 72–9.

Khaira HS, Brown JH. Excision and primary suture of pilonidal sinus. *Ann. R. Coll. Surg. Engl.* 1995; 77: 242–4.

Khatri VP, Espinosa MH, Amin AK. Management of recurrent pilonidal sinus by simple V Y fasciocutaneous flap. *Dis. Colon Rectum* 1994; 37: 1232–5.

Khubchandani IT, Reed JF. Sequelae of internal sphincterotomy for chronic fissure in ano. *Br. J. Surg.* 1989; 76: 431–4.

Klotz HP, Buchmann P. Sliding flap-plasty in treatment of anal fistula: a prospective study. *Helv. Chir. Acta* 1993; 60: 287–9.

Kortbeek JB, Langevin JM, Khoo RE, Heine JA. Chronic fissure-in-ano: a randomized study comparing open and subcutaneous lateral internal sphincterotomy. *Dis. Colon Rectum* 1992; 35: 835–7.

Krasznay P. Ambulatory cryotherapy of anal fissures. *Orvosi Hetilap.* 1990; 132: 1761–2.

Kronborg O. To lay open or excise a fistula-in-ano: a randomized trial. *Br. J. Surg.* 1985; 72: 97–8.

Kufahl JW, Andreasen JJ. Microbiology related to anal abscess complicated with fistula formation. *Ugeskrift Laeger* 1992; 154: 1428–9.

Latteri M, Grassi N, Salanitro L, Pantuso G, Bottino A, Gitto C, Farro G. Surgical treatment of hemorrhoids using Milligan–Morgan technique. Survey of 366 cases. *Minerva Chir.* 1991; 46: 1119–218.

Leff EI. Hemorrhoidectomy—laser vs. nonlaser: outpatient surgical experience. *Dis. Colon Rectum* 1992; 35: 743–6.

Leong AF, Seow-Choen F. Lateral sphincterotomy compared with anal advancement flap for chronic anal fissure. *Dis. Colon Rectum* 1995; 38: 69–71.

Lewis WG, Finan PJ, Holdsworth PJ, Sagar PM, Stephenson BM. Clinical results and manometric studies after rectal flap advancement for intralevator trans-sphincteric fistula-in-ano. *Int. J. Colorectal Dis.* 1995; 10: 189–92.

Lin JK. Anal manometric studies in hemorrhoids and anal fissures. *Dis. Colon Rectum* 1989; 32: 839–42.

London NJ, Bramley PD, Windle R. Effect of four days of preoperative lactulose on post haemorrhoidectomy pain: results of placebo controlled trial. *Br. Med. J. (Clin. Res.)* 1987; 295: 363–4.

Lund JN, Armitage NC, Scholefield JH. Use of glyceryl trinitrate ointment in the treatment of anal fissure. *Brit. J. Surg.* 1996; 83: 776–7.

Lund JN, Scholefield JH. A randomised, prospective, double-blind, placebo-controlled trial of glyceryl trinitrate ointment in treatment of anal fissure. *Lancet* 1997; 349: 11–4.

Lunniss PJ, Barker PG, Sultan AH, Armstrong P, Reznek RH, Bartram CI, *et al.* Magnetic resonance imaging of fistula in ano. *Dis. Colon Rectum* 1994; 37: 708–18.

Lunniss PJ, Sheffield JP, Talbot IC, Thomson JP, Phillips RK. Persistence of idiopathic anal fistula may be related to epithelialization. *Br. J. Surg.* 1995; 82: 32–3.

Lyngdorf P, Frimodt-Moller C, Jeppesen N. Voiding disturbances following anal surgery. *Urol. Int.* 1986; 41: 67–9.

MacDonald A, Smith A, McNeill AD, Finlay IG. Manual dilatation of the anus. *Br. J. Surg.* 1992; 79: 1381–2.

MacRae HM, McLeod RS. Comparison of hemorrhoidal treatment modalities. A meta analysis. *Dis. Colon Rectum* 1995; 38: 687–94.

MacRae HM, McLeod RS, Cohen Z, Stern H, Reznick R. Treatment of rectovaginal fistulas that has failed previous repair attempts. *Dis. Colon Rectum* 1995; 38: 921–5.

Mann CV, Clifton MA. Re-routing of the track for the treatment of high anal and anorectal fistulae. *Br. J. Surg.* 1985; 72: 134–7.

Mann CV, Motson R, Clifton M. The immediate response to injection therapy for first-degree haemorrhoids. *J. R. Soc. Med.* 1988; 81: 146–8.

Marks CG, Ritchie JK, Lockhart-Mummery HE. Anal fistulas in Crohn's disease. *Br. J. Surg.* 1981; 68: 525–30.

Marsh GD, Huddy SP, Rutter KP. Bupivacaine infiltration after haemorrhoidectomy. *J. R. Coll. Surg. Edinburgh* 1993; 38: 41–2.

Marti MC, Koscinski T. Mucosal flaps in the treatment of anal fistula. *Chirurgie* 1992; 129: 232–5.

Maskow G, Kirchner H. Knot sutures in the treatment of hemorrhoids—a conservative and modern method. *Rozhl. Chir.* 1990; 69: 329–31.

Matos D, Lunniss PJ, Phillips RK. Total sphincter conservation in high fistula in ano: results of a new approach. *Br. J. Surg.* 1993; 80: 802–4.

Mathai V, Ong BC, Ho YH. Randomized controlled trial of lateral internal sphincterotomy with haemorrhoidectomy. *Brit. J. Surg.* 1996; 83: 380–2.

Mattana C, Maria G, Pescatori M. Rubber band ligation of hemorrhoids and rectal mucosal prolapse in constipated patients. *Dis. Colon Rectum* 1989; 32: 372–5.

Mazier WP, Senagore AJ, Schiesel EC. Operative repair of anovaginal and rectovaginal fistulas. *Dis. Colon Rectum* 1995; 38: 4–6.

McCourtney JS, Finlay IG. Setons in the surgical management of fistula in ano. *Br. J. Surg.* 1995; 82: 448–52.

McNamara MJ, Percy JP, Fielding IR. A manometric study of anal fissure treated by subcutaneous lateral internal sphincterotomy. *Ann. Surg.* 1992; 211: 235–8.

Medich DS, Fazio VW. Hemorrhoids, anal fissure, and carcinoma of the colon, rectum, and anus during pregnancy. *Surg. Clin. North Am.* 1995; 75: 77–88.

Melange M, Colin JF, Van Wymersch T, Vanheuverzwyn R. Anal fissure: correlation between symptoms and manometry before and after surgery. *Int. J. Colorectal Dis.* 1992; 7: 108–12.

Morgado PJ, Suarez JA, Gomez LG, Morgado PJ Jr. Histoclinical basis for a new classification of hemorrhoidal disease. *Dis. Colon Rectum* 1988; 31: 474–8.

Mortensen PE, Olsen J, Pedersen IK, Christiansen J. A randomized study on hemorrhoidectomy combined with anal dilatation. *Dis. Colon Rectum* 1987; 30: 755–7.

Mosquera DA, Quayle JB. Bascom's operation for pilonidal sinus. *J. R. Soc. Med.* 1995; 88: 45–46.

Myers SR. Tuberculous fissure in ano. *J. R. Soc. Med.* 1994; 87: 46.

Myhr GE, Myrvold HE, Nilsen G, Thoresen JE, Rinck PA. Perianal fistulas: use of MR imaging for diagnosis. *Radiology* 1994; 191: 545–9.

Nelson RL, Prasad ML, Abcarian H. Anal carcinoma presenting as a perirectal abscess or fistula. *Arch. Surg.* 1985; 120: 632–5.

Nelson RL, Abcarian H, Davis FG, Persky V. Prevalence of benign anorectal disease in a randomly selected population. *Dis. Colon Rectum* 1995; 38: 341–4.

Neto JA, Quilici FA, Cordeiro F, Reis Junior JA. Open versus semi-open hemorrhoidectomy: a random trial. *Int. Surg.* 1992; 77: 84–9.

Nino-Murcia M, Friedland GW. Unusual fistulae between the rectum and the lower urinary tract: simple techniques for diagnosis. *Urol. Radiol.* 1988; 9: 240–2.

Notaras MJ. Anal fissure and stenosis. *Surg. Clin. North Am.* 1988; 68: 1427–41.

Nyam DC, Wilson RG, Stewart KJ, Farouk R, Bartolo DC. Island advancement flaps in the management of anal fissures. *Br. J. Surg.* 1995; 82: 326–8.

O'Holleran TP. Infrared photocoagulation of hemorrhoids. *Nebr. Med. J.* 1990; 75: 307–8.

Oh C, Divino CM, Steinhagen RM. Anal fissure. 20 year experience. *Dis. Colon Rectum* 1995; 38: 378–82.

Parkash S, Lakshmiratan V, Gajendran V. Fistula-in-ano: treatment by fistulectomy, primary closure and reconstitution. *Aust. N.Z. J. Surg.* 1985; 55: 23–7.

Parks AG, Stitz RW. The treatment of high fistula-in-ano. *Dis. Colon Rectum* 1976; 19: 487–92.

Pernikoff BJ, Eisenstat TE, Rubin RJ, Oliver GC, Salvati EP. Reappraisal of partial lateral internal sphincterotomy. *Dis. Colon Rectum* 1994; 37: 1291–5.

Pescatori M, Interisano A, Mascagni D, Bottini C. Double flap technique to reconstruct the anal canal after concurrent surgery for fistulae, abscesses and haemorrhoids. *Int. J. Colorectal Dis.* 1995; 10: 19–21.

Petros JG, Rimm EB, Robillard RJ. Clinical presentation of chronic anal fissures. *Am. Surg.* 1993; 59: 666–8.

Piazza DJ, Radhakrishnan J. Perianal abscess and fistula-in-ano in children. *Dis. Colon Rectum* 1990; 33: 1014–6.

Pines A, Shemesh E, Bat L. Prolonged rectal bleeding associated with hemorrhoids: the diagnostic contribution of colonoscopy. *South Med. J.* 1987; 80: 313–4.

Poenaru D, Yazbeck S. Anal fistula in infants: etiology, features, management. *J. Pediatr. Surg.* 1993; 28: 1194–5.

Pons L, Muntada J. Internal lateral sphincterectomy. Results. *Rev. Esp. Enferm. Aparato Dig.* 1989; 75: 589–92.

Pople IK, Ralphs DN. An aetiology for fistula in ano. *Br. J. Surg.* 1988; 75: 904 5.

Prohm P, Bonner C. Is manometry essential for surgery of chronic fissure in ano? *Dis. Colon Rectum* 1995; 38: 735–8.

Purkiss SF. Decision making in surgery: a pilonidal sinus. *Br. J. Hosp. Med.* 1993; 50: 554–6.

Quevedo-Bonilla G, Farkas AM, Abcarian H, Hambrick E, Orsay CP. Septic complications of hemorrhoidal banding. *Arch. Surg.* 1988; 123: 650–1.

Recondo G, Sella A, Ro JY, Dexeus FH, Amato R, Kilbourn R. Perianal ulcer in disseminated histoplasmosis. *South Med J.* 1992; 84: 931–2.

Richman IM. Use of Toradol in anorectal. *Surg. Dis. Colon Rectum* 1993; 36: 295–6.

Robinson AM, Smith LE, Perciballi JA. Outpatient hemorrhoidectomy. *Military Med.* 1990; 155: 299–300.

Romano G, Rotondano G, Santangelo M, Esercizio L. A critical appraisal of pathogenesis and morbidity of surgical treatment of chronic anal fissure. *J. Am. Coll. Surg.* 1994; 178: 600–4.

Romano G, Rotondano G, Esposito P, Pellecchia L, Novi A. External anal sphincter defects: correlation between pre-operative anal endosonography and intraoperative findings. *Brit. J. Radiol.* 1996; 69: 6–9.

Rudd WW. Ligation and cryosurgery of all hemorrhoids. An office procedure. *Int. J. Surg.* 1989; 4: 148–51.

Rudin EP, Ragimov NS. Selection of the method of treatment of complicated hemorrhoids. *Khirurgiya* 1990; 7: 86–90.

Rutten H, Buth J. Treatment of high anorectal fistulas by anoplasty. *Neth. J. Surg.* 1988; 40: 93–6.

Saad AM, Omer A. Surgical treatment of chronic fissure-in-ano: a prospective randomised study. *East Afr. Med. J.* 1992; 69: 613–5.

Sainio P. A manometric study of anorectal function after surgery for anal fistula, with special reference to incontinence. *Acta Chir. Scand.* 1985; 151: 695–7.

Sainio P, Husa A. A prospective manometric study of the effect of anal fistula surgery on anorectal function. *Acta Chir. Scand.* 1985; 151: 279–88.

Saleeby RG, Jr Rosen L, Stasik JJ, Riether RD, Sheets J, Khubchandani IT. Hemorrhoidectomy during pregnancy: risk or relief? *Dis. Colon Rectum* 1991; 34: 260–1.

Scarpa FJ, Hillis W, Sabetta JR. Pelvic cellulitis: a life-threatening complication of hemorrhoidal banding. *Surgery* 1988; 103: 383–5.

Schneider IH, Thaler K, Kockerling F. Treatment of pilonidal sinuses by phenol injections. *Int. J. Colorectal Dis.* 1994; 9: 200–2.

Schouten WR, Briel JW, Auwerda JJ, De Graaf EJ. Ischaemic nature of anal fissure. *Brit. J. Surg.* 1996; 83: 63–5.

Schouten WR, Briel JW, Auwerda JJ. Relationship between anal pressure and anodermal blood flow. The vascular pathogenesis of anal fissures. *Dis. Colon Rectum* 1994; 37: 664–9.

Semelka RC, Hricak H, Kim B, Forstner R, Bis KG, Ascher SM, Reinhold C. Pelvic fistulas: appearances on MR images. *Abdominal Imaging* 1997; 22: 91–5.

Senagore A, Mazier WP, Luchtefeld MA, MacKeigan JM, Wengert T. Treatment of advanced hemorrhoidal disease: a prospective, randomized comparison of cold scalpel vs. contact Nd:YAG laser. *Dis. Colon Rectum* 1993; 36: 1042–9.

Senapati A, Nicholls RJ. A randomised trial to compare the results of injection sclerotherapy with a bulk laxative alone in the treatment of bleeding haemorrhoids. *Int. J. Colorectal Dis.* 1988; 3: 124–6.

Seow-Choen F, Low HC. Prospective randomized study of radical versus four piles haemorrhoidectomy for symptomatic large circumferential prolapsed piles. *Br. J. Surg.* 1995; 82: 188–9.

Seow-Choen F, Ho YH, Ang HG, Goh HS. Prospective, randomized trial comparing pain and clinical function after conventional scissors excision/ligation vs. diathermy excision without ligation for symptomatic prolapsed hemorrhoids. *Dis. Colon Rectum* 1992; 35: 1165–9.

Seow-Choen F, Leong AF, Goh HS. Results of a policy of selective immediate fistulotomy for primary anal abscess. *Aust. N.Z. Surg.* 1993; 63: 485–9.

Serdev N. The surgical treatment of hemorrhoids. Their suturing ligation without excision. *Khirurgiia* 1990; 43: 65–8.

Shafer AD, McGlone TP, Flanagan RA. Abnormal crypts of Morgagni: the cause of perianal abscess and fistula-in-ano. *J. Pediatr. Surg.* 1987; 22: 203–4.

Shafik A. Role of hemorrhoids in the pathogenesis of recurrent bacteriuria with a new approach for treatment. *Eur. Urol.* 1985; 11: 392–6.

Shemesh EI, Kodner IJ, Fry RD, Neufeld DM. Endorectal sliding flap repair of complicated anterior anoperineal fistulas. *Dis. Colon Rectum* 1988; 31: 22–4.

Shouler PJ, Grimley RP, Keighley MR, Alexander-Williams J. Fistula-in-ano is usually simple to manage surgically. *Int. J. Colorectal Dis.* 1986; 1:113–5.

Shukla HS, Gupta SC, Singh G, Singh PA. Tubercular fistula in ano. *Br. J. Surg.* 1988; 75: 38–9.

Silverman WB, Marmolya G. Endoscopic placement of a Foley catheter across a stricture and rectovaginal fistula to perform a barium enema. *Am. J. Gastroenterol.* 1989; 86: 99–101.

Simkovic D. Personal experience with the treatment of chronic anal fissures using internal lateral sphincterotomy. *Rozhl. Chir.* 1989, 68: 536–40.

Smith LE. Hemorrhoidectomy with lasers and other contemporary modalities. *Surg. Clin. North Am.* 1992; 72: 665–79.

Smith RB, Moodie J. Comparative efficacy and tolerability of two ointment and suppository preparations ('Uniroid' and 'Proctosedyl') in the treatment of second degree haemorrhoids in general practice. *Curr. Med. Res. Opinion* 1988; 11: 34–40.

Solomon MJ, McLeod RS, Cohen EK, Cohen Z. Anal wall thickness under normal and inflammatory conditions of the anorectum as determined by endoluminal ultrasonography. *Am. J. Gastroenterol.* 1995; 90: 574–8.

Sondenaa K, Andersen E, Nesvik I, Soreide JA. Patient characteristics and symptoms in chronic pilonidal sinus disease. *Int. J. Colorectal Dis.* 1995; 10: 39–42.

Sorf M, Krislo V, Skovajsova T, Lackovicova V. Ambulatory therapy of internal hemorrhoids using infrared photocoagulation and elastic ligature. *Vnitrni Lekarstvi* 1993; 39: 38–42.

Stephens FO, Stephens RB. Pilonidal sinus: management objectives. *Aust. N.Z. J. Surg.* 1995; 65: 558–60.

Stolz E, Vuzevski VD, van der Stek J. General perianal skin problems. *Neth. J. Med.* 1990; 37 (Suppl. 1): S43–6.

Sultan AH, Kamm MA, Talbot IC, Nicholls RJ, Bartram CI. Anal endosonography for identifying external sphincter defects confirmed histologically. *Br. J. Surg.* 1994; 81: 463–5.

Sun WM, Peck RJ, Shorthouse AJ, Read NW. Haemorrhoids are associated not with hypertrophy of the internal anal sphincter, but with hypertension of the anal cushions. *Br. J. Surg.* 1992; 79: 592–4.

Sweeney JL, Ritchie JK, Nicholls RJ. Anal fissure in Crohn's disease. *Br. J. Surg.* 1988; 75: 56–7.

Tajana A. Hemorrhoidectomy according to Milligan–Morgan: ligature and excision technique. *Int. J. Surg.* 1989; 74: 158–61.

Tanaka S. Cryosurgical treatment of hemorrhoids in Japan. *Int J Surg* 1989; 74: 146–7.

Tio TL, Kallimanis GE. Endoscopic ultrasonography of perianorectal fistulas and abscesses. *Endoscopy* 1994; 26: 813–5.

Van Beers B, Grandin C, Kartheuser A, Hoang P, Mahieu P, Detry R, *et al.* MRI of complicated anal fistulae: comparison with digital examination. *J. Comput. Assist. Tomogr.* 1994; 18: 87–90.

Van Beers B, Grandin C, Kartheuser A, Hoang P, Mahieu P, Detry R, *et al.* MRI of complicated anal fistulae: comparison with digital examination. *J. Comput. Assist. Tomogr.* 1994; 18: 87–90.

Van Beers BE, Kartheuser A, Delos MA, Grandin C, Detry R, Jamart J, Pringot J. MRI of the anal canal: correlation with histologic examination. *Magnetic Resonance Imaging* 1996; 14: 151–6.

Varma JS, Chung SC, Li AK. Prospective randomised comparison of current coagulation and injection sclerotherapy for the outpatient treatment of haemorrhoids. *Int. J. Colorectal Dis.* 1991; 6: 42–5.

Vasilevsky CA, Gordon PH. Results of treatment of fistula-in-ano. *Dis. Colon Rectum* 1985; 28: 225–31.

Walker AJ, Leicester RJ, Nicholls RJ, Mann CV. A prospective study of infrared coagulation, injection and rubber band ligation in the treatment of haemorrhoids. *Int. J. Colorectal Dis.* 1990; 5: 113–6.

Watson SJ, Kamm MA, Nicholls RJ, Phillips RK. Topical glyceryl trinitrate in the treatment of chronic anal fissure. *Brit. J. Surg.* 1996; 83: 771–5.

Weinshel E, Chen W, Falkenstein DB, Kessler R, Raicht RF. Hemorrhoids or rectal varices: defining the cause of massive rectal hemorrhage in patients with portal hypertension. *Gastroenterology* 1986; 90: 744–7.

Weinstein SJ, Rypins EB, Houck J, Thrower S. Single session treatment for bleeding hemorrhoids. *Surg. Gynecol. Obstet.* 1987; 165: 479–82.

Weisman RI, Orsay CP, Pearl RK, Abcarian H. The role of fistulography in fistula-in-ano. Report of five cases. *Dis. Colon Rectum* 1992; 34: 181–4.

Williams N, Scott NA, Irving MH. Effect of lateral sphincterotomy on internal anal sphincter function. A computerized vector manometry study. *Dis. Colon Rectum* 1995; 38: 700–4.

Wiltz O, Schoetz DJ Jr, Murray JJ, Roberts PL, Coller JA, Veidenheimer MC. Perianal hidradenitis suppurativa. The Lahey Clinic experience. *Dis. Colon Rectum* 1990; 33: 731–4.

Winslett MC, Allan A, Ambrose NS. Anorectal sepsis as a presentation of occult rectal and systemic disease. *Dis. Colon Rectum* 1988; 31: 597–600.

Wolkomir AF, Luchtefeld MA. Surgery for symptomatic hemorrhoids and anal fissures in Crohn's disease. *Dis. Colon Rectum* 1993; 36: 545–7.

Xynos E, Tzortzinis A, Chrysos E, Tzovaras G, Vassilakis JS. Anal manometry in patients with fissure-in-ano before and after internal sphincterotomy. *Int. J. Colorectal Dis.* 1993; 8: 125–8.

Yabe T, Furukawa M The origin of pilonidal sinus: a case report. *J. Dermatol.* 1995; 22: 696–9.

Zinberg SS, Stern DH, Furman DS, Wittles JM. A personal experience in comparing three nonoperative techniques for treating internal hemorrhoids. *Am. J. Gastroenterol.* 1989; 84: 488–9.

19 Anal tumours

Clinically, carcinoma of the anal region comprises tumours arising in the anal canal and those of the anal margin. It is recommended that the anal verge be taken as the distal limit of the anal canal, as this correlates with lymphatic drainage and clinical course of the tumour (Hermanek and Sobin 1987). Tumours arising at or above the anal transitional zone may contain varying proportions of squamous or adenocarcinoma, while only squamous carcinoma is found below this level. However, the limit of the transitional zone does not correspond with the dentate line, being found anywhere from 0.5 cm below to 2 cm above this landmark (see Chapter 1).

Incidence

Anal tumours are rare, being 20–30 times less common than colon cancer. Anal margin tumours comprise only 15% of all anal tumours. The annual age-adjusted incidence per 100 000 population for squamous cell carcinoma is 1.4 for females and 0.7 for males (Goldman *et al.* 1989). Time trend studies suggest the incidence of anal tumours has risen over the last 30 years (Melbye *et al.* 1994).

Age and sex distribution

The mean age at presentation of anal tumours is about 60 years but the age range is wide. Tumours in the anal canal show a marked female predominance. The female to male ratio varies from 1.5:1 up to as much as 9:1 (Cho *et al.* 1991; Fisher *et al.* 1997). In contrast, tumours of the anal margin are more frequent in males, showing a male to female ratio of about 4:1 (Greenall *et al.* 1985).

Geographical distribution

Tumours of the anal canal occur throughout the world. The incidence is particularly high in North-East Brazil and India, where the incidence of anal cancer is closely related to that of carcinoma of the cervix, penis, and vulva. This reflects regional variations in human papilloma virus (HPV) infection.

Aetiology (Table 19.1)

The exact cause of anal tumours is unknown but environmental factors, particularly those related to HPV infection appear important.

Smoking is an environmental factor especially in male homosexuals (Frisch *et al.* 1994). Other environmental factors include radiotherapy for pruritis and chronic inflammation related to anal fistulas, especially if associated with Crohn's disease (Lumley and Stitz 1991). Another major risk factor is sexual orientation. Homosexuality is consistently found to be associated with anal cancer, accounting for up to 79% of cases of anal atypia and all cases of giant tumours (Palefsky 1991). The relative risk of anal cancer for male homosexuals is 12.4, although this fell to 2.7 when adjusted for other variables (Holly *et al.* 1989). Anal intercourse is a

Table 19.1 Aetiological factors in anal neoplasms

Aetiological factor	Comment
Environmental factors	
Human papilloma virus	Found in 90% of anal warts and about 70% of anal tumours
	Associated with anal intraepithelial neoplasia
Sexual orientation	Homosexuality (increases risk 3–12 fold)
	Anal intercourse (increases risk 2-fold for women and up to 30-fold for men)
	Increasing number of sexual partners
Smoking	Increases risk 7–10 times
Radiotherapy	Formerly for pruritis
Chronic inflammation in anal fistulas	Usually associated with Crohn's disease
Genetic factors	
Chromosomal	Deletion of chromosome 11 (11q22)
	Deletion short arm chromosome 3

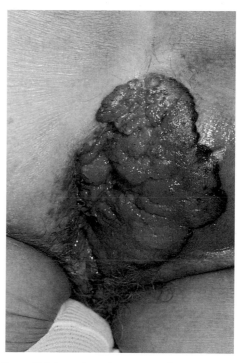

Figure 19.1 Large fungating tumour at the anal margin.

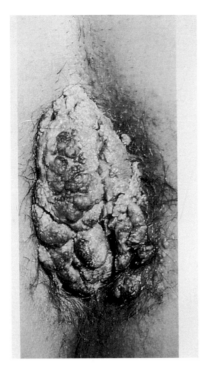

Figure 19.2 Extensive anal warts.

highly important factor in men (relative risk 33.1) and women (relative risk 1.8) (Palefsky 1991). There is also a strong link between anogenital warts and anal cancer (Frisch *et al.* 1994; Noffsinger *et al.* 1995) (Figure 19.2) It is suggested that HIV-related immunodeficiency allows reactivation of HPV resulting in simultaneous or subsequent development of epithelial abnormality (Carter *et al.* 1995; Schutz *et al.* 1996).

The common aetiological factor in many cases is infection with (HPV). HPV is found in 33–90% of squamous cell carcinomas, most reports quoting figures about 70% (Palefsky 1991). HPV is a double-stranded DNA virus that can be subtyped by various DNA *in situ* hybridization techniques. HPV subtypes 6 and 11 are principally associated with condylomata accuminata, being found in 90% of such warts (Bradshaw *et al.* 1992). HPV subtypes 6 and 11 may also occur in the premalignant conditions of Bowenoid papillosis, Buschke–Lowenstein lesions, or in invasive verrucous carcinoma. The principal subtype associated with squamous cell carcinoma is HPV 16, being found in one-half of all cases of anal intra-epithelial neoplasia grade III or frank invasion (Palefsky *et al.* 1991). HPV 16 is reported to occur in 16–80% of squamous or cloacogenic carcinomas, most series quoting figures about 50% (Deans *et al.* 1994). It is suggested that HPV 16/18, as opposed to 6/11, infection results in an endogenous modification and accumulation of mutational events, which leads to chromosomal instability and the conversion of premalignant into invasive growth (Zur Hausen 1991).

Clinical presentation

The symptoms and signs of anal carcinoma are non-specific, occurring in many other anal conditions. Consequently, almost 80% of anal cancers are initially diagnosed as a benign condition (Edwards *et al.* 1991).

Symptoms

The most frequent symptom is bright red rectal bleeding, being found in over half of cases. The mean size for both anal canal and

anal margin tumours at presentation is 3–4 cm, prejudicing the success of conservative treatment. Pruritis and discharge are also very common and may be the principal presenting complaint (Radentz *et al.* 1992). Symptoms such as incontinence, change of bowel habit, pelvic pain, or rectovaginal fistula suggest advanced lesions with malignant infiltration of the sphincters. Anal discomfort is common in anal margin tumours and may be present for some years before the diagnosis is made. The predominant symptoms of anal gland tumours are anal pain (58%), rectal bleeding (40%), and perianal mass (37%) (Abel *et al.* 1993).

Signs

Anal tumours present as indurated, painless, slow growing masses with a nodular, ulcerated, plaque-like, or verrucous pattern (Figure 19.3). In the upper part of the anal canal (40–60% of cases), tumours frequently remain as an area of submucosal nodular infiltration, while tumours in the lower canal tend to develop infiltrating ulcers. Tumours in the middle or lower canal may become visible by growing through the anal orifice. In such circumstances only part of the orifice is involved in contrast to margin tumours which tend to be circumferential. Involvement of the sphincters and the lower 2–3 cm of rectal submucosa is common. Extension into the vagina, bladder, or prostrate occurs in one-fifth of cases. Eventually annular stenosis occurs in both the anus and vagina, although vaginal mucosal ulceration occurs very late, with the vulva usually being spared.

Diagnosis

As the symptoms and signs are non-specific, a high index of suspicion is necessary. Rectal examination, if necessary under anaesthesia should identify the characteristic infiltrating nature of anal cancer (Tanum 1992). It is essential that any suspicious area is biopsied. The difficulty in diagnosis is compounded by the frequent coexistence of other anal conditions (Figure 19.4). These include condylo-

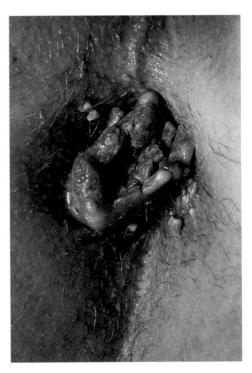

Figure 19.3 Anal tumour with an ulcerating appearance.

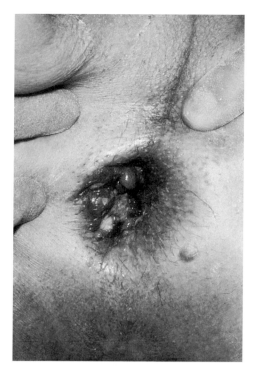

Figure 19.4 Anal carcinoma that was referred as possible thrombosed haemorrhoids.

Table 19.2 Pathological classifications of anal tumours	
Tumour classification	Tumour types
Epithelial tumours	Squamous cell carcinoma (includes small cell variety and verrucous tumours) Adenocarcinoma (includes anal clear cell tumours) Cloacogenic (includes tumours with varying proportions of squamous and adenocarcinoma, such as mucoepidermoid tumour)
Non-epithelial tumours	Tumours of the: Epidermis Dermis Subcutaneous fat Nerves Smooth muscles Striated muscles
Malignant melanoma	
Miscellaneous tumours	Carcinoid tumour Basal cell carcinoma Haematological malignancies Cutaneous secondary deposits
Pre-malignant lesions	Perianal Paget's disease Bowenoid papillosis Bowen's disease Buschke–Lowenstein lesions

mata accuminata, Paget's disease, Bowen's disease, abscesses or fistulas, and Crohn's disease (Lumley and Stitz 1991).

Pathological classification

The International Histological Classification proposed by the WHO for cancers of the anal canal and anal margin is shown in Table 19.2 (Morson and Sobin 1976). Tumours consisting of a mixture of histological types should be classified according to the predominant cell type (Tanum *et al.* 1994). In such cases, examination of only a small biopsy may lead to an incorrect classification. The WHO classification divides anal cancer into epithelial tumours, non-epithelial tumours, malignant melanoma, and premalignant conditions.

Epithelial tumours

These consist of squamous cell (including cloacogenic) and adenocarcinoma.

Squamous cell carcinoma (epidermoid tumour)

This type accounts for more than 80% of tumours of the anal region, comprising equal numbers of pure squamous cell tumours and cloacogenic carcinoma. There is a strong association with anal warts and HPV, especially subtype 16. Typical histological features are of infiltrating sheets and islands of variably differentiated squamous epithelium showing differing degrees of mitotic activity (Figure 19.5). The degree of differentiation depends on the extent of keratinization. Anal canal and anal margin tumours tend to differ in their degree of differentiation. Over half of anal canal tumours are non-keratinizing, while 80% are poorly differentiated. In con-

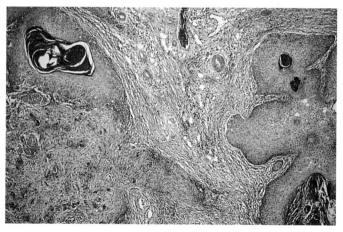

Figure 19.5 Squamous cell carcinoma of the anus showing characteristic keratinization. H&E×40

trast, up to 80% of anal margin tumours show keratinization, with 85% being well differentiated (Greenall *et al.* 1985).

Cloacogenic tumours

These tumours exhibit varying proportions of squamous carcinomas and adenocarcinomas (frequently mucinous), but behave clinically as squamous carcinomas (Figure 19.6). The terms basaloid, cloacogenic, and transitional carcinoma are synonymous. Cloacogenic tumours are now believed to be derived from the anal transitional zone, although the basal epithelium and the anal glands may also be sources of origin. They comprise about 40% of anal tumours.

Other types of epidermoid tumours have been identified (Table 19.2). Mucoepidermoid tumour is a rare variant of cloacogenic

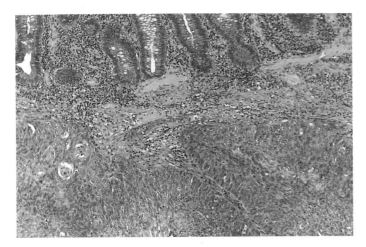

Figure 19.6 Cloacogenic form of anal tumour. H&E×100.

carcinoma, derived from the transitional epithelium at the opening of the anal gland ducts. It consists of an intimate mixture of squamous, mucinous and intermediate tumour types. An anal clear cell tumour similar, to renal clear cell tumours, has also been described (Watson 1990). Verrucous carcinoma is commoner in middle-aged men and is particularly associated with the giant warts of Buschke–Lowenstein lesions. The small cell epidermoid tumour is a rapidly growing anaplastic tumour similar to the small cell tumour of the lung or oesophagus (Boman *et al.* 1984). It may be associated with anal Paget's disease, and has a poor prognosis characterized by rapid visceral metastases.

Adenocarcinoma

Adenocarcinoma of the anus is most often due to a down-growth from a rectal adenocarcinoma. This should be readily detectable on rectal examination (Dawson 1991). More rarely it arises from ectopic islands of glandular mucosa or from the sebaceous glands of the perineum or from an anal fistula. Tumours associated with a fistula are often found in association with perianal Paget's disease and tend to be low grade, well differentiated, and metastasize late to inguinal nodes (Basik *et al.* 1995).

Spread of anal epithelial tumours

Metastases to the inguinal lymph glands occurs in about 10% of anal epithelial tumours. Inguinal node spread is more common in tumours below the dentate line, although figures vary widely from 8% to 42% (Deans *et al.* 1994). It is now recognized that about 20% of anal margin tumours will have inguinal lymph node involvement at presentation. Bilateral involvement occurs in about one-quarter of cases in which the nodes are involved. Salmon *et al.* (1984) reported nodes in 23 of 183 cases of anal carcinoma, 18 having unilateral and five bilateral nodal involvement. In addition to the normal sites of metastases for anal tumours, cloacogenic lesions have been found to metastasize to the brain, spinal cord, penis, perineum, and multiple skin sites (Deans *et al.* 1994).

Prognostic classifications of anal epithelial tumours

Dukes' classification of colorectal tumours is not applicable to anal tumours as it does not relate to inguinal, para-aortic or iliac lymph node involvement. However, histological grading classifying tumours as well, moderate or poorly differentiated, is beneficial. Well differ-

entiated tumours have squamous epithelium showing obvious and abundant keratinization. In moderately differentiated tumours the keratin formation is limited to 'pearls' (concentric laminated whorls of keratinized squames). In poorly differentiated tumours it may be difficult to establish the squamous origin unless intracellular bridges or foci of keratinization are found. Electron microscopy may then be beneficial by identifying desmosomes or tonofilaments.

The extent of tumour spread is related to prognosis. The original TNM system was criticized as it proved difficult to distinguish tumours confined to the internal (T1) from those involving the external sphincter (T2) (Papillon 1982). Subsequent modifications of the TNM system have not become widely used. The current most widely accepted classification is that of the UICC, combining clinical, radiographic, and endoscopic assessments (Hermanek and Sobin 1987) (Tables 19.3 and 19.4). In this, tumours, of the anal canal (ICD-0154.2) and perianal skin (ICD-0173.5) are clearly separated, while invasion of the sphincter muscles does not classify as a T4 lesion. Clinical examination under anaesthesia can assess the size of the lesion and involvement of the mesorectal or inguinal nodes. The latter can be confirmed, if necessary, by fine needle aspiration. Transanal ultrasound (Herzog *et al.* 1994) or computerized tomography (CT) scanning may prove beneficial in the assessment of lymph node involvement (Goodman and Halpert 1991). Another, principally clinical, classification has been derived from centres employing radiotherapy extensively (Papillon 1982). This takes into account almost all the factors needed for conservative treatment of anal

Table 19.3 TNM classification of anal canal tumours

T—Primary tumour
TX Primary tumour cannot be assessed
T0 No evidence of primary tumour
T1 Tumour 2 cm or less
T2 Tumour 2–5 cm in greatest dimension
T3 Tumour greater than 5 cm in greatest dimension
T4 Invasion of adjacent organs irrespective of tumour size

N—Regional lymph nodes
NX Regional nodes cannot be assessed
N0 No regional node metastasis
N1 Metastasis in perirectal lymph nodes
N2 Metastasis in unilateral internal iliac and/or inguinal lymph nodes
N3 Metastasis in perirectal and inguinal lymph nodes and/or bilateral internal iliac and/or inguinal lymph nodes

M—Distant metastasis

G—Pathological grade
GX Grade of differentiation cannot be assessed
G1 Well differentiated tumour
G2 Moderately differentiated tumour
G3 Poorly differentiated tumour
G4 Undifferentiated tumour

Stage

Stage	T	N	M
Stage 0	Tis	N0	M0
Stage I	T1	N0	M0
Stage II	T2/T3	N0	M0
Stage IIIA	T4	N0	M0
	T1–3	N1	M0
Stage IIIB	T4	N1	M0
	Any T	N2,3	M0
Stage IV	Any T	Any N	M1

Table 19.4 TNM classification of anal margin tumours

T designation as for anal canal tumours except:
    T4 Tumour invades deep extradermal structures
N designation
    N1 Ipsilateral inguinal nodes
M designation
    M1 Distant metastasis
Stage as for anal canal tumours except stage III (no stage IIIA or B):

III	T4	N0	M0
	Any T	N1	M0

tumours. In this classification, T1 and T2 tumours are those up to 4 cm in diameter, T3 tumours are those greater than 4 cm in diameter and which are freely mobile with no genital or urological involvement. T4a tumours have ulceration of the vaginal mucosa, while T4b tumours show involvement of the rectum, vagina or perianal skin.

Other assessments of prognosis do not appear to offer consistent improvement over these classifications. The value of DNA flow cytometry as an independent prognostic indicator is unclear (Deans *et al.* 1994). Tumour markers (carcino-embryonic antigen and squamous cell carcinoma antigen) are also of dubious benefit.

Treatment of anal epithelial tumours

Adenocarcinoma of the anus may be considered as analogous to rectal adenocarcinoma (Basik *et al.* 1995). Local control is best obtained by abdominoperineal resection and the prognosis is similar to that of rectal tumours. If local excision is attempted, it must be complete and the patient must be followed closely for many years. Recurrence after local excision can be treated by abdominoperineal resection (Basik *et al.* 1995). The role of pre-operative radiotherapy and chemoradiotherapy in the treatment of anal adenocarcinoma is not yet defined (Abel *et al.* 1993).

Squamous cell tumours of the anus may be treated by radiotherapy, combined radiochemotherapy or surgery, consisting of either local, or abdominoperineal, excision (Myerson *et al.* 1995). The optimum treatment, however, depends on whether the tumour is situated in the anal canal or anal margin.

Anal canal tumours

1. *Radiotherapy alone.* Formerly, interstitial implants, external irradiation, or a combination of the two, had a poor reputation as difficulties with orthovoltage radiation or with accurate placement of the interstitial needles resulted in unacceptable toxicity. Modern megavoltage treatment gives a 5-year survival of 55%, but with limiting toxicity (acute dermatitis, diarrhoea) occurring in 14–34% of cases (Papillon 1982). Toxicity may be reduced by interrupting the radiation course with a rest period. Toxicity is currently reduced by giving a large field treatment to the primary site, pelvic and inguinal nodes, followed 6 weeks later by a booster dose to the primary site, as recommended in the United Kingdom Co-ordinating Committee for Cancer Research's (UKCCR) anal cancer trial protocol. Local failure can thereby be reduced from 25% to 8%, major complications requiring surgery occurring in 5–15% of cases (Papillon 1982).

Anal sphincter function is preserved in about 60% of all cases, being 85% and 75% for tumours less than, and greater than, 4 cm in size respectively (Touboul *et al.* 1994). Local control and 5-year survival for T1 and T2 tumours is about 75% (T1, 100%; T2

59%), while for T3 or T4 tumours, it varies from 40% to 70% (Touboul *et al.* 1994). If there is no nodal involvement, cancer-specific 5-year survival is 64%, compared with 25% when nodal metastases are present (Otim-Oyet *et al.* 1990). Overall 5-year disease-free survival is 65%, with about 20% of patients dying of anal cancer and 15% from other causes (Papillon 1982). From 50% to 80% of treatment failures following radiotherapy can be satisfactorily salvaged by surgery.

2. *Combined radiotherapy and chemotherapy.* Adding chemotherapy to radiotherapy has been suggested and, although regimens vary, results are remarkably constant (Schlag and Hunerbein 1995). These combined modality regimens have been tested as phase II trials using a chemotherapy protocol based on that pioneered by Nigro *et al.* (1974). A 24-h infusion of 5-fluorouracil is given over 4–5 days for one to two courses, mitomycin C being given on day 1 of each course. This has been combined with radiotherapy to the primary tumour and adjacent tissues using variable target volumes and fraction regimens. The 5-year survival rate of 70% is similar to radiotherapy alone. However, primary control may be higher (93% compared with 60% for radiotherapy alone) despite increased haematological and intestinal toxicity.

Toxicity of combined therapy includes dermatitis, mucositis, alopecia, and reversible haematological disorders. Toxicity can be expected in about 20% of cases, but severe toxicity is uncommon (Tanum *et al.* 1993). Late incontinence, intestinal obstruction and chronic pelvic pain occur in 15% of patients. Anal sphincter function is preserved in about 80% of cases (Deans *et al.* 1994), although there is a significant increase in the mean minimal sensory threshold but not in the resting pressure or mean maximal squeeze pressure with treatment (Birnbaum *et al.* 1994). Age is not a contraindication to multi-modality treatment, but sterility is virtually inevitable and young patients should be counselled (de Gara *et al.* 1995).

Complete response rates are in the region of 70–90% being 85% and 73% for tumours less than, and greater than 4 cm, respectively (Deans *et al.* 1994). Approximately 15% of patients will have persistent disease initially, while a further 15% will develop late loco-regional recurrence (Cho *et al.* 1991). The 5-year survival figures of 60–80%, along with an 80% preservation of anal function, makes non-surgical management an attractive therapy in anal canal tumours (Tanum *et al.* 1993; Deans *et al.* 1994) (Table 19.5).

3. *Local surgery.* It is now accepted that local excision of anal canal tumours should only be performed if the tumour is less than 2 cm in diameter and is not touching the dentate line (Touboul *et al.* 1995). This selects patients with a reduced risk of nodal metastases, while allowing a minimum 1 cm tumour clearance with limited risk of subsequent stricture formation. Fewer than 10% of anal canal tumours will satisfy these criteria (Greenall *et al.* 1985), but if they are adhered to, 95% of patients can obtain loco-regional control (Bowman *et al.* 1984). With less strict selection criteria, local recurrence rates have varied between 7% and 65% (Greenall *et al.* 1985) and 5-year survival figures were about 65%. Therefore, local excision can only rarely be recommended for anal canal tumours (Touboul *et al.* 1995).

4. *Abdominoperineal resection.* Radical surgery was formerly considered the treatment of choice for anal canal tumours (Table 19.6). It is a major procedure which results in loss of the anal sphincters and permanent colostomy formation. About 15% of patients will be unsuitable while an operative mortality in the region of 5% can be expected. Sexual function can be maintained in 70% of patients. 5-year survival varies between 23% and 71%, reflecting differences

Table 19.5 Studies of combined chemoradiotherapy for anal canal tumours

Author(s)	Year	No. patients	Local control (%)	Survival (%)
Sischy	1982	29	90	90
Michaelson et al.**	1982	37	81	78
Cummings et al.	1984	30	93	90
Nigro et al.**	1984	104	85	85
Greenall et al.	1985	18	66	88
John et al.	1987	22	100	100
Papillon and Montbarbon*	1987	70	87	N/A
Beck and Karulf	1994	29	90	89

*Chemoradiotherapy and interstitial iridium.
**Pre-operative chemoradiotherapy.
N/A = not available.

Table 19.6 Results of trials of radical surgery in anal canal tumours

Authors	Year	No. patients	Local control (%)	5-year survival (%)
Klotz et al.	1967	94	N/A	50
Hardcastle and Bussey	1968	83	N/A	48
O'Brien et al.	1982	21	N/A	38
Loygue et al.	1980	109	73	62
Singh et al.	1981	47	N/A	53
Schraut et al.	1983	24	46	54
Boman et al.	1984	118	73	71
Frost et al.	1984	109	73	62
Greenall et al.	1985	103	79	58
Merlini and Eckbert	1985	69	N/A	23
Pyper and Parks	1985	37	N/A	42
Clark et al.	1986	61	41	42

N/A = not available.

in patient selection (Deans *et al.* 1994). Most series report 5-year survival about 60%, depending on tumour size, grade, depth of invasion, and nodal involvement. Virtually all the failures are due to loco-regional recurrence. Postoperative radiotherapy in node positive patients reduces local recurrence from 25% to 17% (Frost *et al.* 1984). Recurrence after abdominoperineal resection is associated with a poor prognosis, the median survival following recurrence being 9 months (range 1–48 months) (Greenall *et al.* 1985). Palliative radiotherapy or chemotherapy may prolong mean survival to 14 months, but complete responses are rare, only one in five patients being alive after 3 years (Longo *et al.* 1994).

Anal margin tumours

Interstitial implants and high-dose radiotherapy can give satisfactory results in anal margin tumours, with combined radiochemotherapy achieving local cure in 80–100% of selected cases (Cutuli *et al.* 1988). Mild complications (perineal telangiectasis or fibrosis) occur in 25% of cases, while severe complications requiring a colostomy or intervention for femoral neck fractures, occur in up to 10% of cases (Cutuli *et al.* 1988). T3 or T4 tumours have a 5-year survival of under 50% with 30% local recurrence rate. Half of these can be salvaged by surgery (Longo *et al.* 1994).

In contrast to anal canal cancers, up to 60% of anal margin tumours may be satisfactorily treated by local excision. Local exci-

sion is suitable for anal margin tumours that show superficial, *in situ* or micro-invasive disease. Tumours involving more than half of the anal circumference are not suitable, as poor sphincter function results. Cancer-specific 5-year survival varies from 65% to 100% (Greenall *et al.* 1985). Frozen section and skin grafting allows wider excision and reduces local recurrence rates. Combined local excision and radiotherapy, or abdominoperineal resection should be restricted to T2 or T3 tumours or the rare histological subtypes of mucoepidermoid adenocarcinoma and verrucous carcinoma (Papillon and Chassard 1992).

Lymph node metastases

Anal canal tumours

The morbidity of prophylactic inguinal lymph node dissection outweighs the benefit. Synchronous inguinal nodes, even if locally controlled, are associated with a poor 5-year survival of less than 20% (Greenall *et al.* 1985). In highly selected cases, the addition of radiotherapy to either block dissection or node picking prevents nodal ulceration, with a 5-year survival of 58% being achieved. If metachronous nodes occur (usually within 18 months), combined groin dissection and radiotherapy, together with chemotherapy if the nodes are fixed, has a better prognosis, with 5-year survival in the range of 40–70% (Frost *et al.* 1984).

In surgical series, involvement of the mesorectal or pelvic nodes decreases the 5-year survival from 70% to 30% (Deans *et al.* 1994). The importance of postoperative irradiation in node positive surgically treated cases is therefore apparent (Papillon 1982). However, there seems little place for prophylactic radical pelvic nodal clearance at the time of operation.

Anal margin tumours

Approximately 20% of anal margin tumours will present with inguinal lymph node involvement. Synchronous nodal involvement should be treated by excision of the involved glands combined with groin radiotherapy as 5-year survival of 33–66% can be expected (Cutuli *et al.* 1988). In contrast to anal canal tumours, metachronous inguinal lymph gland involvement from anal margin tumours has an universally poor prognosis, such that for all but the smallest lesion, radiotherapy of involved nodes has been advocated.

Non-epithelial tumours

Benign and malignant lesions of non-epithelial tissue which occur elsewhere in the body may also, athough rarely, be found in the perianal region. These may be classified as lesions of the epidermis, dermis, subcutaneous tissue, nerves and muscle.

Tumours of the epidermis and dermis

These include epidermoid and dermoid cysts, hidradenoma papilliferum, and endometriosis, all of which are benign. Epidermoid cysts may occur after trauma and result in implantation of squamous epithelium into the dermis. They appear as smooth-domed cysts a few millimetres to a few centimetres across. Dermoid cysts are unilocular subcutaneous nodules associated with hair follicles or sebaceous glands and lined with stratified squamous epithelium. Hidradenoma papilliferum appears as a 1–2 cm solitary asymptomatic nodule in the female genitalia or perianal region. Endometriosis has been reported in the anal region following an episiotomy scar. It appears as a bluish painful nodule with cyclical variation in size and symptoms.

Tumours of the subcutaneous fat

These consist principally of lipomas and liposarcomas. As elsewhere in the body, perineal lipomas appear as well circumscribed, slow growing, mobile, painless lumps. They are always benign. Liposarcoma presents clinically as a slow growing painless, deep-seated mass. There are five histological types; adipocytic, sclerosing, myxoid, lipoblastic, and pleomorphic. The larger the lesion the poorer the prognosis. Recurrence approaches 100%, with over a third of the lesions metastasizing in the lipoblastic or pleomorphic varieties. The overall 5-year survival is about 50%. As in other parts of the body, angiolipomas, fibrosarcoma, and fibrous histiocytoma may occasionally be seen in the perineum.

Nerve tumours

Traumatic neuroma and malignant nerve sheath tumours may very rarely occur in the perineum. Anal neurofibromas are common and although maybe solitary, are mostly associated with Von Recklinghausen's neurofibromatosis (Figure 19.7).

Smooth muscle tumours

Leiomyoma arises from the errector pili muscle and tends to affect young adults with a slight male predominance (Bauer and Lubonski 1993). The epidermis is typically unaffected. Leiomyomas of the anal region occur in the submucosa, and vary in size from 1 to 7 cm (average 2.1 cm). Occasionally they may be an incidental finding,

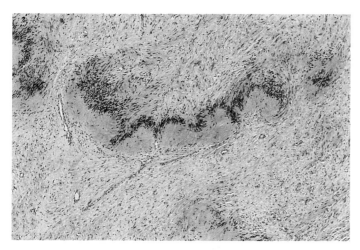

Figure 19.7 Neuroleminoma of the subcutaneous tissue. H&E×100.

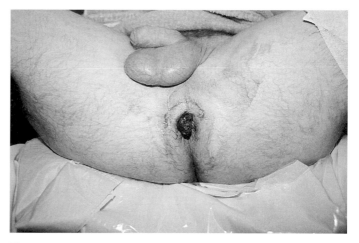

Figure 19.8 Leiomyosarcoma of the anus that was referred as a 'prolapsed haemorrhoid'.

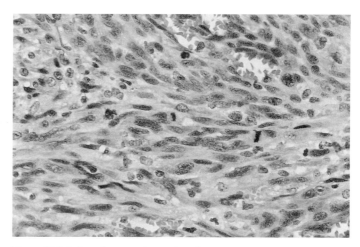

Figure 19.9 Pallasading smooth muscle cells with frequent mitoses suggesting leiomyosarcoma (same patient as Figure 19.8). H&E×250.

having given rise to no clinical symptoms. Despite their benign appearance, however, some may behave like a sarcoma (Figures 19.8 and 19.9). Leiomyosarcoma accounts for 0.1% of all anorectal malignancies. They arise from the errector pili muscles or blood vessels, are commonest in the sixth to seventh decades and show a slight male predominance. Symptoms, consist of bleeding, pain or altered bowel habit, the average size being 5 cm, with a range of 1–11 cm. Recurrence is common (33%) and 5-year survival is 50–75%.

Striated muscle tumours

Rhabdomyoma or sarcoma are rare tumours occurring in infants or middle age and are more common in males.

Malignant melanoma

Incidence and aetiology

Anal malignant melanoma accounts for about 0.01% of all anorectal cancers and 1.3% of all malignant melanomas (Longo *et al.* 1995). However, in developing countries anorectal melanoma accounts for 15% of all melanomas and 45% of non-cutaneous melanomas. It was thought that in the anal region malignant melanoma always develops at the dentate line and transitional mucosa, rectal involvement being due to spread from the anus. However, melanocytes have recently been demonstrated in all three zones of the anal canal, suggesting that malignant melanoma may arise above, as well as below, the dentate line (Clemmensen and Fenger 1991). Although some have reported a female to male ratio of about 2:1 others have noted an equal incidence or only a slight female predominance (Knysh *et al.* 1990). The mean age at presentation is about 60 years, with a range of 21–85 years.

Clinical presentation

Symptoms
Symptoms resemble other anal conditions, namely pain, mucus discharge, passage of blood and alteration in bowel habit. Consequently, late presentation with inguinal metastases is frequent, one-third of patients presenting with synchronous and 88% developing metachronous node metastases.

Signs
Clinically, anal malignant melanoma appears as a polypoid or nodular mass often greater than 4 cm in diameter at presentation (Figure 19.10). A pelvic mass or pulmonary nodules may also be noted at presentation. The majority of tumours range between 2 and 5 cm and all invade into the submucosa (Nakhleh *et al.* 1990). This, and the bluish appearance, result in it being easily mistaken for a haemorrhoid or a rectal carcinoma (Nicholson *et al.* 1993). This is compounded by the occasional rectal adenocarcinoma that may contain melanin. Conversely, pigmentation in anal malignant melanoma is absent in one-third of cases, the diagnosis being made as an incidental finding on biopsy of a supposedly benign lesion. In unpigmented cases electron microscopy and S100 protein staining may be of benefit (Figure 19.11). Alternatively, it may appear as a papillomatous ulcerating and indurated lesion which spreads rapidly into the rectum and perirectal tissue with early inguinal lymph node involvement.

Classification

Breslow's classification, in which the thickness of the tumour is measured from the most superficial aspect of the granular cell layer to the deepest part of the tumour invasion, is of prognostic significance. However, occasional thick tumours or node positive tumours may also do well. Clarke's classification is also related to survival; level I represents an *in situ* tumour; level 2, invasion of the papillary dermis by single cells; level 3, tumour abutting onto the dermal interface; level 4, invasion of the reticular dermis; and level 5, invasion of the subcutaneous fat. Tumours of Clarke's classification II and III or less than 0.76 mm in thickness (Breslow's classification) have a good prognosis, while those of Clarke's classification IV or V or greater than 1.5 mm in thickness have a poor outlook (Table 19.7). CT scanning can be beneficial in staging (Buzaid *et al.* 1993).

Prognosis

In most cases, the late presentation of anal malignant melanoma results in an almost universally abysmal prognosis, irrespective of the method of treatment. Mean survival for anal malignant melanoma is in the region of 6–32 months. The mean survival is 18 months and is related to the depth of tumour invasion and the number of giant multinucleated cells but not to treatment or histology. The 5-year survival is 10%. The mean survival of those not undergoing surgical treatment is 22 months. Loco-regional recurrence is inevitable if local excision is inadequate, although even radical surgery does not improve long-term survival. The outlook is so poor that non-radical treatment has been advocated while others advise surgery, either local excision or abdominoperineal resection

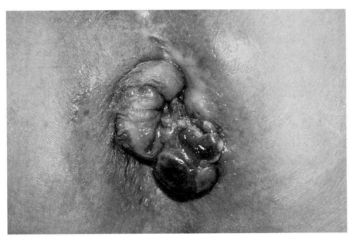

Figure 19.10 Malignant melanoma of the anus referred as a possible thrombosed haemorrhoid. H&E×100 (see colour plates).

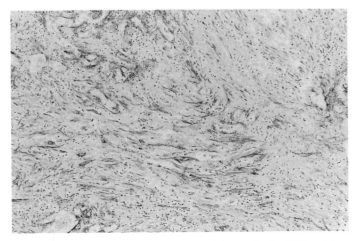

Figure 19.11 Malignant melanoma of anus staining positive for S100 protein.

Table 19.7 Prognostic classifications of malignant melanoma

Classification	Features
Breslow	
Tumour thickness measuring	
0–0.76 mm	metastases exceedingly rare
0.77–1.49 mm	good prognosis
1.5–3.5 mm	intermediate prognosis
> 3.5 mm	poor prognosis
Clark	tumour thickness involving:
Level 1	*in situ* melanoma
Level 2	early invasion of the papillary dermis
Level 3	extensive invasion of the papillary dermis
Level 4	invasion into the reticular dermis
Level 5	invasion into the subcutaneous fat

(Ross *et al.* 1990). Abdominoperineal resection may be preferred in small tumours less than 2 mm thick in the absence of visceral metastases, because in these circumstances, local excision is associated with a higher local recurrence (Brady *et al.* 1995; Konstadoulakis *et al.* 1995). Radiotherapy to extensive tumours is only palliative and chemotherapy has not been found to be effective to date.

Carcinoid tumour

Incidence

This arises from neuroendocrine cells in the anal transitional zone. It accounts for about 0.5% of anorectal tumours. The mean age at presentation is 55 years (range 20–80), with an equal sex incidence (Ponz de Leon *et al.* 1990; Nwiloh *et al.* 1990).

Clinical presentation

Symptoms

Symptoms are uncommon if the tumour is less than 1.5 cm in size but bleeding with or without ulceration occurs if the tumour is greater than 2 cm in diameter (Federspiel *et al.* 1990). Pain and alteration in bowel habit suggest involvement of the anal sphincters. Right upper quadrant pain with weight loss implies hepatic metastases, although the full carcinoid syndrome is rare, even in the presence of hepatic secondaries.

Signs

Clinically, anorectal carcinoid may present as a very hard submucosal nodule with a yellow-orange colour apparent through the mucosa. Most occur less than 10 cm from the anal verge and should therefore be detectable on rectal examination.

Pathology

In the St Mark's experience of 35 anal carcinoids, 31 were benign and four were malignant. Histologically, it presents as a variably sized nodule of regular, round to oval cells containing vesicular nuclei with a tendency towards peripheral pallisading (Figures 19.12 and 19.13). Malignant transformation is suggested by increase in size, lymphochromatosis, or muscular invasion (Federspiel *et al.* 1990; Moesta *et al.* 1990). Anal carcinoid may be associated with other tumours such as synchronous or metachronous polyps (10%), rectal carcinoma (3%), colonic carcinoma (3%), vulva carcinoma

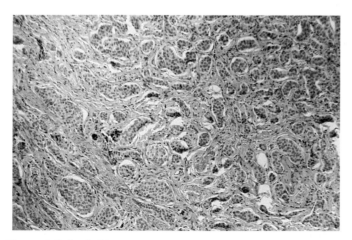

Figure 19.12 Carcinoid tumour showing islands of cells within the bowel wall. H&E×100.

(3%), or other malignancies (5%). Five-year survival is in the region of 80%. An anorectal anaplastic carcinoma of neuroendocrine origin similar to the pulmonary anaplastic tumour has been reported. It has rapid blood and lymphatic spread with no patients surviving beyond the first year.

Treatment

On account of the small size of most anal carcinoids, proctoscopy with deep biopsy is often sufficient to remove the lesion completely (Sauven *et al.* 1990). Carcinoids in the upper part of the canal or rectum can be treated by local excision using a trans-sphincter technique. Metastases can be detected by radioisotope (MIBG) imaging (Watanabe *et al.* 1995).

Basal cell carcinoma

Anal basal cell carcinoma accounts for less than 0.1% of anorectal neoplasms (Quan 1988). The occurrence of a squamous cell carcinoma of the tongue with a perineal basal cell carcinoma is known as Cowden's disease. Clinically, it may appear as an ulcer at or touching the anal margin with an irregular hard and slightly raised edge, 1–2 cm in diameter. Consequently, it may be misdiagnosed as an anal ulcer or haemorrhoid. Inguinal nodes are not involved unless infection supervenes and deep invasion is extremely uncommon. Local excision is normally curative, although crude 5-year survival is only 75% due to the advanced age of many of the patients.

Haematological malignancies

Haematological tumours may also occasionally present in the anorectum. Lymphoma may occur as a perianal infection or abscess, while cases of anorectal lymphoma have been noted in HIV-positive patients (Melbye *et al.* 1994; Schulz *et al.* 1996). Anorectal leukaemia deposits have also been reported.

Cutaneous secondary deposits

Metastases to the skin occur in 0.5% of internal malignancies. The perineum may be involved by direct spread from a pelvic or rectal neoplasm or by haematological or lymphatic spread from more distant tumours. Adenocarcinoma or mucoid carcinomas may metastasize to the anorectal region from the breast or colon.

Tumour-like conditions

Perianal Paget's disease

This is an erythematous skin rash associated with an intra-epithelial adenocarcinoma (Robin 1991). Perianal Paget's disease is rare, less than 100 cases being reported in the literature (Shlatze and Gleysteen 1990; Goldman *et al.* 1992). The average age at presentation is about 60 years, the sex incidence being equal (Beck and Fazio 1987). Perianal Paget's disease appears to be biologically different from that seen in the breast (Nakamura *et al.* 1995). Up to 50% of cases represent a metastasis from a perianal sweat gland carcinoma, or more rarely, from carcinoma of the rectum, prostate, cervix, or stomach (Lertprasertsuke and Tsutsumi 1991). Pruritis ani is a predominant feature which can be present for several years prior to diagnosis (Beck and Fazio 1987). Pain occurs occasionally. Clinically, perianal Paget's disease appears as an erythematous, erosive, or eczematous rash which may be multicentric. Alternatively, it may be found incidentally in 'haemorrhoidectomy' specimens. Tumour nodules may be apparent if presentation is late. Although spontaneous regression has been noted following partial

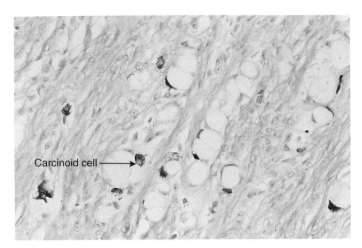

Figure 19.13 Anorectal carcinoid tumour. Grimelius stain reveals scattered positive of mucinous carcinoid.

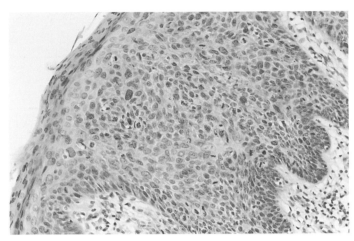

Figure 19.14 Bowen's disease of the anus showing anal intra-epithelial neoplasia (AIN) grade III. H&E×250.

excision (Archer *et al.* 1987), it is important to screen for an underlying carcinoma (Beck and Fazio 1987; Quan 1988).

Mucin and immunohistochemistry can assess malignant potential, recurrence, and distinguish anorectal from sweat gland tumours (Hurt *et al.* 1992; Miller *et al.* 1992). Survival is related to stage of the underlying carcinoma. If no tumour is identified, survival approaches 100%, whereas 5-year survival maybe less than 10% in cases associated with an underlying tumour (Lingam and O'Dwyer 1997).

Bowenoid papillosis

Bowenoid papillosis is a relatively new diagnosis which is probably best considered as being potentially malignant. The exact incidence is unknown, those in the 20–40 year age group being most commonly affected. Condylomata accuminata or herpes simplex virus may coexist, with HPV 16 or 18 being found in 11% of cases (Balazs 1991). Clinically, it presents as multiple elevated reddish and sometimes scaly papules ranging from 0.2 to 1 cm in diameter (LaVoo 1987). The main differential diagnoses are condylomata accuminatum, lichen planus and psoriasis. Histological appearance varies from non-specific findings through dysplasia to carcinoma *in situ*, which can be indistinguishable from Bowen's disease.

Bowen's disease

This is a rare condition of intra-epithelial squamous neoplasia, analogous to the intra-epithelial columnar neoplasia of Paget's disease (Quan 1988). Atypia occurs in 7% of surgically removed anal specimens; 6% of patients with atypia will have Bowen's disease and 80% of these will be male homosexuals. The average age is about 55 years the male to female ratio being 5:1.

Ninety-five per cent of anal Bowen's disease arise near condylomata accuminata (Ribiere 1987) often associated with HPV types 16, 18, and 33 (Yeong *et al.* 1992). It has been described in ulcerative colitics with anal warts or Crohn's disease (Balazs 1991). Like anal Paget's disease, anal Bowen's disease is often associated with an underlying synchronous or metachronous cancer, particularly a multicentric carcinoma of the vulva or anus. Up to 95% of females will have vulva carcinoma *in situ*, while invasive vulval or perineal carcinoma occurs in 50% (Fenger and Nielson 1986).

Pruritis ani may be a marked symptom. Bowen's disease appears as persistent, discrete, irregular, erythematous, or crusted lesions, half of which arise above the dentate line in the transitional zone

(Fenger and Nielson 1986). Bowen's disease is distinguished from Bowenoid papillosis in that it presents as single lesions in elderly patients and anal atypia is invariable. In contrast to Bowenoid papillosis, Bowen's disease appears as a steadily slow growing plaque which progresses to invasive carcinoma.

Histologically, dysplasia affects the entire epidermis and mitoses are frequent (Figure 19.14). Bowenoid cells are large and contain irregular hypochromatic nuclei with conspicuous nucleoli and abundant (occasionally vacuolated) cytoplasm. Immunohistochemistry can distinguish difficult cases of Bowen's disease from Paget's disease and superficial spreading melanoma (Watanabe *et al.* 1993). Bowen's disease of the anus is usually treated by wide local excision areas if random biopsies show dysplasia. Skin grafting or V–Y plasty is often necessary as areas of macroscopic dysplasia may be found a considerable distance from the grossly affected site. Mortality of anal Bowen's disease ranges from 0 to 10%, and recurrence from 9% and 19% (Quan 1988; Boynton and Bjorkman 1991). A more conservative approach of local excision of the grossly affected area only, without skin grafting has been justified as it appears equally effective. Other conservative techniques such as phototherapy or laser therapy may also be suitable for Bowen's disease in inaccessible sites or for particularly large lesions (Boynton and Byorkman 1991).

Buschke–Lowenstein lesions

These present as giant condylomata accuminata. They appear to be an intermediate lesion in a pathological continuum from condylomata accuminata to squamous cell carcinoma. Approximately 30 cases have been reported, squamous cell carcinoma developing in one-third (Bertram *et al.* 1995). They are associated with HPV types 6 and 11 (Schwartz *et al.* 1991; Bertram *et al.* 1995). Clinically, they appear as a craggy malignant looking mass. Despite the clinical appearance of malignancy, they are benign in two-thirds of cases. Local invasion and focal cytological atypia suggests transformation into a verrucous carcinoma. Repeated deep biopsies are required to distinguish the infiltrating pattern of verrucous carcinoma from the exophytic appearance of warts and condylomas. Recurrence may occur but metastases are relatively rare. Giant tumours measuring 10–17 cm have been identified in homosexuals (Cobb *et al.* 1990). CT is useful in assessing the extent of Buschke–Lowenstein lesions.

References

Balazs M. Bowenoid change in perianal condyloma acuminatum associated with ulcerative colitis. *Hepatogastroenterology* 1991; 38: 311–3.

Basik M, Rodriguez Bigas MA, Penetrante R, Petrelli NJ. Prognosis and recurrence patterns of anal adenocarcinoma. *Am. J. Surg.* 1995; 169: 233–7.

Bauer P, Luboinski J. Leiomyoma of the anal canal. A case. *Presse Med.* 1993; 22: 255–7.

Beck DE, Karulf RE. Combination therapy for epidermoid carcinoma of the anal canal. *Dis. Colon Rectum* 1994; 37: 1118–25.

Bertram P, Treutner KH, Rubben A, Hauptmann S, Schumpelick V. Invasive squamous cell carcinoma in giant anorectal condyloma (Buschke Lowenstein tumor). *Langenbecks Arch. Chir.* 1995; 380: 115–8.

Birnbaum EH, Myerson RJ, Fry RD, Kodner IJ, Fleshman JW. Chronic effects of pelvic radiation therapy on anorectal function. *Dis. Colon Rectum* 1994; 37: 909–15.

Boman BM, Moertel CG, O'Connell MJ, Scott M, Weiland LH, Beart RW. Carcinoma of the anal canal. A clinical and pathologic study of 188 cases. *Cancer* 1984; 54: 114–25.

Boynton KK, Bjorkman DJ. Argon laser therapy for perianal Bowen's disease: a case report. *Lasers Surg. Med.* 1991; 11: 385–7.

Bradshaw BR, Nuovo GJ, DiCostanzo D, Cohen SR. Human papillomavirus type 16 in a homosexual man. Association with perianal carcinoma *in situ* and condyloma acuminatum. *Arch. Dermatol.* 1992; 128: 949–52.

Brady MS, Kavolius JP, Quan SH. Anorectal melanoma. A 64 year experience at Memorial Sloan Kettering Cancer Center. *Dis. Colon Rectum* 1995; 38: 146–51.

Buzaid AC, Sandler AB, Mani S, Curtis AM, Poo WJ, Bolognia JL, Ariyan S. Role of computed tomography in the staging of primary melanoma. *J. Clin. Oncol.* 1993; 11: 638–43.

Carter PS, de Ruiter A, Whatrup C, Katz DR, Ewings P, Mindel A, Northover JM. Human immunodeficiency virus infection and genital warts as risk factors for anal intraepithelial neoplasia in homosexual men. *Br. J. Surg.* 1995; 82: 473–4.

Cho CC, Taylor CW 3d, Padmanabhan A, Arnold MW, Aguilar PS, Meesig DM, *et al.* Squamous cell carcinoma of the anal canal: management with combined chemo radiation therapy. *Dis. Colon Rectum* 1991; 34: 675–8.

Clark J, Petrelli N, Herrera LM, Helmann A. Epidermoid carcinoma of the anal canal. *Cancer* 1986; 57: 400–6.

Clemmensen OJ, Fenger C. Melanocytes in the anal canal epithelium. *Histopathology* 1991; 18: 237–41.

Cobb JP, Schecter WP, Russell T. Giant malignant tumors of the anus. A strategy for management. *Dis. Colon Rectum* 1990; 33: 135–7.

Cummings B, Keane TJ, Thomas G, Harwood A, Rider W. Results and toxicity of the treatment of anal canal carcinoma by radiation therapy or radiation therapy and chemotherapy. *Cancer* 1984; 54: 2062–8.

de Gara CJ, Basrur V, Figueredo A, Goodyear M, Knight P. The influence of age on the management of anal cancer. *Hepatogastroenterology* 1995; 42: 73–6.

Deans GT, McAleer JJ, Spence RA. Malignant anal tumours. *Br. J. Surg.* 1994; 81: 500–8.

Edwards AT, Morus LC, Foster ME, Griffith GH. Anal cancer: the case for earlier diagnosis. *J. R. Soc. Med.* 1991; 84: 395–7.

Federspiel BH, Burke AP, Sobin LH, Shekitka KM. Rectal and colonic carcinoids. A clinicopathologic study of 84 cases. *Cancer* 1990; 65: 135–40.

Fisher G, Harlow SD, Schottenfeld D. Cumulative risk of second primary cancers in women with index primary cancers of uterine cervix and incidence of lower anogenital tract cancers, Michigan, 1985–1992. *Gynecol. Oncol.* 1997; 64: 213–23.

Frisch M, Olsen JH, Melbye M. Malignancies that occur before and after anal cancer: clues to their etiology. *Am. J. Epidemiol.* 1994; 140: 12–9.

Frost DB, Richards PC, Montague ED, Giacco GG, Martin RG. Epidermoid cancer of the anorectum. *Cancer* 1984; 53: 525–30.

Goldman S, Glimelius B, Glas U, Lundell G, Pahlman L, Stahle E. Management of anal epidermoid carcinoma––an evaluation of treatment results in two population based series. *Int. J. Colorectal Dis.* 1989; 4: 234–43.

Goldman S, Ihre T, Lagerstedt U, Svensson C. Perianal Paget's disease: report of five cases. *Int. J. Colorectal Dis.* 1992; 7: 167–9.

Goodman P, Halpert RD. Invasive squamous cell carcinoma of the anus arising in condyloma acuminatum: CT demonstration. *Gastrointest. Radiol.* 1991; 16: 267–70.

Greenall MJ, Quan SH, De Cosse JJ. Epidermoid cancer of the anus. *Br. J. Surg.* 1985; 72: 597.

Hardcastle JD, Bussey HJR. Results of surgical treatment of squamous cell carcinoma of the anal canal and anal margin seen at St Mark's Hospital 1928–66. *J. R. Soc. Med.* 1968; 61: 629–30.

Herzog U, Boss M, Spichtin HP. Endoanal ultrasonography in the follow up of anal carcinoma. *Surg. Endosc.* 1994; 8: 1186–9.

Hurt MA, Hardarson S, Stadecker MJ, Santa Cruz DJ. Fibroepithelioma like changes associated with anogenital epidermotropic mucinous carcinoma. Fibroepitheliomatous Paget phenomenon. *J. Cutan. Pathol.* 1992; 19: 134–41.

John MJ, Flam M, Lovalvo L, Mowry PA. Feasibility of non-surgical definitive management of anal canal carcinoma. *Int. J. Radiat. Oncol. Biol. Phys.* 1987; 13: 299–303.

Klotz RG, Pamukoglu T, Souillard DH. Transitional cloacogenic carcinoma of the anal canal. Clinicopathological study of 373 cases. *Cancer* 1967; 20: 1727–47.

Knysh VI, Parshikova SM, Timofeev IM, Perevoshchikov AG, Dudarova RG, Babaev DI. Melanomas of the anorectal region. *Vopr. Onkol.* 1990; 36: 940–4.

Konstadoulakis MM, Ricaniadis N, Walsh D, Karakousis CP. Malignant melanoma of the anorectal region. *J. Surg. Oncol.* 1995; 58: 118–20.

Lingam M, O'Dwyer P. Clinicopathological study of perineal Paget's disease. *Br. J. Surg.* 1997; 84: 231–2.

Longo WE, Vernava AM 3rd, Wade TP, Coplin MA, Virgo KS, Johnson FE. Recurrent squamous cell carcinoma of the anal canal. Predictors of initial treatment failure and results of salvage therapy. *Ann. Surg.* 1994; 220: 40–9.

Longo WE, Vernava AM 3rd, Wade TP, Coplin MA, Virgo KS, Johnson FE. Rare anal canal cancers in the U.S. veteran: patterns of disease and results of treatment. *Am. Surg.* 1995; 61: 495–500.

Loygue J, Laugier A, Parc A, Weisgerber G. Cancer epidermoide de l'anus. A propos de 149 observations. *Chirurgie* 1980; 6: 710–16.

Lumley JW, Stitz RW. Crohn's disease and anal carcinoma: an association? A case report and review of the literature. *Aust. N.Z. J. Surg.* 1991; 61: 76–7.

Melbye M, Cote TR, Kessler L, Gail M, Biggar RJ. High incidence of anal cancer among AIDS patients. The AIDS/Cancer Working Group. *Lancet* 1994; 343: 636–9.

Merlini M, Eckert P. Malignant tumors of the anus. *Am. J. Surg.* 1985; 150: 370–2.

Michaelson RA, Maginn GB, Quan SHQ, Leaming RH, Nikrui M, Stearns MW. Preoperative chemotherapy and radiation therapy in the management of anal epidermoid cancer. *Cancer* 1982; 51: 390–5.

Miller LR, McCunniff AJ, Randall ME. An immunohistochemical study of perianal Paget's disease. Possible origins and clinical implications. *Cancer* 1992; 69: 2166–71.

Moesta KT, Schlag P. Proposal for a new carcinoid tumour staging system based on tumour tissue infiltration and primary metastasis; a prospective multicentre carcinoid tumour evaluation study. West German Surgical Oncologists' Group. *Eur. J. Surg. Oncol.* 1990; 16: 280–8.

Morson BC, Sobin LH. Histological typing of intestinal tumours. In: *International Histological Classification of Tumours* No. 15. Geneva: World Health Organization. 1976: 67–9.

Myerson RJ, Shapiro SJ, Lacey D, Lopez M, Birnbaum E, Fleshman J, *et al.* Carcinoma of the anal canal. *Am. J. Clin. Oncol.* 1995; 18: 32–9.

Nakamura G, Shikata N, Shoji T, Hatano T, Hioki K, Tsubura A. Immunohistochemical study of mammary and extramammary Paget's disease. *Anticancer Res.* 1995; 15: 467–70.

Nakhleh RE, Wick MR, Rocamora A, Swanson PE, Dehner LP. Morphologic diversity in malignant melanomas. *Am. J. Clin. Pathol.* 1990; 93: 731–40.

Nicholson AG, Cox PM, Marks CG, Cook MG. Primary malignant melanoma of the rectum. *Histopathology* 1993; 22: 261–4.

Nigro MD. An evaluation of combined therapy for squamous cell carcinoma of the anal canal. *Dis. Colon Rectum* 1984; 27: 763–6.

Noffsinger AE, Hui YZ, Suzuk L, Yochman LK, Miller MA, Hurtubise P, *et al.* The relationship of human papillomavirus to proliferation and ploidy in carcinoma of the anus. *Cancer* 1995; 75: 958–67.

Nwiloh JO, Pillarisetty S, Moscovic EA, Freeman HP. Carcinoid tumors. *J. Surg. Oncol.* 1990; 45: 261–4.

O'Brien PH, Jenrette JM, Wallace KM, Metcalf JS. Epidermoid carcinoma of the anus. *Surg. Gynecol. Obstet.* 1982; 155: 745–51.

Otim Oyet D, Ford HT, Fisher C, Crow J, Horwich A. Radical radiotherapy for carcinoma of the anal canal. *Clin. Oncol. R. Coll. Radiol.* 1990; 2: 84–9.

Palefsky JM. Human papillomavirus associated anogenital neoplasia and other solid tumors in human immunodeficiency virus infected individuals. *Curr. Opin. Oncol.* 1991; 3: 881–5.

Palefsky JM, Holly EA, Gonzales J, Berline J, Ahn DK, Greenspan JS. Detection of human papillomavirus DNA in anal intraepithelial neoplasia and anal cancer. *Cancer Res.* 1991; 51: 1014–9.

Papillon J, Montbarbon MD. Epidermoid carcinoma of the anal canal. *Dis. Colon Rectum* 1987; 30: 324–34.

Papillon J. *Rectal and Anal Cancers.* 1982; Berlin: Springer.

Papillon J, Chassard JL. Respective roles of radiotherapy and surgery in the management of epidermoid carcinoma of the anal margin. Series of 57 patients. *Dis. Colon Rectum* 1992; 35: 422–9.

Ponz de Leon M, Sacchetti C, Sassatelli R, Zanghieri G, Roncucci L, Scalmati A. Evidence for the existence of different types of large bowel tumor: suggestions from the clinical data of a population based registry. *J. Surg. Oncol.* 1990; 44: 35–43.

Pyper PC, Parks TG. The results of surgery for epidermoid carcinoma of the anus. *Br. J. Surg.* 1985; 72: 712–14.

Quan SH. Anal cancers. Squamous and melanoma. *Cancer* 1992; 70 (Suppl.): 1384–9.

Radentz WH, Wall K, Daines MC. An unusual case of pruritus ani. Anal margin squamous cell carcinoma (SCC). *Arch. Dermatol.* 1992; 128: 1115, 1118.

Ribiere O, Fidalgo P, Crickx B, Grossin M, Benhamou G, Vilotte J. A case of Bowen's disease of the anus associated with condylomata acuminata having developed into an epidermoid carcinoma. *Gastroenterol. Clinique Biologique* 1987; 11: 830–1.

Ross M, Pezzi C, Pezzi T, Meurer D, Hickey R, Balch C. Patterns of failure in anorectal melanoma. A guide to surgical therapy. *Arch. Surg.* 1990; 125: 313–6.

Salmon RJ, Fenton J, Asselain B, Mathieu G, Girodet J, Durand JC. Treatment of epidermoid anal canal cancer. *Am. J. Surg.* 1984; 147: 43–8.

Sauven P, Ridge JA, Quan SH, Sigurdson ER. Anorectal carcinoid tumors. Is aggressive surgery warranted? *Ann. Surg.* 1990; 211: 67–71.

Schlag PM, Hunerbein M. Anal cancer: multimodal therapy. *World J. Surg.* 1995; 19: 282–6.

Schraut WH, Wang C, Dawson PJ, Block GE. Depth of invasion, location and size of cancer of the anus dictate operative treatment. *Cancer* 1983; 51: 1291–6.

Schultz TF, Boshoff CH, Weiss RA. HIV infection and neoplasia. *Lancet* 1996; 348: 587–91.

Schwartz RA, Nychay SG, Lyons M, Sciales CW, Lambert WC. Buschke Lowenstein tumor: verrucous carcinoma of the anogenitalia. *Cutis* 1991; 47: 263–6.

Shutze WP, Gleysteen JJ. Perianal Paget's disease. Classification and review of management: report of two cases. *Dis. Colon Rectum* 1990; 33: 502–7.

Singh R, Nime F, Mittelman A. Malignant epithelial tumors of the anal canal. *Cancer* 1981; 48: 411–15.

Sischy B. The use of radiation therapy combined with chemotherapy in the management of squamous cell carcinoma of the anus and marginally resectable adenocarcinoma of the rectum. *Int. J. Radiat. Oncol. Biol. Phys.* 1982; 11: 1587–97.

Tanum G. Diagnosis and treatment of anal carcinoma. An overview. *Acta Oncol.* 1992; 31: 513–8.

Tanum G, Tveit KM, Karlsen KO. Chemoradiotherapy of anal carcinoma: tumour response and acute toxicity. *Oncology* 1993; 50: 14–7.

Tanum G, Hannisdal E, Stenwig B. Prognostic factors in anal carcinoma. *Oncology* 1994; 51: 22–4.

Touboul E, Schlienger M, Buffat L, Lefkopoulos D, Pene F, Parc R, *et al.* Epidermoid carcinoma of the anal canal. Results of curative intent radiation therapy in a series of 270 patients. *Cancer* 1994; 73: 1569–79.

Touboul E, Schlienger M, Buffat L, Ozsahin M, Belkacemi Y, Pene F, *et al.* Conservative versus nonconservative treatment of epidermoid carcinoma of the anal canal for tumors longer than or equal to 5 centimeters. A retrospective comparison. *Cancer* 1995; 75: 786–93.

Watanabe N, Seto H, Ishiki M, Shimizu M, Kageyama M, Wu YW, *et al.* I 123 MIBG imaging of metastatic carcinoid tumor from the rectum. *Clin. Nuclear Med.* 1995; 20: 357–60.

Watanabe S, Ohnishi T, Takahashi H, Ishibashi Y. A comparative study of cytokeratin expression in Paget cells located at various sites. *Cancer* 1993; 72: 3323–30.

Watson PH. Clear cell carcinoma of the anal canal: a variant of anal transitional zone carcinoma. *Hum. Pathol.* 1990; 21: 350–2.

Yeong ML, Wood KP, Scott B, Yun K. Synchronous squamous and glandular neoplasia of the anal canal. *J. Clin. Pathol.* 1992; 45: 261–3.

Zur-Hausen H. Viruses in human cancers. *Science* 1991; 254: 1167–73.

Index

Note: page numbers in *italics* refer to figures and tables.